Contraception and Office Gynecology
choices in reproductive healthcare

Commissioning Editor: Miranda Bromage
Project Development Manager: Rachel Robson
Senior Production Controller: Helen Sofio

Contraception and Office Gynecology
choices in reproductive healthcare

Edited by

Ali Kubba MBChB MFFP FRCOG
Consultant Community Gynaecologist; Honorary Senior Lecturer, Department of Obstetrics and Gynaecology, Guy's, King's and St Thomas' School of Medicine, King's College, London, UK

Joseph Sanfilippo MD FACOG
James and Marjorie Gilmore Professor of Obstetrics and Gynecology, MCP–Hahnemann School of Medicine; Chairman, Department of Obstetrics and Gynecology, Allegheny General Hospital, Pittsburgh, Pennsylvania, USA

and

Naomi Hampton BSc MBBS MRCOG MFFP
Consultant in Reproductive Healthcare and Community Gynaecology, Enfield Community Care NHS Trust, Enfield, UK

W B Saunders
LONDON • EDINBURGH • NEW YORK • PHILADELPHIA • SYDNEY • TORONTO

WB SAUNDERS
An imprint of Harcourt Publishers Ltd

© Harcourt Publishers Ltd 1999

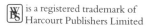 is a registered trademark of
Harcourt Publishers Limited

The right of A. Kubba, J. Sanfilippo and N. Hampton to be
identified as author/s of this work has been asserted by them
in accordance with the Copyright, Designs and Patents Act
1988

First published 1999

ISBN 0-7020-2361-2

British Library Cataloguing in Publication Data
A catalogue record for this book is available from the British
Library

Library of Congress Cataloging in Publication Data
A catalog record for this book is available from the Library of
Congress

Note
Medical knowledge is constantly changing. As new
information becomes available, changes in treatment,
procedures, equipment and the use of drugs become
necessary. The editors/authors/contributors and the
publishers have, as far as it is possible, taken care to ensure that
the information given in this text is accurate and up-to-date.
However, readers are strongly advised to confirm that the
information, especially with regard to drug usage, complies
with the latest legislation and standards of practice.

The
Publisher's
policy is to use
**paper manufactured
from sustainable
forests**

II

Typeset by Phoenix Photosetting, Chatham, Kent, England
Printed in China

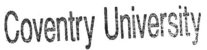

Contents

Preface

What will decide the shape of reproductive healthcare in the early decades of the third millennium? The global need is so great that anything other than community-based care will not do. Our path has been charted by the Cairo Conference on Population and Development. The scope of services designed to meet societal and, more importantly, individual needs is best summarized by action point 7.6 of the Cairo declaration:

'All countries should strive to make accessible through the primary healthcare system, reproductive health to all individuals ... Reproductive health care in the context of primary healthcare should *inter alia*, include: family planning counselling ..., education and services for prenatal care, safe delivery and post-natal care, ... prevention and appropriate treatment of infertility, abortion ..., treatment of reproductive tract infections, sexually transmitted diseases ...; and information, education and counselling, as appropriate, on human sexuality. Referral for family planning services and further diagnosis and treatment for ... infertility, ... breast cancer and cancer of the reproductive systems...'.

This book is the natural product of the dizzy highs of the mid-1990s with 'Cairo', the establishment of a Faculty of Family Planning in the UK and the inexorable move worldwide towards primary care gynaecology. The contributors list includes individuals whose work shaped and continues to influence progress in women's healthcare in different parts of the world.

The topics covered in the 35 chapters and their format aim to meet the needs of many: the academic gynaecologist, the clinical specialist in his or her 'office', and the front line reproductive health provider be it a doctor, a nurse or a field worker. All of us want to deliver within our resources evidence-based care and information. Where evidence exists the authors have striven to identify it. Where evidence is lacking, an opinion has been stated clearly (e.g. progestins in HRT).

We envisaged each chapter as a combination of a referenced text and an easy-to-use manual for the busy clinician. The authors obliged, worked with us as a team and taught us so many things. Our thanks go to them for their enthusiasm and patience faced with our idiosyncrasies and obsessions.

Our thanks also go to our families for their love and support and for enduring long and recurrent periods of 'family exclusion'. We thank our publishing team for keeping faith in the project and seeing it through. Most importantly our thanks go to you, our readers for making contact with us through this publication.

Ali Kubba
Joseph Sanfilippo
Naomi Hampton

Contributors

Janet Barter MBChB MRCOG MFFP
Consultant in Community Gynaecology, Department of Community Gynaecology, Royal Free Hospital, London, UK

Roger Beech BSc(Hons) MSc PhD MFPHM(Hons)
Senior Research Fellow in Health Operational Research, Centre for Health Planning and Management, Darwin Building, Keele University, Keele, UK

Toni Belfield BSc FRSH
Director of Information, Family Planning Association, London, UK

Lori A. Boardman MD
Assistant Professor, Department of Obstetrics and Gynecology, Women and Infants Hospital, Brown University School of Medicine, Providence, RI, USA

George Creatsas MD
Professor of Obstetrics and Gynaecology, University of Athens Alexandra Hospital, Athens, Greece

Mitchell D. Creinin MD
Associate Professor, Department of Obstetrics, Gynecology and Reproductive Sciences, University of Pittsburgh School of Medicine, Magee-Womens Hospital, Pittsburgh, PA, USA

Philip Darney MD MSc
Professor and Chief, Department of Obstetrics, Gynecology and Reproductive Sciences, San Francisco General Hospital, University of California, San Francisco, CA, USA

Max Elstein FRCOG
Executive Director, Institute of Medicine, Law and Bioethics, University of Manchester, Manchester, UK

Tommaso Falcone MD
Head, Section of Reproductive Endocrinology and Infertility, Department of Gynecology and Obstetrics, The Cleveland Clinic Foundation, Cleveland, OH, USA

Sebastian Faro MD PhD
Professor and Chairman, Department of Obstetrics and Gynecology, Rush Presbyterian St Luke's Medical Center, Chicago, IL, USA

G. Marcus Filshie DM FRCOG MFFP
Reader/Consultant in Obstetrics and Gynaecology, Department of Obstetrics and Gynaecology, Queen's Medical Centre, Nottingham, UK

The late Anna Flynn MB BCH BAO NUI FRCOG
Formerly Senior Research Fellow in Natural Family Planning, Birmingham Women's Hospital, Edgbaston, Birmingham, UK

Hilary Furniss MRCOG
Research Fellow, Institute of Medicine, Law and Bioethics, University of Manchester, Manchester, UK

R. Don Gambrell Jr MD FACOG
Clinical Professor, School of Medicine, Department of Physiology and Endocrinology, Medical College of Georgia, Augusta, GA, USA

Deirdre S. Gifford MD MPH
Assistant Professor, Department of Obstetrics and Gynaecology, Women and Infants Hospital, Brown University School of Medicine, Providence, RI, USA

Anna Glasier BSc MD FRCOG
Consultant/Director, Family Planning and Well Woman Services, Lothian Primary Care NHS Trust, Edinburgh, UK

Jeffrey M. Goldberg MD
Section of Reproductive Endocrinology and Infertility, Department of Gynecology and Obstetrics, Cleveland Clinic Foundation, Cleveland, OH, USA

Raymond E. Goodman MSc MRCS LRCP DRCOG CBiol MIBiol
Member, Institute of Psychosexual Medicine (London); Honorary Clinical Teacher, Department of Medicine, University of Manchester; Consultant in Psychosexual Medicine, Manchester, UK

John Guillebaud MA FRCSE FRCOG
Professor of Family Planning and Reproductive Health, University of London; Medical Director of the Margaret Pyke Centre, London, UK

Kate A. Guthrie BSc MB FRCOG MFFP
Honorary Consultant Gynaecologist, Centre for Metabolic Bone Disease, H.S. Brocklehurst Building, Hull Royal Infirmary, Hull, UK

Naomi Hampton, BSc MBBS MRCOG MFFP
Consultant in Reproductive Healthcare and Community Gynaecology, Enfield Community Care NHS Trust, Enfield, UK

Paula Adams Hillard MD
Associate Professor, Department of Obstetrics and Gynecology, University of Cincinatti, Cincinatti, OH, USA

William H. Hindle MD
Professor of Clinical Obstetrics and Gynecology; Director, Breast Diagnostic Center, Women's and Children's Hospital, Los Angeles County and University of Southern California Medical Center, Los Angeles, CA, USA

Barbara A. Hollingworth MBChB DRCOG MFFP
Clinical Lead in Reproductive Health for Redbridge, Barking, Havering and Brentwood, Hertfordshire, UK

Arjun Jeyarajah MA MRCOG
Consultant Gynaecological Oncologist, Department of Gynaecological Oncology, St Bartholomew's Hospital, London, UK

John Kelly FRCS FRCOG
Consultant, Birmingham Women's Hospital, Edgbaston, Birmingham, UK

Athol Kent MBChB MPhil FRCOG
Honorary Lecturer, Department of Obstetrics and Gynaecology, University of Cape Town, Cape Town, South Africa

Valerie S. Kitchen MBChB FRCP
Senior Lecturer/Consultant, Department of Genito-Urinary Medicine and Communicable Diseases, St Mary's Hospital Medical School, London, UK

Ali Kubba MBChB MFFP FRCOG
Consultant Community Gynaecologist, Honorary Senior Lecturer, Department of Obstetrics and Gynaecology, Guy's, King's and St Thomas' School of Medicine, King's College, London, UK

Roni Liyanage MA
Youth Officer Vision 2000 Fund Management, International Planned Parenthood Federation, Regent's College, London, UK

Linda F. Lucas BS MD
Associate Professor; Director of Pain Management Services, Department of Ansthesiology, University of Louisville, School of Medicine, Louisville, KY, USA

Laura MacIssac MD MSc
Assistant Professor of Obstetrics and Gynecology, New York University, School of Medicine, New York, NY, USA

David Oram FRCOG
Consultant Gynaecological Oncologist, Department of Gynaecological Oncology, St Bartholomew's Hospital, London, UK

Jeffrey Peipert MD MPH
Director of Clinical Research; Associate Professor, MPH Department of Obstetrics and Gynecology, Women and Infants Hospital, Brown University School of Medicine, Providence, RI, USA

Walter Prendiville MAO FRCOG FRACOG
Associate Professor, Department of Obstetrics and Gynaecology, Royal College of Surgeons in Ireland, Coombe Women's Hospital, Dublin, Ireland

John P. Pryor MS FRCS
Consultant Uroandrologist; ex-Dean, Institute of Urology, London, UK

David W. Purdie MD FRCOG FRCP(Ed)
Consultant, Centre for Metabolic Bone Disease, H.S. Brocklehurst Building, Hull Royal Infirmary, Hull, UK

Fran Reader FRCOG MFFP BASRTaccred
Consultant in Family Planning and Reproductive Health Care, Ipswich Hospital NHS Trust, Ipswich, Suffolk, UK

Margaret Rees MA DPhil MRCOG
Honorary Senior Clinical Lecturer, Nuffield Department, Obstetrics and Gynaecology, John Radcliffe Hospital, Women's Centre, Headington, Oxford, UK

Benjamin M. Rigor MD
Department of Anesthesiology, University of Louisville School of Medicine, Louisville, KY, USA

Helen Roberts MB MPH
Senior Lecturer in Womens' Health, Department of Obstetrics and Gynaecology, National Women's Hospital, Auckland, New Zealand

Gillian E. Robinson MD MRCOG MFFP
Department of Community Gynaecology, The Royal Free Hospital, London, UK

Sam Rowlands MRCGP MFFP DCH DRCOG
Medical Director, EPIC, Regeneration House, London, UK

Joseph Sanfilippo MD FACOG
James and Marjorie Gilmore Professor of Obstetrics and Gynaecology, MCP Hahnemann School of Medicine; Chairman, Department of Obstetrics and Gynecology, Allegheny General Hospital, Pittsburgh, PA, USA

Jill L. Schwartz MD
Assistant Professor, Department of Obstetrics, Gynecology and Reproductive Sciences, University of Pittsburgh School of Medicine, Magee-Women's Hospital, Pittsburgh, PA, USA

Pramilla Senanayake MBBS DTPH PhD FRCOG
Assistant Director General, International Planned Parenthood Federation, Regent's College, London, UK

Talha Shawaf MBChB FRCS(Ed) FRCOG
Consultant in Reproductive Medicine at St Bartholomew's and Royal London Hospitals, St Bartholomew's Hospital, London, UK

Ronald S. Swerdloff MD
Professor of Medicine, Clinical Study Center, UCLA School of Medicine, Torrance, CA, USA

Christina Wang MD
Director and Professor of Medicine, Clinical Study Center, UCLA School of Medicine, Torrance, CA, USA

Kaye Wellings MA MSc
Senior Lecturer, Department of Public Health and Policy, London School of Hygiene and Tropical Medicine, London, UK

Christopher Wilkinson MFFP
Consultant in Women's Sexual Health, Department of Sexual Health, The Caldecot Centre, King's College Hospital, London, UK

Charles D.A. Wolfe MD FRCOG FFPHM
Reader/Consultant in Public Health Medicine, Guy's, King's and St Thomas' School of Medicine, King's College, London, UK

Section 1:
Fundamental concepts

Sexuality, sexual behaviour and sexual health

Kaye Wellings MA MSc

There have been major changes in sexual behaviour over the past few decades, and in the social backcloth against which sexuality is allowed expression. This chapter examines trends in sexual attitudes and lifestyles in the recent past, the context in which they occur, and some of their implications for sexual health and sexual satisfaction. Most, though not all, of the data for this chapter are drawn from the National Survey of Sexual Attitudes and Lifestyles (NSSAL), a survey undertaken in the early 1990s based on a random probability sample of nearly 19 000 people aged 16–19 years in Britain [1,2].

Age at sexual debut

Perhaps the most dramatic change over the past 50 years has been in the age at first sexual experience. The last few decades have seen a progressive reduction in the age at which sexual intercourse first takes place and an increase in the proportion of young people who have had intercourse before the age of sexual consent. Between the 1950s and the 1980s, the median age at first intercourse fell by 4 years for women from 21 to 17, and by 3 years for men, from 20 to 17. Among women born in the 1930s, fewer than 1% had had sexual intercourse at 15 years or younger, while among those born in the 1970s, the proportion had risen to nearly 20%. Initiation into sexual experience in the wider sense – kissing, cuddling, petting – also occurs at an earlier age.

At the same time, premarital sex has become the norm. By the late 1980s, none of the men interviewed and fewer than 1% of women were married at the time of first intercourse, and less than 1% of men and 3% of women were engaged to be married [1,2]. This was not the case a generation ago. Nearly 40% of women aged 45–59 at the beginning of the 1990s were married at the time of first intercourse and a further 14% were engaged; the figures for men were 14% and 6%, respectively. In the 1950s and early 1960s, more than half of women lost their virginity to their husband or fiancé, and around one in five men did so to wives or fiancées.

Some degree of gender convergence is also apparent in the data on first intercourse. There are signs in Britain that the gap between the age at which young women have sexual intercourse for the first time and the age at which young men do so has been closing with successive birth cohorts. For those over the age of 25 at the time of interview, median age for men is 1 year earlier than it is for women, whilst for those under the age of 25 it is the same for both sexes. The gap between men and women is also narrowing with respect to the proportions reporting first intercourse before the age of 16. The ratio of men to women who had experienced sexual intercourse before the age of 16 has narrowed from 7:1 in the oldest age group (55–59 at the time of interview) to 3:2 in the youngest (16–19).

There has been a widespread belief that men differ from women in sexual behaviour, that they have a higher sex drive, lower tolerance of sexual abstinence and are more easily sexually aroused [3]. However, a recent shift towards greater convergence between the sexes is documented in literature on the subject, particularly that from the USA. Several studies in the past two decades have shown a decline in differences in attitudes and behaviour between men and women, towards a single standard for both [4–6]. Changes in age at first intercourse among men compared with women would seem consistent with these trends.

Age at first intercourse varies

markedly with social class, particularly for men. Overall, across all age groups, age at first sexual intercourse is higher for those in higher social class groups compared with those in lower social class groups. The median age at first intercourse for men of all ages in social class I is 19, which is 3 years later than for men in social class V; for women in social class I it is 20, which is 2 years later than for women in social class V. Age at first sexual intercourse also increases with educational level. Median age at first intercourse for graduates is 1 year higher than for non-graduates for both men and women, and for non-graduates with qualifications it is 1 year higher than for those with no qualifications at all. Educational level may influence age at first intercourse, but in many cases, young people will have experienced first intercourse before completing their education, and it might equally be hypothesised that the age at which the event occurs might itself wield an effect on level of educational achievement.

The need for sex education

Research evidence reveals that regret over the timing of the early experience is not uncommon among young people [1,7]. Most people (more than two-thirds of women and more than three-quarters of men) judge the timing of their first coitus to have been acceptable. Yet more than a third of women aged 16–24 considered the experience to have happened too soon, and the figure rises to 50% if they were under 16 at the

time. For men, the comparable proportions are roughly half of these figures.

Peer pressure may be a factor here, and alcohol is certainly implicated, but the evidence is that ignorance is also a problem. Despite the assumed sexual sophistication of the young, the evidence is that they are still not as well informed about sexual matters as they might be. More than two-thirds of young people see themselves as inadequately prepared in terms of information at the time of first intercourse. School-based sex education lessons are not the main source of sexual information for most people: sexual knowledge is still apparently more likely to be gained from friends, although this trend is becoming less marked. Yet preferred sources tend to be those which are more authoritative, such as teachers or parents. More than a third of women and more than half of all men say they would have preferred to have learned more from school.

Given the proportion of young people who have had sex before the age of 16, it is hard to escape the conclusion that sex education at 14 or 15 is too late. Concern is sometimes expressed that the provision of school sex education might hasten the onset of sexual experience. There is no evidence to support this supposition. The evidence is rather that soundly based information about sexuality might help young people to postpone sexual activity until they are ready for it. NSSAL data showed that those whose main source of sex education was school-based lessons were less likely to have had intercourse before the age of 16 than those citing boy or girlfriends, friends or

another source. These conclusions are reinforced by data from other sources. The results of a review of 35 studies carried out by the World Health Organisation (WHO) Global Programme on AIDS revealed that in no study was there evidence of sex education leading to earlier or increased sexual activity in the young people exposed to it; in six studies, sex education appeared to be associated with either a delay in the onset of sexual activity or to a decrease in sexual activity overall [8].

Sexual practices

Vaginal intercourse

Vaginal intercourse is the mainstay of the sexual repertoire and, for those of mainly heterosexual orientation, is virtually synonymous with the term sex. Among those who are sexually active, the experience of vaginal intercourse is near universal and, given the traditional emphasis on the procreative functions of sex, this is perhaps not surprising. The frequency with which couples have intercourse varies with age and with the length of the relationship. Younger people are considerably more active than those older than themselves, and newly matched lovers have sex more frequently than those more habituated to one another.

Oral sex

Evidence from NSSAL shows oral sex also to be a commonplace experience. Although not quite as widespread as vaginal intercourse, three-quarters of men and almost as many women report having experienced oral sex at some time in their lives, and roughly one in four men and one in five women as recently as in the last week. According to these findings, both men and women report slightly greater experience of cunnilingus than fellatio; oral sex seems to be more commonly practised by men to women than by women to men. Some of the American literature suggests that oral sex is quite commonly practised among young people, and that this experience quite often precedes intercourse.

Anal sex

Anal sex is a fairly uncommon sexual activity, and there is no sign that it is becoming less so. According to NSSAL data, although a minority of people (14% of men and 13% of women) had experienced heterosexual anal sex in their lifetime, little more than 1 in 20 men and women had experienced it in the more recent period of the last year. Anal sex between a man and a woman has been illegal in England and Wales since the 16th century. In France, where it is not legislated against, research shows it to be twice as common as in Britain. However, British society is not the only society to have outlawed anal intercourse: Jesuits recorded that it was an act punishable by hanging among 16th century Incas.

Safer sex

The focus here is on sexual behaviour that is likely to reduce the risk of adverse health consequences of sexual activity. It has to be said there is a good deal more potential for safer sex practice in the extension of our repertoire of sexual acts. Non-penetrative sex (when practised separately from intercourse) is not widespread, at least not among those reporting heterosexual relationships. While heterosexual sex is nearly synonymous with penetrative sex, there is far more evidence of diversification in terms of practices among men reporting male sexual partners. Gay men have adapted their behaviour in ways which reduce the risk of infection with HIV and other sexually transmitted infections (STIs). The range of possible sexual activity is far wider than the range of behaviour most people experience in their lives. Human beings are born with myriad possibilities for satisfying their sexual urges and the possibilities actually explored are fairly narrow. Cross-cultural studies of sex show that sexual customs vary markedly from one society to another.

Sexual partnerships

The number of partners and the type of relationship, i.e. whether exclusive or not, is of interest in the context of sexual health. Some evidence of temporal change in sexual behaviour is available from the data on lifetime numbers of partners.

A good deal is written and surmised about the assumed increase in so-called promiscuity in modern society. Despite concerns about moral decline, the British sexual behaviour survey showed the population to be predominantly monogamous. When asked with how many partners they had had intercourse in the past 5 years, two-thirds of men and three-quarters of women had had only one partner or none at all. At the other end of the scale, the survey revealed a high level of activity amongst a minority. One per cent of men reported more than 22 partners and 1% of women reported more than eight.

Certainly young people today are likely to have larger numbers of partners than did their parents' generation. The proportion of those aged 16–24 with between 3 and 10 partners in their lifetime to date is already higher than it is for those in middle age, who have had a considerably longer period of time in which to accumulate them. Demographic trends help explain why this might be so. Young people begin their sexual experience earlier than was formerly the case and get married later, or not at all, so that there is a longer period in which to acquire sexual partners. The change in the age at marriage has been dramatic in the past decade. In 1977, nearly half of all men (48%) were married before the age of 25 compared with only 31% a decade later in 1989. Two-thirds of women were married by the age of 25 in 1977 compared with just under a half (46%) a decade later. At the same time, the age at which young people reach sexual maturity has been declining. So, in effect, there is more than a decade between the time at which young people are sexually mature and the time when they enter stable cohabiting relationships.

A sizeable minority of young

people at any one time are celibate. In the past year, more than a quarter of young men report having had no sexual partner and nearly half have had only one. For women, nearly a quarter have had no sexual partner and 60% only one.

There is a clear gender difference in reporting of relationships: men are more likely than women to report larger numbers of sexual partners and are less likely to report having been monogamous in any time period. Overall, only one in five men (21%) claims to have had only one sexual partner in their lifetime to date compared with two in five women (39%). One partner for life is a minority lifestyle pattern for men in *all* age groups, and increasingly so: fewer than one in three men (30.5%) aged 45–59 reported only ever having had one heterosexual partner, a proportion which further decreases to 16.3% for those aged 16–24. By contrast, lifelong monogamy was the dominant pattern for women aged 45–59, the majority of whom (57.7%) reported one lifetime partner, compared with only 30.5% of those aged 16–24.

The gap between the proportion of men and women reporting larger numbers of partners is wide and shows few signs of closing (women in every age range are far less likely to report large numbers of partners in any time period), although there is some evidence of it narrowing a little. Although small, the proportion of respondents reporting ten or more lifetime partners has increased steadily over time, an effect that is more marked for

women than for men. Around 3% of women whose sexual debut occurred in the 1950s reported ten or more lifetime partners compared with 10% for those commencing intercourse in the 1970s.

The general trend then is away from monogamy for both sexes – the proportion of both men and women who claim to have been monogamous in their lifetime decreases with successive cohorts. Again, there is some evidence that the pace of this trend has been faster for women than for men, with the ratio of ever-monogamous men to women narrowing slightly from nearly 2:1 in the oldest age group of respondents to around 5:3 for the youngest, in their late teens and early twenties at the time of interview. This trend is not explained in terms of life stage, since logic dictates that with increasing age the proportion reporting only one partner throughout their lifetime would diminish as the opportunities to gain others increase over time.

The trends away from lifelong monogamy and towards larger numbers of lifetime partners seem to be genuinely secular in origin. Furthermore, in common with the trend towards earlier intercourse, they seem to have been occurring at a faster rate for women than for men, although the acceleration is less marked than it is for onset of sexual activity.

Concurrent partnerships

In the context of sexual health, concurrent relationships may be of greater interest than those

conducted serially because of the greater opportunity for acquiring sexually transmitted infection. The NSSAL data also provide the opportunity to identify men and women who had an additional sexual partner outside a cohabiting relationship in the past 5 years. Although the term 'adultery' (in common with many others used to describe sexual relationships) has moral overtones, it is here used in a purely descriptive sense, and in preference to the more judgemental 'unfaithful' and to the clumsier 'sexually non-exclusive'. In practice, all those who had had more than one partner in the past year were asked to chart the start and, where appropriate, the finish, of these relationships so that it was possible to assess whether or not they were conducted concurrently.

Overall, we see a considerable difference between married and cohabiting men and women in the likelihood of reporting an additional partner to the one with whom they have been living for the past 5 years. Only 4% of women do so compared with 10% of men overall. Older women and men are less likely to have been adulterous: 3% of women aged 45–49 compared with 5% of those age 16–24, and 7% and 5% of men in these age groups, respectively.

The propensity of women to seek an additional sexual relationship shows no clear pattern of variation with social position, fluctuating between 4% and 5% across all social class groups. By contrast, the behaviour of men in this respect varies greatly with social class: 11% of married and cohabiting men in social class I and 13% in social class II have had an affair in the past 5 years, compared with only 2.2% of those in social class V. A factor which strongly determined whether *women* had non-exclusive sexual relationships seems to be whether or not their working lifestyle involves staying away from home overnight.

Sexual attitudes

Sexual attitudes have also changed in recent decades. Premarital sex, for example, is now nearly universally approved: fewer than 5% condemn sex before marriage as wrong. While one in four women and one in seven men in the older age range (45–49) think that sex before marriage is wrong, a smaller proportion (1 in 20) of the youngest age group do so, and the proportion is the same for men and women.

However, less tolerance is extended to extramarital relationships. The dominant lifestyle of serial monogamy rather than concurrent partnerships is reflected in the findings on attitudes towards sexual exclusivity, which show widespread condemnation of sex outside marriage. Young people continue to hold monogamy in very high regard, with some 80% of people believing extramarital relationships to be almost or always wrong. One of the most striking of the NSSAL findings was the universal condemnation of sexual non-exclusivity. The vast majority of both men and women believe sex outside a regular relationship to be wrong. The degree of disapproval varies only slightly with the degree to which the relationship is

institutionalised, and there are no major differences between the sexes: women are only slightly more censorious of such relationships, especially in marriage. Furthermore, again somewhat surprisingly, the proportions pronouncing these transgressions as wrong varies little with age. On the subject of one-night stands (used as an indicator of casual sex), men and women differ more markedly, and here the gender difference over time has increased rather than narrowed.

Factors explaining trends in sexual behaviour

Although it is not possible to attempt any conclusive explanation of the temporal changes in sexual behaviour, some attempt can be made to assess the possible contribution of maturational effects and social influences on sexual behaviour. One possible explanation for the more dramatic lowering of age at first sexual intercourse in women may have been earlier physical maturation, affecting women more than men. There has been a small but significant fall in the mean age of menarche between the oldest age group (45–49) and women under 45, and there is indeed a significant correlation between menarche and first intercourse (median age at first sexual experience and first sexual intercourse for women who first menstruate at 15 or older is one year later than for those who do so under the age of 15). The decline in the age of menarche, however, is not of an order which would explain the dramatic lowering of age at first intercourse, and we

must look to other factors to explain most of this effect.

The trend towards earlier intercourse is often held to be a consequence of the availability of reliable birth control. A common assumption is that the advent of oral contraception and the extension of family planning services preceded and probably facilitated a lowering of the age at first intercourse, by removing one of the most powerful deterrents – the fear of unwanted pregnancy – from the sexual act. Yet the fall of 4 years in the median age at first intercourse did not take place evenly and uniformly over the four decades from 1950 to 1990. Median age at first intercourse fell by 2 years during the single decade of the 1950s, between 1950 and 1960, and by another 2 years during the following three decades up to 1990. In other words, the major decrease occurred before the advent of the contraceptive pill in the early 1960s, and certainly well before it became generally available to all women regardless of marital status or ability to pay, which was not achieved until the 1970s in Britain.

Sexual behaviour may be a biological capacity, but its expression is strongly socially influenced. Given the importance of social factors in determining the start of sexual experience, the historical backcloth against which these changes have taken place is of interest here. The past four decades have been a time of rapid social change, much of which has had a direct impact on sexual behaviour. The 1960s saw the decriminalization of abortion and of homosexuality, and liberalizing reform of laws relating to sexual offences, pornography and divorce. The weakening hold of religion in Britain has further separated sexual expression from a purely reproductive function. Technological advances not only brought about the means by which women could control their fertility, widening the range of reproductive choices, but also created labour-saving devices, increasing leisure. In addition, there has been a growth in international travel and a more open attitude to sexual expression. All these changes affected both sexes, but the effect has been arguably greater on women than men. Some changes have selectively affected women.

Scientific investigation into the sexuality of both genders, but especially women, by researchers such as Masters and Johnson furthered our understanding of sexual expression and sexual satisfaction. The large-scale entry of women into the workplace and the consequent creation of new opportunities for meeting potential sexual partners has permitted freer sexual expression, particularly for women. Greater gender equality has also extended to sexual mores, with some consequent erosion of the so-called 'double standard' and an observable convergence in the sexual behaviour of men and women.

Sexual health implications

These data are not only of sociological interest but, in addition, have clear sexual health implications. The fall in the age at first coitus is a major social trend and has clear policy relevance for the provision of sex education

and sexual health services. Early onset of sexual activity is associated with a larger number of lifetime sexual partners, decreased likelihood of contraceptive use and an increased likelihood of teenage pregnancy, and some degree of regret.

In modern industrialised societies, young people are expected to delay serious mating and stable relationships associated with childbearing until they have completed the relatively lengthy process of socialisation and induction into society and adult life. It is the disjuncture between maturational readiness for sexual activity and the socially approved timing of its occurrence which underlies many of the problems relating to the maintenance of sexual health of young people. A balance has constantly to be sought between, on the one hand, assisting young people by providing the necessary education, information and resources with which they can safeguard their sexual health and avoid unplanned pregnancy and sexually transmitted infection, and on the other hand, avoiding appearing to encourage premature sexual activity.

Evidence of earlier age at first sexual activity, together with a possible delaying effect of sex education, has important implications for the provision of sexual health education, its nature and content. They are clearly important to the presentation of a case for school-based sexual health education.

The increasing interval between onset of sexual activity and settling with a partner will mean longer periods of contraceptive use by the woman.

This is most likely to be the pill. Attention needs to be paid to ensuring that the formulae used present the least risk of adverse side effects with prolonged use.

The relationship between age at first intercourse and sexual behaviour is also of interest in the context of cervical cancer. Epidemiological studies have suggested that the importance of early sexual experience in the aetiology of this disease [9, 10], suggesting that early age at first intercourse, rather than multiple partners, may be a more useful focus in explaining the incidence of cervical cancer in different subgroups in the population [11–13].

The relevance of information about sexual practices relates to their differential capacity for carrying a risk of infection or an unintended pregnancy. There is certainly ample scope for further education of heterosexuals in terms of exploring the means of sexual expression, which involves greater gains in terms of achieving a reduction in risk.

There have clearly been genuine generational changes away from lifelong monogamy and towards greater diversity in sexual partnerships. These behaviours to date have been more characteristic of men but the trend towards them is occurring for both sexes, and the pace of change has in recent decades been more rapid for women. Women are now more common attenders at STD clinics. Young women today are more likely to have visited an STD clinic by their mid-twenties than are those aged 45–59 during their entire lives. While women in the older age range who had visited an STD clinic were outnumbered by men in that group by 2:1, equal proportions of women and men in the 16–24 age range (around 1 in 20) have been to an STD clinic. This is confirmed in the increased incidence of gonorrhoea and other STDs from the early 1960s onwards [14].

References

1. Wellings K, Field J, Johnson A, Wadsworth J. *Sexual behaviour in Britain*. London: Penguin Publications, 1994.

2. Johnson A, Wadsworth J, Wellings K, Field J. *Sexual attitudes and lifestyles*. Oxford: Blackwell Publications, 1994.

3. Bancroft J. *Human sexuality and its problems*, 2nd edn. London: Churchill Livingstone, 1989.

4. Christiansen HR, Gregg CF. Changing sex norms in America and Scandinavia. *J Marriage Family* 1970;32:616–27.

5. Robinson IE, Jedlicka D. Changes in sexual attitudes and behaviour in college students from 1965 to 1980: a research note. *J Marriage Family* 1982;44:237–40.

6. Orr DP, Wilbrandt ML, Brack CJ, Raunch SP, Ingersoll GM. Reported sexual behaviours and self esteem among young adolescents. *Am J Dis Child* 1989;143:86–90.

7. Curtis HA, Lawrence CJ, Tripp JH. Teenage sexual intercourse and pregnancy. *Arch Dis Child* 1988;63:373–9.

8. Baldo M, Aggleton P, Slutkin G. Does sex education lead to earlier or increased sexual activity in youth? PO DO2 3444 *IXth International Conference* on AIDS, Berlin, June 1993.

9. Boyd JT, Doll R. A study of the aetiology of carcinoma of the cervix uteri. *Br J Cancer* 1964;18:419–34.

10. Wynder EL. Epidemiology of carcinoma *in situ* of the cervix. *Obstet Gynaecol Surv* 1969;24:697–711.

11. Harris RWC, Brinton LA, Cowdell RH et al. Characteristics of women with dysplasia or carcinoma in situ of the cervix uteri. *Br J Cancer* 1980;42:359–69.

12. Brown S, Vessey M, Harris R. Social class, sexual habits and cancer of the cervix. *Community Med* 1984;6:281–6.

13. Mant D, Vessey M, Loudon N. Social class differences in sexual behaviour and cervical cancer. *Community Med* 1988;10:52–6.

14. Adler MW. Sexually transmitted disease. In: Miller DL, Farmer RDT (eds) *Epidemiology of diseases*. Oxford: Blackwell Scientific Publications, 1982.

An overview of reproductive epidemiology, statistics and methods for evaluating research

Jeffrey F Peipert MD MPH
Deidre S Gifford MD MPH
Lori A Boardman MD

Introduction

Obstetrician–gynecologists and reproductive health researchers should have a common knowledge base regarding clinical research design in order to review papers in the reproductive health literature critically, and to plan and appropriately perform research projects. As the emphasis on evidence-based medicine increases [1], it is becoming more important to be able to evaluate the quality of medical evidence available. The US Preventive Services Task Force [2] has adopted the criteria outlined in Table 2.1 to evaluate the quality of evidence [3]. Some basic knowledge about research methodology is necessary to interpret studies and to evaluate evidence in the medical literature. The purpose of this review is to outline the various types of clinical research design and to point out their individual advantages, disadvantages and scientific value.

Figure 2.1 illustrates the fact that not all research methods are created equal. The randomized clinical trial is the 'gold standard' of clinical research design and, if performed with sufficient methodologic rigor, is least likely to be subject to serious biases. Observational studies, including cohort, case-control and cross-sectional studies, are common analytic studies used in reproductive health. These methods are more susceptible to multiple types of bias that can be introduced, and can distort the researcher's results and conclusions. Descriptive studies, such as case series and case reports, are often interesting clinical vignettes but have limited scientific merit. This manuscript will review the basic components of these studies and illustrate examples of these methods in reproductive health literature.

Table 2.1 Strength of recommendations as suggested by the Canadian Task Force on the Periodic Health Examination

Strength of recommendations

A. There is good evidence to support the recommendation that the condition be specifically considered in a periodic health examination.

B. There is fair evidence to support the recommendation that the condition be specifically considered in a periodic health examination.

C. There is poor evidence regarding the inclusion of the condition in the periodic health examination, but recommendations may be made on other grounds.

D. There is fair evidence to support the recommendation that the condition be excluded from consideration in a periodic health examination.

E. There is good evidence to support the recommendation that the condition be excluded from consideration in a periodic health examination.

Quality of evidence

I. Evidence obtained from at least one properly designed randomized controlled trial.

II-1. Evidence obtained from well-designed controlled trials without randomization.

II-2. Evidence obtained from well-designed cohort of case-control studies, preferably from more than one center or research group.

II-3. Evidence obtained from multiple time series with or without the intervention. Dramatic results in uncontrolled experiments (such as the results of the introduction of penicillin treatment in the 1940s) could also be regarded as this type of evidence.

III. Opinions of respected authorities, based on clinical experience, descriptive studies or reports of expert committees.

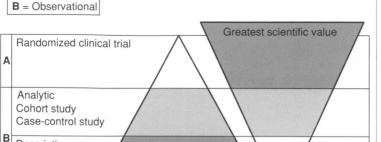

Fig. 2.1 A hierarchy of clinical studies. A = experimental; B = observational. (Reprinted from ACOG PROLOG: Patient management in the office, 2nd edn, Washington, DC: ACOG, 1991, p.21.)

The randomized clinical trial

The randomized clinical trial (RCT) is considered to be the 'gold standard' against which other research methodologies are compared and by which medical interventions should be evaluated [4]. The major advantage of an RCT over an observational study is the strength of causal inference it offers. The RCT is the best design for controlling the influence of known and unknown confounding variables [5]. Historians will surely regard randomized clinical trials as one of the main scientific advances in methods of clinical research in the 20th century [6]. The idea of doing controlled trials, however, is not at all recent or new. In the Bible, Daniel proposed a trial in which youths would eat either royal cuisine or a 'kosher' collection of leguminous plants and water, and the state of health of the two groups would then be compared [7]. The concept of assigning treatment by randomization was proposed by

Fisher in 1923 for application in agricultural research [8].

There are five basic steps in the design of a randomized clinical trial:

1. Assemble the study population.
2. Evaluate baseline characteristics.
3. Randomly assign subjects to two or more study groups.
4. Apply intervention or placebo, preferably in a blinded fashion.
5. Follow the groups and measure outcome variables (blindly, if possible) [5].

Embedded in these five steps are a number of methodologic issues that must be addressed in a properly performed RCT. Inclusion and exclusion criteria that are appropriate to the research question must be carefully determined. Subjects with a contraindication to the intervention must be excluded. An adequate sample size should be determined and plans for recruitment should be consistent

with these calculations. When measuring baseline characteristics, important predictors of the outcome and confounding variables should be considered.

Numerous authorities have pointed out the importance of randomizing patients in a truly 'random' fashion, such as with a random number table or computer-generated random assignment, rather than by hospital number or day of the week, and concealing the assignment in opaque envelopes to avoid foreknowledge of the treatment assignment [9]. In this way, the investigator is unable to 'game' the randomization scheme to move patients into the preferred treatment group. When applying the intervention, it is extremely important to blind the investigator and the subject to the group assignment (double-blind approach). By doing so, the subjects' follow-up and evaluation of the outcome will be performed in a strictly objective manner, uninfluenced by group assignment. When analysing the results of the RCT, an important concept to remember is the principle 'once randomize, analyze'. An RCT in which many of the patients have been 'dropped from the analysis' should be suspect and carefully scrutinized.

The RCT, therefore, offers many advantages. In the hierarchy of clinical research, the RCT provides the greatest strength of causal inference and is the best methodology to test the efficacy of treatment programs. Randomization, if performed properly, protects against selection bias and confounding, if the sample size is adequate. Blinding will help ward off problems of ascertainment bias, diagnostic suspicion bias and detection bias. However, the disadvantages of a randomized trial include expense, feasibility and inability to randomize patients to certain agents for ethical reasons. For example, how can we randomize patients to a specific contraceptive method or to smoking? In addition, RCTs may not be generalizable to the general population owing to strict inclusion and exclusion criteria of the trial, and the fact that patients who consent to participate in an RCT may be different from non-participants.

Observational studies

Cohort (longitudinal or follow-up) study

Since RCTs cannot always be performed because of ethical and feasibility considerations, observational studies are often necessary. Observational studies can be divided into the cohort (longitudinal or follow-up) study, the case-control study and cross-sectional studies. A cohort study is carried out by assembling a group of individuals who have been 'exposed' and by comparing this group to a control group of patients who have not been exposed. These two groups are followed over time and evaluated for a specific outcome of interest. An excellent example in the reproductive health literature is the Nurses Health Study [10,11], one of the most comprehensive cohort studies ever performed. Thousands of nurses are followed over time with comprehensive interviews and medical record reviews to evaluate various risk factors (e.g. oral contraceptive use

or estrogen replacement therapy) and the development of a disease (e.g. breast cancer or cardiovascular disease).

Cohort studies are much weaker than RCTs in establishing causation for two main reasons. First, since a clinician's decision to recommend a specific therapy and a patient's choice to accept therapy are clearly non-random, we have lost the strength (provided by randomization) that the two groups are equal at baseline. For example, women who use oral contraceptives may have very different baseline characteristics than women who use other forms of contraceptives or no contraception, and these characteristics may be related to the outcome of interest. The second major limitation of cohort studies is that women receiving an intervention may be cared for or evaluated differently than women who do not. For example, a woman on oral contraceptives is more likely to be seen on a regular basis than a woman using an over-the-counter contraceptive. As a result, there is an increased chance of

detecting an abnormality. This is called 'diagnostic access' or 'diagnostic suspicion' bias. While cohort studies can attempt to control for differences in baseline characteristics and confounding variables through stratification and multivariate analysis, it is impossible to control for unknown or unmeasured confounding variables. As a result of these major sources of bias, cohort studies cannot provide the strength of association as evidence of causation that well done randomized trials can provide.

Case-control study

The second major class of observational studies is the case-control study. In contrast to the cohort study, the case-control study 'begins at the end' (Figure 2.2) [12]. Cases (patients with a disease) are compared to controls (individuals without the disease) to determine whether there is an association between an exposure and the disease. As a result of the process of selecting individuals based on the outcome or disease,

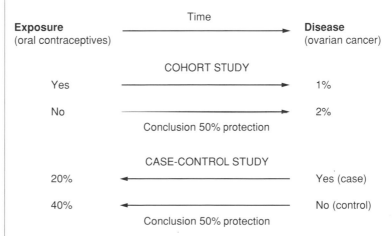

Fig. 2.2 Examples of cohort and case-control studies of relationship between oral contraceptives and ovarian cancer. (Reprinted from Piepert JF, Grimes DA. The case-control study: a primer for the obstetrician-gynecologist. *Obstet Gynecol* 1994;84:140–5.)

2

An overview of
reproductive
epidemiology,
statistics and
methods for
evaluating
research

case-control studies can only study one outcome but may evaluate several exposures. For example, the CASH (Cancer and Steroid Hormone) Study is a case-control study evaluation of the association between cancer (the disease) and the exposure to hormones [13].

Case-control studies are highly efficient; they often require the fewest number of patients to demonstrate an association and can be done in less time and with less money, especially when the disease in question is rare or takes years to develop. Consider how long it would take to evaluate a cohort of women using oral contraceptives (usually at a relatively young age) for the development of ovarian cancer. Despite these advantages, case-control studies are easy to do poorly and are prone to numerous biases [12]. The Women's Health Study, for example, was a multicenter case-control study to evaluate the relationship between pelvic inflammatory disease (PID) and the intrauterine device. A poor choice of control group (condom users) resulted in an inflated estimate of the relationship between the intrauterine device and PID, since condoms are known to protect against sexually transmitted diseases [14]. The control group should be representative of persons at risk for the disease and who have the same opportunity for exposure as the cases. Therefore, the choice of control group is critical in these studies.

Cross-sectional study

The cross-sectional study can be thought of as a 'snapshot' of a group of individuals, some of whom have the disease (outcome) and/or exposure, and some of whom do not. While associations between disease and exposure can be evaluated, the temporal relationship between the two cannot be established. For example, if we assembled a large group of young women, some of whom are using oral contraceptives (exposed) while the remainder are not, and we obtain prolactin levels in all women, we may discover that there is an association between oral contraceptives and elevated prolactin levels. Can we conclude that oral contraceptives 'cause' elevations in prolactin? Or is it possible that women with elevated prolactins are more likely to have irregular bleeding and are more likely to be prescribed oral contraceptives? Since cross-sectional studies often use prevalent cases rather than incident cases (newly discovered cases during a period of follow-up), it may be difficult to establish a temporal relationship and the information provided can be misleading.

Cross-sectional studies are fairly quick and easy to perform. They are often used to evaluate screening and diagnostic tests (see section below). For example, in a recent study to evaluate laboratory tests used to diagnose PID, C-reactive protein was found to be more highly associated with upper genital tract infection than erythrocyte sedimentation rate [15].

Descriptive studies

Descriptive studies, such as case reports and case series, represent the least sophisticated of study designs. As the name implies, the purpose of such studies is to assess and describe a finding in a case or group of cases. While causal inferences cannot be drawn, these studies may generate hypotheses, and may have a valuable role as the basis for future observational studies and clinical trials.

Despite their severe limitations, case reports and case series have some advantages. The data to be analyzed are often already collected or relatively easy to obtain; sources of information include hospital records, laboratory reports, morbidity and mortality documents. Statistical analyses are usually unnecessary. The cost of the study is, therefore, low and ethical problems are minimal.

On the other hand, these studies are flawed by the lack of a comparison group, by the loss of follow-up of study participants and by the potential biases of the investigators. Establishing cause and effect, while often compelling, is not possible in the context of these studies and represents a potential pitfall for both the researcher and reader. Caillouette and Koehler's report of seven women who developed functional ovarian cysts while on phasic contraceptive pills represents a descriptive study [16] which led to further investigation and refutation [17] of these authors' assertion that 'phasic contraceptive pills may be a threat to patient health and safety'.

Screening and diagnostic tests

To interpret and apply the results of screening and diagnostic tests fully, the reader must first understand the concepts of reproducibility and validity. Fulfillment of these criteria is crucial in order for a test to be useful in clinical practice. Ideally a test should consistently give the same result upon retesting (reproducibility) and should either closely correlate with the gold standard test for the presence of a particular disease or, if such a standard is not available, with another objective measure of predictive potential (validity).

Inherent in the concept of validity are the measures of sensitivity, specificity and predictive value. How valid a test is depends on its ability to identify correctly those with the outcome of interest (i.e. sensitivity or the proportion of patients with the disease who will have a positive test) and those without the outcome of interest (i.e. specificity or the proportion of non-diseased individuals who will have a negative test). A 2 × 2 table (Table 2.2) clarifies the possible combinations of test results, and presence or absence of a condition. To determine sensitivity, the number of patients with both a positive test and the presence of a condition (true positives) is divided by the total number of patients with the condition regardless of the test results (true positives + false negatives). In a similar fashion, specificity is determined by dividing the number of patients with both a negative test result and the absence of the condition (true negatives) by the total number of patients without the condition (true negatives + false positives). A good screening or diagnostic test should possess both high sensitivity and

specificity in trials, and be applicable to and reliable in clinical practice. In order for this to occur, a broad spectrum of patients both with and without the condition under study must be tested [18,19].

While finding a test with both high sensitivity and specificity remains a worthy goal, it is often elusive in real practice. Choosing a good screening or diagnostic test will therefore depend on what is being evaluated. In some cases, such as screening for malignancies, high sensitivity with few false negatives is clearly the aim. Conversely, a screening test for a less serious condition may benefit from high specificity by reducing the number of false positives. The 'receiver operating characteristic' (ROC) curve of the test allows the researcher to see the relationship between sensitivity (plotted on the *y*-axis) and 1 − specificity (plotted on the *x*-axis) and then choose cut-off points along the generated curve which best correlate with the desired characteristics of the test being studied (Figure 2.3).

Sensitivity and specificity are predicated upon the presence or absence of a condition or disease.

Predictive values, on the other hand, are based on the test's ability to predict the presence or absence of the disease; they are thus more useful in clinical practice as patients more commonly present not with or without disease, but asking what is their probability of having a condition or disease in the presence of a positive or negative diagnostic test. Again, using the 2 × 2 table (Table 2.2), positive predictive value is expressed as the number of true positives divided by the number of patients with a positive test (true positives + false positives) and negative predictive value as the number of true negatives divided by the number of individuals with a negative test (true negatives + false negatives). Another means of determining predictive values is via Bayes' theorem:

Positive predictive value = (Sensitivity × prevalence)/ [(sensitivity × prevalence) + (1 − specificity) × (1 − prevalence)]   (2.1)

Negative predictive value = (Specificity) × (1 − prevalence)/ {[specificity × (1 − prevalence)] + (1 − sensitivity) × (prevalence)}   (2.2)

Table 2.2 2 × 2 table illustrating the use of C-reactive protein in the diagnosis of pelvic inflammatory disease

Test	PID present	PID absent (normal laparoscopy)	Total
Positive or abnormal (CRP > 20 mg/l)	True positive (74)	False positive (33)	107
Negative or normal (CRP ≤ 20 mg/l)	False negative (26)	True negative (67)	93
Total	100	100	200

PID = pelvic inflammatory disease; CRP = C-reactive protein; TP = true positive; FN = false negative; TN = true negative; FP = false positive.
Sensitivity: TP/(TP+FN) = 74/100 = 74%.
Specificity: TN/(TN + FP) = 67/100 = 67%.
Positive predictive value: TP/(TP + EP) = 74/107 = 69%.
Negative predictive value: TN/(TN + FN) = 67/93 = 72%.
From: Piepert JF, Boardman L, Hogan JW et al. Laboratory evaluation of acute upper genital tract infection. *Obstet Gynecol* 1996;87:730–6.

2

An overview of
reproductive
epidemiology,
statistics and
methods for
evaluating
research

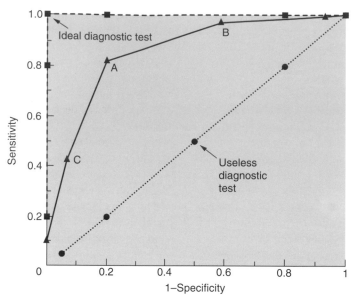

Fig. 2.3   Receiver operating characteristic curve demonstrating various cutoff
points and their impact on sensitivity and specificity. Note; x-axis is 1 – specificity.
Cutoff point A has equal false positives and false negatives, with sensitivity and
specificity of approximately 80%. Point C represents a cutoff point with low
sensitivity and high specificity, whereas point B has a high sensitivity and low
specificity (Reprinted from Grimes DA, Godwin AJ, Rubin A, Smith JA, Lacarra M.
Ovulation and follicular development associated with three low-dose oral
contraceptives: a randomized controlled trial. *Obstet Gynecol* 1994;83:29–34.)

Systematic reviews of medical evidence

Meta-analysis

Meta-analysis is a method of
combining data from several
studies to produce a summary
measure of the effect of a
treatment, intervention or risk
factor on a health outcome. It has
been used to summarize both
experimental [20] and non-
experimental data [21], and is
becoming an increasingly popular
method of summarizing a body
of literature [22]. Meta-analysis is
particularly useful when the
outcome of interest is rare, and
available studies are not large
enough to show significant
differences, or when different
studies of the same question give
conflicting results. It is also
extremely useful to define

deficiencies in the medical
literature in a specific area and to
define methodologic issues which
may improve the study of a
particular question. The field of
obstetrics and gynecology has
been a leader in the development
and dissemination of meta-
analysis [20].

Meta-analysis is a fairly new
method of summarizing data and
there is controversy about the
validity of the method, especially
when it is applied to non-
experimental data [23]. The
consumer of the medical literature
should have some familiarity with
the elements of a good meta-
analysis in order to evaluate the
validity and clinical usefulness of
those which appear in the
literature. It is important to
emphasize that meta-analytic
techniques cannot overcome flaws
in the design and execution of

individual studies, and the results
of a meta-analysis are only as good
as the studies that it contains
('garbage in – garbage out'
phenomenon).

Meta-analysis differs from
traditional literature review in
several important aspects, which
are intended to reduce the
subjectivity inherent in an
unstructured review. First, it uses a
systematic means of finding all the
studies available on a particular
topic. Computer literature
searches are commonly done. The
search terms used by the
investigators should be specified so
that the method of finding the
studies is explicit. Further, hand
searches of bibliographies of
relevant textbooks and journals
should be performed, since
computer literature searches often
fail to identify pertinent studies
[24]. Finally, experts in the field
are often contacted to inquire
about studies which the authors
may have missed. Whatever
methods of literature search are
chosen, they should be explicitly
stated and designed to ensure that
all the available evidence on a
subject is obtained.

Specific criteria for including
and excluding articles in the meta-
analysis are then developed. These
criteria might include particular
dates or languages of publication,
or they may pertain to study
design (e.g. only randomized
trials) or study outcomes. All the
studies found in the literature
search are then subjected to the
established criteria, and studies are
selected for inclusion.

Once a group of studies is
selected, data on study design,
exposure variables, outcomes and
important covariates are
systematically collected. The idea
of meta-analysis is to combine

data from studies in similar populations, which have examined the same relationship between the exposure/intervention and outcome. Obviously, all studies of a particular question are not alike. Therefore, once data on the measure of effect, such as an odds ratio or risk ratio, are available from each study, statistical procedures are used to evaluate for *heterogeneity* between studies. Heterogeneity refers to very divergent results between studies or very different effects of a particular exposure on an outcome. When significant heterogeneity between studies is found, it suggests that the study populations or study designs were different. It is important that appropriate statistical methods are used to deal with such heterogeneity in the meta-analysis. If not, studies may be inappropriately combined and summary results may be invalid.

Once heterogeneity has been addressed, it may be possible to combine study results. A meta-analysis will typically provide a summary measure of effect (such as an odds ratio), which describes the *overall effect* found in the studies included. The overall effect of a meta-analysis may differ from that found in individual studies. This is why meta-analysis can be useful in areas where some studies have shown effects of an exposure on an outcome and others have not. While traditional literature review can describe, in qualitative terms, the findings of a body of literature, it does not provide a method for quantitatively summarizing the results of several studies with possibly conflicting results.

Meta-analysis is an attractive method of summarizing data, but caution should be used as regards overinterpreting the results. Most importantly, a meta-analysis cannot overcome flaws in the design or execution of the studies which are contained within it. Some meta-analysts propose weighting studies with a quality score, so that high-quality studies receive more weight in the summary statistic [25]. Alternatively, measures of study quality, such as blinding or adequate randomization methods, can be used in the inclusion criteria when selecting studies at the outset. One can also explore the effect of quality by doing analyses with and without studies of low quality, and examining the effect on the overall summary statistic. Whichever method is used, some attention to the quality of the studies contained in the meta-analysis is essential for the reader to understand the overall quality of the meta-analysis itself.

Decision analysis and economic analysis

Decision analysis and economic analysis, such as cost–benefit and cost-effectiveness analyses, are additional methods of combining information and systematically reviewing data to arrive at a summary conclusion. Decision analysis is a quantitative approach to assess the relative values of different management options. The process begins by systematically breaking down a clinical problem into its components and creating an algorithm or 'decision tree' to represent the components (parameters) and decision options.

Probability values for each of these parameters are determined from a review of the medical literature and expert opinion. The decision tree is then analysed using statistically based methods, and a net value of the different decision options in relation to each other is determined [26]. A technique called *sensitivity analysis* can be used to test how variations in these probabilities can affect the conclusions of the decision analysis. As an example in the obstetric literature, a decision analysis was performed to evaluate the reductions in cost and cesarean delivery rate with the use of routine external cephalic version for breech presentations [27].

Economic analysis, including cost–benefit and cost-effectiveness analysis, is similar to decision analysis, but focuses on monetary cost. After decision analysis is performed, data on costs of various management options are collected, and the costs of the options are compared. The cost-effectiveness of prenatal carrier screening for cystic fibrosis, for example, was evaluated by Lieu and colleagues [28]. Cost–benefit analysis differs from cost-effectiveness analysis in that the latter method values some of the consequences of the decision options in non-monetary terms, such as years of life saved or disability avoided [26].

Health services research

Health services research is a field of applied research which often combines the work of many disciplines to study an aspect of medical care delivery. Health services research studies can be

2

An overview of
reproductive
epidemiology,
statistics and
methods for
evaluating
research

methodologic, descriptive, analytic or experimental [29]. There is considerable overlap between health services and what is considered as 'traditional clinical research'. In general, health services research studies how health care delivery systems, health policies, payment structure and provider–patient interactions affect health. Although health services methodologies can be used to study more traditional clinical topics, such as the effect of a particular disease or treatment on health, it is often distinct from clinical research in the way that health and disease outcomes are measured and defined. In addition, methodologies such as meta-analysis, decision analysis and cost–benefit analysis are often used to synthesize data and compare different treatment strategies.

One area of health services research examines the variation in health care utilization between different geographic areas. These studies, referred to as studies of 'small area variation', can show wide variation in the use of particular procedures and in hospitalization rates for certain diagnoses between geographic areas [30–32]. Such data led to speculation about overuse or underuse of particular procedures in some areas, and spawned the development of methodologies to examine the appropriateness of medical care [33]. Appropriateness methodologies involve devising clinical scenarios in which procedures are deemed appropriate, equivocal or inappropriate, as rated by expert panels, and then comparing these scenarios to actual practice. Studies have examined the appropriateness of carotid

endarterectomy [34], coronary artery bypass graft surgery [35] and hysterectomy [36], to cite a few. In each case, significant levels of inappropriate use of procedures were found. As a result of the documentation of wide variation in health care utilization and possible inappropriate use of some procedures, guideline development and dissemination has become another important area of health services research [29].

Outcomes research

Measuring the health outcomes of medical intervention is a focus of health services research. Often referred to as 'outcomes research', these studies attempt to define the effectiveness of medical interventions and use a broader definition of outcomes than traditional clinical studies. An important contribution of health services research has been to emphasize the importance of patients' subjective assessment of their own health as an important measure of the effectiveness of medical care. Research methodologies from psychology and other social sciences have been used to devise and refine measures of functional status, psychological well-being, social functioning, general well-being and other patient-rated domains. Many of these tools have proven to be reliable and valid methods for assessing the results of care [37].

Another important aspect of outcomes research is its emphasis on 'real-world' situations, rather than the somewhat artificial conditions of the randomized controlled trial. While

randomized trials usually occur in academic institutions with highly trained physicians and patients who fit stringent inclusion criteria, outcomes research attempts to study the outcomes of care provided by 'regular' doctors to 'regular' patients. This approach is sometimes referred to as the study of effectiveness of care, as opposed to the study of 'efficacy', which is the study of care under ideal conditions. However, the observational nature of outcomes research is both a strength and a limitation. Studies which compare the outcomes of different treatment options in non-randomized populations require detailed data on covariates and co-morbidities in order properly to control for confounding. Although large administrative data sets are often used to perform outcomes research, they are often limited in the availability of important covariates.

The types of studies described above are a few examples of health services research. While they comprise a diverse array of topics and methodologies, they share the common thread of studying the effects of the structure and process of medical care on the health outcomes of individuals and populations.

Statistics in reproductive research

Hypothesis testing

Before we describe the basic concepts of statistical testing, it is helpful to understand some of the terms commonly used to describe data. A term often used to describe a population is the 'normal distribution' (Figure 2.4). In the normal distribution, 95% of the data points fall within (±) 1.96 standard deviations. The mean of a collection of data points is the average (sum of observations/number of observations), while the mode is the 'peak' or most common data point of the frequency curve. If the curve has a single peak, the data are 'unimodal'. The measurements of a continuous variable can be grouped into quarters (25% of the observations). The cut-off points between them are called quartiles, with the middle quartile being the median. Centiles are the product of splitting the data into 100 groups. The median is therefore the 50th centile. The median rather than the mean is used to express the distribution of the data when the distribution is skewed (i.e. not normal). The extremes of the distribution curve would be expressed as the 10th, 90th, 3rd or 97th centiles.

The basis of statistical tests is hypothesis testing. Studies should clearly state their research hypothesis a priori. This is often phrased in the form of null hypothesis (H_0). An example of a null hypothesis is that there is no association between oral contraceptives and the development of ovarian cancer. If one rejects the null hypothesis (H_0), then an alternative hypothesis that some association exists is accepted. An 'association', however, may be clinically important or trivial. Therefore, it is important for the reader to distinguish between statistical significance and clinical significance.

We are all aware that research

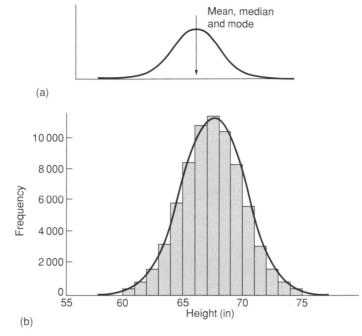

(a)

(b)

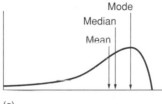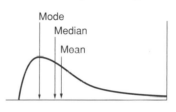

(c)

Fig 2.4   Normal and skewed distributions. (a) The normal distribution is symmetric and bell-shaped. (b) A distribution of heights of young adult males with an approximately normal distribution. (c) Skewed distributions are asymmetric and the mean and median will be quite different.

studies, like diagnostic tests, are fallible. Two specific 'types' of error are of concern to epidemiologists and researchers: the *type I* (or alpha) error and the *type II* (beta) error. Type I errors are analogous to a 'false-positive' study, or the chance that a significant difference was found when in reality there is no difference. The level of type I error is based on where we chose our cut-off for our significance value. A significance value of 0.05 implies that the risk of type I error, or the chance that a positive study finding was due to chance alone, is 5%. Type II error is analogous to a false-negative study, or the chance that no difference was found when a difference really does exist. The chance of a type II error is inversely related to sample size and to the statistical power of the study. The chance of a type II (beta) error is derived from 1−power. Therefore, a 20% chance of a false-negative study translates to 80% power. The only way to reduce the chance of type II or beta error is to increase study sample size. A study's power is its ability to detect an association when one really exists, which is analogous to diagnostic sensitivity. Calculating sample size prior to beginning a study is extremely important to avoid the problem of a type II error [38]. Freiman and colleagues have demonstrated that a large number of clinical trials are discarding a therapy as 'ineffective' when, in reality, the therapy may have a clinically meaningful effect, but the trial was not of sufficient size to detect it [39].

The use of P values and hypothesis testing is firmly entrenched in the medical literature. However, confidence interval estimation and the use of 'point estimates' is more informative for researchers and readers [40]. In fact, many authorities favor the use of point estimates, such as a relative risk or an odds ratio and their 95% confidence interval, over the calculation of P values [40,41]. A relative risk is the risk of outcome in the exposed population relative to that in the unexposed or control population. A relative risk greater than 1.0 implies an increased risk and a relative risk less than 1 implies a protective effect. For example, the relative risk of endometrial cancer in women greater than 50 pounds overweight is 10.0, or a 10-fold increased risk, while the relative risk of endometrial cancer in combination oral contraceptive users is 0.5 or a 50% decreased risk [42]. When the 95% confidence interval excludes 1.0, then the results are statistically significant. The width of the confidence interval provides some estimate of the precision of the effect size. The narrower the confidence interval, the more precise the estimate.

The major difference between relative risks and odds ratios is that relative risks are calculated from prospective data such as a cohort study or a randomized trial, while odds ratios are usually calculated in case–control studies. The odds ratio is a reasonable approximation of the relative risk when the disease under study is rare. The reason why relative risks or odds ratios and their confidence intervals are preferred is that these data provide more than just a test of significance: they also provide a measure of the magnitude of the association and its direction (i.e. whether the exposure results in an increased or decreased risk of the disease).

There are many statistical tests used in reproductive health research, and their indications and uses cannot be fully described in this brief chapter. Interested readers should consult a basic biostatistics text [43,44]. One common problem in epidemiologic research is how to control for covariates or confounding variables in the analysis. Stratification allows the researcher to assess the exposure–disease relationship for each category of relevant covariates. This method is often impractical if more than one or two covariates must be controlled. One of the most commonly used tools employed by epidemiologists and reproductive health researchers is a multivariate mathematical model called logistic regression. Logistic regression is used to control for multiple covariates statistically and thereby improve the chance of obtaining an accurate measure of the exposure–disease relationship [45]. Researchers interested in employing multivariate analysis (MVA) should work closely with a statistician.

Interpreting the medical literature

While epidemiologic studies cannot prove causation, they can be used to determine the likelihood of causation. Criteria to consider to determine a cause and effect relationship include:

- Strength of the association: the stronger the association, the more likely it is to be real.

- Consistency of the study findings over numerous reports (from study to study).

- Temporal relationship: does the cause precede the effect?

- Biological plausibility: does the relationship make biologic sense?

- Biologic gradient: is there a dose–response relationship?

- Is there experimental evidence to support or refute the association?

- Is the association specific?

A critical reader of the medical literature should be able to characterize the methodology of a research study and recognize its scientific value. The US Preventive Services Task Force has outlined specific guidelines to determine the level of evidence of a specific practice (Table 2.1). However, when interpreting the medical literature, the reader should consider not only the methodology (e.g. randomized trial, observational study, etc.), but also the quality of the study. Readers should no longer accept the 'gospel of the expert'. As illustrated in Table 2.1, opinions of authorities and reports of expert committees are no longer acceptable as sound evidence. An educated reader will evaluate the evidence available from quality studies in the medical literature and recognize when evidence to support a specific practice or association is weak and in need of further study.

References

1. Grimes DA. Introducing evidence-based medicine into a department of obstetrics and gynecology. *Obstet Gynecol* 1995;86:451–7.

2. US Preventive Services Task Force. Guide to clinical preventive services, 2nd edn. Baltimore: Williams and Wilkins, 1996.

3. Canadian Task Force on the Periodic Health Examination. The periodic health examination. *Can Med Assoc J* 1979;121:1193–1254.

4. Grimes DA. Randomized controlled trials: 'It Ain't Necessarily So'. *Obstet Gynecol* 1991;78:703–4.

5. Hulley SB, Cummings SR. Designing clinical research: an epidemiologic approach. Baltimore: Williams and Wilkins, 1988.

6. Feinstein AR. Clinical epidemiology: the architecture of clinical research. Philadelphia: WB Saunders, 1985, p.684.

7. Sigerist HS. The university at the crossroads. New York: H Shumann, 1946.

8. Fisher RA, Mackenzie WA. Studies in crop variation: II. The manurial response to different potato varieties. *J Agric Sci* 1923;13:315.

9. Schulz KF, Chalmers I, Grimes DA, Altman DG. Assessing the quality of randomization from reports of controlled trials published in obstetrics and gynecology journals. *JAMA* 1994;272:125–8.

10. Colditz GA, Hankinson SE, Hunter DJ, Willett WC, Manson JE, Stampfer MJ, et al. The use of estrogens and progestins and the risk of breast cancer in postmenopausal women. *N Engl J Med* 1995;332:1589–93.

11. Grodstein F, Stampfer MJ, Manson JE, Colditz GA, Willett WC, Rosner B, et al. Postmenopausal estrogen and progestin use and the risk of cardiovascular disease. *N Engl J Med* 1996;335:453–61.

12. Peipert JF, Grimes DA. The case-control study: a primer for the obstetrician–gynecologist. *Obstet Gynecol* 1994;84:140–5.

13. The Centers for Disease Control Cancer and Steroid Hormone Study. Oral contraceptive use and the risk of endometrial cancer. *JAMA* 1983;249:1600–4.

14. Burkman RT. Association between intrauterine device and pelvic inflammatory disease. *Obstet Gynecol* 1981;57:269–76.

15. Peipert JF, Boardman L, Hogan JW, et al. Laboratory evaluation of acute upper genital tract infection. *Obstet Gynecol* 1996;87:730–6.

16. Caillouette JC, Kochler AL. Phasic contraceptive pills and functional ovarian cysts. *Am J Obstet Gynecol* 1987;156:1538–42.

17. Grimes DA, Godwin AJ, Rubin A, Smith JA, Lacarra M. Ovulation and follicular development associated with three low-dose oral contraceptives: a randomized controlled trial. *Obstet Gynecol* 1994;83:29–34.

18. Peipert JF, Sweeney PJ. Diagnostic testing in obstetrics and gynecology: a clinician's guide. *Obstet Gynecol* 1993;82:619–23.

19. Ransohoff DF, Feinstein AR. Problems of spectrum and bias in evaluating the efficacy of diagnostic tests. *N Engl J Med* 1978;199:926–30.

20. Enkin M, Keirse MJ, Chalmers I. Effective care in pregnancy and childbirth. New York: Oxford University Press, 1969.

21. Longnecker MP, Berlin JA, Orza MJ, et al. A meta-analysis of alcohol consumption in relation to risk of breast cancer. *JAMA* 1988;260:652–6.

22. Sacks HS, Berrier J, Reitman D, et al. Meta-analysis of randomized controlled trials. *N Engl J Med* 1987;316:450–5.

23. Shapiro S. Meta-analysis/shmeta-analysis. *Am J Epidemiol* 1994;140:771–8.

24. Kirpalani H, Schmidt B, McKibbon KA, Haynes R, Sinclair J. Searching MEDLINE for randomized clinical trials involving care of the newborn. *Pediatrics* 1988;83:543–7.

25. L'Abbe KA, Detshy AS, O'Rourke K. Meta-analysis in clinical research. *Ann Intern Med* 1987;107:224–33.

26. Pettiti DB. Meta-analysis, decision analysis, and cost-effectiveness analysis: methods for quantitiative synthesis in medicine. New York: Oxford University Press, 1994, pp.5–6.

27. Gifford DS, Keeler E, Kahn KL. Reductions in cost and cesarean delivery rate by routine use of external cephalic version: a decision analysis. *Obstet Gynecol* 1995;85:930–6.

28. Lieu TA, Watson SE, Washington AE. The cost-effectiveness of perinatal carrier screening for cystic fibrosis. *Obstet Gynecol* 1994;84:903–12.

29. Brook RH. Health services research: Is it good for you and me? *Academic Med* 1989;64:124–30.

30. Wennberg J, Gittelsohn A. Small are variations in health care delivery. *Science* 1973;182:1102–8.

31. Wennberg JE, Freeman JL, Shelton RM, Bubolz TA. Hospital use and mortality among Medicare beneficiaries in

2

An overview of
reproductive
epidemiology,
statistics and
methods for
evaluating
research

Boston and New Haven. *N Engl J Med* 1989;321:1168–73.

32. Wennberg JE Freeman JL, Culp WJ. Are hospital services rationed in New Haven or over–utilized in Boston? *Lancet* 1987;1:1185–9.

33. Chassin MR, Kosecoff J, Park RE, et al. Does inappropriate use explain geographic variations in the use of health care services? A study of three procedures. *JAMA* 1987;258:2533–7.

34. Brook RH, Park RE, Chassin MR, Solomon DH, Keesey J, Kosecoff J. Predicting the appropriate use of carotid endarterectomy, upper gastrointestinal endoscopy and coronary angiography. *N Engl J Med* 1990,323:1173–7.

35. Winslow CM, Kosecoff JB, Chassin M, Kanouse DI, Brook RH. The appropriateness of performing coronary artery bypass surgery. *JAMA* 1988;260:505–9.

36. Bernstein SJ, McGlyn EA, Siu AL, et al. The appropriateness of hysterectomy: a comparison of care in seven health plans. *JAMA* 1993;269:2398–402.

37. National Institutes of Health. Quality of life assessment: practice, problems and promise. Proceedings of a Workshop, 1990.

38. Peipert JF, Metheny WP, Schulz K. Sample size and statistical power in reproductive research. *Obstet Gynecol* 1995;86:302–5.

39. Freiman JA, Chalmers TC, Smith H, Kuebler RR. The importance of beta, the type II error and sample size in the design and interpretation of the randomized control trial. A survey of 71 'negative' trials. *N Engl J Med* 1978;299:690–4.

40. Grimes DA. The case for confidence intervals. *Obstet Gynecol* 1992;80:865–6.

41. Rothman KJ. A show of confidence. *N Engl J Med* 1978;299:1362–3.

42. Rose PG. Endometrial carcinoma. *N Engl J Med* 1996;335:640–9.

43. Rosner B. Fundamentals of biostatistics, 4th edn. Belmont: Wadsworth, 1995.

44. Kramer MS. Clinical epidemiology and biostatistics: a primer for clinical investigators and decision-makers. New York: Springer-Verlag, 1988.

45. Peterson HB, Kleinbaum DG. Interpreting the literature in obstetrics and gynecology: II. Logistic regression and related issues. *Obstet Gynecol* 1991;78:717–20.

Section 2:
Contraception

Contraceptive efficacy and safety

Paula Adams Hillard MD

Introduction

The voluntary control of fertility is an important issue for modern individuals, couples and societies, but this ability to control fertility effectively during the reproductive years is a relatively modern development. Barrier methods of contraception, including male condoms and diaphragms, have been available for a number of years. Hormonal methods define a 'modern era' of contraception. Oral contraceptives were first approved by the Food and Drug Administration (FDA) in the USA in 1960. Couples have available a number of different reversible methods of contraception. These include barrier methods: male condoms, female condoms, the diaphragm, cervical cap and vaginal spermicides. Hormonal methods available today include oral contraceptives, injectable depot medroxyprogesterone acetate, and the implant device containing levonorgestrel. Other reversible methods include the intrauterine contraceptive device. Outside the USA, monthly combined injectables and intrauterine systems are among the available methods. Emergency contraception, usually administered as high-dose combination hormones, is also available, but widely underutilized in the USA because of lack of familiarity by both clinicians and the public. Permanent sterilization in the form of vasectomy for men or bilateral tubal occlusion for women is now the most widely used form of contraception in the USA.

Contraceptive methods

Methods of contraception available can be divided into five categories:

1. Hormonal methods: oral contraceptives, injectables (depot medroxyprogesterone acetate) and the subdermal implant containing levonorgestrel. The hormone-releasing intrauterine system is available in Europe. Combined injectables are available in some countries.
2. Barrier methods: male condoms, female condoms, the diaphragm, cervical cap and where available, the contraceptive sponge.
3. Spermicides: designed to be used either alone or in conjunction with the barrier methods.
4. Other: the intrauterine device (currently available are a copper-containing T and a progesterone-releasing device); natural family planning; emergency contraception.
5. Permanent sterilization: vasectomy for men, and bilateral tubal occlusion for women.

The effectiveness of the barrier methods and spermicides is generally lower than that of the hormonal methods or the intrauterine device (IUD). Their efficacy is dependent upon their correct and consistent use – compliance. The safety of the barrier methods is generally considered to be a significant advantage over hormonal methods; however, when one factors in the lower efficacy, and thus the higher risk of pregnancy with its attendant risks, the equation changes. A graphic representation of the risks of *mortality* associated with various methods of contraception, factoring in the risks of pregnancy by age, as contained in the USA patient package insert of oral contraceptives, is presented in Figure 3.1.

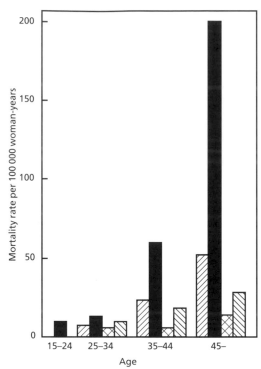

Fig. 3.1 Circulatory disease mortality rates per 100 000 woman-years by age, smoking status and oral contraceptive use. ▨ = ever-users (non-smokers); ▩ = controls (non-smokers); ■ = ever-users (smokers); ▨ = controls (smokers). Adapted from Layde PM, Beral V, Kay CR. Further analysis of mortality in oral contraceptive users' Royal College of General Practitioners' Study. *Lancet* 1981; 1:541–6.

Safety

Contraceptive benefits to health

Most couples in industrialized countries choose to limit the number of children they have. Americans are not very successful in preventing unintended pregnancies: over 50% of all pregnancies in the USA are unintended [1]. The USA has one of the highest abortion rates and one of the highest rates of unintended births in the developed world. About half of those births occur among the 10% of women who are not using a method of contraception; however, the remaining half occur among women who experience a contraceptive

failure. American couples have fewer contraceptive options than do women in other developed countries [2]. Women in the USA are more likely to choose less effective methods of contraception and they also tend to use these methods less effectively. [1]

Many explanations have been given for this phenomenon: lack of access to medical care, cultural attitudes about sexuality, religious factors, lack of information about contraception, fear of side effects of contraception, media attention to the risks of birth control, and a litigious climate [3]. The emphasis that the media place on the potential risks of contraception leads to fears about the use of contraception, which then results in non-use of contraception.

Most couples do not recognize that pregnancy and birth can themselves present significant health risks. Thus, the potential medical risks of contraception should be viewed in comparison with risks associated with unintended pregnancies which would occur if no method, or a less effective method, were used.

Risk of ectopic pregnancy

Most ectopic pregnancies are a consequence of previous pelvic infection with tubal scarring and dysfunction. Use of *any* method of contraception reduces the risk of ectopic pregnancy when compared with the use of *no method*. The interaction between risk of ectopic pregnancy and method of contraception depends on: how likely it is that the woman will contract a sexually transmitted infection (STI); how effective her contraceptive method is in preventing pregnancy; how likely it is that the pregnancy will be ectopic if the method should fail; and whether the method influences her chance of developing an upper genital tract infection [3]. The estimated annual number of ectopic pregnancies with various methods of contraception and by sexually transmitted disease (STD) risk status is shown in Figure 3.2.

Combination oral contraceptives markedly reduce the number of ectopic pregnancies, but even IUDs decrease the risk of ectopic pregnancy over the use of no method of contraception. The use of a contraceptive method prevents an estimated 30–280 annual ectopics per 100 000 women who are in mutually monogamous relationships

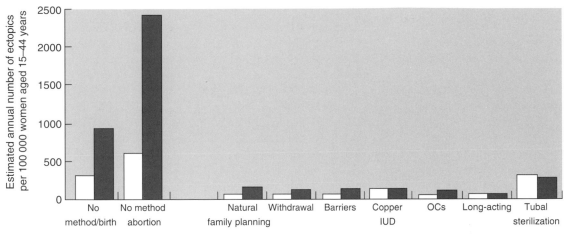

Fig. 3.2 Ectopic pregnancies and STI risk markers. Solid columns = not mutually monogamous; shaded columns = mutually monogamous. Adapted from Harlap S, Kost K, Forrest JD. Preventing pregnancy, protecting health: a new look at birth control choices in the United States. New York: The Alan Guttmacher Institute, 1991: p. 51.

(compared to women using no method who give birth) and an estimated 680–920 annual ectopics per 100 000 in non-monogamous relationships. [3]

Non-contraceptive benefits of birth control methods

The benefits of hormonal methods include menstrual-related effects, as well as other medical benefits such as a decreased risk of cancer. The barrier methods have the primary benefit of decreasing the risks of STDs.

Hormonal methods – oral contraceptives

Oral contraceptives (OCs) have a number of beneficial effects related to the menstrual cycle: a decreased risk of dysmenorrhea, regular cycles and a lighter flow, with a consequent lower risk of anemia. These are quality-of-life issues that are not always appreciated by a significant number of women [4]. Oral contraceptive pills also decrease

the risks of benign breast disease, ovarian cysts, and both ovarian and endometrial cancer [5]. For suppression of ovarian cysts, the risks are lowest with higher estrogen pills, somewhat higher for users of low-dose monophasic pills, and the least protection is offered by multiphasic pills. Women who use OCs have been found in several studies to have a lower risk of toxic shock syndrome, although this has not been a consistent finding in all studies. Women who have ever used the pill have a 40% lower risk of developing ovarian cancer [6]. Women who have used OCs for at least 2 years have a 40% reduction in risk of endometrial cancer. These benefits are also widely underappreciated [4]. Women with acne will benefit from OCs, as noted in the FDA's decision to approve a specific OC for women with acne who need contraception.

It has been estimated that 1614 per 100 000 current pill users avoid being hospitalized each year because of protective effects of the pill [3]. This benefit relates to hospitalizations prevented by

pregnancy and its complications, but also to the beneficial effects of preventing breast disease, ovarian cysts and invasive cancers.

Barrier methods

Barrier methods of contraception, particularly those which are used with or include a spermicide, can help protect against STDs; however, in order for them to be more effective in providing this benefit, they must be used correctly and consistently. The Center for Disease Control (CDC) has stated that 'Latex condoms are highly effective for preventing HIV infection and other STDs when used consistently and correctly' [7]. The benefits which these methods can provide when used consistently are best illustrated by the very low rates of HIV transmission (in one study 0%) which can be achieved between serodiscordant members of heterosexual couples when condoms are used consistently [8]. Clearly, behavioral factors such as having sex with more than one partner or with a partner who has other partners increased the risk for STDs. Condoms, when used correctly for every act of intercourse, can greatly decrease transmission for bacterial STDs and provide some protection for viral STDs such as herpes simplex virus, human papilloma virus and HIV [3]. Contraceptive diaphragms, especially when used with spermicides, can also decrease risk of some infections. *In vitro*, spermicides kill organisms responsible for gonorrhea, chlamydia, HIV and other viruses [9]. The use of barrier methods and spermicides can lead to a decreased risk of genital upper tract infection/pelvic inflammatory disease (PID), even among women who are not in mutually monogamous relationships [3].

Risks of contraceptive methods

Risks of barrier methods

The primary risks of barrier methods relate to their failure rates and thus to the failure in preventing the risks associated with pregnancy, including the risks of ectopic pregnancy, spontaneous abortion or other pregnancy-related complications [3]. Failure rates of barrier methods are due in part to the intrinsic failure of the method itself but also, importantly, to the lack of consistent and correct use (see the discussion of efficacy below). Thus, users of barrier methods are more likely to be exposed to the risks of pregnancy because of the higher failure rates associated with the methods than with hormonal methods. These risks of pregnancy, including complications such as pregnancy-

associated hypertension, genital lacerations with birth, postpartum hemorrhage and cesarean delivery, occur in a quarter of all pregnancies.

Other risks of barrier methods include the risk of latex allergy. Allergy to latex occurs in up to 17% of medical personnel, although in a smaller percentage in the general population [10]. Most current condoms are made of latex and the benefits of condom use in decreasing STD risk have been demonstrated with latex condoms. Diaphragm users have been shown to have an increased risk of urinary tract infection, although most of these infections are treated on an outpatient basis.

Risks of hormonal methods

Oral contraceptives

The risks of oral contraceptives have been divided into 'major' risks and 'minor' risks, although this categorization minimizes the effects that the so-called 'minor' side effects can have on oral contraceptive continuation and compliance [11]. The most common side effects associated with oral contraceptives include bleeding irregularities, occurring in 20–30% of users during the first month of use, but declining in frequency thereafter [12]. Nuisance effects which are not medically serious but which can lead to dissatisfaction with the method include mood changes, headaches, nausea, breast symptoms or changes in libido [13].

The occurrence of medically serious complications with oral contraceptives has been

extensively studied. The overall risk of serious cardiovascular complications is very low in young women, and in non-smokers who are healthy and who have no predisposing factors for cardiovascular disease [3]. Studies addressing the cardiovascular risks of OCs have led to decreased doses of both the estrogen and the progestin components of the pills, with a consequent decrease in risk. In addition, clarification of risk factors such as smoking or other cardiovascular risk factors (such as hypertension, abnormalities of cholesterol metabolism and diabetes) has led to the more selective prescribing of oral contraceptives and to a more careful weighing of risks *vs* benefits, which must be communicated with the user herself.

The incidence of cardio-vascular risks increases with age. Studies of myocardial infarction have led to the conclusion that smoking is the primary risk factor and that this is compounded by the use of OCs. Non-smoking pill users do not have an increased risk of myocardial infarction (MI) over non-pill users. For pill users who smoke and are over the age of 35, the estimated number of deaths associated with pill use is approximately four times higher than the estimated risks of death associated with pregnancy in that age group [14]. For this reason, clinicians discourage the use of oral contraceptives in smokers over 35.

The risks of stroke have been studied in pill users. A recent study found no significant increase in the risk of either hemorrhagic or ischemic stroke among users of low-dose OCs, after adjusting for other risk factors. Smoking, however, markedly increased the risk [15]. Another international case-control study concluded that, for women under 35, the overall risk of stroke is low, and any additional risk attributable to OC use is small, especially in the absence of smoking or hypertension [16].

Venous thrombosis and embolism have been examined recently, as several articles have suggested an increased risk of thromboembolic phenomena among users of pills containing the progestins desogestrel and gestodene [17–22]. These studies have concluded that users of the so-called 'third generation' progestin-containing pills have a risk of non-fatal venous thromboembolism of approximately 20–30 per 100 000 women of childbearing age, compared with a risk of approximately 5 for women who do not take OCs, a risk of approximately 10–14 for women taking older pills and a risk of 60 for pregnancy [23]. Some authors have criticized these studies for including prescribing biases that are not accounted for by the statistics, lacking biologic plausibility [24–26]. The US FDA has reviewed the data and decided that the 'risk is not great enough to justify switching to other products' [19]. The FDA further noted that the risk is still at least twice as high among pregnant women as it would be in women taking pills with gestodene or desogestrel.

The issue of risk of breast cancer for OC users has been extensively studied, but remains somewhat unclear. Overall, it appears that the risk of being diagnosed with breast cancer by

age 55 does not differ between women who have and have not used the pill, when all age groups are considered together [6]. However, the studies of risks for younger women are inconsistent [27]. The Cancer and Steroid Hormones (CASH) study indicated that for women 35 or younger, pill users were 1.4 times more likely to have been diagnosed with breast cancer than those who had never used oral contraceptives, but in older women, pill users had 0.9 the rate of never-users [3,28]. Other studies have noted that women on OCs who develop breast cancer have an earlier stage at diagnosis. More research is needed to clarify these risks.

When all cases of breast, ovarian, endometrial and liver cancers are totaled, pill users will have fewer reproductive cancers than will non-users, and the protection gained is greatest at older ages [3].

Progestin-containing hormonal methods

The levonorgestrel contraceptive implant and the injectable method, depot medroxy-progesterone acetate, have similar side-effect profiles [29]. The most common side effect with both is that of menstrual disturbances [30–32]. Most women have at least some degree of menstrual irregularity, although with the injectable methods, amenorrhea is more likely to be the effect after prolonged use, with 50% of users being amenorrheic at 1 year [32]. Other reported side effects include headaches, mood changes, acne, changes in hair growth and weight gain [32]. Bone density has been studied in users of injectable progestins, and

there are some preliminary data to suggest that there may be a reversible decrease in bone density for users of this method [33]. More recent work refutes this observation (Randall S, personal communication).

Other methods

The IUD

In the USA, the perception of risks associated with IUD use has been colored by the Dalkon Shield experience. Reanalysis of studies which included the Dalkon Shield have concluded that the other types of IUD are not associated with the same magnitude of risk [34]. A number of recent reports have strongly urged that the use of the IUD is significantly safer than previously suspected, particularly for women at low risk of STDs [35–37]. An international World Health Organization (WHO) study indicated that, although there was a slight increase in the risk of PID in the first 20 days after insertion, the overall risk of PID was low and continued to be close to the baseline risk [38]. The levonorgestrel-containing IUD is felt to have a protective effect on the risk of PID, especially in young users [39]. The clinical practice in the USA is to reserve IUD use for women with a low risk of STDs.

Contraceptive efficacy

Contraceptive efficacy has traditionally been measured by the use of the Pearl index. The Pearl index is defined as the number of failures per 100 woman–years of exposure. The denominator becomes the total number of months or cycles of exposure from the time of initiation of method use until the study ends, a pregnancy occurs, or the method is discontinued. The quotient is multiplied by 1200 (if months of exposure are used) or by 1300 (if cycles are used). The Pearl index fails to take into account the fact that failure rates usually decline with time and duration of use, as users become more adept at using the method and as less compliant users get pregnant. Therefore, another method of calculation, the life-table analysis, is now much more frequently used [40].

Life-table analysis calculates a failure rate for each month of use, ultimately allowing the determination of a cumulative failure rate for a given interval of exposure. Pregnancy can occur as a result of 'method failure' or 'user failure', which takes compliance into account. Attempts have thus been made to sort out these two ways of looking at contraceptive failure. However, it is virtually impossible to determine true method failure rates, defined as failure during perfect use, as all clinical trials involve real humans with human foibles. Thus the terms pregnancy rates during 'perfect use' (or the 'lowest expected' pregnancy rates) and the pregnancy rates during 'typical use' were introduced in the 1980s [41]. Table 3.1 shows the failure rates during the first year of use [42].

An additional problem in defining contraceptive efficacy is the term 'failure rate', which refers to the occurrence of a pregnancy, which may or may not be due to method failure

Table 3.1 Percentage of women experiencing an unintended pregnancy during the first year of typical use and the first year of perfect use of contraception, and the percentage continuing use at the end of the first year (USA)

| Method (1) | Percentage of woman experiencing an unintended pregnancy within first year of use | | Percentage of woman continuing use at 1 year* |
	Typical use[a] (2)	Perfect use[b] (3)	(4)
Chance[d]	85	85	
Spermicides[e]	25	6	40
Periodic abstinence	25		68
Calendar		9	
Ovulation method		3	
Sympto-thermal[f]		2	
Postovulation		1	
Withdrawal	19	4	
Cap[g]			
Parous women	40	26	42
Nulliparous women	20	9	56
Sponge			
Parous women	40	20	42
Nulliparous women	20	9	56
Diaphragm[g]	20	6	56
Condom[h]			
Female (Reality)	21	5	56
Male	14	3	61
Pill	5		71
Progestin only		0.5	
Combined		0.1	
IUD			
Progesterone T	2.0	1.5	81
Copper T 380A	0.8	0.6	78
LNg 20	0.1	0.1	81
Depo-Provera	0.3	0.3	70
Norplant and Norplant-2	0.05	0.05	88
Female sterilization	0.5	0.5	100
Male sterilization	0.15	0.10	100

Emergency Contraceptive Pills: Treatment initiated within 72 hours after unprotected intercourse reduces the risk of pregnancy by at least 75%.[i]
Lactational Amenorrhea Method: LAM is a highly effective, *temporary* method of contraception.[j]
Source: Trussell J. Contraceptive efficacy. In: Hatcher RA, Trussell J, Stewart F. (eds) Cates W, Stewart GK, Kowal D, Guest F, Contraceptive Technology: 17th Revised Ed.. New York NY: Ardent Media, 1998.
[a]Among typical couples who initiate use of a method (not necessarily for the first time), the percentage who experience an accidental pregnancy during the first year if they do not stop use for any other reason.
[b]Among couples who initiate use of a method (not necessarily for the first time) and who use it *perfectly* (both consistently and correctly), the percentage who experience an accidental pregnancy during the first year if they do not stop use for any other reason.
[c]Among couples attempting to avoid pregnancy, the percentage who continue to use a method for 1 year.
[d]The percentage becoming pregnant in columns (2) and (3) are based on data from populations where contraception is not used and from women who cease using contraception in order to become pregnant. Among such populations, about 89% become pregnant within 1 year. This estimate was lowered slightly (to 85%) to represent the percentage who would become pregnant within 1 year among women now relying on reversible methods of contraception if they abandoned contraception altogether.
[e]Foams, creams, gels, vaginal suppositories, and vaginal film.
[f]Cervical mucus (ovulation) method supplemented by calendar in the preovulatory and basal body temperature in the postovulatory phases.
[g]With spermicidal cream or jelly.
[h]Without spermicides.
[i]The treatment schedule is one dose within 72 hours after unprotected intercourse, and a second dose 12 hours after the first dose. The FDA has declared the following brands of oral contraceptives to be safe and effective for emergency contraception: Ovral (1 dose in 2 white pills), Alesse or Levlite (1 dose is 5 pink pills), Nordette or Levlen (1 dose is 2 light-orange pills), Lo/Ovral (1 dose is 4 white pills), Triphasil or Tri-Levlen (1 dose is 4 yellow pills).
[j]However, to maintain effective protection against pregnancy, another method of contraception must be used as soon as menstruation resumes, the frequency or duration of breastfeeds is reduced, bottle feeds are introduced, or the baby reaches 6 months of age.

(because of differing degrees of compliance, the varying ability to conceive, and the frequency and timing of intercourse) [40]. Thus, it has been suggested that the term 'failure rate' should be replaced with the more precise term 'pregnancy rate' [40].

'Efficacy' is an epidemiologic term indicating how well something works under ideal conditions; thus with pregnancy, this would be during perfect use. 'Effectiveness is used to denote how well something works under normal or typical use. In order to calculate these values for a contraceptive method, the number of pregnancies prevented by the method must be compared with the number of pregnancies which would have occurred without the method – the number of expected pregnancies. The probability of conception varies by day of the menstrual cycle and the time of intercourse, and several studies have reported these values [43–45]. Steiner et al. have proposed that it would be valuable actually to measure the expected pregnancy rate using a randomized study design [40].

'Contraceptive effectiveness' or use effectiveness is generally defined as one minus the pregnancy rate. Contraceptives can fail only if a pregnancy would have occurred in the absence of contraception: if a method has a 3% pregnancy rate, this does not represent a 3% failure rate (or conversely, a 97% effectiveness rate), as fewer than 100% of women would have become pregnant [46]. Thus it is not accurate to refer to the typical-use and perfect-use pregnancy rates as failure rates. 'Contraceptive failure rate' is, more precisely, the pregnancy rate per 100 woman-years (usually stated for the first year of use, as poorer users may drop out or better users continue). Pregnancy may or may not be due to failure of the method itself. Few couples use contraception perfectly.

Under-reporting of abortion (by approximately two-thirds) also occurs [47]. The issue of cumulative failure rate over time should also be considered. This issue is rarely discussed [48]. Pregnancies among OC users generally decline after the first year of use, as individuals who are poorer pill-takers discontinue using the method. Some individuals discontinue use because they become pregnant, others because they have difficulty using the method owing to side effects; still others may discontinue if they realize they are poor pill-takers. Long-term pregnancy rates can be estimated by multiplying the probabilities of not becoming pregnant in each year of use. If one assumes, for example, a first year failure rate of 8% with OCs with a decline to 5% during the second year, the cumulative likelihood of pregnancy after 3 years would be 17% [46].

Compliance

The differences between the lowest expected and typical use failure rates are due to a variety of factors, including variation in correct and consistent use of the method. Thus issues of contraceptive compliance have been recognized in recent years as a major area of investigation and research.

Contraceptive compliance can be placed in the context of compliance with other medications. The potential consequence of failing to comply with contraception is pregnancy.

Presumably women are using contraception in an effort to avoid pregnancy, but the literature on compliance suggests that there is no consequence of failed compliance that is severe or onerous enough to ensure complete compliance [49]. In addition, surveys of medication use which utilize electronic monitoring to measure the use of medication for a variety of medical disorders suggest that, overall, about 75% of doses are taken [50].

How effective are contraceptives? Pregnancy rates vary not only across different methods, but also for any one method across different populations, and among users within those populations (such as by marital status, age and socioeconomic status) [46]. Potter reviewed 53 articles on effectiveness and identified sociodemographic subgroups – age, poverty level and marital status – which she felt would help to target efforts to increase effective use [46].

Both *correct and continued* use of contraception are components of compliant use. Discontinuation of method and switching from one contraceptive method to another are common. Continuation rates, defined as the percentage of women who continue to use the method for 1 year for various contraceptive methods vary from 90% for users of Norplant contraceptive implants to 75% for IUDs, to approximately 75% or less for oral contraceptives [42]. Some methods are easier for the user to discontinue; IUDs and Norplant cannot easily be discontinued by the user herself. Oral contraceptives are the method of contraception which has been studied best with regard to both correct and continuing use.

The use of oral contraceptives, unlike the longer-acting methods of contraception, requires a daily activity on an ongoing basis. Overall, 27% of users of oral contraceptives discontinue the method and have a need for ongoing contraception, but use no method; the percentage among adolescents is 38% [51]. In one survey of women having an abortion, about half had used a method of contraception during the month in which they conceived [52]. Adolescents and single adults may practice patterns of serial monogamy in which they use oral contraceptives during the months in which they are in a relationship, but discontinue them when they break up with a partner [53]. Unfortunately, when a relationship is resumed, or a new relationship dictates contraception, they may resume using the method after they resume sexual activity, thus placing themselves at risk of unintended pregnancy. Adolescents, particularly inner-city adolescents, can have failure rates with oral contraceptives of 16% [54]; failure rates of up to 38% are seen in inner-city adolescents who have already given birth [55]. These failure rates are due to a variety of problems in taking oral contraceptives: problems in continuing to use a method (including financial problems paying for OCs or making follow-up clinic appointments) or in taking the pill correctly.

Incorrect use of oral contraceptives includes a variety of ways in which the pills can be taken in the wrong order, starting a new package late and missing pills [56]. Such misuse appears to be fairly frequent, although relatively few studies have assessed this issue carefully, and it is not clear how much of a role these problems play in oral contraceptive failure rates. Oakley reported on what she termed 'misbehaviours' – components of correct pill-taking. The results of her work are presented in Table 3.2 [57]. Only 13% of individuals took all pills correctly all the time. Balassone found that adolescents who were 'consistent' pill-takers (i.e. continuing users) missed 2.7 pills/month; 'inconsistent' pill users missed 3.4 pills/month. In this study, the pregnancy rate was 9.9/1000 woman-years [58].

Missed pills, which result in an extension of the hormone-free interval (such as starting a new pack of pills 2–3 days late), may result in escape follicular development, possibly ovulation, and potentially pregnancy [59–61]. These studies have included only small numbers, but the link with ovulation and pregnancy as an outcome has not been shown [62].

Potter argues that 'better than average' users of oral contraceptives can have a pregnancy rate of about 4%; for 'poorer than average' users the pregnancy rate is closer to 8% [46]. The knowledge that failure rates vary can help an individual user to better understand her role in effective contraception. Knowing that failure rates among typical users vary with sociodemographic factors can help lead to selective interventions by clinicians.

Measuring contraceptive use is difficult. A variety of methods have been reported, including the use of indirect measure such as diaries or questionnaires (self-report). Return visits or prescription refills can also serve as a measure of continuing use [54,63]. Biologic assays for contraceptive steroids in, for example, urine or serum have been reported, but are clearly much more cumbersome and not clinically practical [64]. Electronic measures of pill use have been reported, but cannot determine if the pills were actually swallowed [65,66]. When diary data are compared with an electronic pill pack, overall agreement was only 48% [46]. The largest errors were among those who missed the most pills: those who missed three or more hormonally active pills were more likely to report not missing any than were those who had missed only 1 or 2 days [57].

Further study is needed to determine the effects of missing

Table 3.2 Behaviors concerning oral contraceptive use among initial family planning clinic clients in Oakland County, Michigan, USA, from 1987 through 1989

Behavior	Percentage of 1167 pill users
Never took others' pills	99
Always took in same order	98
Took all pills	89
Always used back up if needed	61
Took pill every day	42
Took pill every day, same time	20
Used completely correctly	13

Adapted from Oakley D, Sereika S, Bogue EL. Oral contraceptive pill use after an initial visit to a family planning clinic. *Fam Plann Perspect* 1991; 23: 50–4.

one or more pills, as well as the effects of the time in the cycle in which pills were missed. There may also be a reinforcement of behaviors: if missing a pill does not lead to a pregnancy, the user is more likely to miss another pill, believing that it does not matter. It is not at all clear how much compliance is 'enough' to provide contraceptive effectiveness. However, there may be significant individual variations in hormone metabolism both between and within different populations [67].

Goldzieher has stated that large numbers of patients would need to be studied to determine the effects of compliance and estimated that this would require at least 5000–10 000 cycles of use [68].

Compliance with the use of barrier methods is problematic as well. Oakley has described microbehaviors relating to condom use, and noted that only about one in three adolescents and only 40–60% of older women reported condom use with every act of intercourse [69].

Summary

The use of contraception is, on balance, healthy and safe. Pregnancy itself carries significant risks to health. The use of contraceptive measures, whether hormonal or barrier, is an effective public health measure with preventive value. Planned, intended pregnancies are the goal of responsible societies. The benefits to the individual are significant, and the cumulative effect of contraception is a healthier future.

References

1. Jones EF, Forrest JD. Contraceptive failure in the United States: revised estimates from the 1982 National Survey of Family Growth. *Fam Plann Perspect* 1989;21:193.

2. Anonymous. Obstacles and opportunities. Washington, DC. National Academy Press, 1990.

3. Harlap S, Kost K, Forrest JD. Preventing pregnancy, protecting health: a new look at birth control choices in the United States. New York: The Alan Guttmacher Institute, 1991.

4. Peipert JF, Gutmann J. Oral contraceptive risk assessment: a survey of 247 educated women. *Obstet Gynecol* 1993;82:112–7.

5. Grimes DA. The safety of oral contraceptives: epidemiologic insights from the first 30 years. *Am J Obstet Gynecol* 1992; 166:1950–4.

6. Schlesselmann JJ. Cancer of the breast and reproductive tract in relation to use of oral contraceptives. *Contraception* 1989;40:1.

7. Anonymous. Condoms for prevention of sexually transmitted diseases. *MMWR* 1988;37:133–7.

8. de-Vincenzi I. A longitudinal study of human immunodeficiency virus transmission by heterosexual partners. European Study Group on Heterosexual Transmission of HIV. *N Engl J Med* 1994; 331:341–6.

9. Institute of Medicine. The hidden epidemic: confronting sexually transmitted diseases. Washington, DC. National Academy Press, 1997.

10. Yassin MS, Lierl MB, Fischer TJ, et al. Latex allergy in hospital employees. *Ann Allergy* 1994; 72:245–9.

11. Hillard PJ. The patient's reaction to side effects of oral contraceptives. *Am J Obstet Gynecol* 1989;161:1412–15.

12. Rosenberg MJ, Burnhill MS, Waugh MS, Grimes DA, Hillard PJA. Compliance and oral contraceptives: a review. *Contraception* 1995;52:137–41.

13. Guillebaud J. Practical prescribing of the combined oral contraceptive pill. In: Filshie M, Guillebaud J. (eds) Contraception, Science and Practice. Oxford: Butterworths 1989, p. 87.

14. Ory HW. Association between oral contraceptives and myocardial infarction. A review. *JAMA* 1977;237:2519–22.

15. Petitti DB, Sidney S, Bernstein A, et al. Stroke in users of low-dose oral contraceptives. *N Engl J Med* 1996;335:8–15.

16. WHO Collaborative Study of Cardiovascular Disease and Steroid Hormone Contraception. Haemorrhagic stroke, overall stroke risk, and combined oral contraceptives: results of an international, multicentre, case-control study. *Lancet* 1996;348:505–10.

17. Spitzer WO, Lewis MA, Heinemann LA, et al. Third generation oral contraceptives and risk of venous thromboembolic disorders: an international case-control study. Transnational Research Group on Oral Contraceptives. *Br Med J* 1996;312:83–8.

18. Farmer RD, Lawrenson RA, Thompson CR, et al. Population-based study of risk of venous thromboembolism associated with various oral contraceptives. *Lancet* 1997;349:83–8.

19. Carnall D. Controversy rages over new contraceptive data. *Br Med J* 1995;311:1117–18.

20. World Health Organization Collaborative Study of Cardiovascular Disease and Steroid Hormone Contraception. Venous thromboembolic disease and combined oral contraceptives: results of international multicentre case-control study. *Lancet* 1995;346:1575–82.

21. World Health Organization Collaborative Study of Cardiovascular Disease and

Steroid Hormone Contraception. Effect of different progestagens in low oestrogen oral contraceptives on venous thromboembolic disease. *Lancet* 1995;346:1582–8.

22. Jick H, Jick SS, Gurewich V, et al. Risk of idiopathic cardiovascular death and nonfatal venous thromboembolism in women using oral contraceptives with differing progestagen components. *Lancet* 1995;346:1589–93.

23. Food and Drug Administration. Oral contraceptives and risk of blood clots. FDA Talk Paper 1995;Nov. 4, 1995. Available on internet at www.fda.gov/bbs/topics/ANS WERS/ANS00694.html

24. Farmer RDT, Lawrenson R. Utilization patterns of oral contraceptives in UK general practice. *Contraception* 1996;53:211–15.

25. Westhoff CL. Oral contraceptives and venous thromboembolism: should epidemiologic associations drive clinical decision making? *Contraception* 1996;54:1.

26. Lewis MA, MacRae KD, Bruppacher R, et al. Transnational Research Group on Oral Contraceptives and the Health of Young Women. The increased risk of venous thromboembolism and the use of third generation progestagens: role of bias in observational research. *Contraception* 1996;54:5–13.

27. Collaborative Group on Hormonal Factors in Breast Cancer. Breast cancer and hormonal contraceptives: collaborative reanalysis of individual data on 53 297 women with breast cancer and 100 139 without breast cancer from 54 epidemiological studies. *Lancet* 1996;347:1713–27.

28. Ory HW. Long-term oral contraceptive use and the risk of breast cancer. The Centers for Disease Control Cancer and Steroid Hormone Study. *JAMA* 1983;249:1591–5.

29. Westfall JM, Main DS. The contraceptive implant and the injectable: a comparison of costs. *Fam Plann Perspect* 1995;27:34–6.

30. Shoupe D, Mishell DR. Norplant: subdermal implant system for long-term contraception. *Am J Obstet Gynecol* 1989;160:1286–1292.

31. Cullins VE, Remsburn RE, Blumenthal PD, et al. Comparison of adolescent and adult experiences with Norplant levonorgestrel contraceptive implants. *Obstet Gynecol* 1994;83:1026–32.

32. Kaunitz AM. Long acting injectable contraception with depot medroxyprogesterone acetate. *Am J Obstet Gynecol* 1994;170:1543–9.

33. Cromer BA, Blair JM, Mahan JD, et al. A prospective comparison of bone density in adolescent girls receiving depot medroxyprogesterone acetate (Depo Provera), levonorgestrel (Norplant) or oral contraceptives. *J Pediat* 1996;129:671–6.

34. Sivin I. Another look at the Dalkon Shield: meta analysis underscores its problems. *Contraception* 1993;48:1–12.

35. Fraser IS. A fresh look at IUDs: advancing contraceptive choices. *Med J Aust* 1992;157:582–4.

36. WHO Scientific Groups. Mechanism of action, safety and efficacy of intrauterine devices: report of a WHO Scientific Group. *WHO Tech Rep Ser 753* 1987;1–91.

37. Lee NC, Rubin GL, Burucki R. The intrauterine device and pelvic inflammatory disease revisited: new results from the Women's Health Study. *Obstet Gynecol* 1988;72:1–6.

38. Farley TMM, Rosenberg MJ, Rowe PJ, et al. Intrauterine devices and pelvic inflammatory disease: an international perspective. *Lancet* 1992;339:785–8.

39. Toivonene J, Luukkainen J. Protective effect of intrauterine release of levonorgestrel on pelvic infection: three years' comparative experience of levonorgestrel and copper releasing intrauterine devices. *Obstet Gynecol* 1991;77:261–4.

40. Steiner M, Dominik R, Trussell J, et al. Measuring contraceptive effectiveness: a conceptual framework. *Obstet Gynecol* 1996;88:24S–30S.

41. Trussell J, Kost K. Contraceptive failure in the United States: a critical review of the literature. *Stud Fam Plann* 1987;18:237–83.

42. Trussell J, Hatcher RA, Cates WJ, et al. Contraceptive failure in the United States: an update. *Stud Fam Plann* 1990;21:51–4.

43. Dixon GW, Schlesselman JJ, Ory HW, Blye RP. Ethinyl estradiol and conjugated estrogens as postcoital contraceptives. *JAMA* 1980;244:1336–9.

44. Wilcox AJ, Weinberg CR, Baird DD. Timing of intercourse in relation to ovulation: probability of conception, survival of the pregnancy, and sex of the baby. *N Engl J Med* 1995;244:1336–1339.

45. Vollman RF. Assessment of the fertile and sterile phases of the menstrual cycle. *Int Rev Nat Fam Plann* 1977;1:40–2.

46. Potter LS. How effective are contraceptives? The determination and measurement of pregnancy rates. *Obstet Gynecol* 1996;88:135–235.

47. Jones EF, Forrest JD. Contraceptive failure rates based on the 1988 NSFG. *Fam Plann Perspect* 1992;24:12–19.

48. Ross JA. Contraception: Short-term vs long-term failure rates. *Fam Plann Perspect* 1989;21:275–7.

49. Cramer JA. Compliance with contraceptives and other treatments. *Obstet Gynecol* 1919;88:4–12.

50. Cramer JA. The relationship between medication compliance and medical outcomes. *Am J Health Syst Pharm* 1995; 52:27–29.

51. Pratt WF, Bachrach CA. What do women use when they stop using the pill? *Fam Plann Perspect* 1987;19:257–66.

52. Henshaw SK, Silverman J. The characteristics and prior contraceptive use of U.S. abortion patients. *Fam Plann Perspect* 1988;20:158–68.

53. Hillard PJA. Oral contraception noncompliance: the extent of the problem. *Adv Contracept* 1992:8 (Suppl 1):13–20.

54. Emans SJ, Grace E, Woods ER, Smith DE, et al. Adolescents' compliance with the use of oral contraceptives. *JAMA* 1987;257:3377–81.

55. Polaneczky M, Slap G, Forke C, et al. The use of levonorgestrel implants (Norplant) for contraception in adolescent mothers. *N Engl J Med* 1994;331:1201–6.

56. Hillard PJA. The patient's reaction to side effects of oral contraceptives. *Am J Obstet Gynecol* 1989;21:1412–5.

57. Potter L, Oakley D, Wong E, et al. Measuring oral contraceptive pill taking. *Fam Plann Perspect* 1996;28:154–80.

58. Balassone ML. Risk of contraceptive discontinuation among adolescents. *J Adolesc Health Care* 1989;10:527–33.

59. Killick SR, Bancroft K, Oelbaum S, et al. Extending the duration of the pill-free interval during combined oral contraception. *Adv Contracept* 1990;6:33–40.

60. Landgren BM, Diczfalusy E. Hormonal consequences of missing the pill during the first two days of three consecutive artificial cycles. *Contraception* 1984;29:437–46.

61. Letterie GS, Chow GE. Effect of 'missed' pills on oral contraceptive effectiveness. *Obstet Gynecol* 1992;79:979–82.

62. Molloy BG, Coulson KA, Lee JM, et al. 'Missed pill' conception: fact or fiction? *Br Med J* 1985;290:1474–5.

63. DuRant RH, Jay MS, Linder CW, et al. Influence of psychosocial factors on adolescent compliance with oral contraceptives. *J Adolesc Health Care* 1984;5:1–6.

64. DuRant RH, DuBard MB, Goldenberg RL, et al. Are pill counts valid measures of compliance in clinical obstetric trials? *Am J Obstet Gynecol* 1993;169:3273–7.

65. Cramer JA, Mattson RH, Prevey ML, et al. How often is medication taken as prescribed? A novel assessment technique. *JAMA* 1989;261:3273–7.

66. Cramer JA. Identifying and improving compliance patterns: a composite plan for health care providers. In: Cramer JA, Spilker B (eds) Patient compliance in medical practice and clinical trials. New York: Raven Press, 1991.

67. Goldzieher JW. Pharmacology of contraceptive steroids: a brief review. *Am J Obstet Gynecol* 1989;160:1260–4.

68. Edelman DA, Goldzieher JW. Evaluating efficacy and safety. In: Goldzieher JW, Fotherby K (eds) Pharmacology of the contraceptive steroids. New York: Raven Press, 1994:427–37.

69. Oakley D, Sereika O, Bogue EL. Quality of condom use as reported by female clients of a family planning clinic. *Am J Public Health* 1995;85:1526–30.

The menstrual cycle, ovulation and fertility awareness

Anna Flynn* MB BCH BAO NUI FRCOG
John Kelly FRCS FRCOG

The menstrual cycle

Women menstruate cyclically from the menarche to the menopause, apart from during pregnancy and lactation or in the presence of disease. The cycle lengths were believed to approximate to the lunar month of 28 days; in 1858, Clos, a Belgian physician, claimed to have definitely demonstrated a statistical association between the phases of the moon and menstrual cycle lengths [1]. In the 19th century, the determination of the menstrual cycle length seemed a favourite theme for research among scientists, physicians and philosophers over several decades [2,3]. Today, with our detailed knowledge of reproductive physiology and endocrinology, we have more reliable and factual information about the menstrual cycle and a 'regular cycle' is anything between 23 and 35 days [4].

Physiology of the menstrual cycle

A female baby is born with several thousand primordial oocytes present in the ovaries – her complement for life. These immature ova lie dormant until puberty. From then a complex interplay of hormones acting on the female reproductive organs ensures that, at approximately monthly intervals, an ovum is released from the ovary for possible fertilization. The cycle begins when, at the end of the menstrual flow, low plasma levels of oestrogen and progesterone trigger the release of follicle stimulating hormone (FSH) from the anterior pituitary gland. The FSH stimulates the development of three or four follicles (containing the immature ova) in the ovaries. As the follicles grow, one (or occasionally two) becomes dominant while the others regress. This dominant follicle, as it grows, secretes increasing amounts of oestrogen into the circulation with a bimodal feedback to the anterior pituitary.

This rising level of oestrogen has three effects:

- Less FSH is produced by the anterior pituitary in order to inhibit the development of any more ova.

- The endometrial lining of the uterus begins to develop in preparation for a possible future implantation.

- The crypts of the uterine cervix begin to produce an alkaline mucous secretion which is favourable to sperm transport and survival [5].

As the developing ovum reaches* maturity (after 5 or 6 days) the oestrogen blood level rises sharply, reaching a peak which triggers a surge of luteinizing hormone (LH) from the anterior pituitary. The LH peak causes the follicle to rupture, releasing the ovum, which is picked up by the fimbria of the fallopian tube. This rupture and release of the mature ovum is known as *ovulation*.

Immediately after ovulation, the progesterone-secreting cells present in the base of the empty follicle rapidly increase, forming the corpus luteum. The corpus luteum produces increasing quantities of progesterone causing secretory activity in the endometrium (previously primed by oestrogen) to facilitate implantation should fertilization

---

*Dr Anna Flynn died in 1997.

occur. The high circulating levels of progesterone inhibit the further production of FSH and LH, thus impeding any further ovulations in the current cycle; mucus in the cervical crypts changes to a thick sticky plug under the influence of progesterone.

Should the ovum be fertilized (in the outer third of the fallopian tube), it develops and travels down the tube to implant in the prepared endometrium. The corpus luteum (of pregnancy) develops further in size, producing increased amounts of progesterone to assist the implantation and development of the embryo over the first 3 months of the pregnancy until the placenta takes over this function.

If the ovum is not fertilized, it dies within 18–24 hours, travels along the tube and is shed from the uterus. The corpus luteum begins to degenerate, progesterone levels fall over the next 10 days, the secretory endometrium breaks up and is shed vaginally in what constitutes *menstruation*. The low levels of oestrogen and progesterone in the circulation stimulate the anterior pituitary to begin FSH production once more and a new menstrual cycle begins [6,7] (Figure 4.1).

Fertility during the menstrual cycle

It has been established that the fertilizable life of the ovum is no longer than 24 hours. By contrast, the fertilizing life of the sperm is uncertain. Although it appears to be quite short, i.e. 2–3 days, under optimal conditions in the female

reproductive tract a fertilizing capacity of 6 or even 7 days has been postulated in exceptional circumstances [8,9]. This combined fertilizing capacity of the sperm and ovum constitutes the fertile phase, during which sexual intercourse could potentially result in a pregnancy. One can therefore divide the menstrual cycle into fertile and infertile phases (Figure 4.1).

Phase one

The preovulatory infertile phase: this covers the time from the start of menstruation until the onset of cervical mucus production, which creates conditions favourable to sperm transport and survival whether in the cervical crypts or in the fallopian tube. This preovulatory infertile phase varies in length depending on the rapidity of the follicular response to FSH.

Phase two

The fertile phase: this extends from the onset of cervical mucus until the time after ovulation, when the ovum is no longer fertilizable [10]. Before ovulation, fertility depends on the capacity of the spermatozoa to survive in cervical mucus. After ovulation, the ovum is only fertilizable for 12–24 hours. However, since the moment of ovulation cannot be clinically identified exactly, potential fertility must be assumed for 48 hours [11]. The fertile phase in the cycle refers to the combined fertility of the couple.

Phase three

The postovulatory infertile phase: this extends from the end of ovulation until the onset of the next menstruation and ranges in duration from 10 to 16 days, with a mean of 14 days [12, 13]. This

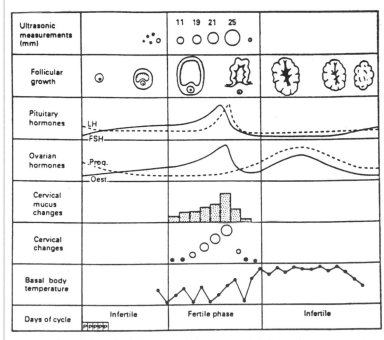

Fig. 4.1 The relationship during the cycle between serial ultrasonic measurements, hormonal control and clinical indicators of fertility. Reproduced with permission from Flynn AM, Bonnar J. Contraception, science and practice. London: Butterworths 1989: 205.

phase is defined as being absolutely infertile because the rapid rise of the luteal hormones after ovulation inhibits any further ovulation, thus rendering conception impossible (Figure 4.1).

Fertility awareness

Oestrogen and progesterone affect target organs in the body, producing a variety of signs and symptoms which women can observe for themselves and use as clinical indicators of fertile and infertile phases in the cycle. This process is known as fertility awareness. There are three main observable changes which are always present in ovulatory cycles and these are referred to as major indicators.

Major indicators
- Changes in the quantity and quality of the mucus produced by the cervical crypts. (cervical mucus patterns)
- Changes in the uterine cervix.
- Changes in basal body temperature (BBT).

Changes in cervical mucus

In a typical 28-day cycle, hormone levels are low after menstruation and no mucus is produced. As the follicle develops and oestrogen increases, the cervix is stimulated to produce increasing amounts of mucus, which changes from an initial thick, rubbery consistency to a watery, stretchy, transparent secretion as the oestrogen peaks and ovulation approaches.

After ovulation, the high levels of progesterone cause an abrupt drying of the mucus, which rapidly reverts to being thick and rubbery, forming a plug in the cervix. Observations of cervical mucus should be made during the day and recorded on a chart at night. If the mucus changes during the day, the most fertile signs should be recorded. Mucus is observed in three ways.

External observations

Sensation
This is the feeling a woman experiences at the vulva; it can be dry, moist/damp or wet/slippery. Dry indicates infertility, moist/damp indicates potential fertility and wet indicates high fertility.

Mucus quality
Women are taught to wipe their vulva with a tissue on each visit to the toilet and observe any mucus collected. They should record on a chart:

- Appearance – cloudy, white, yellow, clear or transparent.

- Consistency – creamy, pasty, rubbery, flaky, watery, stretchy or slippery.

Internal observations
Mucus is secreted in the cervix and may take some hours to appear at the vulva. It is therefore helpful to check for mucus internally on the cervical os and in the fornices. Any mucus found should be recorded as for the external observations, but a note made that the observations were made internally.

Changes in the uterine cervix

In the fertile phase, the cervix is drawn upwards (a cephalad shift of 1–3 cm), the os becomes soft and opens to admit sperm. At all other times of the cycle, the cervix remains lower in the vagina, firm to the touch with the os relatively closed. [14, 15] (Figure 4.2).

By inserting a finger into the vagina and palpating the cervix, a

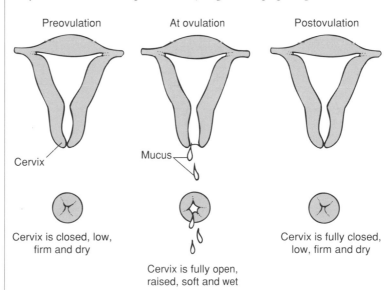

Preovulation   At ovulation   Postovulation

Cervix   Mucus

Cervix is closed, low, firm and dry

Cervix is fully open, raised, soft and wet

Cervix is fully closed, low, firm and dry

Fig. 4.2 Cervical changes during the cycle.

woman can assess whether the position of the cervix in the pelvis is low (nearer to the vulva) or has moved upwards in the vagina; whether the os is open, closed or intermediate; and whether the cervix around the os is firm to touch, like the tip of a nose, or soft like a chin.

Observations are made daily at about the same time, later in the day preferably, either in a squatting position or with one foot raised on a stool. In recording these observations on the chart, a dot widening to a circle indicates openness while placing it high or low indicates position (Figure 4.1).

Changes in the basal body temperature

The BBT is the temperature of the body after at least 3 hours' rest. Oestrogen has no appreciable effect on the BBT, but the progesterone surge after ovulation causes a sudden increase in the BBT of approximately between 0.2°C and 0.6°C. The temperature remains at this higher level during the luteal phase and returns to baseline at the end of the cycle with onset of menses. If pregnancy occurs, the temperature remains elevated.

To record the BBT shift, the temperature is taken in the morning in bed, after a night's sleep and before any metabolic activity takes place. A mercury thermometer requires 3 minutes (orally or rectally) to record BBT, a digital one takes 1 minute. Women are taught to recognize disturbed readings caused by fever, stress, alcohol, disturbed nights and varying times.

The BBT detects neither the onset of the fertile phase nor ovulation. It merely indicates to the woman that ovulation has occurred and, after 3 days of raised temperature, the rest of the cycle is infertile [16] (Figure 4.1).

The minor indicators

These indicators are specific to individual women and do not occur in all ovulatory cycles. The most common signs are ovulation pain, midcycle bleeding, breast symptoms, acne, bloating, vulval swelling and mood changes. For those who experience them they are an important component of body language and can be used as backup to the major indicators.

The methodologies of fertility awareness

Historical background

The problem of fertility control has taxed people's imagination for centuries. Among primitive societies fertility was controlled by traditional customs and taboos, and these methods still continue in some parts of the world. In the Old Testament, the book of Leviticus and others make frequent references to a woman's fertile period, correctly identified as about the middle of the cycle. This is in distinct contrast to the centuries which followed when the physiological misconception of equating menstruation with ovulation and fertility was the norm until the early part of the century [17]. Independent studies by Ogino

[18] in Japan and Knaus [19] in Austria in the 1930s demonstrated that conception can only occur during a brief period between menses around the time of ovulation. They also showed that, regardless of the length of the menstrual cycle, the time from ovulation to the next menstruation remains fairly constant with a mean of about 14 days. Using this discovery, both Ogino and Knaus developed formulae to determine the fertile and infertile days in the cycle and this formed the basis for the calendar or rhythm method (also known as the Ogino–Knaus method) of natural family planning. However, this was not found to be very effective. Research in the field of reproductive medicine between 1940 and 1980 opened the way for a more scientific approach to natural methods: indicators of fertility – cervical mucus, BBT and cervical changes – were introduced with apparent increasing efficacy. In the 1990s these newer indicators were added to the calendar calculations, resulting in the highly efficient double-check natural method in use today.

Natural family planning methods

The clinical indicators already described can be used singly or in combination to determine the fertile phase in the cycle. Five natural methods are used at present: four single-index and the multiple-index methods of which there are several different combinations.

Single-index methods

Cervical mucus method (Billings method)

The onset of the fertile phase is detected as the earliest cycle day in which mucus is perceived at the vulva either by sensation or by appearance. The last day of watery, stretchy mucus before it reverts back to a thick plug is defined as the **peak** mucus day, the peak of fertility. The fourth evening after the peak mucus day marks the end of the fertile phase. To achieve a pregnancy, intercourse is advised around the peak mucus day when conditions are optimal for conception [8, 20]. Couples wishing to avoid a pregnancy are advised to practise abstinence during the fertile phase [21]. Some couples choose to use barriers during the fertile phase [22].

Cervix method

The onset of the fertile phase is detected by the first discovery of any degree of openness, softness or upward movement (cephalad shift) of the cervix. The end of the fertile phase is the fourth day after the peak cervix day, that is, the day on which the openness, softness and cephalad shift are maximal. The indicator is seldom used alone, but it may form a part of the multiple-index approach [23].

Basal body temperature method

This method cannot detect the beginning of the fertile phase but is a reliable indicator of the end of it. The morning of the third day after the BBT shift, provided the elevation was maintained over 3 consecutive days, indicates the onset of postovulatory infertility. Consequently, this method cannot be used to achieve a pregnancy and, if used as a single-index method to avoid conception, intercourse has to be restricted to the postovulatory infertile phase. For this reason, the temperature method is nowadays seldom used on its own, but plays a dominant role in the multiple-index methods.

Lactational amenorrhoea method (LAM)

This is an efficient natural method in the fully or nearly fully breastfeeding woman over the first 6 months postpartum, providing she remains amenorrhoeic [24]. To be successful LAM requires that:

- The mother is fully, or almost fully, breastfeeding by both day and night.
- The infant is not receiving regular supplementation.
- Menstruation has not returned (bleeding before the 56th postpartum day is ignored).
- The woman is within 6 months of delivery.

If all of these conditions are met, breastfeeding provides 98% protection from pregnancy. If any of these criteria are no longer present, the woman should consider herself potentially fertile.

The multiple-index methods

In this approach, several clinical indicators are combined to demarcate the onset and end of the fertile phase. Thus, the deficiency in one method is balanced by the advantage of another, thereby resulting in greater efficiency. Initially, the woman observes several indicators during the learning phase. From this initial combination, women can freely change to other combinations that are more effective and convenient for their particular circumstances, thus tailoring the method to the individual [23].

The three most usual combinations are given below.

The double-check method

In order to determine the first fertile day of the cycle, the mucus symptom is cross-checked with the calendar calculations. The woman takes her shortest cycle of the previous 12 and subtracts 20 from it, giving her the last infertile day if still dry. To determine the end of the fertile time, the woman counts 4 days after the peak of the mucus symptom and cross-checks it by charting three consecutive raised temperatures.

The mucothermal method

This method uses the mucus symptom to detect the beginning of the fertile phase and the BBT shift to determine the end.

The calculothermal method

This method uses the calendar calculation (shortest cycle length minus 19) to determine the onset of fertility and the BBT shift to detect the end of the fertile phase.

The effectiveness of natural family planning (NFP) methods

Historically, natural methods have had a bad press consequent on a wide variation in efficiency rates for published NFP studies prior to 1990. It must be stated, however, that one of the main problems in assessing the effectiveness of NFP methods lies in the difficulty of how to interpret the various factors that can influence the results (as illustrated in Tables 4.1 and 4.2). For comparative purposes the Pearl index is used in these tables. In Table 4.1 we see that, where intercourse is restricted to the postovulatory infertile phase, the pregnancy outcome for both method and total rates is considerably better than when women are exposed to pregnancy risk in both the preovulatory and postovulatory infertile phases [25]. Table 4.1 also illustrates that the motivation of the user is another important variable. Couples who are spacing their family (less motivated) have a significantly higher pregnancy rate than those who are limiting [26]. The influence of a third variable, the quality of the NFP teaching/instruction of the user, is also shown (Table 4.1). It can be seen that, among couples taught

by inexperienced teachers, the pregnancy rate was significantly higher than that for couples taught by experienced instructors [27].

It was becoming apparent to programme developers and NFP researchers in Europe in the late 1980s that, even when teaching was standardized and the couples were well motivated, the efficiency of NFP methods was critically dependent on the method used. The single-index mucus method was associated with the highest pregnancy rate [28]; the mucothermal method resulted in only a slight improvement in the efficiency [22], whereas the double-check method has a pregnancy rate comparable to current contraceptive methods [22]. Since the double-check method can determine the limits of the fertile phase with great precision and accuracy [29], intercourse does not have to be restricted to the postovulatory phase and, consequently, compliance and acceptability are satisfactory, with a low user-failure rate [22].

NFP prevalence, advantages and disadvantages

In a survey of contraceptive use [30], 10% of the world's population used some form of a natural method for fertility control. In the same survey, on average, 25% of couples in the reproductive age group in developed countries relied on 'non-supply' methods (i.e. rhythm and withdrawal) for contraception, the figure for the UK being 7% [30]. For NFP alone, the use in developed countries is up to 5% and in developing countries up to 20%. The increasing trend in Western countries to live more in harmony with nature may favour NFP as women move away from invasive drugs and devices. Natural methods are being successfully used by motivated couples for reasons of ecology and health, rather than solely for moral or religious reasons as is commonly believed.

Advantages of natural methods

The perceived advantages of natural methods are the absence

Table 4.1 Factors influencing the efficiency of natural methods – timing of coitus, motivation of client and quality of teaching received

| Authors Year | NFP method used | Volunteers | Months of exposure | Failure rate[a] | | | | |
				Method related	Teaching related	Combined method – user failure	For those spacing	For those limiting
Marshall 1968 [25]	BBT postovulation	321	4739	1.2	—	6.6		
Marshall 1968 [25]	BBT – calendar (pre- and postovulation)	255	3545	5.0	—	19.3		
Rice et al. 1981 [26]	Symptothermal (pre- and postovulation)	1022	21 736	0.93	—	7.47	14.56	4.13
Perez et al. 1983 [27]	Ovulation method (pre- and postovulation)	5140	21 660	2.8	—	13.3	16.8 (inexperienced instructors, 4.7 experienced instructors)	

NFP = natural family planning; BBT = basal body temperature;
[a] Pearl formula: pregnancies per 100 woman-years.

Table 4.2 Factors Influencing the efficiency of natural methods – the particular natural method used

Authors and Year	Method	Months of exposure	Method failure rate	Practice/user failure rate
Marshall (1968) [25]	Basal body temperature	4739	1.2	5.4
World Health Organization (1981) [28]	Cervical mucus ovulation	10 215	2.2	22.3
Freundl et al. (European Multicenter (1993) [22]	Mucothermal (method B)	1352	1	10.6
Freundl et al. (European Multicenter (1993) [22]	Double-check	7404	0	2.5

of medical complications and other side effects; they are holistic and can be used autonomously in harmony with the natural bodily rhythms; they are readily reversible and can be used to achieve as well as to avoid a pregnancy. They promote shared responsibility, communication between partners and the involvement of men [31]. Couples, once they become autonomous users of a natural method, do not require any further expenditure on medication or medical follow-up, and this guarantees long-term cost-effectiveness [32,33].

Disadvantages

Natural methods require a learning phase of about 3 months supervised by trained instructors who are not as yet readily available within all health systems; to be successful they demand a stable relationship and the co-operation of both partners. Efficacy also appears to be trainer dependent. The methods are associated in many minds with the inefficient calendar/rhythm method and with the Catholic Church. Like other methods, apart from barriers, natural

methods offer no protection against sexually transmitted diseases (STDs). However, the fact that they require stability in the partnership may reduce exposure to these. The chore of observations and charting, which poses a difficulty for some women, is presently being addressed by the development of technology to determine the fertile phase reliably and home kits/devices are already on the market which can do this. There is a long-held belief that the abstinence required to avoid a pregnancy is a major obstacle to the use of natural methods. However, abstinence was found to be a problem in only 10% of couples using NFP in England and Wales in 1984 [31], and in more recent larger studies, abstinence is seen as a major problem among users (Freundl, 1996, personal communication). The psychological problems related to periodic abstinence need further study.

The method may not be suitable for perimenopausal women, those with lower genital tract infection and couples with risk-taking behaviour. Any disease condition or medication

that affects the menstrual cycle makes this method unreliable.

The possibility of chromosomal abnormalities arising from fertilization between 'aged gametes' and leading to miscarriages or congenital abnormalities has been studied, but no adverse association was confirmed beyond doubt [34,35]. Few studies address the discontinuation rates for NFP. A small number show high discontinuation, which is not surprising, as the methods require mutual motivation.

Other methods of monitoring ovulation

What of the future?

Although present-day natural methods can be used very efficiently for fertility control, they still have some limitations both in precision and in that they are not always seen to be user friendly. Rapid developments in medical technology over the past decade have led to the production of simple tests and devices for the prediction and detection of ovulation. Women having difficulties in observing or interpreting the clinical indicators, either because they are not clearly evident or because the woman's lifestyle is not conductive to detailed charting, may find that these new technological methods enable them to use NFP successfully, whereas before many had to discontinue. Two of these new technologies, the Bioself electronic thermometer and Persona, the Unipath personal contraceptive system, have been tested for reliability by clinical trials and are available over the counter (OTC) in pharmacies or from distributors in the UK. One important area for development is that of counselling couples on communication, sexuality and living with the demands of periodic abstinence to improve the acceptability of these methods.

The Bioself 110 fertility indicator

This is a hand-held electronic computerized thermometer (Figure 4.3) used as an aid to couples using periodic abstinence. It measures the BBT and relates it to the woman's menstrual cycle length (which is logged in by the user). Thus, it identifies her safe (infertile) and unsafe (fertile) phases. In studies, it correctly identified the postovulatory infertile phase in 93% of cycles [36]. The method has not had a significant impact on family planning programmes in spite of being available for some years.

Persona®

Persona® is a further advance in electronic monitoring of ovulatory indices (Figure 4.4). It combines the features of a microprocessor and a minilaboratory. The hand-held device was launched in the UK in 1996 [37].

The user feeds the device information about her menstrual cycle by logging in the first day of menses. She then tests her urine using disposable dipsticks. The machine tests simultaneously for oestrone-3-glucuronide (E_2-3-G), the main urinary metabolite of oestradiol, and for LH. The start of the rise of E_2-3-G is taken as the start of the fertile phase. The device's testing threshold detects E_2-3-G levels corresponding to the 5th or 6th preovulation day, which covers over 95% of sperm survival. Levels tend to mirror cervical mucus change. The identification of the LH surge is used to calculate the start of the postovulation infertile phase.

The safe (infertile) menstrual/postmenstrual phase is indicated by a green light. A yellow light shows further on in the preovulatory phase to alert the woman to the need to test her urine using the disposable dipstick. Once the urine test is 'read', a green or red light will show and the woman continues to test daily until a green light is displayed denoting the start of the postovulation 'safe' period. Sixteen tests are required in the first cycle and 8 tests for all subsequent cycles. The device has a failure rate of 6% per year based on pre-launch data from the manufacturer. The impact of Persona® may be limited by its

Fig. 4.3 The Bioself 110 fertility indicator.

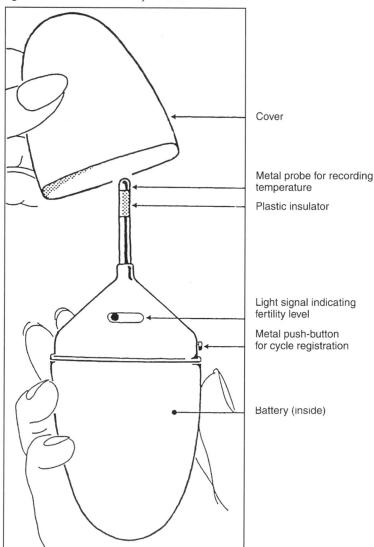

Cover

Metal probe for recording temperature

Plastic insulator

Light signal indicating fertility level

Metal push-button for cycle registration

Battery (inside)

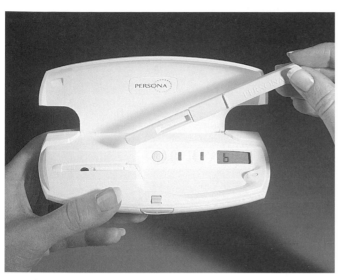

Fig. 4.4 The Persona® personal contraceptive system.

excludes this method for the time being.

- Urinary LH – the LH surge is easily diagnosed by any of many dipsticks. The problem is that this test is limited by its ability to detect only the postovulatory 'infertile' phase, and it is expensive.

- Other urinary or salivary assays of oestrogen and progesterone metabolites – ratios of metabolites have been tried but are unlikely in practice to be user friendly.

Conclusion

Attempts to develop some natural form of family planning are evident from the beginning of history. However, efficient natural methods, comparable to modern artificial methods, were only developed in the 1980s and 1990s. Intensive technological research has also resulted in the availability of simple techniques to detect the fertile phase in the cycle suitable for home use by non-medical persons, which greatly improves the ease of use of these methods. The scarcity of trained instructors, particularly in existing family planning clinics and general practitioners' surgeries, still creates a problem for would-be users and one hopes that this difficulty will be addressed in the future. Used perfectly, fertility awareness and natural family planning has high efficacy but, like other methods, it is unforgiving when used imperfectly.

cost and by a failure rate which is higher than some methods.

The requirements and rules for Persona® use are:

- Women must have cycles of 23–35 days.

- After pregnancy, breastfeeding or hormone contraception use Persona® use can only be started after two cycles of 23–35 days.

- Persona® use is contraindicated for women taking tetracycline (which may affect the dipstick reading in a few women), but not minocycline or oxytetracycline.

The advantages of Persona® are that it can be used to plan a pregnancy and it is an effective, non-invasive method of contraception. There is also a very clear educational manual accompanying the device. The disadvantages of Persona® are that it is not suitable during lactation, or for women with long cycles and, like other non-barrier methods, Persona® offers no protection against STIs and HIV.

Other methods of monitoring/predicting ovulation

- Ultrasonography is an accurate but expensive method to monitor ovarian activity. Tracking follicular activity from early in the cycle in the futuristic home with an ultrasound monitor next to the television set is still only a theoretical possibility. Ovulation is likely to occur when follicular size is 18 mm or over. The end of the fertile phase can therefore be defined as 7 days after an 18 mm follicle is picked up by ultrasound. The practicality of ultrasound for universal use

Resource list

- The Natural Family Planning and Fertility Clinic, The Hospital of St John and St Elizabeth, St John's Wood, London NW8 9NH, UK. Tel. 0207-286 5126.

- The Fertility Awareness Kit – Wisebody 1995 – available by mail order from UK Family Planning Sales. Tel. 01865 749333.

- Fertility- by Dr. Elizabeth Clubb and Jane Knight, The NFP Centre, Clitherow House, 1 Blythe Mews, Blythe Road, London W14 0NW.

References

1. Clos JA. De l'influence de la lune sur la menstruation. *Bull Acad Roy Sci* (Belgique) 1858;2 serie 4:108–60.

2. Goodman J. The menstrual cycle. *Trans Am Gynecol Soc* 1877;2:650–62.

3. Foster EP. The periodicity and duration of the menstrual flow. *N Y Med J* 1889;49:610–11.

4. Vollman RF. The length of the menstrual cycle. In: Friedman EA (ed.) The menstrual cycle. Philadelphia: WB Saunders, 1977.

5. Odeblad E. The functional structure of human cervical mucus. *Acta Obstet Gynecol Scand* 1968;47:58.

6. Keltzky OA, Nakamura RM, Thorneycroft IH, et al. Log distribution of gonadotrophins and ovarian steroid values in the normal menstrual cycle. *Am J Obstet Gynecol* 1975; 121:688–94.

7. Kerin JF, Edmonds DK, Warnes GM, et al. Morphological and functional relations of graafian follicle growth to ovulation in women using ultrasonic, laparoscopic and biochemical measurements. *Br J Obstet Gynaecol* 1981;88:81–90.

8. Wilcox AJ, Weinberg CR, Baird DD. Timing of sexual intercourse in relation to ovulation. *N Engl J Med* 1995;333:1517–21.

9. Barrett JC, Marshall J. The risk of conception on different days of the menstrual cycle. *Population Stud* 1969;23:455.

10. Schwartz NB, Hoffman JC. Ovulation, basic aspects. In: Balin H, Glasser S (eds) Reproductive biology. Amsterdam: Excerpta Medica, 1972:438.

11. Oritz ME, Croxatto BB. Observations on the transport, ageing and development of ova in the human genital tract. In: Talwar GP (ed.) Recent advances in reproduction and regulation of fertility. New York: Elsevier/North Holland Biochemical Press, 1979: 307–17.

12. Hartman GG. Science and the safe period. Baltimore: Williams and Wilkins, 1962:226–34.

13. Vollman RF. The phases of the menstrual cycle. In: Friedman EA (ed.) The menstrual cycle. Philadelphia: WB Saunders, 1977:91–149.

14. Keefe EF. Self-observation of the cervix to distinguish days of possible fertility. *Bull. Sloane Hosp. Women* 1962;8:129–36.

15. Keefe EF. Cephalad shift of the cervix uteri: sign of the fertile time in women. *Int Rev Nat Fam Plann* 1977;1:55.

16. Marshall J. Thermal changes in the normal menstrual cycle. *Br Med J* 1963;1:102.

17. Du Mas B. Description des moyens a employer par les epoux pour n'avoir pas d'enfants ou pour en limiter le nombre a volonté. Villeurbanne, 1895, author's edition.

18. Ogino K. Ovulationstermin und Kinzeptionstermin. Zentralbl Gynäkol 1930;54:464.

19. Knaus H. Die Periodische Frucht-und Unfruchtbarkeit des Weibes. *Zentralb Gynäkol* 1933;57:1393.

20. World Health Organisation. A prospective multicenter trial of the ovulation method of natural family planning 111. Characteristics of the menstrual cycle and of the fertile phase. *Fertil Steril* 1983;40:773–7.

21. Billings JJ. The ovulation method. Melbourne: Advocate Press, 1964.

22. Freundl G. Prospective European multicenter study of natural family planning (1989–1992). *Adv Contraception* 1993;9:269–83.

23. Flynn AM, Brooks M. Muliple-index methods. In: The manual of natural family planning. London: Thorsons, 1996:74–93.

24. Kennedy K, Rivera R, McNeilly A, et al. Consensus statement on the use of breastfeeding as a family planning method. *Contraception* 1989;39:477–96.

25. Marshall J. A field-trial of the basal body temperature method of regulating births. *Lancet* 1968;2:8–10.

26. Rice FJ, Lanctot CA, Garcia-Devesa C. Effectiveness of the symptothermal method of natural family planning. An international study. *Int J Fertil* 1981;26:222–30.

27. Perez A, Zabala A, Larrain A, et al. The clinical efficiency of the ovulation method (Billings). *Rev Chilena Obstet Ginecol* 1983;48:97.

28. World Health Organisation, Task Force on Methods for the determination of the Fertile Period. Special Programme of Research Development and Research Training in Human Reproduction. A prospective multicentre trial of the ovulation method of natural family planning. 2 – effectiveness phase. *Fertil Steril* 1981;36:591–8.

29. Flynn AM, Docker M, Morris R, et al. The reliability of women's subjective assessment of the fertile period relative to

urinary gonadotrophins and follicular ultrasonic measurements during the menstrual cycle. In: Bonnar J, Thompson W, Harrison RF (eds) Studies in fertility and sterility: research in family planning. Lancaster: MTP Press, 1984;3–11.

30. World Health Organisation: Entre-nous No. 13. Denmark: Sexuality and Family Planning Unit of the Regional Office for Europe of WHO, March 1989:16–17.

31. Flynn AM, von Fragstein M, Royston JP. Analysis of a representative sample of natural family planning users in England and Wales (1984–1985). *Int J Fertil* 1988;33:70–77.

32. Kambic RT, Lanctot CA, Wesley R. Trial of a new method of natural family planning in Liberia. *Adv Contraception* 1994;10:111–19.

33. Flynn AM. Natural family planning in developing countries. *Lancet* 1992, 340:309.

34. World Health Organisation. A prospective multicentre study of the ovulation method of natural family planning. IV. The outcome of pregnancy. *Fertil Steril* 1984;41:393–8.

35. Simpson JL, Gray R, Queenan J, et al. Cohort study of natural family planning users to assess fetal outcome associated with ageing gametes. *Adv Contraception* 1995;11:116.

36. Labrecque M, Drouin J, Rious JE, et al. Validity of the Bioself 110 fertility indicator. *Fertil Steril* 1989;52:604–8.

37. Bonnar J, Flynn AM, Freundl G, Kirkman R, Royston P, Snowden R. Personal hormone monitoring for contraception. *Br J Fam Plan.* 1999; 24:128–34.

Combined oral contraceptives: epidemiological studies and risk–benefit analysis

Helen Roberts MB MPH

Epidemiological studies of combined oral contraceptives

Apart from the potential ethical problems in using randomized trials for investigating the oral contraceptive pill, observational case-control and cohort studies are useful in investigating rare outcomes such as cardiovascular disease and cancer. Case-control studies compare oral contraceptive (OC) use in cases with the disease under investigation with OC use in control group(s), chosen either from the general population or from admissions to the same hospital as the cases. To clarify the possible association, most studies will also attempt to control for confounding variables which may be associated with the pill and also independently with the disease under investigation. A common confounder in pill studies is age, which is associated with both pill use and the majority of diseases. However, this type of study can suffer from the problem of bias. For example, if pill users were more likely to be investigated for possible thrombosis than other women in the population, there would be the issue of diagnostic or referral bias. Information bias may be manifest if cases and controls differed in the accuracy of recall of past contraceptive use.

A cohort study prospectively follows a group of OC users over time and directly observes the incidence of disease. Bias, although still present, is less likely with cohort studies. The main problem is the need for large numbers of women, investigated for long periods of time, with the resultant loss to follow-up or change of method.

Systematic reviews have recently become more common in the literature and can help clarify consistency of results. Meta-analysis, where the results of different studies are combined can, with larger numbers, help to detect effects more precisely. The difficulty is to ensure the inclusion of all relevant data and their combinability.

Cohort studies measure relative risk – the ratio of incidence of disease among exposed women to that in unexposed women. In case-control studies, the odds ratio is used as an estimate of the relative risk. Confidence intervals (CI) are usually given for a relative risk, most studies using a 95% CI; if the CI includes 1.0, the results are not statistically significant.

Studying relative risks will tell us the likelihood of an association as long as we can rule out that it is not due to chance, bias or confounding. We then need to assess whether the association is causal. This becomes more likely with relative risks further away from 1.0, when there is consistency among studies, when the risk shows a time or dose dependency, and when there is a possible biological explanation for the risk association. Relative risks, however, do not help us to assess the clinical or public health importance of associations: a large relative risk for a disease that has a low incidence in the population may not be a concern. Absolute risks, which depend on both the incidence of the disease in question and the relative risk of that disease with pill use, give real awareness of the impact of associations.

Non-contraceptive benefits of oral contraceptives

The validity of comparing the mortality from pill use with that of pregnancy has often been questioned, as non-use may not necessarily result in that outcome.

5

Combined oral
contraceptives:
epidemiological
studies and
risk–benefit
analysis

However, the fact that the oral contraceptive pill is an effective method of contraception needs to be included in the benefit–risk equation. It can prevent many of the medical problems associated with wanted and unwanted pregnancy, including a decreased risk of ectopic pregnancy. The Alan Guttmacher Institute has calculated that, for sexually active women aged 15–44, the annual pregnancy-related mortality rate is 0.4 per 100 000 women using the pill compared to 6.5 per 100 000 women using no method [1]. However, there are other health benefits of the pill.

Menstrual problems

Early studies in the 1970s showed a 50% reduction in menorrhagia, and about a 30% reduction in intermenstrual bleeding and irregular menses when pill users were compared to controls. The risk of iron deficiency anaemia was also about half for pill users, the effect lasting for several years after pill discontinuation [2]. Pill use in women with dysmenorrhoea decreases the amount of prostaglandin in menstrual fluid. A 25% decrease in hospital admissions for menstrual problems is apparent with current use of more modern low-dose pills [3].

Benign breast disease

A 25% decreased risk for all types of benign breast disease (fibroadenoma and fibrocystic disease without atypia) has been found in both case-control and cohort studies [4]. Most show a decreasing risk with duration of use and two have found that pills

with the greatest progestogen content provide higher protection. Some recent studies have found a smaller protective effect, with the suggestion that this may be due to the lower dosage of currently available pills [5].

Pelvic inflammatory disease (PID)

The incidence of acute salpingitis is halved for oral contraceptive users compared to women using no method. An even lower risk for pill users (RR 0.24) was found when the salpingitis was laparoscopically confirmed; women who were taking the pill and had a gonorrheal or chlamydial infection of the cervix were less likely to have salpingitis than were women who were not using the pill but also had a positive culture. Oral contraceptive users with salpingitis are also more likely to have milder disease laparoscopically than non-users [6]. A more recent study has found a similar protective effect for PID in pill users compared to women using no method of contraception, the association in this study being only for chlamydial infection [7]. There seems to be no clear dose relationship. Although oral contraceptives are associated with increased detection of cervical chlamydia, it has been suggested that this may be influenced by the degree of cervical ectopy.

Functional ovarian cysts

The results of past cohort studies using high-dose monophasic pills

showed a decreased risk of functional ovarian cysts. The Oxford/Family Planning Association study found half the risk of follicular ovarian cysts in current pill users and one-fifth the risk of corpus luteal cysts when compared to women who had never taken the pill or who had used it in the past [8]. A more recent study of hospital admissions, with surgical confirmation, found a 76% decreased risk of developing functional ovarian cysts in high-dose pill users, a 48% reduction for women using low-dose monophasic pills, and a non-significant reduction with multiphasic formulations [9]. These findings have not been repeated in other studies.

Endometrial cancer

For endometrial cancer, the relative risk for pill users is 0.8 after 1 year of use decreasing to 0.4 after 4 or more years of use. A study in developing nations also found a 50% decreased risk. The large Cancer and Steroid Hormone (CASH) Study in the USA showed ongoing protection after the pill was discontinued – a 70% reduction 15 years after the pill was stopped [6]. Schlesselman's review of the data found that, regardless of the oestrogen/progestagen ratio of combined pill used, the risk of endometrial cancer is reduced by about 50% in women who had ever used the pill [10].

Ovarian cancer

Both case-control and cohort studies have shown the

protective effect of the pill against epithelial cancers of the ovary. The reduction in risk is related to the duration of pill use, with about a 50% reduction after 5 or more years of use [4]. In the CASH Study the relative risk for 10 or more years of pill use was 0.2. Past use of the pill was also protective, with a relative risk of 0.5 for women who had used the pill 10 or more years ago. Further data are required regarding use for more than 20 years. There was similar protection for both nulliparous and multiparous women, and most studies show the protective effect for both younger and older women. Some studies have found this protective effect for both high-dose and low-dose pills [11]. Nulliparity and family history are risk factors for ovarian cancer which can be reduced by pill use: 5 years of continuous use for a nulliparous woman decreases her risk to that of a woman who has had children, and 10 years of pill use will balance the risk from a positive family history of ovarian cancer [12].

Risks of combined oral contraceptives

Cardiovascular disease (Tables 5.1 and 5.2)

Combined oral contraceptive pills can, for some women, increase the risk of venous thromboembolism (VTE), myocardial infarction (MI) and ischaemic stroke. The risk is for current use and disappears after the pill is stopped. The risk of VTE has in the past been related to the oestrogen content of the pill, and the majority of studies have shown decreasing risk with lower-dose pills with no effect of duration of use or smoking. Compared to other blood groups, women with blood group O are at decreased risk of VTE. Case-control and cohort studies since the 1980s have included lower-dose pills and have found relative risks for fatal VTE and pulmonary embolism of 2.1 (CI 0.8–5.2) for current users compared to non-users, and 3.8 (CI 2.4–6.0) for non-fatal DVT [13]. Carriers of an inherited clotting defect, Factor V Leiden

mutation, found in about 20% of cases of DVT, have an eightfold increased risk of thrombosis. Its presence will escalate the fourfold increased risk for non-carrier pill users to 30–50-fold for pill users who are also carriers [14]. Four recent studies have suggested that the risk of VTE may also be related to the type of progestagen in the pill, with doubling of the risk for those containing gestodene and desogestrel compared with those containing levonorgestrel [13].

Although some of the studies controlled for many of the confounding issues in this relationship, such as personal and family history of thrombosis and body mass index, there has been ongoing discussion about the influence of other issues in the studies, such as referral, and diagnostic and prescribing bias. A control only study suggested that women with familial thrombotic disposition were four times more likely to be prescribed third-generation rather than second-generation pills and that this confounding issue had not been corrected for in three out of the

Table 5.1 Combined oral contraceptives (COCs) and the risk of cardiovascular disease

Condition	Background risk (per year)	Magnitude of COC-associated risk	Overall attributable risk[a]	Risk in pregnancy	Case fatality
VTE	80/1 000 000	3–6×	160/1 000 000	600/1 000 000	2%
IS	10/1 000 000	2.5×	15/1 000 000	80/1 000 000	25%
HS	27/1 000 000	1.5×	14/1 000 000		30%
AMI < 35	Non-smoker 1/1 000 000 Smoker 8/1 000 000	3–6×	Non-smoker 3/1 000 000 Smoker 35/1 000 000	100/1 000 000	30%[b]
AMI > 35	Non-smoker 10/1 000 000 Smoker 88/1 000 000	3–6×	Non-smoker 31/1 000 000 Smoker 396/1 000 000		

VTE = venous thromboembolism; IS = ischaemic stroke; HS = haemorrhagic stroke; AMI = acute myocardial infarction.
[a]Except where indicated, these figures include women with risk factors.
[b]Case fatality is highest in < 25 (36%) than > 35 (17%).
Data taken from several studies and models.

5

Combined oral
contraceptives:
epidemiological
studies and
risk–benefit
analysis

Table 5.2 What are the risk factors for individual cardiovascular conditions?

Condition	Age	Smoking	FH of VTE	FH of AMI	FH of stroke	Obesity	Hypertension	Diabetes	Varicose veins	Other
VTE	?+	?−	+	−	−	+	−	?−	+	
IS	+	+	+	+	+	?−	+	+	−	Migraine
HS	−	?−	−	−	?+	−	+	?−	−	
AMI	+	+++	+	+	+	?+	+	+	−	Severe hyperlipidaemia

FH = family history
For explanation of other abbreviations, see footnote to Table 5.1.
+ = association; − = no association; +++ = strong association; ?+ = weak association; ?− = probably no association.

four studies [15]. On the other hand, causal support for the effect of different progestogens on thrombosis was found in a study looking at the effect of thrombin generation in plasma; third-generation pill users had a significantly lower sensitivity to activated protein C when compared to second-generation users [16]. The relative risk differences are small but the important issue is to look at the absolute risks under discussion. If the baseline population risk of DVT is one in 10 000 women per year, the use of a second-generation pill would increase the risk to 3.6 in 10 000 and the use of third-generation to about 5 in 10 000. The event rate for women who are pregnant is 6–7 per 10 000 women per year [17]. The majority of DVTs are non-fatal, the risk of death being 1–2%. Another way of presenting the data is to look at the percentage of women free of thrombosis – 99.985% on third-generation pills as opposed to 99.993% on second-generation pills [18]. Prescribing guidelines, by the Faculty of Family Planning and Reproductive Health Care in the United Kingdom, advised that having been given the information, the woman herself should choose if she had no contraindications or risk factors [19].

Any increase in cardiovascular risk with pill use is now thought to be due to thrombosis not atherogenesis. Recent studies with low-dose pills have found an increased risk of myocardial infarction only for those women who use the pill and have other risk factors [20,21] (see Chapter 16). Smoking interacts with pill use synergistically and pill users who smoke have a 30-fold excess risk of acute myocardial infarction (AMI) compared to non-smokers not using the pill. The risk of AMI has been found to be less for the third-generation progestogen pills than the second-generation pills. Although this difference was initially not statistically significant [22], final analysis of the Transnational Study did show a statistically significant reduction, but this was based on a small number of cases [23].

Unlike older studies, the most recent have not shown an overall increased risk of ischaemic stroke with low-dose pills containing either second- or third-generation progestogens [24].

The WHO Collaborative Study found a non-significant increase among European low-dose pill users, but an odds ratio of 3.26 (2.19–4.86) in users of these pills in developing countries [25]. Likewise low-dose pill users

in Europe had no increased risk of haemorrhagic stroke, although an increased risk was found for developing countries (odds ratio 1.76) [26]. For both types of stroke smoking had a synergistic effect, and a history of hypertension markedly increased the risk. Although other work has not shown any significant increased risk of thrombotic stroke with pill use, a recent Danish study found a relative risk of 1.8; this was one-third of the risk found for users of higher-dose pills. For a 20-year-old woman, the absolute attributable risk of low-dose pill use is about 4/100 000/year. As the absolute risk of cerebral thrombosis increases with age, a 40-year-old woman will have 10 times this risk [27].

Benign liver tumours

Two case-control studies have shown an increased risk of this condition in pill users with higher risks with longer duration and also perhaps for pills with high oestrogen potency [4]. However, this condition is very rare in women of reproductive age, and for long-term pill users the estimated annual incidence of hepatocellular adenoma is 3–4 per 100 000.

Breast cancer

There have been a large number of prospective and case-control studies looking at the relationship between oral contraceptive use and breast cancer. The Collaborative Group on Hormonal Factors in Breast Cancer has carried out a reanalysis of both published and unpublished data from 54 studies in 25 countries worldwide using studies that included at least 100 women with breast cancer [28]. Their findings were that, while women were taking the pill, and in the 10 years after stopping, they have a small increased relative risk of having breast cancer diagnosed – RR 1.24 in current users, 1.16 at 1–4 years after stopping and 1.07 at 5–9 years after stopping. All confidence intervals were greater than one. However, the cancers diagnosed in women who had used the pill were less advanced clinically. Family history of breast cancer, varying reproductive history of the women and different ethnic backgrounds resulted in similar results. There was no significant risk of having breast cancer diagnosed 10 or more years after stopping the pill, although there is still little information beyond 20 years after cessation of use. There were no significant trends with duration of use among women who had used low-, medium or high-dose preparations. Calculation showed that, for a given duration of use, earlier use did not lead to a greater number of cancers being diagnosed. The authors conclude that the observed relationship between breast cancer risk and the pill is unusual, and it is not possible to infer whether it is due to an earlier diagnosis of breast cancers in ever-users, the biological effects of the pill on tumour growth, or a combination of reasons.

Cervical cancer

The relationship between pill use and cervical cancer still remains uncertain, despite extensive research, as many studies have not controlled for confounding issues such as cigarette smoking, sexual behaviour or exposure to human papilloma virus (HPV). Since 1990, case-control and cohort studies showing a positive association between invasive squamous cervical cancer and the pill had a relative risk of between 1.3 and 2.2 [29]. Only two of the eight studies looking at this relationship have confidence intervals above one. This potential excess risk for pill users is much lower than the risk difference that exists geographically between countries with high and low incidences. Increased risk seems to be mainly for current or recent users with 5 or more years of use; however, there is no agreement as to whether age of first use of the pill influences risk. Similarly, the extent of any difference in risk between high-dose and low-dose pills is unclear. There is no strong support for the concern that the development of invasive cervical cancer has a shorter time frame for younger pill users. The WHO have commented that it is not clear whether a biological relationship explains this increased risk as we do not have enough information on the role of HPV. Women with documented HPV infection who are pill users have a higher relative risk of invasive cancer than those not using the pill: up to six times the risk in one study, suggesting that the pill may promote carcinogenesis by interaction with HPV [30]. This increase in risk may also apply to adenocarcinoma of the cervix, which is responsible for less than 20% of cervical cancer and has been less thoroughly studied. The 1994 Los Angeles study found that ever-use of the pill doubled the risk of adenocarcinoma, with a fourfold increase in risk for long-term users – more than 12 years [31]. The larger WHO collaborative study of neoplasia found a relative risk of adenocarcinoma of 1.6 for ever-users and 2.4 for long-term users – more than 8 years [32]. The risk was highest in current and recent users, and declined with cessation of use. Recommendations for screening are generally considered to be the same for pill users as for other women.

Liver cancer

The small number of cases of this disease in studies looking at the effects of the pill may lead to imprecise relative risk estimations. The largest study published before 1990 shows a relative risk of 1 for ever use but 4.4 for 8 or more years of use [4]. A 1992 publication with a larger number of cases showed non-significant increases in pill users between 25 and 49 years for ever-users (OR 1.6) or long-time users (OR 2.0) [33]. Case-control studies carried out in high-risk populations, where hepatitis B virus is endemic, have shown no effect of the pill, although the study was of short-term use only [4].

5

Combined oral
contraceptives:
epidemiological
studies and
risk–benefit
analysis

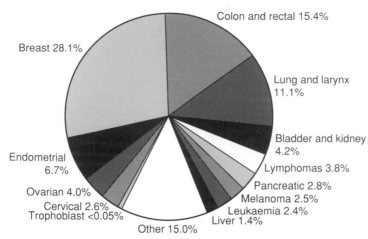

Fig 5.1 Cancers diagnosed among women of all ages in the USA, 1989 (505 000). Adapted with permission from Harlap S, Kost K, Darroch Forrest J. Preventing pregnancy, protecting health: a new look at birth control choices in the United States. New York: The Alan Guttmacher Institute, 1991.

Figure 5.1 shows the incidence of cancer diagnosis in women in the USA.

Other effects of combined oral contraceptives

There is now consensus that the combined pill does not cause premature closure of the epiphyses or inhibit skeletal growth in adolescent users.

Endometriosis

Multiple risk factors for endometriosis have been suggested, with agreement that the condition occurs less often in women who have shorter period duration and longer cycles. There appears, however, to be less consensus regarding the role of oral contraceptives: a recent review of eight papers on the possible relationship between oral contraceptives and endometriosis found a reduction in risk in four studies, an increase in risk in two

and no effect in the remainder [34]. The Oxford/FPA Study found a decreased risk (RR 0.4) in current pill users with an increased risk in previous users (RR 1.8), a pattern similar to that found in the Walnut Creek study [35]. Comparison of a low-dose cyclic pill with a gonadotrophin-releasing agonist found reduction in deep dyspareunia, non-menstrual pain and dysmenorrhoea, with a similar return of symptoms when both treatments were discontinued [36]. The suggestion is that, while endometriosis may be suppressed by pill use, hormonal treatment does not cure endometriosis: ectopic endometrium survives in an atrophic form ready for reactivation once treatment is suspended.

Uterine fibroids

The Royal College of General Practitioners (RCGP) and the Oxford Family Planning Association studies found a

protective effect of the pill for leiomyomas; however, the Walnut Creek found a non-significant increase in risk [4]. More recent case-control studies suggest that fibroids are unrelated to the use of the pill, but that makers of access to medical care contribute to the detection of fibroids [37,38]. In a non-randomized study of women with fibroids those taking the pill had no significant change in uterine size (as measured by ultrasound) compared to women not on the pill [39]. However, period duration decreased.

Gallstones

Early studies suggested that the risk of symptomatic gallbladder disease was increased but more recent studies have found this only at the beginning of pill use, with the possibility that the pill may accelerate presentation in predisposed women. Further data from the RCGP study found that the development of gallbladder disease in oral contraceptive users was not significantly different from that in non-users; current users had a relative risk of 1.15 (CI 0.99–1.34) for symptomatic gallbladder disease, and former users a relative risk of 1.03 (CI 0.9–1.18) [40].

Rheumatoid arthritis

A recent meta-analysis combined the results of past observational studies and evaluated the discrepancies found in previous meta-analyses looking at the association between the pill and rheumatoid arthritis [41]. A protective effect (RR 0.5) was found when considering only the hospital-based control studies; however, the studies that used population-based controls had an average relative risk of approximately 1.0. The conclusion was that, although there is some evidence that the pill might be protective against more severe forms of rheumatoid arthritis, other explanations are possible and additional research is required.

Human immunodeficiency virus (HIV)

A recent review of studies looking at the association between pill use and HIV was unable to find any consistent outcome, and further research with larger numbers and longer duration of use are needed [42]. The current consensus sees no incompatibility in pill usage by HIV-positive women.

Osteoporosis

Although several studies have shown oral contraceptive use to stabilize or increase bone mass, others have not confirmed this association. This difference may be due to small sample size, the methodology used for measuring bone density or, more likely, to the large number of confounding variables that may affect bone density, e.g. body mass index and smoking. One of the largest, most comprehensive studies found a significant increase in bone density with more than 10 years of use of the pill; however, there was no correction for smoking, exercise or different pill formulations. A recent review has concluded that, while it appears that premenopausal use of the pill allows women to enter the menopause with a bone density 2–3% higher than non-users, we do not yet know the clinical importance of this change [43].

Inflammatory bowel disease

Equivocal evidence exists for an association between oral contraceptive use and Crohn's disease and ulcerative colitis. Bias may have arisen owing to the lack of adjustment for cigarette smoking or the particular control groups used in study design. A recent population-based case-control study found an increased risk of both Crohn's disease (RR 2.6) and ulcerative colitis (RR 2.0) in pill users, the risk of Crohn's disease increasing with duration of use [44]. There were no firm conclusions about the relationship of pill dose and the authors point out that potential mechanisms for the role of contraceptives in inflammatory bowel disease must be speculative as the aetiology of these disorders is unknown.

Colorectal cancer

There has been no consistent pattern in studies looking at the relationship between oral contraceptive use and colorectal cancers. The largest work to date, a hospital case-control, found that pill use did not increase the risk of these cancers and indeed may decrease it with a relative risk of 0.58 (CI 0.36–0.92) [45].

However, even in this study, the number of cases and controls exposed were limited and there was no consistent time–risk relationship.

Hydatidiform mole

Concern regarding an increased incidence of choriocarcinoma for users of the pill after mole evacuation has led to differing advice. A recent review has taken into consideration previous study weaknesses and concluded hormonal methods of contraception are appropriate post mole evacuation [46]. In the UK, expert opinion continues to maintain that starting the combined oral contraceptive prior to return of human chorionic gonadotrophin (hCG) to normal increases the risk of choriocarcinoma and trophoblastic disease remains a contraindication to steroidal contraception until hCG levels return to normal [47]. The American College of Obstetricians and Gynecologists allows the use of the pill immediately post molar evacuation. It takes the view that oral contraceptives do not increase the incidence of postmolar gestational trophoblastic disease or affect the pattern of regression of hCG levels [48].

Other cancers

Studies do not suggest any statistical increase in the risk of gallbladder cancer, pituitary tumours or cutaneous melanoma for oral contraceptive users.

5

Combined oral
contraceptives:
epidemiological
studies and
risk–benefit
analysis

Risk–benefit perspective

One way of presenting the risks and benefits of the pill is to look at the overall net effect. Although the relative risks used in the estimations have varied between studies, overall pill users will have fewer gynaecological cancers diagnosed than non-users [49].

The 20-year follow-up of the RCGP Oral Contraceptive Study found that the relative risk of mortality in ever-users compared with never-users was 1.10 (CI 0.96–1.25) for all causes, 0.93 (CI 0.77–1.11) for all cancers and 1.57 (CI 1.18–2.09) for all circulatory diseases [50]. Tracing those women who were no longer attending their general practitioner did not change the overall relationship of oral contraceptive use with mortality.

Although the presentation of net effects with pill use is reassuring, most health professionals and women wish to have more detailed information on risk. Studies in the past tended to present their findings in terms of relative risk. However, the incidence of the disease in question is needed in order for relative risks to have any real meaning. Indeed, recent studies have shown that, when physicians were presented with the same study results, benefits presented in relative risk terms were thought to be greater than when presented in absolute risk terms [51]. It is little wonder then that women and the media have difficulties in assessing risks and benefits of pill taking. The Alan Guttmacher Institute has helped clarify this by presenting disease incidence at various ages and the effects of pill use [52]. These results are presented in Tables 5.3–5.5, the absolute attributable annual risk of the pill being the difference in incidence between users and non-users. It may also be useful to compare pill risks with other everyday risks that we accept in our daily lives. For example, the annual risk of death for a non-smoker under age 35 is 1 in 77 000, increasing to 1 in 2000 for a smoker; for car drivers in the UK it is 1 in 6000 [53].

Cost-effectiveness of combined oral contraceptives

Cost may influence whether a contraceptive is used at all, not only by the individual but its access by social service systems. Comparison of different methods of contraception has shown the pill (combined and progestogen only) to be the second most cost-effective method after the injectable method for the first year of use in a private payment system [54]. Assuming use continuation, long-term methods such as vasectomy and subdermal implants become more cost-effective after 5 years of use.

Although the pill was the fourth most cost-effective method after the intrauterine device (IUD), injectable and the condom in the first year of use in the public system, assuming an ability to purchase pills at $5 per cycle showed the pill to provide more cost savings at 5 years than all other methods except the IUD, vasectomy and the implant.

Costs included those of the method and visit, the costs of side effects and the costs of unintended pregnancies. For highly effective methods, such as female sterilization, the method costs are 96% of the total costs, whereas for less effective methods such as the condom, the costs of unintended pregnancy are 85% of the total. Cardiovascular side effects of the pill were included in the analysis but not the effects on cancer, as the assumption was made that

Table 5.3 Effect of pill use on cancer and cardiovascular disease for 100 000 women per year aged 15–19 years

Condition	Non-use		Pill use	
Ovarian cancer[a]	2		0	
Endometrial cancer[a]	0		0	
Breast cancer[a]	0		0	
	Non-smoker	Heavy smoker[>25]	Non-smoker	Heavy smoker [>25]
Myocardial infarction[b]	0	0	0	3 (1)
Venous thrombosis and embolism[c]	1 (0)	7 (0)	3 (0)	22 (0)

[a]Estimated annual number of newly diagnosed cases with non-use and use.
[b]Estimated annual number of newly diagnosed cases and deaths (in brackets) with non-use and ever-use.
[c]Estimated annual number of newly diagnosed cases with current use and ever-use.
[>25] = more than 25 cigarettes per day.
Adapted with permission from Harlap S, Kost K, Darroch Forest J. Preventing pregnancy, protecting health: a new look at birth control choices in the United States. New York: The Alan Guttmacher Institute, 1991.

Table 5.4 Effect of pill use on cancer and cardiovascular disease for 100 000 women per year aged 20–39 years

Condition	Non-use		Pill use	
Ovarian cancer[a]	23		5	
Endometrial cancer[a]	14		7	
Breast cancer[a]	89		108	
	Non-smoker	**Heavy Smoker [>25]**	**Non-smoker**	**Heavy Smoker [>25]**
Myocardial infarction[b]	6 (1)	27 (6)	11 (3)	260 (60)
Venous thrombosis and embolism[c]	27 (0)	195 (1)	83 (0)	584 (6)

[a]Estimated annual number of newly diagnosed cases with non-use, 10 or more years of use, or use from age 15 if less than 25 years old.
[b]Estimated annual number of newly diagnosed cases and deaths (in brackets) with non-use and ever use.
[c]Estimated annual number of newly diagnosed cases with current use and ever use.
[>25]-more than 25 cigarettes per day
Adapted with permission from Harlap S, Kost K, Darroch Forest J. Preventing pregnancy, protecting health: a new look at birth control choices in the United States. New York: The Alan Guttmacher Institute, 1991.

any increased costs of cervical, breast and liver cancer would be exactly offset by the decreased risk of ovarian and endometrial cancers.

The emergency contraceptive pill (ECP) can also be cost-effective when used after unprotected intercourse [55]. Advance provision of ECP to women using barriers, spermicides, withdrawal or periodic abstinence results in even higher cost savings.

The message is simple: contraception saves money as preventing unintended pregnancy is very cost-effective. The high cost of non-use, $3000 per year for a woman not using contraception, justifies investment in outreach.

However, to be cost-effective, methods need to be used correctly and consistently. Most studies use a typical pill failure rate of 3%. Decreasing the delivery cost of the pill in combination with improved use-effectiveness resulted in further savings [56].

Policy and provision changes

The awareness of the economic benefits of contraceptive provision has led to some proposals for change in insurance coverage. Although the majority of Health Maintenance Organisations in the USA have covered reversible

contraception, only a third of typical indemnity policies include oral contraception in the coverage. Early 1997 saw the sponsoring of a US bill to provide equity in insurance coverage for contraception. Under this legislation, plans already covering prescription drugs and devices must include equal coverage for contraceptive drugs and devices, and outpatient contraceptive services. The FDA had previously in 1989 deleted health warnings for older, healthy, non-smoking pill users and in 1993 modified the requirement for physical examination prior to pill use. In 1997 they endorsed the use of certain combinations of pill as emergency contraceptives and

Table 5.5 Effect of pill use on cancer and cardiovascular disease for 100 000 women per year aged 40–44 and 45–54 years

Condition	Age 40–44		Age 45–54	
	Non-use	Pill use	Non-use	Pill use
Ovarian cancer[a]	17	3	60	12
Endometrial cancer[a]	19	8	91	36
Breast cancer[a]	112	123	398	358
	Non-smoker	Heavy smoker [>25]	Non-smoker	Heavy smoker [>25]	Non-smoker	Heavy smoker [>25]	Non-smoker	Heavy smoker [>25]
Myocardial infarction[b]	10 (2)	49 (10)	20 (5)	470 (115)	N/A		N/A	
Venous thrombosis and embolism[c]	16 (0)	113 (2)	48	338 (3)	N/A		N/A	

[a]Estimated annual number of newly diagnosed cases with non-use or 10 or more years of use.
[b]Estimated annual number of newly diagnosed cases and deaths (in brackets) with non-use and ever-use.
[c]Estimated annual number of newly diagnosed cases with current use and ever-use.
[>25] = more than 25 cigarettes per day.
Adapted with permission from Harlap S, Kost K, Darroch Forest J. Preventing pregnancy, protecting health: a new look at birth control choices in the United States. New York: The Alan Guttmacher Institute, 1991.

5

Combined oral
contraceptives:
epidemiological
studies and
risk–benefit
analysis

have called for pharmaceutical manufacturers to submit new applications which would enable them to label and market pills for this purpose. This may help to resolve some of uncertainty regarding the medicolegal implications, which until now may have limited its use.

One month's supply of low-dose pills today contains about the same amount of hormone as one pill 25 years ago. While cardiovascular risks with modern-day pills have decreased, the protective effect on some cancers still remains in spite of the lower dose. However, over 40% of women in a 1994 British study were concerned about the risk of cardiovascular disease and cancer with pill use [57]. In addition, unless providers take time to explain that the short-term side effects of the pill, such as nausea, breast tenderness and breakthrough bleeding, are self-limiting, women, fearing associated risks to their health, may stop using contraception without returning to discuss their problems. The women who are more aware of the advantages of the pill are more likely to use it, and it has been suggested that the continuing need for provider input is not just to obtain the prescription but, more importantly, to offer a psychological advisory service [58].

The requirement for increasing physician and nursing advice has often not been considered in the recent discussions regarding pharmacy pill supply. Recognizing that ease of access is an important consideration in pill use, availability over the counter, without the need for

prescription, is one solution. The medical safety of this approach has been accepted by many health care professionals and the main concern has been that women who depend on subsidized access for pill prescriptions may also lose the reproductive health care received at the visit. The ability of nurses to prescribe the pill also has the potential to improve access. Swedish midwives have had this ability for many years, yet the clarification for midwives in New Zealand took place only recently, at the end of 1996.

The need for prevention of sexually transmitted disease (STD) as well as pregnancy is a reality for many women but the likelihood of one method that can effectively do both is not imminent. The financial and resource difficulties of further merging of contraceptive and STD services needs to be addressed. Involvement of men and peer education will improve the social marketing of contraceptives.

Some pharmaceutical companies have introduced condoms to their pill starter packaging as a reminder of this need. Other issues of packaging are more problematic. The need for standardized package inserts that present risks and benefits in a way that can be easily understood, has been widely recognized. The existence of the European Medicines Evaluation Agency should facilitate this happening but it is still a long way from becoming a reality. Although the USA has had fairly standardized patient inserts for the last decade, it is only in the last few years that these have included a shortened summary

along with instructions for pill taking. Attention is now being paid to simplifying the language to improve understanding.

Application to developing countries

In the developing world more than 120 million married women are estimated to have an unmet need for contraception. Lack of access and information, opposition from husbands and concerns about associated risks and side effects all play a part. This can have devastating outcomes, such as the 20 000 deaths from illegal abortion for women in Romania, during two decades of removal of contraceptive and abortion services.

Variations exist in the incidence of disease in developing countries and in the prevalence of risk factors which may alter the absolute risk of cardiovascular disease or cancer with pill use. In addition the risk of maternal mortality may need to be considered if contraception is not used. Women in Western Europe have a high incidence of breast, ovarian and endometrial cancer with a low incidence of cervical cancer. Cancer patterns are different for women in Asia (low incidence of breast, ovarian and endometrial cancer) and Central/South America (high incidence of cervical cancer; intermediate incidence of breast, ovarian and endometrial cancer). Despite these differences, current evidence does not change the mainly favourable assessment of the benefits of the pill.

References

1. Kost K, Forrest JP, Harlap S. Comparing the health risks and benefits of contraceptive choices. *Fam Plann Perspect* 1991;23:54–61.

2. Mishell D. Noncontraceptive benefits of oral contraceptives. *Am J Obstet Gynecol* 1982;142:809–16.

3. Brown S, Vessey M, Stratton I. The influence of method of contraception and cigarette smoking on menstrual patterns. *Br J Obstet Gynaecol* 1988;95:905–10.

4. WHO Scientific Group. Oral contraceptives and neoplasia. WHO Technical Report Series no. 817. Geneva: World Health Organisation, 1992:1–46.

5. Vessey MP. The Jephcott lecture, 1989. An overview of the benefits and risks of combined oral contraceptives. In: Mann RD (ed.) Oral contraceptives and breast cancer. New Jersey: Parthenon 1990:121–35.

6. Mishell D. Noncontraceptive benefits of oral contraceptives. *J Reprod Med* 1993;38:1021–9.

7. Wolner-Hansen P. Relationship between oral contraceptives and pelvic inflammatory disease and associated sexually transmitted diseases. In: Hannaford PC, Webb AMC (eds) Evidence-guided prescribing of the pill. Carnforth, UK: Parthenon 1996:175–180.

8. Vessey M, Metcalfe A, Wells C, McPherson K, Westhoff C, Yeates D. Ovarian neoplasms, functional ovarian cysts and oral contraceptives. *Br Med J* 1987;294:1518–20.

9. Lanes SF, Birmann B, Walker AM, Singer S. Oral contraceptive type and functional ovarian cysts. *Am J Obstet Gynecol* 1992;166:956–61.

10. Schlesselman JJ. Oral contraceptives and neoplasia of the uterine corpus. *Contraception* 1991;43:557–9.

11. Franceschi S. Oral contraceptive use and risk of cancer of the ovary and corpus uteri. In: Hannaford PC, Webb AMC (eds) Evidence-guided prescribing of the pill. Carnforth, UK: Parthenon, 1996:135–44.

12. Gross TP, Schlesselman JJ. The estimated effect of oral contraceptive use on the cumulative risk of epithelial ovarian cancer. *Obstet Gynecol* 1994;83:419–24.

13. Bloemenkamp KWM, Rosendaal FR, Helmerhorst FM, et al. Evidence that currently available pills are associated with vascular disease, venous disease. In: Hannaford PC, Webb AMC (eds) Evidence-guided prescribing of the pill. Carnforth, UK: Parthenon, 1996:61–76.

14. Vandenbroucke JP, Koster T, Briet E, et al. Increased risk of venous thrombosis in oral contraceptive users who are carriers of factor V Leiden mutation. *Lancet* 1994;244:1453–7.

15. Lidegaard O. The influence of thrombotic risk factors when oral contraceptives are prescribed. *Acta Obstet Gynecol Scand* 1997;76:252–60.

16. Rosing J, Tan SG, Nicolas GA, et al. Oral contraceptives and venous thrombosis: different sensitivities to activated protein C in women using second and third generation oral contraceptives. *Br J Haematol* 1997;97:233–8.

17. Lewis MA, Heinemann LA, Macrae KD, Bruppacher R, Spitzer, W. The increased risk of venous thromboembolism and the use of third generation progestagens: role of bias in observational research. *Contraception* 1996;54:5–13.

18. Hall M. Perception of risk is affected by presentation. *Br Med J* 1995;311:1065.

19. Mills AM, Wilkinson CL, Bromham DR, et al. Guidelines for prescribing combined oral contraceptives. *Br Med J* 1996;312:121–2.

20. Chasen-Taber L, Stampfer MJ. Oral contraceptives and risk of arterial disease: epidemiological evidence on acute and long-term effects. In: Hannaford PC, Webb AMC (eds) Evidence-guided prescribing of the pill. Carnforth, UK: Parthenon, 1996:49–60.

21. WHO Collaborative Study of Cardiovascular Disease and Steroid Hormone Contraception. Acute myocardial infarction and oral contraceptives; results of an international multicentre case-control study. *Lancet* 1997;349:1202–9.

22. Lidegaard O, Milsom I. Oral contraceptives and thrombotic diseases: impact of new epidemiological studies. *Contraception* 1996;53:135–9.

23. Lewis MA, Spitzer WO, Heineman LA, Macrae KD, Bruppacher R. Lowered risk of dying of heart attack with third generation pills may offset risk of dying of thromboembolism (letter). *Br Med J* 1997;315:679–80.

24. Petitti DB, Sidney S, Bernstein A, et al. Stroke in users of low-dose oral contraceptives. *N Engl J Med* 1996;335:8–15.

25. WHO Collaborative Study of Cardiovascular Disease and Steroid Hormone Contraception. Ischaemic stroke and combined oral contraceptives: results of an international, multicentre, case-control study. *Lancet* 1996;348:498–505.

26. WHO Collaborative Study of Cardiovascular Disease and Steroid Hormone Contraception. Haemorrhagic stroke, overall stroke risk and combined oral contraceptives: results of an international, multicentre, case-control study. *Lancet* 1996;348:505–10.

27. Lidegaard O. Oral contraception and risk of a cerebral thromboembolic attack: results of a case-control study. *Br Med J* 1993;306:956–63.

28. Collaborative Group on Hormonal Factors in Breast

5

Combined oral
contraceptives:
epidemiological
studies and
risk–benefit
analysis

Cancer. Breast cancer and hormonal contraceptives; collaborative re-analysis of individual data on 53 297 women with breast cancer and 100 239 women without breast cancer from 54 epidemiological studies. *Lancet* 1996;347:1713–27.

29. Irwin K. The association between oral contraceptive use and neoplasia of the cervix, vagina and vulva. In: Hannaford PC, Webb AMC (eds) Evidence-guided prescribing of the pill. Carnforth, UK: Parthenon, 1996:145–56.

30. Bosch FX, Munoz N, de Sanjose S, et al. Risk factors for cervical cancer in Colombia and Spain. *Int J Cancer* 1992;52:750–8.

31. Ursin G, Peters RK, Henderson BE, et al. Oral contraceptive use and adenocarcinoma of cervix. *Lancet* 1994;344:1390–4.

32. Thomas DB, Ray RM. Oral contraceptives and invasive adenocarcinomas and adenosquamous carcinomas of the uterine cervix. The World Health Organisation Collaborative Study of Neoplasia and Steroid Contraception. *Am J Epidemiol* 1996;144:281–9.

33. Hsing AW, Hoover RN, McLaughlin JK, et al. Oral contraceptives and primary liver cancer among young women. *Cancer Causes Control* 1992;3:43–8.

34. Vercellini P, Ragni G, Trespidi L, Oldani S, Crosignani PG. Does contraception modify the risk of endometriosis? *Hum Reprod* 1993;8:547–51.

35. Vessey M, Villard MacKintosh L, Painter R, et al. Epidemiology of endometriosis in women attending Family Planning Clinics. *Br Med J* 1993;306:182–4.

36. Vercillini P Tresidi L, Colombo A, et al. A gonadotrophin-releasing hormone agonist versus a low dose oral contraceptive for pelvic pain associated with endometriosis. *Fertil Steril* 1993;60:75–9.

37. Parazzini F, Negre E, La Vecchia C, et al. Oral contraceptive use and the use of uterine fibroids. *Obstet Gynecol* 1992;79:430–3.

38. Samadi AR, Lee NC, Flanders WD, et al. Risk factors for self reported uterine fibroids: a case control study. *Am J Public Health* 1996;86:858–62.

39. Friedman AJ, Thomas PP. Does low-dose combination oral contraceptive use affect uterine size or menstrual flow in premenopausal women with leiomyomas? *Obstet Gynecol* 1995;85:631–5.

40. Murray FE, Logan RF, Hannaford PC, et al. Cigarette smoking and parity as risk factors for the development of symptomatic gall bladder disease in women: results of the Royal College of General Practitioners' Oral Contraceptive Study. *Gut* 1994;35:107–11.

41. Pladevall-Vila M, Delchos GL, Varas C, et al. Controversy of oral contraceptives and risk of rheumatoid arthritis: meta-analysis of conflicting studies and review of conflicting meta-analysis with special emphasis on analysis of heterogeneity. *Am J Epidemiol* 1996;144:1–14.

42. Taitel HF, Kafrissen ME. A review of oral contraceptive use and risk of HIV-transmission. *Br J Fam Plann* 1995;20:112–6.

43. Corson SL. Oral contraceptives for the prevention of osteoporosis. *J Reprod Med* 1993;38:1015–20.

44. Boyko EJ, Theiss MK, Vaughan TL, Nicol-Blades B. Increased risk of inflammatory bowel disease associated with oral contraceptive use. *Am J Epidemiol* 1994;140:268–78.

45. Fernandez E, La Vecchaic, D'Avanzo B. Oral contraceptives, hormone replacement therapy and the risk of colorectal cancer. *Br J Cancer* 1996;73:143–5.

46. IMAP Statement on contraception for women with medical disorders. *IPPF Med Bull* 1995;29:2.

47. Store M, Dent J, Kardana A, Bagshawe KD. Relationship of oral contraception to development of trophoblastic tumour after evacuation of hydatidiform mole. *Br J Obstet Gynaecol* 1976;83:913–6.

48. American College of Obstetrics and Gynecology. Management of gestational trophoblastic disease. *ACOG Tech Bull* 1993;178:1–7.

49. Schlesselman JJ. Net effect of oral contraceptive use on the risk of cancer in the United States. *Obstet Gynecol* 1995;85:793–801.

50. Beral V, Herman C, Kay C, et al. Mortality in relation to method of follow-up in the Royal College of General Practitioners' Oral Contraception Study. In: Hannaford PC, Webb AMC, (eds) Evidence-guided prescribing of the pill. Carnforth, UK: Parthenon, 1996:327–39.

51. Fahey T, Griffiths S, Peters T. Evidence based purchasing: understanding results of clinical trials and systematic reviews. *Br Med J* 1995;311:1056–60.

52. Harlap S, Kost K, Darroch Forest J. Preventing pregnancy, protecting health: a new look at birth control choices in the United States. New York: The Alan Guttmacher Institute, 1991.

53. Fraser IS. A health perspective of hormonal contraceptives. *Acta Obstet Gynecol Scand* 1986;134(suppl):33–43.

54. Trussell J, Levegne JA, Koenig JD. The economic value of contraception: a comparison of 15 methods. *Am J Public Health* 1995;85:494–503.

55. Trussell J, Keonig J, Ellertson C, Stewart F. Preventing unintended pregnancy: the cost-effectiveness of three methods of emergency contraception. *Am J Public Health* 1997;87:932–7.

56. Ashraf T, Arnold SB, Maxfield M Jr. Cost-effectiveness of levonorgestrel subdermal implants, comparison with other contraceptive methods available in the United States. *J Reprod Med* 1994;39:791–8.

57. Oddens BJ, Visser AP, Vemer HM, Everaerd WT, Lehert P. Contraceptive use and attitudes in Great Britain. *Contraception* 1994;49:73–86.

58. Oddens BJ. Current accessibility and perceptions about the pill in Western Europe. In: Hannaford PC, Webb AMC (eds) Evidence-guided prescribing of the pill. Carnforth UK: Parthenon, 1996:27–42.

Combined oral contraceptives: metabolic effects and practical prescribing

Hilary Furniss MRCOG
Max Elstein FRCOG

Background and development of combined oral contraceptive pills

Since the first combined oral contraceptive pill (COC), Enovid®, was marketed in 1960, there has been a great deal of research within both the pharmaceutical industries and the medical profession, which aims to provide COCs which remain effective, but with fewer adverse effects. Nowadays, there are over 70 million users of COCs worldwide and, consequently, there are significant public health implications of the use of such a potent pharmacological agent in healthy women.

The primary aim has always been for any COC to provide fail-safe effectiveness, hence the earlier high-dosage formulations. However, the fact that the major desired action of suppression of ovulation, via the inhibition of pituitary–ovarian function, was possible with lower steroid dosage, which maintained the ancillary contraceptive actions of genital tract changes (endometrial and cervical), enabled the development of lower dosage products. Ideally, 'the pill' should have no undesired effects and the progestogen should also have a significant 'anti-oestrogenic' activity. By 1963 there had been over 300 reports of thromboembolism connected with the usage of the first COC, Enovid, in the USA. This pill contained a dosage of 150 µg mestranol and this high oestrogen content was implicated. During the 1960s and 1970s, the development of COCs saw the gradual reduction in dosage of the oestrogenic component and the emergence of ethinyloestradiol (EE_2) as the oestrogen of choice, replacing its pro-drug mestranol. Pills containing 50 µg EE_2 were recommended [1]. Subsequently, still lower dose formulations containing 35 µg and 30 µg were developed with an enhanced safety profile [2,3]. Latterly, the dose of oestrogen has been further reduced to 20 µg, the concern being to ensure adequate contraceptive effectiveness while maintaining the non-contraceptive benefits [4], the proviso for acceptability of these lower dose formulations being adequate cycle control [5].

Pharmacology

Ethinyloestradiol (EE_2) is the synthetic oestrogen in most combined oral contraceptives. Mestranol is a pro-drug of EE_2 and, dose for dose, would be considered weaker. EE_2 is absorbed within 2 hours of ingestion, and passes through the hepatic circulation (the first-pass effect), where it is glucuronated. The inactive conjugated oestradiol is excreted with bile and has to be reactivated by large bowel bacterial flora and reabsorbed (the so-called enterohepatic circulation). Most of the progestins in currently available COC formulations are 19–nortestosterone derivatives, notable exceptions being cyproterone acetate and chlormadinone acetate, which are 17-hydroxyprogesterone derivatives.

By the early 1980s, the progestogenic component of COCs was also implicated, particularly with regard to arterial disease [6]. Attention was thus turned to the development of newer, more potent progestogens. The estrane progestogen, norethisterone, was thus superseded by the gonanes, initially levonorgestrel, sometimes referred to as a 'second-generation progestogen', and, latterly, the 'third-generation progestogens' gestodene,

6

Combined oral
contraceptives:
metabolic
effects and
practical
prescribing

Table 6.1 Progestational activity of various progestogens on the pituitary–ovarian axis and on the endometrium in female volunteers

Progestogenic component of COC	Dosage to inhibit ovulation (mg/day)	Dosage to transform the endometrium (mg/cycle)
Progesterone	300	100–150
Norethisterone	0.5	50–60
Norgestimate	0.25	a
Desogestrel	0.06	2.5
Levonorgestrel	0.05	5–6
Gestodene	0.04	2–3

a No published data.
Adapted from Dusterberg B, Beier S, Schneider WHF, Spona J. Pharmacological features of gestodene in laboratory animals and man. In: Gestodene, a new direction in oral contraception, Vol. 1. Carnforth, UK: Parthenon, 1988: 13–30.

desogestrel and norgestimate, and more recently dienogest. Also used are the pregnanes (C-19 steroids), such as cyproterone acetate, which has a particularly useful anti-androgenic activity, and chlormadinone acetate in some countries, e.g. Germany. The difference in potency between different progestogens is measured by certain end-organ effects in both human females and in some animal models (Table 6.1) and also their anti-oestrogenic effects [8]. The more potent or selective a progestogen is, the greater its progestogenic activity at relatively low concentrations or doses. The potential for undesirable androgenic effects would only become manifest at relatively higher concentrations or doses.

Another way to 'classify' progestogens is by their binding affinity to the progestogen receptor, thereby reflecting their cycle control and contraceptive potential, and to the androgen receptor, reflecting their androgenicity. Table 6.2 shows the relative binding affinity to androgen receptors and clearly demonstrates the low androgenicity of norgestimate and 3-ketodesogestrel. Collins described the measure of progestogen selectivity as the ratio of the affinity for progesterone receptors to the affinity for androgen receptors: the selectivity index [9]. Apart from its inhibitory and antigonadotrophic action with regard to ovulation, the progestogenic component of COCs has the important 'progestational' effect on the endometrium of transforming the proliferative epithelium, resulting from the oestrogenic effect to a secretory endo-metrium.

Norethisterone and the gonane levonorgestrel produce androgen-related metabolic effects when used in higher doses in COCs. The newer gonanes, gestodene, norgestimate and desogestrel, have higher selectivity indices, i.e. they have more specific end-organ effects with minimal systemic androgen-related action (and consequently fewer unwanted side effects). Norethisterone and levonorgestrel COCs with the lowest dose of the 'second-generation' progestogens are comparable to third-generation pills in overall metabolic impact. Gestodene is the most selective of the progestogens with its desired progestogenic and suppressive effects at a relatively low dosage; levonorgestrel and desogestrel follow, then norgestimate followed by norethisterone (Table 6.1).

Triphasic COCs were introduced in the late 1960s and early 1970s. These provide a dosage profile closely resembling that of the physiological menstrual cycle, but allow the total hormone content per cycle to be reduced from that utilized in some of the previous marketed monophasic products [10].

Undesirable effects of COCs

Unfortunately, there is no pharmacological agent that is devoid of undesirable side effects. The aim is to reduce these effects to an absolute minimum, especially, as in the case of COCs, when the users are generally fit,

Table 6.2 Relative binding affinities for rat prostatic androgen receptors

Progestogen	Relative androgen binding a
Progesterone	0.005
Norgestimate	0.003
17-Deacylated norgestimate	0.013
Levonorgestrel	0.220
Gestodene	0.154
3-Ketodesogestrel	0.118
Dihydrotestosterone	1.000

a As assessed by relative ability to displace radiolabelled dihydrotestosterone from rat prostatic receptors.
Adapted from Phillips A, Demarest K, Hahn DW et al. Progestational and androgenic receptor binding affinities and in vivo activities of norgestimate and other progestins. Contraception 1989; 41: 399–410.

healthy young women. Improving user acceptability is particularly important when the 'use effectiveness' of 'the pill' is to a major extent dependent on patient compliance. Side effects can be divided into the following categories:

- Metabolic adverse effects
- Abnormalities of cycle control
- Nuisance side effects
- Acne.

These effects and their influence on the further development of COCs are considered below.

Metabolic adverse events

Lipoproteins

High blood lipid concentrations have been shown to be associated with an increased risk of cardiovascular disease: the higher the ratio of low-density lipoprotein (LDL) and total cholesterol to high-density lipoprotein (HDL), the greater the risk. A dose-dependent effect of both oestrogens and progestogen on lipids is seen with COCs. This effect is modulated by the type of progestogen (P) and the balance of EE_2 to P in the particular formulation. Progestogens elevate LDL-C and reduce HDL-C. Oestrogens have the opposite effect and also raise triglyceride levels. The net effect for low-dose pills is a balancing off of lipid levels within normal limits [11].

The progestogenic component of COCs has for some time been implicated as a possible factor in the development of arterial disease through its effect on the

plasma lipid profile. Arterial disease remains the leading cause of death in women in the developed world [12], although its prevalence in women under 35 is rare. British data showing an association of arterial disease with the progestin component of the pill applied to higher progestin content pills that are no longer in routine clinical use. This mirrors the effect of COCs on a woman's lipid profile, with high progestin content pills altering the LDL/HDL ratio unfavourably. The combination of better patient selection (safer prescribing) and lowering the EE_2 and P doses of COCs (safer pills) means that present-day women who are healthy have a minuscule risk of cardiovascular disease. Age and smoking exert a more profound effect than the COC itself [6,13]. Levonorgestrel (LNG) and norethisterone (NET) pills, which have less than 150 µg of LNG and less than 1 mg of NET, have a neutral effect on the lipid profile. Also, the 'atherogenic' effect of androgenic progestins on the arterial wall is likely to be counteracted by the direct protective vasoactive effect of EE_2 on the arterial wall, which is similar to the effect of natural oestrogen. This explains the fact

that, in the small number of studies performed in humans and animals, pill users seem to have 'cleaner' arteries [14,15].

The newer gonane progestogens (gestodene, desogestrel and norgestimate) have been found to have more favourable effects on the lipid profile (Table 6.3); whether this would be translated into a less adverse effect on arterial disease risk is the subject of intense epidemiological work. The first such work [16] raised the possibility that gestodene and desogestrel low-dose combined pills may minimize the risk of cardiovascular disease (in the form of acute myocardial infarction) compared to levonorgestrel/norethisterone. Indeed, in 1991, Engel [15] reported on angiographic findings in women under 50 years of age after they had suffered an acute myocardial infarct (AMI) and related these findings to their COC usage. He found that 60% of the women who sustained an AMI during COC medication did not have angiographic evidence of coronary atherosclerosis, whereas in non-users 80% had angiographically demonstrable atherosclerosis. This may be due partly to the pill

Table 6.3 Effect of various progestogens on plasma lipoproteins (composite picture based on literature as of 1998)

Progestogen and dosage (µg)	Total cholesterol	HDL	LDL	HDL/LDL	Triglycerides
Levonorgestrel 150 EE₂ 30	0	–	+	–	0
Gestodene 75 EE₂ 30	0	0/+	0	0/+	+
Norgestimate 250 EE₂ 35	0	0/+	0	0/+	+
Desogestrel 150 EE₂ 30 or EE₂ 20	0	+	0	+	+

HDL = high-density lipoprotein; LDL = low-density lipoprotein; 0 = no significant change; + = increased levels; 0/+ = slight increase in some reports; – = decreased levels.

6

Combined oral
contraceptives:
metabolic
effects and
practical
prescribing

having an antioxidant effect on LDL. Smoking appeared to be the most important factor in the pathogenesis of AMI. This provides some evidence that the cardiovascular disease observed in pill users is more likely to be related to a thrombotic pathogenetic process rather than one of atherogenesis and, consequently, it is likely that the effect of COCs on coagulation factors/fibrinolysis is the more telling. COC users have raised triglyceride levels (an oestrogen effect balanced by a negative influence of the progestogen).

Coagulation factors/haemostasis

The 'pill' was associated with thromboembolism at a very early stage in its development. The oestrogen and, to a lesser extent, the progestogenic component have been implicated. The effect is manifest for pills containing 50 µg of EE_2 or more. With sub-50 µg pills, this dose–dependent effect on thrombosis risk disappears (i.e. there is no difference epidemiologically between 35, 30 or 20 µg pills). COCs alter the haemostatic balance of the coagulation and fibrinolytic system, as demonstrated by Winkler et al. in 1991 (Figure 6.1) [17]. Reducing the steroid dosage leads to a

reduction in the overall imbalance created by a COC but the thromboembolic risk may persist in predisposed women due to an idiosyncratic response to the pill. With increasing age there is increased fibrin turnover in women taking COCs, especially current users who smoke [18], but generally the overall balance between generation and resolution of fibrin is maintained. However, there may be an increased susceptibility to the evolution of thrombosis in older women taking COCs when they are exposed to the 'trigger' of thrombosis, leading to a decompensated balance. Predisposition may be due to specific disorders of blood coagulation leading to thrombophilic tendencies, such as activated protein C (APC) resistance (Box 6.1), and protein C and S deficiencies [19]. It would be ideal if these women could be identified prior to receiving COC treatment, as 80% of such people may experience thromboembolic events before the age of 40 years [20] without the added risk factor of COC usage. However, given the 5% prevalence of Factor V Leiden carriers in the general population, there is no evidence to favour a generalized screening policy in all potential COC users.

The guidelines indicating those women who should be screened are as follows:

- Cases with familial thrombophilia.

- Women with a thrombotic event during COC use, not only to evaluate the future risk in these patients, but also to elucidate mechanisms of risk.

The presence of thrombophilia may be a contraindication to COCs. However, individual risks have to be assessed taking into account the potential benefits of the pill and the increased risk of venous thromboembolism (VTE) in pregnancy.

The greatest risk factor for arterial disease in women is smoking and this therefore remains one of the most important factors to evaluate when prescribing COCs. Hypertension is another risk factor. There is no epidemiological evidence that smoking is a risk for VTE. The risk factors for VTE include a body mass index greater than 30 kg/m², parents or siblings with VTE, and severe varicose veins [21]. They must all be taken into account when evaluating the VTE risk for a particular patient (see Table 6.4 for risk factors for arterial and venous disease).

Carbohydrate metabolism

Glucose tolerance is reduced by and insulin levels rise with the use of COCs. The effect is thought to be that of both oestrogen and progestogen, with the latter having the greater impact. However, lower dose COCs have such minor effects on insulin levels, and little or no impact on

---

Box 6.1   Characteristics of APC resistance

- It is due to a genetic mutation of Factor V (Leiden factor).
- It affects 5% of European women.
- It accounts for 40% of familial VTE and 20% of all VTE.
- Heterozygotes for Factor V Leiden mutation have an eight-fold higher risk of VTE.
- Homozygotes for Factor V Leiden mutation have 80-fold higher risk of VTE.
- Acquired APC resistance is seen in pregnancy and to a lesser extent in COC users.
- Heterozygote carriers of Factor V Leiden mutation who use COCs have a 30-fold higher risk of VTE [19].

6

Combined oral
contraceptives:
metabolic
effects and
practical
prescribing

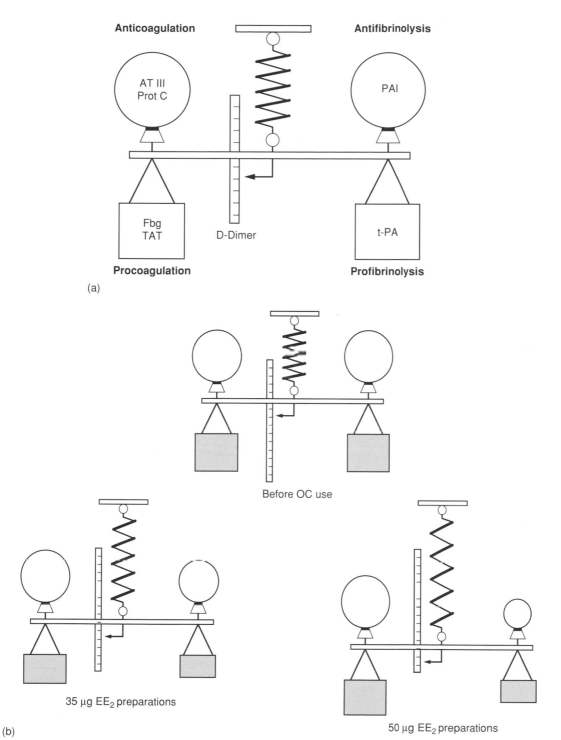

Fig. 6.1 Winkler's hypothesis: the dynamic balance of haemostasis. At III = antithrombin III; Prot C = protein C; PAI = plasminogen activator inhibitor; Fbg = fibrinogen; TAT = thrombin–antithrombin III complexes; t-PA = tissue plasminogen activator. EE_2 = ethinyloestradiol; OC = oral contraceptive. Adapted from Winkler UH, Koslowski S, Oberhoff C, Schindler EM, Schindler AE. Changes in the dynamic equilibrium of haemostasis associated with the use of low-dose oral contraceptives: a controlled study of cyproterone acetate containing oral contraceptives combined with either 35 or 50 μg ethinyl estradiol. *Adv Contracept* 1991 7(suppl 3): 273–284.

6

Combined oral
contraceptives:
metabolic
effects and
practical
prescribing

Table 6.4 Risk factors for arterial and venous disease among COC pill users

Risk factors for arterial disease	VTE risk factors
1. Smoking > 15 cigarettes/day – maximum risk < 15 cigarettes/day – still high risk	1. FH of VTE/genetic predisposition
2. Hypertension	2. Acquired predisposition (e.g. antiphospholipid syndrome)
3. Diabetes	3. Obesity (BMI > 30)
4. Android obesity	4. Severe varicose veins
5. FH of arterial or venous thrombosis	5. Dehydration
6. Age – background risk of AMI and IS rises after 35, synergism with smoking	6. Trauma and immobilization (e.g. postoperative)
7. Hyperlipidaemia	7. Age? If has an effect, it is likely to be small

FH = family history VTE = venous thromboembolism; AMI = acute myocardial infarction;
IS = ischaemic stroke; BMI = body mass index.

glucose tolerance [22], as to make such changes of no clinical significance. Significant glucose intolerance may occasionally occur in susceptible individuals and in insulin-dependent diabetics; however, there is no increased risk of clinical diabetes in pill users. Once assessed and considered suitable for a COC from the viewpoint of their cardiovascular status, a minority of insulin-dependent diabetics (less than 10%) may require adjustments in their insulin dosage.

Abnormalities of cycle control

While women obviously have great concerns regarding the more serious side effects of COC usage, which are usually related to their metabolic/haematological action, abnormalities of cycle control, such as the absence of withdrawal bleeding, breakthrough bleeding and spotting, are significant factors influencing adherence and continuation of usage. The bleeding irregularities experienced with low-dose pills might be caused by failure of conversion of the endometrium to a secretory phase or unstable angiogenesis within the endometrium or endometrial atrophy (all so-called end-organ effects). The low-dose gonane combination COCs show acceptable cycle control, with a suggestion that gestodene preparations may have lower rates of breakthrough bleeding compared with desogestrel and norgestimate pills [23]. It is important for the prescribing physician to stress to the pill user that the tendency is for any bleeding irregularities to settle over the first 6 months of use and to discuss this in detail with the woman, reinforcing the fact that such irregularities are not in themselves dangerous, so that the rate of discontinuation and potential pill failure is minimized. The causes of breakthrough bleeding are listed in Box 6.2.

Nuisance side effects

Together with disturbances of cycle control and irregular bleeding, the minor or nuisance side effects such as headaches, nausea, breast tenderness, mood changes, weight gain and hirsutism are important reasons for COC discontinuation [24]. These side effects have been shown to account for discontinuation rates of up to 50% within the first year of usage in new users and up to 37% may switch to another COC within that same time span, largely because of perceived side effects or unacceptable cycle control [25,26]. With modern low-dose pills, all side effects are rare and disappear with continued use. Side effects are anecdotally ascribed to either a progestogen or an oestrogen effect (Table 6.5).

> **Box 6.2 Causes of breakthrough bleeding**
>
> Organic causes – excluded by examination and tests:
>
> - Cervical bleeding – ectropion, cervicitis, cervical carcinoma
> - *Chlamydia trachomatis* endometritis
> - pregnancy, complications of pregnancy (miscarriage, trophoblastic disease).
>
> User/bioavailability causes:
>
> - missing pills
> - use of interacting drugs (see Chapter 16)
> - vomiting
> - severe diarrhoea
> - vegetarianism – which may reduce the recycled EE_2 because of low bowel bacterial flora
> - disorders of absorption, e.g. coeliac disease (not very likely to cause loss of bioavailability)
> - smoking – reduces bioavailability of EE_2 by 20%.

Table 6.5 Side effects and their relationship to the component steroids of COCs

Side effects attributed to oestrogen	Side effects attributed to progestogen
Breast tenderness/tension	Fluid retention and 'bloatedness'
Nausea	Seborrhoea and acne (in androgenic
Headaches	susceptible subjects)
Vaginal discharge	Mastalgia
Premenstrual syndrome/fluid retention	Lassitude/depression
	Loss of libido

6

Combined oral
contraceptives:
metabolic
effects and
practical
prescribing

Acne

Sexual activity often starts at a time in a young woman's life when acne is common. Users' concerns about the effect of COCs on acne are therefore real and legitimate. Most low-dose COCs tend to improve acne as they suppress ovarian biosynthesis of androgens. Moreover, oestrogen-dominant pills such as triphasic LNG pills or lowest dose NET pills raise sex hormone binding globulin (SHBG), thereby 'mopping up' excess testosterone, and are suitable alternatives for acne sufferers. On the other hand, progestin-dominant pills with relatively higher content of the androgenic progestogens LNG and NET can induce or cause worsening of acne. Users of COCs containing the selective potent progestogens desogestrel and gestodene are less likely to have problems with acne and, with COCs such as the 30/150 desogestrel combination or triphasic levonorgestrel, acne tends to improve over a period of 3–6 months of use. Another product is the combined pill of 35 µg EE_2 and 2 mg cyproterone acetate, an anti-androgen; this has a therapeutic role in the treatment of not only acne but also of hirsutism. Chloasma is now a rare side effect of low-dose COCs. It fades slowly after discontinuation. Switching to a non-oestrogen contraceptive is the only option.

Risk–benefit assessment

Non-contraceptive benefits

There are significant health benefits to users of COCs, quite apart from the obvious benefit of pregnancy prevention. The two major health benefits often overlooked and overshadowed by the rare adverse effects are those of a reduction of 50% in the incidence of endometrial and epithelial ovarian cancers [27]. The lowering of risk of uterine carcinoma appears to be mediated by the suppression of the oestrogenic proliferation of the endometrium. The reduction in epithelial ovarian cancers is attributed to the inhibition of ovulation and elimination of surface inclusion cysts. The protective effect is long lasting, incremental and universal with low-dose as well as high-dose pills. It is maximal in nulliparous women. It is apparent within the first year of use and persists up to 15 years after cessation of use.

Other health benefits include a reduction in benign breast disease, fewer functional ovarian cysts, prevention of ectopic pregnancies, less pelvic inflammatory disease, menorrhagia and anaemia and a lower incidence of fibroids, which, if they do occur, tend to be much smaller and isolated [27,28] (see also Chapter 5).

Adverse clinical effects (see Chapter 5)

The established risks associated with COC usage (in susceptible women) are those of venous thromboembolism, acute myocardial infarction and ischaemic stroke. It is now well accepted that <50 µg oestrogen COCs carry a lower risk for an arterial thrombotic event, the AMI risk being concentrated in smokers. This risk is absent in non-smoking pill users under 35. Box 6.3 lists the adverse effects of smoking on arterial disease. The risks appear to be related to current use only (no ex-use effect), but are not eliminated by the lower doses of oestrogen (see the earlier section on Metabolic adverse events). Four large epidemiological studies looking at VTE and AMI associated with COC use were published at the end of 1995 and led to a pill scare in some European countries, with women precipitately stopping their pills, partly due to the sensationalistic media coverage of the reports. These reports showed a differential in VTE risk, with COCs containing gestodene (GSD) and desogestrel (DSG) having a higher VTE risk than those containing levonorgestrel. It is possible that this differential is at least partly due to prescribing bias, healthy user effects and other epidemiologic confounders, as pills containing GSD and DSG were perceived as being safer and were consequently prescribed for women with potential risk factors for VTE. However, one study [14] showed that AMI appeared to occur less often in the gestodene and desogestrel group than in the levonorgestrel group.

6

Combined oral
contraceptives:
metabolic
effects and
practical
prescribing

Box 6.3   Smoking and COCs

- Smoking is an established risk factor for coronary artery disease and ischaemic stroke.
- Smoking and the COC have a synergistic effect on the risk of coronary artery disease and ischaemic stroke; this risk becomes unacceptable from 35 years onwards.
- Women over 35 who smoke are at significant risk of coronary artery disease and ischaemic stroke. They should avoid COCs.
- Women who stop smoking can be considered 'non-smokers' 1–2 years after discontinuation.
- Users of nicotine patches should be classified as 'smokers'.
- Smoking raises plasma fibrinogen levels and impairs endothelial nitric oxide synthesis (causing vasoconstriction).
- Nicotine and carbon monoxide induce arterial endothelial damage, cause platelet aggregation and activation, increase catecholamine release, decrease HDL, increase LDL, decrease oestradiol plasma levels and increase the vasoconstrictor endothelin 1 levels.
- Nicotine can acutely raise blood pressure.
- Smokers show increased thromboxane A_2 consistent with increased platelet activity.
- Smokers attain their menopause 2 years earlier through a dose-related effect on oestradiol levels (reduced) and possible direct toxic effect on oocytes.
- Reduced oestradiol levels are seen because of a smoking-induced rise in sex hormone binding globulin and increased 2-hydroxylation of oestradiol to the less potent 2-hydroxyoestradiol.
- There is no evidence that smoking increases the risk of VTE.

Hypertension

The COC can influence blood pressure via its effects on the renin–angiotensin system. Renin substrate (plasma angio-tensinogen) tends to rise in COC users. In addition, there is some increase in cardiac output in some COC users. COC users should expect a 2–3 mmHg rise in their systolic and diastolic blood pressures. The high-dose pills of the 1960s and 1970s were associated with hypertension in 5% of users. Lower-dose pills are less likely to have this impact, but may still cause an increase in blood pressure from the user's baseline reading. Blood pressure returns to baseline after discontinuation, although this may take 3–6 months. As hypertension is an important risk factor for stroke and coronary artery disease, it is vital that the baseline blood pressure is checked in any prospective pill user and that blood pressure is monitored regularly (at least every 6 months), especially since an idiosyncratic iatrogenic hypertensive event may still be a complication of a low-dose pill. Research on the use of 'selective' progestogens with anti-mineralocorticoid action may provide a pill suitable for 'borderline' hypertensives.

Breast cancer

In 1988 the Royal College of General Practitioners' Study suggested that COC usage may accelerate the clinical presentation of breast carcinoma in predisposed at-risk subjects, especially in the young nulliparous woman. Also, women delaying their first full-term pregnancy put themselves at higher risk of breast cancer [29]. A more recent collaborative worldwide study identified current users of COCs as being at greatest risk, but the risk declines after pill discontinuation (Table 6.6). The risks are not associated with the duration of usage, the dosage or type of hormone within the COC, parity, ethnicity or being a woman in the developing world, and there is no synergism with other risk factors for breast cancer (e.g. family history). A reassuring finding in the collaborative study was that breast cancer diagnosed in women who have used COCs is clinically less advanced than in those who have never used the pill and is less likely to have spread beyond the breast. The possibility of the identification of an at-risk individual in due course would enable selective prescription and avoid exposure of the at-risk population. Age is a risk factor for breast cancer (Table 6.7)

Cervical cancer

The evidence of a moderately increased risk of cervical intraepithelial neoplasia may be related to the increased frequency of cervical smears which are taken during COC usage, or may reflect the sexual behaviour or poor use of barrier contraception in COC users. COC-associated ectropion

Table 6.6   Relative risk of breast cancer related to COC usage

COC usage	Relative risk	Comments
Current users	1.24	1.59 for starters <20 years old
1–4 years after stopping	1.16	1.49 for starters <20 years old
5–9 years after stopping	1.07	
10+ years after stopping	1.01	

Adapted from Collaborative Group on Hormonal Factors in Breast Cancer (Beral V). Breast cancer and hormonal contraceptives: collaborative reanalysis of individual data on 53, 297 women with breast cancer and 100, 239 women without breast cancer from 54 epidemiological studies. *Lancet* 1996, 347: 1713–1727.

Table 6.7 Cumulative risk of breast cancer in women who used the pill for 5 years and were followed up for 10 years after stopping, compared with non-users (number of cases per 10 000 women)

Age while using the pill (years)	15–20	20–25	25–30	30–35	35–40	40–45
Age at end of follow-up (years)	30	35	40	45	50	55
Breast cancer risk (number of cases)	4.0	16.0[a]	44.0	100.0	160.0	230.0
Never-users	4.5	17.5[b]	49.0	110.0	180.0	260.0
Number of extra cases of breast cancer	0.5	1.5[c]	5.0	10.0	20.0	30.0

[a]6.0 in developing countries.
[b]6.5 in developing countries.
[c]0.5 in developing countries.
Adapted from Statement on Hormonal Contraceptives and Breast Cancer Faculty of Family Planning and Reproductive Healthcare. 1996, London.

and reserve cell hyperplasia may increase the 'vulnerability' of the cervix to oncogenes. There is also evidence to suggest an interaction between human papilloma virus (HPV) infection and COC usage [31]. Ross reported a significant 70% higher risk of genital warts in COC users [32]. Therefore, screening for intraepithelial abnormalities and HPV infection to identify those at risk is to be encouraged. Adenocarcinomas of the cervix are less likely to be identified with cytological screening, but fortunately are relatively rare. There may also be an increased incidence of such tumours in COC users [33].

Fertility and pregnancy

The many gynaecologically protective effects of COCs work towards enhancing fertility and preventing primary subfertility. Fertility drops with increasing age and women who delay their attempt at a first pregnancy beyond age 30 may experience some delay. 'Post-pill amenorrhoea' affects under 1% of pill users and is no different in causation to spontaneous secondary amenorrhoea (e.g. weight related, polycystic ovarian syndrome, etc.). Pituitary microadenomas do not seem to grow with the use of low-dose COCs. Exposure to COCs in the cycle of conception and early

pregnancy is associated with an excess risk of congenital defects of 1/1000 over the accepted risk of 20/1000 in the general population. The literature is inconsistent regarding the type of abnormalities associated with the pill used. There is no increase in miscarriage rates in pill users in future pregnancies.

Guidelines for choice of COC formulation and selection of users

Identification of the 'at-risk' subject

Before prescribing any COC, there should be a full assessment

of the potential user by a trained medical officer. A full personal history should be taken from the woman, including any intercurrent illness or medication, any gynaecological problems and, in particular, any history suggestive of venous thromboembolism or similar in a first-degree relative. If there are any factors in the history suggesting a thrombophilic tendency, then the possibility of thrombophilia screening should be considered. A full clinical examination is desirable. Measurement of the blood pressure is mandatory. Cervical cytological screening should be performed if indicated following local policies. The subject may

Table 6.8 WHO classification of potential contraceptive use – for COCs

Classification	COC usage	Examples of situation
1	Yes	No restriction for the use of COCs – normal, healthy, menstruating women, those with a dysfunctional menstrual cycle (e.g. PCOS) or where enhancement of endocrine function is desirable
2	Yes – generally, with caution	Conditions where the advantages of COC generally outweigh the theoretical or proven risks – careful follow-up is required
3	Use of COC not usually recommended – consider alternative contraceptive methods	Conditions where the theoretical or proven risks usually outweigh the advantages of COCs – careful clinical judgement is required, taking into account the severity of the condition and the availability, practicality and acceptability of an alternative method
4	No – do not use COCs	Conditions which represent an unacceptable health risk if COC is used

PCOS = polycystic ovarian syndrome.

Table 6.9 Conditions present in the subject and the consequential classification according to the above WHO classification (NB. A dynamic situation, which should be continually reassessed)

WHO category			
1	2	3	4
<40 years age	≥40 years age	Light smoking and ≥35 years	Heavy smoker (>20 cigarettes/day) ≥35 years
Obesity (with no other risk factors)	Smoking and age <35 years	Unexplained vaginal bleeding	Vascular disease
Previous PET or gestational diabetes		Family history of VTE	History of DVT or PE
Varicose veins			Current DVT or PE
Minor surgery without immobilization	Major surgery without prolonged immobilization		Major surgery with prolonged immobilization (anticoagulate in emergency)
Headaches – mild	Superficial thrombophlebitis		Active viral hepatitis
Benign breast disease		Cirrhosis – mild	Severe cirrhosis
Family history of breast carcinoma	Post cholecystectomy	Current gallbladder disease	Liver tumours – benign or malignant
Endometrial/ovarian carcinoma	History of cholestasis	Past COC cholestasis	
Cervical ectopy			
PID – current/past	Valvular heart disease (uncomplicated)		Complicated valvular heart disease (especially with pulmonary hypertension or AF)
HIV/AIDS			
Fibroids			
Previous ectopic pregnancy	Headaches (including migraine with no focal neurological symptoms)		Headache (including migraine) with focal neurological symptoms (with aura)
Trophoblastic disease[a]			
Thyroid disease	Hyperlipidaemias	Hyperlipidaemias	IHD
Epilepsy			Stroke
Endometriosis	Hypertension (140–159/90–99 mmHg)	History of essential hypertension 160–179/100–109 mmHg	Hypertension >180 systolic and >110 mmHg diastolic
Benign ovarian tumour			
Dysmenorrhoea			
Iron deficiency anaemia	Diabetes (NIDDM or IDDM) with no vascular disease		Diabetes with nephropathy ± retinopathy ± neuropathy DM + vascular disease or diabetes over 20 years' duration
Malaria			
TB	Pituitary microadenoma[b]		
Schistosomiasis	Breast disease – undiagnosed mass	Past history of breast carcinoma but no evidence of current disease for 5 years	Current breast carcinoma
Sickle cell trait	CIN	Microinvasive carcinoma of cervix	Porphyria[b]
	Cervical cancer awaiting treatment	Microinvasive carcinoma of cervix	Pemphigoid gestationis[b]
	Thalassaemia	Breast feeding 6 weeks to 6 months post-partum	Haemolytic uraemic syndrome[b]
		Sickle cell disease	
	Breast feeding over 6 months post-partum		Pregnancy
			Breast feeding <6 weeks post-partum

[a]Would be in category 3 in the UK (authors' addition); [b]authors' additions.
PET = pre-eclamptic toxaemia; VTE = venous thromboembolism; PE = pulmonary embolism; DVT = deep vein thrombosis;
PID = pelvic inflammatory disease; AF = atrial fibrillation; IHD = ischaemic heart disease; NIDDM = non-insulin dependent diabetes mellitus;
IDDM = insulin dependent diabetes mellitus; DM = diabetes mellitus; TB = tuberculosis; CIN = cervical intraepithelial neoplasia.

then be classified according to the WHO classification of medical eligibility criteria for contraceptive use classes 1 to 4 (Tables 6.8 and 6.9).

Low-risk women

Those women who fall into WHO category 1 are suitable for any low-dose COC. This group includes all normal, healthy, non-smoking women with a normal menstrual cycle, as well as women with polycystic ovarian syndrome (PCOS). Also included are those subjects who again are healthy, but who may gain other significant health benefits from COCs other than contraception and protection against the aforementioned diseases, such as those with acne or hirsutism (COCs containing desogestrel or cyproterone acetate may be more suitable). Women without 'androgenic predisposition' could well be at an added advantage using LNG/NET pills with their perceived lesser risk of venous thromboembolism. Obesity, without any other identifiable conditions which may place a subject in an 'at-risk' group, is not an absolute contraindication to COC usage, unless the body mass index is over 40.

'At-risk' women

These are the women who fall into WHO categories 2 and 3. Each case has to be assessed individually and with great care by the prescribing physician. In certain situations, further screening tests may be useful to assess the degree of risk in addition to the basic history and examination. For instance, a family history suggestive of thrombophilia may prompt screening for such abnormalities [34]. Those women with risk factors for VTE who choose the COC after counselling should be prescribed a LNG/NET preparation (Table 6.10). Alternative contraceptive methods should be considered and discussed with the subject as to their potential acceptability.

Subject information, follow-up monitoring and troubleshooting

Contraceptive service providers should be aware of guidelines for screening clients for the conditions in which the use of COCs would carry unacceptable health risks. Likewise, the clients themselves should be provided with adequate information so that they may make an informed, voluntary choice of a contraceptive method. This should include information regarding the efficacy of the various COCs and their correct usage, especially with regard to instructions for missed pills, switching pills and potential side effects. Both the health risks and benefits of the COCs should be given, as well as any signs or symptoms which would necessitate a return to the clinic (Box 6.4). As with any contraceptive, advice regarding sexually transmitted diseases should be given and information on the return to fertility after pill discontinuation.

All COC users should be instructed at the initiation of treatment concerning when they should reattend for review, usually after the first 2–3 months of use. At this visit, side effects are reviewed and careful attention paid to any changes in the medical history, especially with regard to any signs or symptoms which may be suggestive of the development of a significant health risk. Adherence should be assessed and support

Table 6.10 Choice of progestogen within COC

Progestogen	Attributes	Problems
Norethisterone (NET)	Longstanding usage – safe Risk of VTE ×2	Androgenic effects in high doses (seborrhoea, acne), fluid retention, premenstrual syndrome
Levonorgestrel (LNG)	Longstanding usage – safe Risk of VTE ×2	Androgenic in high doses
Newer gonanes (gestodene, desogestrel)	More potent – lower doses required AMI risk not raised	Greater risk of thromboembolism than with LNG/NET (RR ×3–4)
Norgestimate	Highly selective	To be identified as relatively new
Cyproterone acetate	Anti-androgenic – useful in PCOS, hirsutism, acne, etc.	Fluid retention
Dienogest	Anti-androgenic as above	Fluid retention
Drospirenone [34] (not yet marketed)	Antimineralocorticoid – useful in those with tendency for weight gain ± hypertension. Slightly anti-androgenic	Yet to be identified

VTE = venous thromboembolism; PMS = premenstrual syndrome; AMI = acute myocardial infarction; PCOS = polycystic ovary syndrome.

6

Combined oral
contraceptives:
metabolic
effects and
practical
prescribing

Box 6.4   COC users should seek medical advice if they develop the following symptoms

M   Migraine (especially with aura/focal neurological deficit)
U   Unilateral pain or swelling in a lower limb
C   Chest pain or haemoptysis

maintained, encouraging continuation of use despite nuisance side effects, which will usually regress within the first 6 months of usage. The pattern of bleeding should be noted and any cycle irregularities assessed: they may well settle spontaneously with perseverance. The patient should be examined, paying particular regard to weight and blood pressure. Details of any missed pills should be discussed and instructions given for switching to an alternative preparation should be provided as necessary. Further monitoring visits should occur on a 6-monthly basis and the above details reviewed again (Table 6.11).

Future prospects and developments

'Fine tuning' of COCs

The ongoing research in the field of COCs aims to provide preparations with fewer adverse effects, reduced nuisance side effects and better cycle control. This should allow for tailoring of the COC to the user's individual needs. For instance, the development of progestogens with antimineralocorticoid activity will provide a useful alternative for those women with a predisposition to hypertension and weight gain [35]. Experimentation into COCs with oestrogen–priming regimens during the traditional pill-free phase, or shortening of this phase, may help reduce the follicular activity which can occur at this time in the cycle,

Table 6.11   COC troubleshooting – nuisance side effects and pill-taking irregularities

Problem	Action
Persistent early breakthrough bleeding/spotting (lasting > 6 months)	Consider 1. COC with increased progestogen content; if it fails, consider COC with increased ethinyloestradiol content 2. Switch to a different progestogen with high progesterone receptor affinity 3. Exclude organic and user cause – see Box 6.2 4. Stop smoking
Persistent late breakthrough bleeding/spotting (lasting > 6 months)	1. Consider triphasic products 2. Stop smoking
Absent withdrawal bleed	1. Exclude pregnancy 2. Switch to an oestrogen-dominant pill
Weight gain	Document and exclude fluid retention, recommend dietary modification, consider lower dose pill. Rarely may require change of method
PMS, fluid retention, bloatedness	Change to preparation containing gestodene, desogestrel or norgestimate
Depression	1. Exclude other causes 2. Consider vitamin B_6
Androgenic side effects, e.g. acne	COC containing cyproterone acetate/desogestrel – see section on Acne
Loss of libido	COC not a recognized cause; use an oestrogen-dominant pill
Persistent mild headaches, nausea, breast tenderness	Consider COC with reduced ethinyloestradiol content
Headaches in withdrawal phase	Consider prolonged regimens, e.g. 9 weeks continuous use with 1 week withdrawal, or add natural oestrogen in pill-free week
Missed pill, tablet taken <12 h late	No further action required, continue COC administration as normal
Missed pill, tablet taken >12 h late	*The '7 day rule'[a]* • If one pill is forgotten for >12 h • If vomiting or diarrhoea >12 h • If taking other interacting drugs User should continue to take tablets as usual and additional contraceptive precautions must be taken for the next 7 days *But*, if these 7 days run beyond the end of the current 21-day pack, the next pack must be started as soon as the current one is finished (i.e. no 'pill-free phase'; this usually defers bleed until end of second pack).
Switching from one COC to another	Commence first tablet of new pack on day after the last pill of previous cycle, i.e. omit pill-free phase

PMS = premenstrual syndrome.
[a]Applies to monophasic 21-day preparations.

hence improving efficacy at the same time as potentially reducing breakthrough bleeding and withdrawal migraines. Oestradiol may be used instead of ethinyloestradiol in COCs, although preliminary studies have shown unacceptable bleeding patterns. A formulation containing oestradiol with low doses of ethinyloestradiol (10 μg) with dienogest seems to overcome these problems. Other possibilities include the antiprogestogens, which have been shown to be well tolerated and effective as postcoital contraceptives.

Tips for safe practice

Criteria for safe practice – checklist

- Careful history and examination (screening tests if indicated).
- Selection of low-risk acceptors – WHO category 1 – discuss COC choice.
- Careful monitoring of acceptors with potential risk factors – WHO category 2.
- Higher-risk group – WHO category 3 – seek alternative method of contraception.
- High risk – WHO category 4 – COC contraindicated.
- Continuing reassessment of client throughout COC use according to WHO categories.

Enhancement of continuation of use

- Minimize/eliminate nuisance side effects.
- Lowest effective dose.
- Selective progestogens are more acceptable to some users.
- Correlation of metabolic disturbance.
- Androgenic manifestations – change to anti-androgenic preparation.
- Other adverse effects – explore alternative progestogens and other formulations.
- Cardiovascular effects, e.g. hypertension – monitor, consider alternatives.

References

1. Inman WHW, Vessey PH, Westerholm B, Engelund A. Thromboembolic disease and the steroidal content of oral contraceptives. A report to the committee of safety of drugs. *Br Med J* 1970;2:203–9.

2. Bye P, Elstein M. A clinical assessment of a low-oestrogen combined oral contraceptive. *Br Med J* 1973;2:203–9.

3. Meade TW, Greenberg G, Thompson SG. Progestogens and cardiovascular reactions associated with oral contraceptives and a comparison of the safety of 50 and 30 μg oestrogen preparations. *Br Med J* 1980;280:1157–61.

4. Elstein M. Consensus paper: Low dose contraceptive formulations: is further reduction in steroid dosage justified? *Adv Contracept* 1994;10:1–4.

5. Fruzzetti F, Ricci C, Fioretti P. Haemostasis profile in smoking and non-smoking women taking low-dose oral contraceptives. *Contraception* 1994;49:579–2.

6. Kay CR. Progestogens and arterial disease – evidence from the Royal College of General Practitioners' Study. *Am J Obstet Gynecol* 1982;142:762–5.

7. Dusterberg B, Beier S, Schneider WHF, Spona J. Pharmacological features of gestodene in laboratory animals and man. In: Gestodene, a new direction in oral contraception, Vol. 1. Carnforth, Parthenon, UK: 1988:13–30.

8. Phillips A, Demarest K, Hahn DW et al. Progestational and androgenic receptor binding affinities and in vivo activities of norgestimate and other progestins. *Contraception* 1989;41:399–410.

9. Collins DC. Sex hormone receptor binding, progestin selectivity, and the new oral contraceptives. *Am J Obstet Gynecol* 170:1508–13.

10. Lachnit-Fixson U, Aydinlik S, Lehnert J. Clinical comparison between a monophasic preparation and a triphasic preparation, In: Advances in fertility, control and treatment of sterility. Lancaster: MTP Press, 1984:71–9.

11. Petersen KR, Skouby SO, Pedersen RG. Desogestrel and gestodene in oral contraceptives: 12 months' assessment of carbohydrate and lipoprotein metabolism. *Obstet Gynecol* 1991;78:666–72.

12. Kaffrissen ME, Corson SL. Comparative review of third generation progestins. *Int J Fertil* 1992;37(suppl. 2):104–15.

13. Meade TW. Risks and mechanisms of cardiovascular events in users of oral contraceptives. *Am J Obstet Gynecol* 1988;158:1646–52.

14. Engel HJ. Angiographic findings after myocardial infarctions in young women: role of oral contraceptives. *Adv Contracept* 1991;7 (suppl 3):235–243.

15. Adams MR, Wagner JD, Washburn SA and Clarkson TB. The effects of contraceptive steroids on atherosclerosis: experimental evidence. *Adv Contracept* 1991;7(suppl 3):227–234.

16. Lewis MA, Spitzer WO, Heinemann LAJ, MacRae KD, Bruppacher R, Thorogood M. on behalf of the Transnational Research Group on Oral Contraceptives and the Health of Young Women. Third generation oral contraceptives and risk of myocardial infarction:

6

Combined oral
contraceptives:
metabolic
effects and
practical
prescribing

an international case-control study. *Br Med J* 1996;312:88–90.

17. Winkler UH, Koslowski S, Oberhoff C, Schindler EM, Schindler AE. Changes in the dynamic equilibrium of hemostasis associated with the use of low-dose oral contraceptives: a controlled study of cyproterone acetate containing oral contraceptives combined with either 35 or 50 µg ethinyl estradiol. *Adv Contracept* 1991;7(suppl 3):273–284.

18. Jespersen J. Plasma resistance to activated protein C: an important link between venous thromboembolism and combined oral contraceptives – a short review. *Eur J Contracept Reproduct Health Care* 1996;1:3–11.

19. Vandenbroucke JP, Koster T, Briet E, et al. increased risk of venous thrombosis in oral contraceptive users who are carriers of factor V Leiden mutation. *Lancet* 1994; 344:1453–7.

20. Rabe Th, Runnebaum B. Update on oral contraception. *Eur J Obstet Gynecol Reproduct Biol* 1993;49:10–12.

21. Lidegaard O, Milson I. Oral contraceptives and thrombotic diseases: impact of new epidemiological studies. *Contraception* 1996;53:135–139.

22. Petersen KR, Skouby SO, Jespersen J. Contraception guidance in women with pre-existing disturbances in carbohydrate metabolism. *Eur J Contracept Reproduct Health Care* 1996;1:53–9.

23. Brill K, Muller C, Schnitker J, Albring M. The influence of different modern low-dose oral contraceptives on intemenstrual bleeding. *Adv Contracept* 1991;7(suppl 2):51–61.

24. Rosenberg MJ, Long SC. Oral contraceptives and cycle control: a critical review of the literature. *Adv Contracept* 1992;8(suppl 1):35–45.

25. Serfaty D. Medical aspects of oral contraceptive discontinuation. *Adv Contracept* 1992;8(Suppl 1):21–33.

26. Oddens BJ, Visser APh, Vemer UM, Everaerd WThAM, Lehert Ph. Contraceptive use and attitudes in Great Britain. *Contraception* 1994;49:73–86.

27. Thorneycroft IH. Non-contraceptive benefits of modern low-dose oral contraceptives. *Adv Contracept* 1992;8 Suppl 1:5–12.

28. Thorogood M, Villard-Mackintosh L. Combined oral contraceptives: risks and benefits. *Br Med Bull* 1993;49:124–139.

29. Kay CR, Hannaford PC. Breast cancer and the pill – a further report from the Royal College of General Practitioners' Oral Contraception Study. *Br J Cancer* 1988;58:675–80.

30. Collaborative Group on Hormonal Factors in Breast Cancer (Beral V). Breast cancer and hormonal contraceptives: collaborative reanalysis of individual data on 53,297 women with breast cancer and 100 239 women without breast cancer from 54 epidemiological studies. *Lancet* 1996; 347:1713–1727.

31. Irwin KL. The association between oral contraceptive use and neoplasia of the cervix, vagina and vulva. In: Hannaford P, Webb A (eds) Evidence-guided prescribing of oral contraceptives. Carnforth, UK: Parthenon, 1996:Ch. 16.

32. Ross JDC. Is oral contraception associated with genital warts? *Genitourinary Med* 1996; 72:330–333.

33. Fitzgerald C, Elstein M. The oral contraceptive pill and cervical neoplasia. *Br J Fam Plann* 1995;20:79–81.

34. Machin SJ, Mackie LJ, Guillebaud J. Factor V Leiden mutation, venous thromboembolism and oral contraceptive usage. *Br J Fam Plann* 1995;21:13–14.

35. Foidart JM, Dombrowicz N, Heithecker A, Oelkers W. Clinical tolerance and impacts on blood pressure, the renin–aldosterone system, glucose and lipid metabolism of a new oral contraceptive containing an anti-mineralocorticoid progestogen drospirenone. *Int J Gynecol Obstet* 1994;46(suppl 3):11.

Progestin-only contraception

Laura MacIsaac MD
Philip Darney MD MSc

Progestin-only methods in general

Definition, mechanism, efficacy

Progestin-only methods, particularly the sustained-release systems such as subdermal implants, provide promising advances in contraceptive technology. These methods do not employ oestrogen, thereby avoiding oestrogen-associated health risks and side effects. This chapter will outline the major progestin-only systems in use and under investigation: the progestin-only 'minipill', injectable contraception, implant systems and vaginal rings. Definitions, mechanisms, efficacy rates, advantages, disadvantages and tips for practice – in general and for each method – will be presented. Lastly, a discussion of future areas of research is provided.

Progestin-only contraceptives rely, at the lower doses provided by pills and implants, on the sensitivity of cervical mucus glands to small changes in serum progestin concentration. Sustained levels, even when too low to inhibit follicular growth, make cervical mucus so viscous that sperm cannot penetrate it. In addition, the absence, in many users, of cyclic estrogen, blocks the normal maturation of the endometrium, causing the endometrium to involute and become unfavourable for implantation. At higher doses, such as after Depo-Provera, or in the first months after implant insertion, gonadotrophins are inhibited, ovarian follicles do not develop and ovulation is inhibited. The combination of a consistently viscous cervical mucus, atrophic endometrium and variable dose-dependent inhibition of ovulation makes progestin-only methods highly effective. Progestins also affect fallopian tube motility and ciliation.

For the sustained release and depot systems that minimize user requirements, the efficacy rates of progestin-only methods are comparable to sterilization. Women on progestin-only pills who take their pills every day at the same time have similar failure rates to women on combined oral contraceptives (Table 7.1).

Usage of progestin-only methods

Injectable progestins have been used by over 14 million women worldwide. Depo-Provera constitutes the bulk of this experience, but Noristerat is used by 1–2 million women worldwide. Progestin-only pills are poorly used, with a worldwide use of under 1 million. In the UK, under 10% of hormonal contraceptive users take the progestin-only pill; in the USA, this is likely to be under 1%.

Advantages of progestin-only contraception

There are two main advantages of the progestin-only methods: the absence of oestrogen and, depending on the delivery system, low pregnancy rates. A progestin-only method is ideal for women who have contraindications to the use of oestrogen-containing oral contraceptives, such as patients with systemic lupus erythematosus (SLE), hypercoagulability or history of thromboembolism, and women over 35 years who smoke, have diabetes or other cardiovascular risk factors (Box 7.1). Progestin-only contraception (POC) has not been associated with clinically significant changes in carbohydrate or lipid metabolism, coagulation, liver or kidney function, or immunoglobulin levels. Depo-Provera can transiently lower high-density lipoprotein (HDL), and elevate LDL and total cholesterol immediately after injection; the clinical significance of these changes is unclear. The sustained-release implants and the injectables both offer theoretical effectiveness nearly equal to use effectiveness – when pregnancy poses a health hazard, or when elective abortion is unacceptable, their high use efficacy is important. In addition, because there is no increased risk of thromboembolism, the minipill, injectables and implants can all be used postpartum and can enhance breastfeeding [1] (see Table 7.1 and Box 7.1).

Disadvantages of progestin-only contraception

There are no life-threatening side effects of progestin-only methods; however, they share disadvantages which can be reasons for patient dissatisfaction (Table 7.2) but which can often be easily treated. Patient education and reassurance are essential for managing many of the side effects and preventing early discontinuation.

STD prevention

Every prospective user must know that the progestin-only methods do not offer the protection against sexually transmitted disease (STD), including HIV, that are provided by condoms and other barrier methods.

Irregular bleeding

Owing to their unpredictable effect on ovulation, the progestin-only methods can cause irregular bleeding. Over the first year of use, up to 80% of Norplant users, 50–70% of Depo-Provera users and 40% of minipill users have abnormal bleeding patterns. This problem discourages some women, but despite the increased number of days of bleeding in the first year, hemoglobin levels rise as a result of overall less blood loss. If, after reassurance, the irregular bleeding is still intolerable, there are two treatments to offer: hormonal therapy or a trial of non-steroidal anti-inflammatory agents. The more effective treatment is hormonal [2]. A short course of oral estrogen: conjugated estrogens (1.25 mg) or estradiol (2 mg) is administered daily for 7 days (some recommend up to 21 days). Low-dose oral contraceptives (OCs) given from 14 to 21 days are an alternative. In one study, a combined levonorgestrel (250 μg) and ethinylestradiol

---

Box 7.1 Indications for progestin-only contraception

Contraindications to oestrogen
- previous venous thromboembolism
- conditions aggravated by oestrogen (e.g. systemic lupus erythematosus)
- risk factors for venous thrombosis (e.g. severe obesity)

Risk factors for arterial disease
- women over 35 years who smoke
- hypertension
- diabetes mellitus
- history of migraine headache with aura or severe migraine

Non-compliance with oral hormonal contraception

Breastfeeding
- injectable progestins enhance milk volume and content [1]. Other POCs have no effect on milk volume or content

---

Table 7.1 Progestin-only contraception

System	Progestin	Dose	Efficacy – ideal use failure (pregnancies per 100 woman-years)	Efficacy – typical-use failure (pregnancies per 100 woman-years)
Progestin-only pill (POP)/minipill, e.g. Micronor	Norethindrone (norethisterone)	0.350 mg	0.3	5
Injectable progestins, e.g. Depo-Provera	Medroxy-progesterone acetate	150 mg (3 months)	0.3	0.3–1
Subdermal implants, e.g. Norplant[a]	Levonorgestrel	80 μg/24 h	0.2	1.1
Vaginal rings	Levonorgestrel	20 μg/24 h	3.5	Not available

[a]5-year cumulative pregnancy rate 3.9/100 woman-years.
By comparison the ideal-use failure rate for the combined oral contraceptive pill is 0.2/100 woman-years and the typical-use failure rate is 3/100 woman-years.

Table 7.2 Advantages and disadvantages of Progestin-only contraceptives (POPs)

	POP	DMPA	Noristerat[a]	Norplant	Vaginal rings
User compliance required	Yes +++	Minimal	Minimal	Negligible	Moderate
Lipid and carbohydrate metabolism	No clinically significant effects	HDL reduced, LDL increased in long-term users Increases glucose intolerance and insulin levels within normal range[b]	Less effect on lipids than DMPA Greater effect on carbohydrate metabolism	No clinically significant changes Further studies required	No clinically significant changes Further studies required
Haemostasis	No effect	No clinically significant effects	No clinically significant effects	No clinically significant effects	No clinically significant effects
Return of fertility	Immediate	Delayed for up to 18 months from last injection	Return of fertility faster than DMPA	Immediate	Immediate
Reduced efficacy with liver-enzyme inducers	Yes – alternatives advised	No – but reduce injection interval to 10 weeks	Yes – advise backup method	Yes – recommend alternative or backup method up to 2 months after stopping the liver-enzyme inducer	Data limited Advise backup method
Effect on breast feeding	None	Increased volume	Less excreted in milk than DMPA	No effect	No data
Cancer risk	No increase or decrease – likely to be neutral	80% reduction in endometrial cancer No overall increase in breast or cervical cancer Slight increase in risk of breast cancer in recent users (RR = 1.21)	No data	No data	No data
Cycle pattern	40% have irregular bleeding 10% experience amenorrhoea	50% amenorrhoeic at 1 year (33% at 6 months) Irregular bleeding in first 3–6 months in 50–70% of users	Less cycle disruption than DMPA Amenorrhoea 14% at 6 months	Irregular bleeding in up to 86% users Type of bleeding cannot be predicted and may vary with time	As for POP
Progestogenic side effects	Limited data About 20% of users affected Mastalgia is the commonest followed by headache and bloating	5–15% of users have at least one side effect	7% of users experience symptoms	5–10% of users experience symptoms Include acne and mastalgia	Data are sparse
Weight gain	Rare	Average gain 1–3 kg in years May be progressive More likely in 'underweight users'	Less likely to cause weight gain than DMPA	Only 1.7% of discontinuations due to weight gain, i.e. very uncommon Responds to dieting	No data
STD protection	None Cervical mucus effect may protect against PID	As for POP	As for POP	As for POP	As for POP
Functional ovarian cysts	30% of users	No increase	No increase	<20% of users	30% of users
First-year continuation	40–50%	50–80%	Similar to DMPA	76–90%	50%

Table 7.2 Continued

	POP	DMPA	Noristerat[a]	Norplant	Vaginal rings
Special advantages/uses	Diabetes Lactation Women over 40 years (high efficacy)	To cover major surgery as replacement for COC Post-vasectomy or risk of teratogenicity Medical disorders such as renal, hepatic and some cardiac diseases Inflammatory bowel disease HIV Epilepsy Menorrhagia, fibroids, endometriosis, dysmenorrhoea Learning difficulty Hemoglobin–opathies Previous ectopic pregnancy	Less likely to cause amenorrhoea or weight gain than DMPA	As an alternative to sterilization in women unsure about the decision	Initiation and discontinuation under woman's control
Special disadvantages/side effects	Reduction in efficacy in women > 70 kg in weight Some cite ectopic pregnancy as a contraindication	Galactorrhoea in some women Inadvertent use in pregnancy may lead to transient clitoral enlargement 1–2% of users may get heavy irregular bleeding Not a first choice for under-16s as best to avoid any effect on bone density		Headaches in 25–50% Infection at site < 1% Extrusion of implant 0.4%	

DMPA = depot medroxyprogesterone acetate; HDL = high-density lipoprotein; LDL = Low-density lipoprotein; STD = sexually transmitted disease; PID = pelvic inflammatory disease.
[a]Noristerat is not marketed in the USA.
[b]The impact of long-term oestrogen deprivation, as seen in some Depo-Provera users, is unknown. Any risk is likely to apply to arterial disease only, but it is reassuring that no significant increase in coronary artery disease has been shown so far.
[c]No verified association has been found between these methods, and venous or arterial disease including hypertension.

(50 μg) pill provided quicker and longer cessation of bleeding in Norplant users seeking treatment for excessive bleeding compared to ethinylestradiol (50 μg) alone or placebo [3]. The difference in mean duration of bleeding and spotting days between the combined pills and estradiol-alone pills was statistically significant. The second approach, a trial of a non-steroidal anti-inflammatory agent, often diminishes flow, but may not stop spotting entirely. A 5-day course of ibuprofen (800 mg three times a day) or ketoprofen (200 mg,

extended release, once a day) is an effective option.

Although many progestin–only methods are highly effective, pregnancy must always be considered in a patient who was having a normal menstrual pattern and suddenly becomes amenorrheic [4].

Weight gain
Some Depo-Provera and Norplant users complain of weight gain, but verification has been inconsistent. Although the androgenic activity of levonorgestrel could explain an

increase in appetite, it is unlikely that the low serum progestin levels in Norplant users have any clinical impact. A total of 75% of Norplant users in the Dominican Republic experiencing a change in weight lost weight, while in San Francisco, two–thirds gained weight. Only 2.1% of Depo-Provera users cite weight gain as their reason for discontinuation [6], yet documentation of weight gain attributable to Depo-Provera is inconsistent [7,8]. Weight change is difficult to evaluate without a review of each patient's diet and exercise habits.

Follicular cysts

The low-dose progestin-only contraceptives, Norplant and the minipill, do not completely inhibit the hypothalamic–pituitary–ovarian axis, allowing some follicle-stimulating hormone (FSH) activity and, therefore, ovarian follicular stimulation. Users of these methods develop more functional ovarian cysts [9]. Most, if not all cysts, regress spontaneously or on discontinuation. Because these are simple, functional cysts, they need not be sonographically or laparoscopically evaluated unless they become large, painful, or fail to regress. Women who have experienced recurrent or painful cysts may be happier with methods that suppress follicular development, such as combined oral contraceptives or Depo-Provera.

Ectopic pregnancy

Progestin-only contraceptives that work primarily at the level of the endometrium and cervical mucus, and not on the hypothalamic–pituitary–ovarian axis (Norplant and the minipill), do not prevent ectopic pregnancy as effectively as they do intrauterine pregnancy. Because ovulation is not consistently inhibited, and factors affecting implantation are altered, the few eggs that are fertilized have a greater likelihood of ectopic implantation than with methods that always suppress ovulation (such as Depo-Provera or combined OCs). About 30% of Norplant pregnancies are ectopic, for example, but the rate (0.13/100 woman-years) is still lower than in women not using contraception at all [10].

Acne

Acne is another side effect reported with progestin-only contraception. The androgenic activity of levonorgestrel in Norplant and some minipills (Ovrette, Microval, Neogest) may decrease the circulating levels of sex hormone binding globulin (SHBG). Free androgen steroid levels (both levonorgestrel and testosterone) consequently increase despite the low dose of progestin. In contrast, the oestrogen in combined OCs increases SHBG, resulting in a decrease in free androgens. Common therapies for acne include dietary change, good skin hygiene with the use of soaps or skin cleansers, and the application of topical antibiotics (e.g. 1% clindamycin solution or gel, or 1% topical erythromycin solution).

Cancer risks

Research on progestin-only systems is reassuring but definite conclusions will have to await larger user samples. Depo-Provera is the most thoroughly studied progestin-only contraceptive. In large (50 times the dose per weight), continuous doses, medroxyprogesterone produces breast tumours in beagle dogs (perhaps because in dogs progestins stimulate growth hormone secretion, known to be a mammotropic agent in dogs). This effect is unique to dogs and has not appeared in women after many years of use. A very large, hospital-based case-control World Health Organization (WHO) study conducted over 9 years in three developing countries indicated that exposure to Depo-Provera is associated with a very slightly increased risk in breast cancer in the first 4 years of use, but there was no evidence for an increased risk with increased duration of use [11]. The results were interpreted to suggest that growth of already existing tumours is enhanced. The number of cases was not large, so the confidence intervals were wide. A pooled analysis of the WHO and other data indicated that the highest risk was in women who had received a single injection [12]. The risk, if real, is very slight, and it is equally possible that studies suggesting increased risk suffer from small numbers of cases and confounding variables. Because recent use seems to be the key factor, it is appropriate to emphasize that these studies did not find evidence for an overall increased risk of breast cancer in Depo-Provera users, and the risk did not increase with duration of use – only recent short term users were at risk. However, clinicians should consider informing patients that Depo-Provera might accelerate the growth of an already-present occult cancer.

Studies looking at associations between Depo-Provera and other cancers have been inconsistent as well. An increased risk of cervical dysplasia cannot be documented even with long-term use [13]. The WHO collaborative study failed to detect any increased risk of invasive squamous cell cancer of the cervix [14]. However, the risk of cervical carcinoma *in situ* was slightly elevated in one case-control study [15]. It is not clear if this is a real finding or a consequence of unrecognized bias or confounding factors. Nevertheless, it is prudent to recommend regular Pap smears in all users of contraception, no matter what their method. Where annual Pap smears are feasible (e.g. in US practice), they should be recommended. In the USA, women at higher risk for cervical cancer, because of their sexual behavior, are advised to have a Pap smear every 6 months.

Depo-Provera is associated with a reduction in the risk of endometrial cancer. One would expect a reduction in ovarian cancer similar to that seen in OC users; however, the WHO study failed to show such a reduction [16].

Bone density

Long-term use of Depo-Provera results in decreased estrogen levels, which could lead to adverse effects on bone density. Initial studies suggested that Depo-Provera users may lose bone density to some degree over years of use [17]; this effect is reversible on discontinuation [18]. Two recent reports of ongoing long-term studies have failed to find changes in bone mineral density in women using Depo-Provera for up to 8 consecutive years [19,20]. Given the evidence to date, the possibility of bone density changes is not a reason to discourage women from choosing or continuing with Depo-Provera.

Individual progestin-only systems

Minipill/progestin-only pill (POP)

The minipill contains a small dose of a progestin and must be taken every day. The low concentration of progestin in the circulation (about 25% of that in combined OCs) is not enough to suppress the hypothalamic–pituitary–ovarian axis consistently: approximately 40% of women will ovulate normally. The contraceptive effect is at the level of the uterus: cervical mucus thickens and becomes impermeable to sperm penetration and the endometrium becomes resistant to implantation. The progestin effect on cervical mucus is very sensitive to serum concentration: it clears after 24 hours of administration. Unless a new pill is taken, sperm penetration returns to normal. *Thus it is imperative that the minipill be taken at the same time every day.*

There are a variety of formulations of minipills available worldwide (Table 7.3); they do not have any clinical differences. Failure rates range from 1.1 to 9.6 per 100 women in the first year of use [21]. The failure rate is higher in younger, more fertile women (3.1 per 100 woman-years) compared with women over 40 (0.3 per 100 woman-years) [22]. In consistent users, the failure rate is similar to that seen with combination oral contraceptives (less than 1 per 100 woman-years) [23,24].

The advantages of the minipill are as follows:

- It is immediately reversible.
- It is suitable for short- or long-term use.
- Its low dose of progestin is excellent for use in breastfeeding women.

The disadvantages of the minipill are:

- the rigidity of the pill-taking schedule
- the increased risk of functional ovarian cysts
- the increased ectopic pregnancy rate over intrauterine pregnancy rate, but decreased ectopic pregnancy rate compared with a woman using no contraception
- the higher failure rates compared with other progestin-only methods
- menstrual irregularities.

Tips for safe practice

The minipill should be started on the first day of menses or immediately postpartum. UK current practice recommends starting within 21 days of delivery. If started on a day other than the first day of menses, a backup method (such as a condom) is necessary for the next 48 hours. If a patient is more than

Table 7.3   Minipills – progestin-only pills (POPs)

Proprietary name	Generic name	Dose in single daily pill
Micronor, Nor-QD, Noriday, Norod	Norethindrone (norethisterone)	0.350 mg
Microval, Microlut, Noregeston, Ovrette	Levonorgestrel	0.030 mg
Neogest	Norgestrel	0.075 mg
Excluton	Lynestrenol	0.500 mg
Femulen	Ethynodial diacetate (pro-drug for NET)	0.500 mg

NET = norethisterone.

3 hours late in taking a pill, or gastrointestinal illness impairs absorption, the late pill should be taken as soon as remembered and the next pill taken at the regular time. A backup method should be used for 48 hours (see also Chapter 2). US current practice recommends that, if two pills are missed in succession, a backup method should be used in place of the minipill for the remainder of that cycle, and a pregnancy test performed if no menses occur in 4–6 weeks.

Careful medication review is mandatory in prospective minipill users, because the minipill may be subject to a first-pass effect in the liver, where a significant proportion of an absorbed steroid may be metabolized. Thus, the circulating steroid level is affected by medications that induce hepatic enzymes, such as rifampin, phenytoin, phenobarbital, carbamazepine and others (Chapter 16). These medications may increase hepatic enzymes sufficiently to decrease the progestin level below that which is required to maintain cervical mucus viscosity. Concomitant use of broad-spectrum antibiotics has a negligible effect on progestin bioavailability as there is little gut recycling of progestins.

Counselling issues

The following points are derived from the revised text for the progestin-only package inserts [25]:

- the necessity of taking pills at the same time each and every day

- the need to use backup methods such as condoms for the next 48 hours whenever a progestin-only oral contraceptive is taken 3 hours or more late

- the potential side effects of progestin-only oral contraceptives, particularly menstrual irregularities

- the need to inform the clinician of prolonged episodes of bleeding, amenorrhea or severe abdominal pain

- the importance of using a barrier method in addition to progestin-only oral contraceptives if a woman is at risk of contracting or transmitting STDs or HIV.

Injectable progestin-only systems

The injectable progestin-only systems rely on microcrystals suspended in an aqueous solution administered as a deep intramuscular injection. The mechanism of action is different from other lower-dose systems because the higher serum progestin concentrations effectively suppress gonadotrophins, inhibiting folliculogenesis, the luteinizing hormone (LH) surge and ovulation. In addition, the complementary effects on cervical mucus and endometrium are maintained. Injectable contraceptives come in a variety of formulations and dosing schedules (Table 7.4).

Depo-Provera

The efficacy of Depo-Provera is equal to sterilization and higher than other reversible hormonal methods [26] with a failure rate of 1 pregnancy per 100 women after 5 years of consistent use [7,27]. Depo-Provera is approved by more than 90 countries and has over 5 million users worldwide [28].

The advantages of injectable progestin-only systems are as follows:

- There are few compliance problems.

- It increases the quantity of breast milk.

- It decreases the risk of endometrial cancer and possibly ovarian cancer (Table 7.5).

- It is non-oral and therefore useful in patients with bowel disease.

Table 7.4   Injectables (progestin alone and combined estrogen–progestin)

Product name	Generic name	Dose (mg)	Frequency of injection
Depo-Provera	Depot-medroxyprogesterone acetate (aqueous solution)	150	Every 12 weeks ± 7 days
Noristerat, Norigest	Norethindrone/ norethisterone enanthate (oily solution)	200	Every 8 weeks ± 5 days
Cyclofem	Medroxyprogesterone acetate and estradiol cypionate	25 5	Every month ± 3 days
Mesigyna	Norethindrone enanthate and oestradiol valerate	50 5	Every month ± 3 days

Table 7.5 DMPA and reproductive tract cancers (based on WHO studies)

Type of cancer	Relative risk	95% confidence interval
Breast	1.21	0.96–1.52 (ns)
Endometrium	0.21	0.06–0.79 (s)
Ovary	1.07	0.6–1.8 (ns)
Cervix	1.11	0.96–1.29 (ns)

DMPA = depot-medroxyprogesterone acetate.
s = significant; ns = not statistically significant.

- It is private – there is no visible evidence of usage.

- It has an improved hematological profile (higher hematocrit, fewer sickling crises) in sickle cell disease patients [29].

- It provides improvement in seizure control in patients with seizure disorders [30].

- It produces less endometriosis, fibroids, PID, PMS, ectopic pregnancy, dysmenorrhoea and menorrhagia.

- It is extremely effective.

- It is independent of coitus.

The disadvantages and side effects of injectable progestin-only systems are:

- regular injections are required

- it cannot be removed

- menstrual irregularities

- a delayed return of fertility, up to 18 months with Depo-Provera

- mood changes: depression can occur in 1.5% of users and accounts for under 1% of discontinuations [31]. (It responds to vitamin B_6 supplementation in some patients. No causal link has been established.)

- weight gain

- vaginal dryness may be a problem

- other nuisance progestogenic side effects, e.g. headaches, dizziness, bloating, occur in 5–15% of users

- a possible increased risk of breast cancer in patients with already existing tumours.

Tips for safe practice

The injection should be given within the first 5 days of the current menstrual cycle (before a dominant follicle emerges), otherwise a backup method is necessary for 2 weeks (1 week in UK). The injection must be given deeply into the gluteal or deltoid muscle by the Z-track technique and not massaged (massaging may shorten the duration of action). Avoid areas at risk for massage by exercise or other daily activities. If overlying fat makes an 'intramuscular' injection into the gluteal muscle difficult, the deltoid should be utilized.

Counselling issues

The following points should be considered:

- injection interval 12 weeks ± 1 week

- discuss side effects, especially menstrual cycle disturbance

- the most important non-menstrual side effect is weight gain

- delay in return to fertility, but no permanent effect on fertility

- there are no mutagenic or teratogenic effects following inadvertent exposure of the embryo or fetus to depot medroxyprogesterone acetate (DMPA).

Implant contraception

Progestin-only implant contraception employs a non-biodegradable sustained-release system using a membrane permeable to steroid molecules (such as silastic tubing, or ethinyl vinyl acetate; EVA) to provide stable circulating levels of synthetic progestin over years of use. These systems provide long-acting, low-dose, reversible progestin-only contraception, lasting up to 7 years for some systems. The Norplant subdermal implant system, the first new contraception approved in the USA since the 1960s, has been the most studied. It has been chosen by over 1 million women in the USA and another 2 million worldwide. Norplant consists of six flexible silastic capsules, 34 mm long and 2.4 mm in diameter, containing 36 mg of crystalline levonorgestrel each; and can provide effective contraception for up to 7 years, although the current licence is for 5 years. Norplant II, with only two slightly longer (44 mm) levonorgestrel (LNG) capsules, releasing 30 µg LNG/day, offers easier insertion and removal, and confers 3–5 years of protection. Other types of implant systems under development are listed in Table 7.6; they use different types

Table 7.6 Subdermal progestin implants

Trade Name	Number of capsules	Type of progestin	Duration of efficacy
Norplant	6 Silastic capsules	Levonorgestrel	5 years
Norplant II	2 Silastic capsules	Levonorgestrel	3 years
Uniplant	1 Silastic capsule	Nomegestrel	1 year
ST-1435	1 Silastic capsule	Nestorone	2 years
Implanon	1 EVA capsule	3-keto-desogestrel	3 years

EVA = ethinyl vinyl acetate.

of progestins and different delivery vehicles (some biodegradable).

The mechanisms of action of subdermal progestin implants are the same as for the other progestin–only methods. The absorbed progestin circulates systemically and acts at the hypothalamus and pituitary at a dose that only sometimes blocks ovulation. During the first 2 years of use only about 10% of women are ovulatory, but by 5 years of use more than 50% are [32]. As with other progestin-only methods, the constant presence of progestin thickens cervical mucus and prevents normal maturation of the endometrium, eventually causing atrophy.

Norplant is a highly effective method of contraception with a pregnancy rate of 0.2 per 100 woman-years in the first year. The duration of protection of the Norplant system is still under investigation, but is at least 5 years. A recent study of the Norplant system in Thai women found a decreasing efficacy rate with increasing duration of use [33]. The cumulative pregnancy rate for the third year was 1.1%, comparable to other studies. However, in year four, the cumulative pregnancy rate was 2.0% and the fifth, 4.2%. The unwanted pregnancies occurred in a subgroup of slightly heavier women, but the difference was

not statistically significant. This study suggests that Norplant efficacy may decline slightly with prolonged use and this decline may be more rapid in heavier women. The weight-related reduction in efficacy is thought to apply to the older, dense Norplant tubes with lower release rates; in 1988, these were replaced with less dense polymer. In contrast to these data, the effectiveness of Norplant through 7 years of use was demonstrated in a large study in China of 3600 women who maintained their Norplant for 7 years [34]. Pregnancy rates increased with weight and decreased with age, but in years 6 and 7 combined, the pregnancy rate was still less than 1 per 100 woman-years in any group. Cumulative life-table pregnancy rates at the end of 5 and 7 years were 1.53% and 2.32%, respectively – nearly as effective as female sterilization. Continuation rates were high in the first year (over 75%) and acceptable at 3 years (50%).

The advantages of Norplant are as follows:

• No compliance is required.

• There is an immediate return of fertility after discontinuation.

• It is extremely effective.

The disadvantages of Norplant are:

• it requires a surgical procedure to insert and remove

• menstrual irregularities

• implants are visible under skin as raised lines, very occasionally, when the arm is extended

• weight gain

• acne and breast tenderness

• functional ovarian cysts

• headache is the second most common side effect, occurring in 25–50% of women and accounting for 3% of removals

• mood changes, depression and anxiety.

Tips for safe practice

Insertion can be performed at any time during the menstrual cycle as long as pregnancy can be ruled out. Protection is immediate if inserted on day 1 of the cycle. Within 24 hours after Norplant insertion, plasma concentrations of levonorgestrel range from 0.4 to 0.5 ng/ml, high enough to prevent conception [35]. If insertion occurs within the first 7 days of menses, a backup method is only needed for the first 24 hours after insertion. UK practice recommends a backup method for 7 days from insertion; 7 days of a backup method are advised if Norplant is placed at other times of the cycle. Norplant can also be inserted immediately postpartum, and should be initiated no later than the third postpartum week, because ovulation can resume early in women who are not fully breastfeeding.

The need for a surgical procedure for insertion and removal is a cause of concern about Norplant and other implants. Implant systems with fewer capsules, or biodegradable capsules, may help to solve this problem, but it will remain a negative aspect for some. The reader is directed to other sources for extensive discussion of insertion and removal techniques and complications [36]. Some helpful tips for insertion and removal techniques are provided.

Insertion tips

- Implants are placed subdermally, just under and parallel to the skin in the inner aspect of the upper arm.

- The proximal tips should be near the insertion site, close together and with their opposite ends far apart in a fan-shaped distribution.

- The patient should be positioned with her arm flexed and externally rotated, with a firm support (such as a phone book) under the arm.

- Strict aseptic technique and adequate local anesthesia are required.

- The trocar should elevate the skin at all times, and should not be forced into the skin. If resistance is met, a slightly different angle to the left or right should be tried, along with rotation of the trocar under the skin.

- If dimpling is seen, the trocar is *in* the skin, not *under* it, and needs to be pulled back and repositioned *slightly* deeper.

- When placing the implant, the obturator should be held completely stationary and the trocar pulled back. Pushing on the obturator while withdrawing the trocar will push the implant in too far,

resulting in poor alignment and difficult removal.

- The tips of each capsule just placed should be protected with a finger when repositioning the trocar/obturator to place the next capsule.

- The trocar should not be removed from the skin until all implants have been placed, otherwise the implants may be placed in different planes, causing difficult removal.

- A pressure dressing should be applied for 24 hours, or longer if a hematoma occurred during insertion.

- The placements of the capsules should be documented immediately after insertion with a drawing in the patient's chart.

- Information about signs of infection (seen in up to 1% of cases) should be given.

Removal tips

There are more than six methods of removing Norplant capsules. The Population Council (Figure 7.1) and pop-out techniques

Fig 7.1 Norplant removal – Population Council technique.
The patient is placed in a supine position with her arm flexed and externally rotated. All six of the implants should be palpated before starting. The skin is cleansed with antiseptic solution and the arm draped with sterile towels.
Wearing sterile gloves, an incision site is selected by pressing down on the proximal ends of the capsules and palpating their distal tips with a finger. The best incision site is right at the distal tips, midway between the most medial and lateral implants. Generally the removal site is a few millimetres higher up on the arm than the insertion site.
The implant that is the most superficial and closest to the incision is removed first. This implant is pushed gently toward the incision with the fingers until the tip is visible and can be grasped with a curved mosquito clamp.
The fibrous sheath covering the implant is dissected away using a finger covered with an opened gauze sponge. Once the sheath is opened and the white tip of the first implant is exposed, it is grasped with the straight clamp. The curved clamp is released and the implant is gently pulled out. The procedure is repeated with the remaining implants. (From Speroff L, Darney P. A Clinical Guide for Contraception (2nd ed.) Baltimore: Williams & Wilkins, 1996;143–163.)

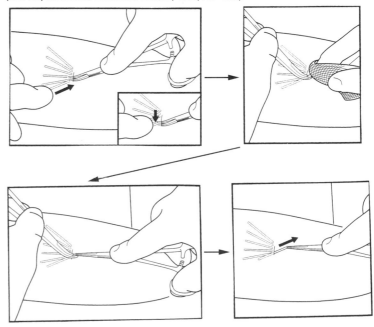

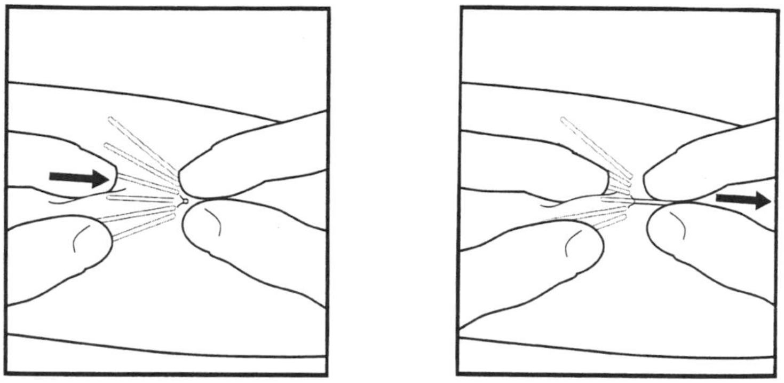

Fig. 7.2 Norplant removal – 'pop-out' technique.
Implants can be removed with less pain and bleeding and through a smaller incision if the use of instruments is avoided. This approach may take longer and may not be successful for implant that are poorly aligned or those placed too deeply.
After preparation, the most centrally located implant is identified. Up to 0.5 ml of buffered lidocaine with epinephrine is injected into the dermis immediately over the most prominent cluster of implant tips. The area should be massaged to disperse the anaesthetic. Pressure is applied with fingers on the proximal (axillary) ends of the implants so that the distal tips press up against the skin. A 3–4 mm incision is made through the skin on to the tips of the implants and the fibrous sheath is incised. As the sheath is opened, the implant comes into view and, with finger pressure on the other end, can be pushed through the incision until it can be grasped and pulled out. (From Speroff L, Darney P. A Clinical Guide for Contraception (2nd ed.) Baltimore: Williams & Wilkins, 1996; 143–163.

(Figure 7.2) employ a 'base of fan' incision, while the U technique (Figure 7.3) employs an incision parallel to and between the third and fourth capsules in the lower third. Removal takes up to 30 minutes with the former and 20 minutes with the latter. Insertion and removal should only be carried out by trained health professionals.

- The patient should be properly positioned with firm arm support, as for insertion.
- All six implants should be palpated before starting.
- If at least some portion of every implant cannot be felt, an imaging study such as sonography or radiography is recommended to localize the non-palpable ones. Compression mammography may also be a useful technique to visualize 'lost' Norplant capsules [37].
- Selection of the incision site is a critical step. The best site is right at the distal (i.e. closest to the elbow) tips, midway between the most medial and lateral implants.
- A removal site may be the same as the insertion site, but generally the optimal site is a few millimeters higher up on the arm.
- No more than 0.5 ml of anesthetic should be injected at the site of the incision; too much will make it difficult to locate the implant tips under the skin. The bulk of the anesthetic is injected across the lower third of the 'fan' in such a way as to 'lift' the implants.

Fig. 7.3 Norplant removal – 'U' technique.
This instrumental technique employs a modified vasectomy forceps and is very useful for removing deeply or asymmetrically placed capsules. It requires a larger incision made in the centre of the field of implants. The vasectomy forceps is advanced under the skin toward the mid-portion of the implants. Those in the centre are grasped first (in the middle of each implant), pulled into the incision and cleaned free of their fibrous sheath as in the Population Council technique. The implant is then extracted, bending it in the middle in a 'U' shape. (From Speroff L, Darney P. A Clinical Guide for Contraception (2nd ed.) Baltimore: Williams & Wilkins, 1996; 143–163.

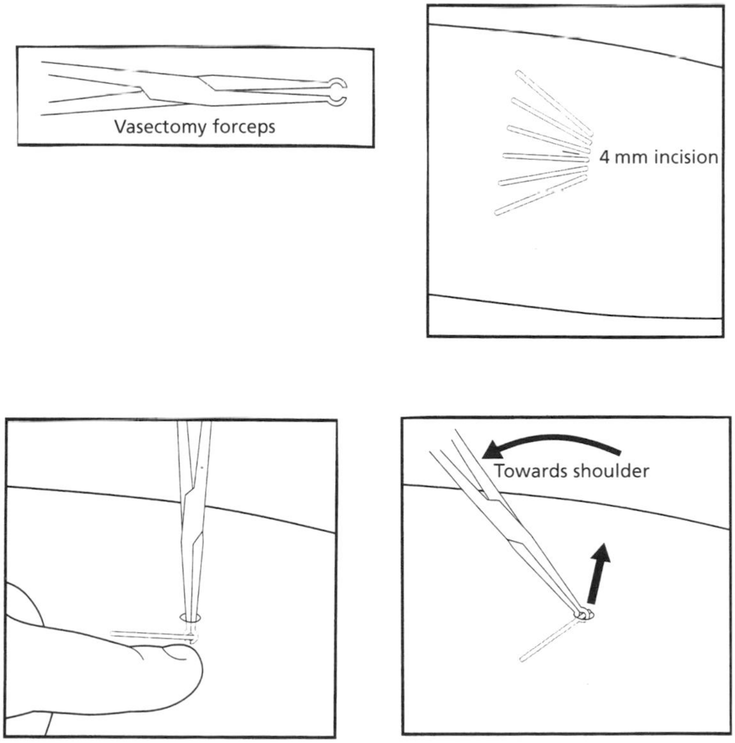

- The implant that is most superficial and closest to the incision should be removed first.

- Use the fingers–only technique [36] to remove as many implants as painlessly as possible.

- When using instruments for removal, we prefer the modified vasectomy clamp (MVC) to the mosquito clamp to grasp the implant.

- Blunt dissection is preferred to release the implant from its fibrous sheath. When incising the fibrous sheath with the scalpel, attempts should be made to cut only at the thick silastic plug at each end. If it is necessary to incise the sheath with the scalpel blade, the cut should be made along, not across, the implant, otherwise the implant itself can be severed and require removal in two portions.

- At the completion of the procedure, the implants should be counted, to ensure that all have been removed, and shown to the patient so that she knows they are all out.

- If removal of some of the implants is difficult, painful or prolonged, the procedure can be interrupted and the patient should return a few weeks later to complete the removal. The remaining implants will be easier to remove after bleeding and swelling have subsided. A new incision can be made closer to the implants that were difficult to remove the first time. Even if some implants remain, the patient should immediately begin to use another method of contraception.

Counselling issues

Frank information about negative factors such as irregular bleeding and possible weight changes is essential, and will avoid surprise and disappointment. It will also encourage women to continue use long enough to enjoy the positive attributes, such as convenience, safety and efficacy. The importance of appropriate counselling cannot be overemphasized. Identifying those women who will not be disturbed by irregular bleeding is most important. Physicians may underestimate the impact of this inconvenience because the irregular bleeding does not cause medical risks. On the contrary, the implant-induced bleeding changes are often associated with improvement of anaemia as the overall amount of bleeding is reduced. Assessing how each potential user will feel about the side effects and how well she will be able to tolerate them will result in less discontent, less wasted time and money, and fewer early removals. Some questions and answers to be prepared for, and which should be openly discussed, are (answers in italic):

- Is it effective? *Highly.*

- How is it inserted and removed? How long do these procedures take? Does it hurt? Will it leave scars? *See above. The scar is tiny unless there is a tendency to form keloid.*

- Will the implants be visible under the skin? *Not usually, but hyperpigmentation of the skin above the capsule may occur and is said to disappear after removal.*

- Will the implants be uncomfortable or restrict movement of the arm? *No.*

- Will the implants move in the body? *No.*

- Will the implants be damaged if they are touched or bumped? *No.*

- Will this contraceptive change sexual drive and enjoyment? *Unlikely.*

- What are the short- and long-term side effects? *See above.*

- Are there any effects on future fertility? *None.*

- What do the implants look and feel like? *Soft matchsticks.*

- What happens if pregnancy occurs during use? *Implants should be removed.*

- How long will it take for the method to be effective after insertion? *See above.*

- Can a partner tell if this method is being used? *Implants can be felt under the skin.*

Box 7.2 gives details of the management of menstrual side effects associated with progestin-only contraception.

Vaginal rings

The contraceptive action of vaginal rings is provided by the sustained release of hormones (either a progestin alone or in combination with estrogen) through the silastic ring. The hormones are absorbed through the lining of the vaginal walls. Progestin-only rings induce the usual changes in endometrium and cervical mucus associated with exposure to low, constant levels of progestin. The levonorgestrel vaginal ring contains 6 mg levonorgestrel

Box 7.2   Management of menstrual side effects associated with progestin-only contraception

- Pre-use counselling essential
- Reassurance, support and exclusion of organic causes and accidental pregnancy
- Hormonal manipulation – sparse data from controlled trials. In many, placebo is as effective as 'treatment'
- Natural estrogens alone
  - Equine estrogens 1.25–2.5 mg
  - Estrone sulfate 2 mg for 7–21 days – oestradiol (oral or transdermal)
- Ethinylestradiol – 10, 20, 50 µg for 14–21 days
- Progestins alone
  - For DMPA, give next injection early
  - For Norplant, give oral LNG for 10–21 days
  - For minipill give a 'haemostatic' dose of progestin
- Low-dose COC, if not contraindicated
- NSAID – see text
- If persistent and not tolerated, switch to alternative method of contraception

DMPA = depot medroxyprogesterone acetate; LNG = levonorgestrel; COC = combined oral contraceptive; NSAID = non-steroidal anti-inflammatory drug.

combined with silastic and an outer silastic shell. The ring is placed transversely across the upper part of the vagina and releases about 20 µg levonorgestrel per day; it can be left in place providing continuous contraception for 3 months. It prevents ovulation in 20–50% of cycles. The vaginal rings were developed to give the same long-acting, low-maintenance, progestin-only system found in Norplant but without a surgical procedure being required. Thus initiation and termination of use would be controlled by the user, have fewer complications and be less expensive. Efficacy rates are similar to the minipill, with a failure rate of about 3.5–4.5 per 100 woman-years [38]. Recent phase III trials revealed that one in six users develop erythematous patches in the upper vagina [39]. Further research is required to elucidate the cause of this finding as a prerequisite for wider use of vaginal rings.

The advantages of vaginal rings are as follows:

- There is an immediate return of fertility.

- The timing and duration of use is controlled by the user.

- It has a low dose but steady plasma levels, and no hepatic first-pass effect.

- It has one size that does not require special 'fitting'. The ring can be taken out for up to 2 hours without affecting efficacy.

The disadvantages of vaginal rings are:

- vaginal discharge/vaginal odor/irritation (in a minority of users)

- expulsion of the ring with urination or defecation (more likely with increased age, body weight and parity)

- insertion and removal may be difficult for some

- discomfort with intercourse is feared by users but is exceptionally uncommon

- lower efficacy than injectables or implants

- irregular bleeding.

Once a month combined injectable contraceptives (CICs)

These are combinations of long-acting progestin depotmedroxyprogesterone acetate (DMPA) or norethisterone enanthate (NET-EN) and a short-acting 'natural estrogen' given by intramuscular injection every 30 days (±3). Their mechanism of action is by ovarian suppression and cervical mucus and endometrial suppression. The main advantages are their high efficacy (similar to combined oral contraceptives; COCs), the fact that they are not user dependent (unlike COCs) and their acceptable menstrual patterns (unlike injectable or implant progestins). The contraindications are similar to those of COCs. The main disadvantage is the need for monthly injections. Of the two developed combined injectables, Cyclofem has had wider clinical use.

Other features of CICs include:

- a first-year pregnancy rate of 0.2% for Cyclofem/Cycloprovera

- the lipid, carbohydrate and haemostatic effects are reassuring, although the data are limited

- they are probably more suitable than injectable progestins for <16-year-olds

- there are no data on effect on breastfeeding

- irregular or prolonged bleeding may occur in the first three cycles.

Future research

Implant systems are an active area of contraception research. New developments are under way in the delivery material (silastic, EVA, biodegradable polymers) and the type and amount of progestin, alone or combined with different oestrogens. The original Norplant system with six implants may soon be joined by the Norplant II system, with two implants, and Implanon or Uniplant, with only one. Implanon and Uniplant are both single implant systems containing newer, less androgenic progestogens, 3-ketodesogestrel and nomegestrol acetate, respectively.

In a randomized 3-year clinical trial comparing Norplant to Norplant II with 600 women in each group, efficacy, side effects and continuation rates were not significantly different between the two systems [40]. There were no pregnancies in either group of women over the 3 years. The only difference seen was in time required for removals: removals of Norplant II were accomplished in about half the time required for removal of Norplant capsules. In another trial of Norplant compared to Norplant II, Norplant II was removed in about half the time with a smaller incision, fewer complications and less pain [41]. Bleeding patterns and return to fertility with Norplant II in studies over a 5-

year period also showed no difference compared to Norplant [42].

Uniplant, containing nomegestrol, offers effective contraception for 1 year. Studies to date show no clinically significant changes in lipoproteins, carbohydrate metabolism, insulin levels and on hepatic function in women using Uniplant for 2 consecutive years (any variations were within the normal range) [43]. In addition, during the same 2-year study with Uniplant, total testosterone and androstenedione *decreased* over the 2 years of use, but remained within the normal range. Furthermore, no significant difference in SHBG or acne vulgaris was noted [44]. The mechanisms of action of Uniplant appear to be the same as for the other progestin-only methods. In one study, Uniplant blocked ovulation in 86% of cycles studied, cervical mucus was scanty and viscous in all women throughout the study, and endometrial thickness, measured by ultrasound, supported a direct, atrophic effect [45].

Capronor is a single capsule, biodegradable, levonorgestrel-releasing subdermal implant composed of the polymer E-caprolactone. The capsules provide contraception for 1 year. The levonorgestrel escapes from the caprolactone at a rate 10 times faster than from the silastic in Norplant, thus allowing a smaller implant. When exposed to tissue fluids, E-caprolactone slowly breaks down into E-hydroxy-caproic acid, then to carbon dioxide and water. The capsule remains intact during the first year, allowing easy removal if necessary, then starts to disappear.

The advantage over Norplant is that no removal is needed or, if required, it is easy. A new implant, good for another year, can simply be placed next to the old one, which disappears over the ensuing months. The disadvantages are the same as Norplant and other continuous progestin-only methods, namely the disturbance in menstrual pattern [46]. Efficacy and other potential side effects are still being studied.

Biodegradable norethindrone/norethisterone (NET)-c cholesterol contraceptive implants (Annuelle) are currently under study. Four or five pellets the size of rice grains are inserted subcutaneously in the upper arm. Their main advantage is that they can be removed during their life span of 1–2 years. Irregular bleeding remains a major problem, persisting in 50% of users for up to 2 years. Different doses and numbers of implants are still being evaluated; the efficacy rates found in the 2–3-year preliminary studies are encouraging [47].

The vaginal ring is also an evolving system. Rings containing natural progesterone are being refined for use in the postpartum lactating woman. The dose of progesterone recommended by recent studies is 20 mg/24 h [48], with rings lasting for 3 months. However, the local irritation caused by continuous progestin exposure, combined with no improvement in abnormal bleeding patterns and relatively high expulsion rates, has led most research to focus on rings containing both estrogen and a progestin [49]. The vaginal ring containing an estrogen and a progestin is placed in the vagina for the first 3 weeks of each cycle and removed for 1 week for menses to occur, or used continuously for its 3-month life, thereby avoiding withdrawal bleeding. Because this regimen minimizes changes in bleeding patterns and the local irritation that occurs with progestin-only rings, it is better tolerated [50,51].

The new progestin Nesterone (ST1435) is being evaluated by the Population Council as an implant, vaginal ring and transdermal cream. It has no effect on lipid or carbohydrate metabolism. Another new progestin is levonorgestrel butanoate (HRPOOZ). It is on trial as a 3-month injectable likely to have a faster return to fertility than DMPA. A *progesterone* vaginal pessary replaced daily is being tested as a postpartum contraceptive. A transdermal progestin or combined patch/bracelet is in phase III trials. New injectables include microspheres in which the progestin is enclosed in a polymer capsule that controls release and helps maintain constant levels.

References

1. Zacharias S, Aguilena J, Assanzo JR, Zanutu J. Effects of hormonal and non-hormonal contraceptives on lactation and incidence of pregnancy. *Contraception* 1986;33:203.

2. Diaz S, Croxatto H, Pavez M, Belhadj H, Stern J, Sivin I. Clinical assessment of treatments for prolonged bleeding in users of Norplant implants. *Contraception* 1990; 42:97–104.

3. Alvarez-Sanches F, Brache V, Thevenin F, Cochon L, Faunder A. Hormonal treatment for bleeding irregularities in Norplant implant users. *Am J Obstet Gynecol* 1996;174: 919–22.

4. Shoupe D, Mishell DR Jr, Bopp B, Fielding M. The significance of bleeding patterns in Norplant implant users. *Obstet Gynecol* 1991;77:256.

5. Darney P, Klaisle C, Tanner A, Alvarado A. Sustained-release contraceptives. *Curr Prob Obstet Gynecol Fertil* 1990;XIII:103.

6. World Health Organization (WHO) Multinational comparative clinical evaluation of two long-acting injectable contraceptive steroids: norethisterone enanthate and medroxyprogesterone acetate. Final report. *Contraception* 1983;28:1.

7. Moore LL, Valuck R, McDougall C, Fink W. A comparative study of one year weight gain among users of medroxyprogesterone acetate, levonorgestrel implants and oral contraceptives. *Contraception* 1995;52:215.

8. Mainwaring R, Hales HA, Stevenson K, Hataska HH, Poulson AM, Jones KP, Peterson CM. Metabolic parameters, bleeding and weight changes in US women using progestin only contraceptives. *Contraception* 1995;51:149–53.

9. Tayob Y, Adams J, Jacobs HS, Guillebaud J. Ultrasound demonstration of increased frequency of functional ovarian cysts in women using progestogen only oral contraception. *Br J Obstet Gynaecol* 1985;92:1003.

10. Franks AI, Beral V, Cates W Jr, Hogue CJ. Contraception and ectopic pregnancy risk. *Am J Obstet Gyncecol* 1990;163:1120.

11. WHO Collaborative Study of Neoplasia and Steroid Contraceptives. Breast cancer and depot-medroxyprogesterone acetate: a multinational study. *Lancet* 1991;338:833.

12. Skegg DCG, Noonan EA, Paul C, Spears DFS, Meirik O, Thomas DB. Depot medroxyprogesterone acetate and breast cancer: a pooled analysis of the World Health Organization and New Zealand studies. *JAMA* 1995;273:799–804.

13. The New Zealand Contraception and Health Study Group. History of long-term use of depot-medroxyprogesterone acetate in patients with cervical dysplasia; case controlled analysis nested in a cohort study. *Contraception* 1994;50:443.

14. WHO Collaborative Study of Neoplasia and Steroid Contraception. Depot-medroxyprogesterone acetate (DMPA) and risk of invasive squamous cell cervical cancer. *Contraception* 1992;45:299.

15. Thomas DB, Ye Z, Ray RM and the WHO Collaborative Study of Neoplasia and Steroid Contraception. Cervical carcinoma *in situ* and the use of depot-medroxyprogesterone acetate (DMPA). *Contraception* 1995;51:25.

16. Stanford JL, Thomas DB. Depot medroxyprogesterone acetate (DMPA) and risk of epithelial ovarian cancer. *Int J Cancer* 1991;49:191–5.

17. Cundy T, Evans M, Roberts H, Wattie D, Ames R, Reid IR. Bone density in women receiving depot medroxyprogesterone acetate for contraception. *Br Med J* 1991; 303:13.

18. Cundy T, Cornish J, Evans MC, Roberts H, Reid IR. Recovery of bone density in women who stop using medroxyprogesterone acetate. *Br Med J* 1993;308: 247–8.

19. Ellis S, Randall S. Bone density and depot medroxyprogesterone acetate (free communication). *Eur J Contracept Reprod Health Care* 1996;1:135.

20. Kirkman RJE, Gbolade BA, Murby B. Cross sectional study of bone mineral density in long term users of depot medroxyprogesterone acetate (DMPA) (free communication).

Eur J Contracept Reprod Health Care 1996; 1:144.

21. Trussell J, Kost K. Contraceptive failure in the United States: a critical review of the literature. *Stud Fam Plann* 1987;18:237.

22. Vessey MP, Lawless M, Yeates D, Mc Pherson K. Progestogen only contraception: findings in a large prospective study with special reference to effectiveness. *Br J Fam Plann* 1985;10:117.

23. Broome M, Fotherby K. Clinical experience with the progestogen-only pill. *Contraception* 1990;42:489.

24. Bisset AM, Dingwall-Fordyce I, Hamilton MJK. The efficacy of the progestogen-only pill as a contraceptive method. *Br J Fam Plann* 1990;16:84.

25. Corfman P. Labelling guidance text for progestin-only oral contraceptives. *Contraception* 1995;52:71–76.

26. Harlap S, Kost K, Forrest DJ. Preventing pregnancy, protecting health: a new look at birth control choices in the United States. New York. The Alan Guttmacher Institute, 1991.

27. WHO. A multicentered phase III comparative clinical trial of depotmedroxyprogesterone acetate given three monthly at doses of 100 mg or 150 mg: contraceptive efficacy and side effects. *Contraception* 1986; 34:223.

28. Rabe T, Grunwald K, Runnebaum B. Injectable contraceptives (abstract). *Eur J Contracept Reprod Health Care* 1996;1:75.

29. De Ceular K, Gruber C, Hayes R, Serjeant G. Medroxy-progesterone acetate and homozygous sickle cell disease. *Lancet* 1982;2:229.

30. Mattson R, Cramer J, Caldwell B, Siconolfi B. Treatment of seizures with medroxy-progesterone acetate: preliminary report. *Neurology* 1984;34:1255.

31. Westoff C, Wieland D, Tiezzi L. Depression in users of Depo medroxyprogesterone acetate. *Contraception* 1995;51:351.

32. Brache Z, Alvarez-Sanchez F, Faundes A, Tejada AS, Cochon L. Ovarian endocrine function through five years of continuous treatment with Norplant subdermal contraceptive implants. *Contraception* 1990;41:169.

33. Chompootaweep S, Kochagarn E, Sirisumpan S, Tang-usaha J, Theppitaksak, Dusitsin N. Effectiveness of Norplant implants among Thai women in Bangkok. *Contraception* 1996;53:33–36.

34. Gu S, Irving S, Mingkun D, et al. Effectiveness of Norplant implants through seven years: a large scale study in China. *Contraception* 1995;52:99–103.

35. Brache V, Faundes AJ, Hohansson E, Alvarez F. Anovulation, inadequate luteal phase and poor sperm penetration in cervical mucus during prolonged use of Norplant implants. *Contraception* 1985;31:261.

36. Darney P, Speroff L. Implant contraception. In: Darney P, Speroff L. (eds) A clinical guide for contraception, 2nd ed. Baltimore: Williams and Wilkins, 1996;143–64.

37. Letterie G, Garnaas M. Localization of 'lost' Norplant capsules using compression film screen mammography. *Obstet Gynecol* 1995;85:886–887.

38. WHO. Microdose intra-vaginal levonorgestrel contraception: a multicenter clinical trial. Contraceptive efficacy and side effects. *Contraception* 1990; 41:105.

39. Bounds W, Szarewski A, Lowe D. et al. Preliminary report of unexpected local reactions to a progestogen-releasing contraceptive vaginal ring. *Eur J Obstet Gynecol Reprod Biol* 1993;48(2):123–125.

40. Sivin I, Viegas O, Compodonico I, et al. Clinical performance of a new two-rod levonorgestrel contraceptive implant: a three-year randomized study with Norplant implants as controls. *Contraception* 1997;55:73–80.

41. Darney P, Klaisle C, Zeiman M. Patient and provider experience with removal of two levo-norgestrel rods (Norplant II) compared to 6 capsules (Norplant), (free communication). *Eur J Contracept Reprod Health Care* 1996;1:91–5.

42. Biswas A, Leong W, Rantam S, Viegas O. Menstrual bleeding patterns in Norplant II users. *Contraception* 1996;54:91–5.

43. Barbosa I, Coutinho E, Athayde C, Lapido O, Olsson S, Ulmsten U. The effects of nomegestrol acetate subdermal implant (Uniplant) on carbohydrate metabolism, serum lipoproteins and on hepatic function in women. *Contraception* 1995;52:111–4.

44. Barbosa I, Coutinho E, Athayde C, Lapido O, Olsson S, Ulmsten U. Androgen levels in women using a single implant of nomegestrol acetate. *Contraception* 1996;53:37–40.

45. Barbosa I, Coutinho E, Athayde C, Lapido O, Olsson S, Ulmsten U. Effects of a single contraceptive Silastic implant containing nomegestrol acetate on ovarian function and cervical mucus production during 2 years. *Fertil Steril* 1996;65:724–9.

46. Darney P, Klaisle C, Monroe S, Cook C, Phillips N, Schindler A. Evaluation of a 1-year levonorgestrel-releasing contraceptive implant: side effects, release rates, and biodegradability. *Fertil Steril* 1992;58:137–143.

47. Raymond EG, Singh M, Archer D, Sarena BB, Baker J, Cole D. Contraceptive eficacy, pharmacokinetics and safety of Annuelle® biodegradable norethindrone pellet implants. *Fertil Steril* 1996;66:954–61.

48. Landgren BM, Jonsson B, Cekan SZ. The effects of small doses of progesterone released from two types of vaginal rings on ovarian activity and bleeding patterns during the first postpartum year. *Contraception* 1995;51:255–60.

49. Roumen F, Boon M, Van Velzen D, Dieben T, Bennink H. Local effects during long term use of a contraceptive vaginal ring (free communication). *Eur J Contracept Reprod Health Care* 1996;1:136.

50. Timmer CJ, Apter D, Voortman G. Pharmokinetics of 3-keto-desogestrel and ethinylestradiol released from different types of contraceptive vaginal rings. *Contraception* 1990;42:629.

51. Olsson SE, Odlind V. Contraception with a vaginal ring releasing 3-keto-deosgestrel and ethinylestradiol. *Contraception* 1990;42:563.

Intrauterine contraception

Sam Rowlands MRCGP MFFP DCH DRCOG
Naomi Hampton BSc MBBS MRCOG MFFP

Historical background

The history of the intrauterine device (IUD) can be traced back to the insertion of pebbles into the uteri of camels to prevent conception during long trips across the desert [1]. Antecedents of human IUDs were the stem pessaries described in 1868 to correct retroversion. In 1909 the first IUD was made from silkworm gut, followed in the 1920s by rings of silver or gold wire, developed separately by Grafenberg in Germany, Haire in Britain and Ota in Japan. Plastics technology allowed a device to be given memory of its shape after being stretched out into a linear form for insertion into the uterus. Zipper, impressed by the antifertility effect of copper in rabbits, introduced copper-bearing IUDs, which proved to be more effective. Copper wire is safe, its action is local, there is no increase in serum copper levels, no evidence of teratogenesis and any copper in the endometrium is shed at menstruation.

Figure 8.1 shows a variety of intrauterine devices. The first of the plastic, non-medicated/inert devices were the Margulies spiral and the Lippes loop. Other plastic devices followed (the Saf-T-coil, Dalkon Shield and Birnberg

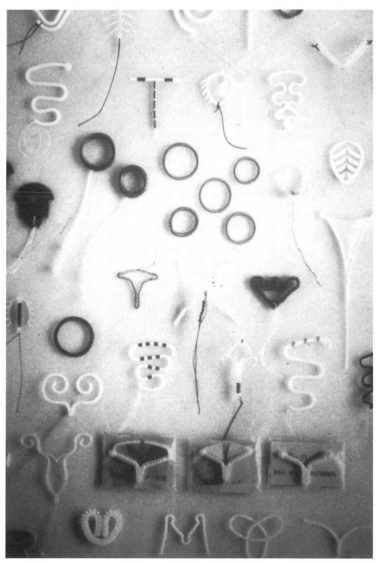

(a)

Fig. 8.1   (a) A variety of IUDs.

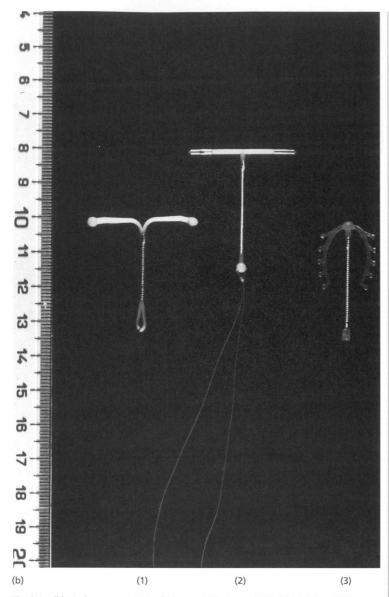

(b) (1) (2) (3)

Fig. 8.1 (b) Modern copper IUDs: (1) Nova-T, (2) Gyne T 380S, (3) Multiload 375.

which is ethylene vinyl acetate. All devices are impregnated with barium sulphate so they show up on X-rays, except the Multiload series.

Modern IUDs

Copper IUDs

Although the inert devices had low expulsion rates and low pregnancy rates associated with a larger surface area of plastic, they were associated with high pain and bleeding rates. The advent of copper-bearing devices allowed a reduction in the girth of the plastic frame. The first-generation copper devices (Copper 7 and Copper T200) had 200 mm^2 of copper. The second-generation devices (Nova T, Copper T 220C and Multiload 250) had 220–250 mm^2 and the third-generation devices (the T380 and Multiload 375) had an even larger copper load. First-generation devices have now been superseded by the newer devices (Figure 8.1b).

T-shaped copper devices are 36 mm long and 32 mm wide. The Nova-T frame is 32 mm long. The Multiload series has a much narrower width (18 mm) and is available in a short version which is 24 mm long. All these devices have two threads.

Another copper-bearing device, called the Cu Safe 300, is now available in some countries. It is quite small (vertical stem 25 mm and width 23 mm), its frame is made of polyethylene and its polypropylene thread is moulded into the stem to minimize the possibility of avulsion. A randomized trial with the Copper T380A over 3 years (300 patients in each group) showed

Bow). Closed devices fell out of favour because of the potential for bowel obstruction should perforation occur. Devices without threads, popular in China, are now less so because removal requires a hook and their advantage regarding pelvic inflammatory disease (PID) is questionable [2]. The Dalkon shield with its multifilament thread was withdrawn from the market in 1975 as it was found to be associated with an increased risk of mid-trimester septic abortion and consequent fatalities in the USA. The problem was thought to be due to the wick effect of the multifilament thread and consequent ascending infection. Women with a Dalkon Shield are advised to have it removed.

All the frames of currently marketed devices are polyethylene, except Progestasert no significant difference in pregnancy rates, a significantly higher expulsion rate and a significantly lower removal rate for pain/bleeding with the Cu Safe 300 (Figure 8.2) [3].

A recent innovation is the first frameless device, GyneFix®, developed in an attempt to minimize three common drawbacks of IUDs: expulsion, pain and bleeding. It consists of a single polypropylene thread on which six copper cylinders (each 5 mm long) are threaded; the top and bottom cylinders are crimped on to the thread to fix all six cylinders. The total surface area of copper is 330 mm². A knot at the upper end of the thread is 'anchored' into the fundal myometrium using a special stylet. A postabortal version of the device is also available and a postplacental version is being developed.

A randomized trial of the GyneFix® and the Copper T380A over 3 years showed no significant differences in pregnancy rates, removal for pain/bleeding, or discontinuation, but there was a higher expulsion rate with the GyneFix® [4]. Failed insertions were a problem with GyneFix® in some centres; the inserter tube and insertion technique have since been modified. GyneFix® is easily removed and is suitable for emergency contraception.

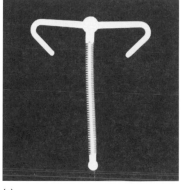

(a)

Fig. 8.2 (a) Cu Safe 300, (b) GyneFix® and (c) GyneFix® *in situ*.

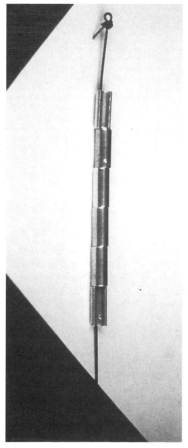

(b)

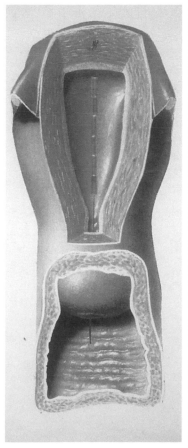

(c)

Hormone-releasing devices

Hormone-releasing intrauterine systems (IUSs) are available in many countries. The Progestasert is a T-shaped device which releases 65 μg progesterone/24 h. It is associated with an increased risk of ectopic pregnancy and has a life span of only 1 year. The levonorgestrel IUS (Mirena®, Levonova®) was introduced in the UK in 1995 (Figure 8.3). The levonorgestrel IUS has been a highly successful innovation and is considered in a separate section below.

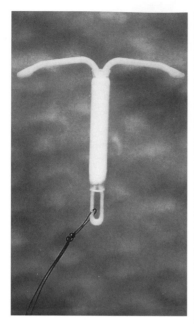

Fig. 8.3 The levonorgestrel-releasing intrauterine system (Mirena®).

Worldwide usage and method acceptability

The IUD is the second most commonly used method in the world, after female sterilization. More than 106 million women worldwide use IUDs, about two-thirds of them in China [2]. Worldwide, about 10% of married women aged 15–44 years use IUDs, but popularity varies enormously from 33% in Vietnam and China to 0% in some African countries. In Western Europe, use in women aged 15–44 years is 7–19%, the highest rates being in Southern Europe and Scandinavia [5]. Usage in the USA had been affected by adverse media publicity in the past, particularly with respect to the Dalkon Shield and subsequent litigation. In Great Britain, use has declined somewhat over the past two decades; in 1995 prevalence of use was 4% among women aged 15–49 [6].

Modes of action of IUDs/IUSs [7]

A sterile 'foreign body' response leads to an increased concentration of white cells, prostaglandins and enzymes. The primary mode of action of copper-bearing IUDs is prevention of fertilization as sperm motility is disrupted and ova development is impeded. Cleaving fertilized ova are not seen in tubal washings in IUD users [8]. The secondary mechanism is prevention of implantation; the implantation process is inhibited and there is also a direct blastocytotoxic effect. Successful implantation, evidenced by beta human chorionic gonadotrophin (βhCG) in blood and urine, is rare in IUD users [9]. Clearly the postcoital IUD does not rely on the first mechanism. IUSs do not prevent fertilization but suppress the endometrium, causing glandular atrophy and decidualization; thickened cervical mucus inhibits sperm migration and, in some women, tubal and ovarian function is also affected. Table 8.1 summarizes the modes of action of IUDs/IUSs.

Efficacy

Compared with the Lippes loop, first-generation copper-bearing

devices performed significantly better with pregnancy rates of less than 2 per 100 woman-years. With the second-generation devices, pregnancy rates were further reduced to 1.0–1.5 per 100 woman-years (see Table 8.2). The third-generation, high-copper-load devices, have failure rates of less than 1 per 100 woman-years, comparable with the efficacy of female sterilization.

Some of the factors responsible for variations in IUD performance are as follows [9]:

- population differences: age, parity, time since last pregnancy
- the skill of the clinician performing the insertion
- the tolerance by patients of side effects
- the attitude of professional staff and the adequacy of counselling
- the use of adjunctive contraceptive methods
- studies with small numbers with an 'exposure' period under 1 year.

Efficacy as emergency contraceptive

Copper-bearing IUDs have the highest efficacy of any available

Table 8.1 Mode of Action of IUDs/IUSs

	Copper-bearing IUDs	IUSs
Foreign body response	+	+
Prevention of fertilization	+	–
Prevention of implantation	+[a]	+[b]
Endometrial suppression	–	+
Cervical mucus thickening	–	+
Ovarian function modification	–	+/–
Tubal motility	+	+
Spermicidal/inhibition of sperm transport	+	?

[a]Effect on enzymes and glycogen metabolism.
[b]Not effective immediately, not suitable for postcoital contraception.

Table 8.2 WHO randomized comparative studies at 3 years of use (cumulative discontinuation rates per 100) of four copper-bearing IUDs

Device	TCu 200C	ML 250	TCu 220C	TCu 380A
Pregnancies				
Total	1.7	2.8	3.4	1.0
Intrauterine	1.7	2.8	3.2	0.9
Ectopic	0	0	0.2	0.1
Expulsion	4.5	3.1	7.7	7.0
Medical removals				
Total	20.8	21.2	12.9	14.6
Pain/bleeding	17.3	17.6	11.9	12.9
Other	4.2	4.3	1.2	1.9
Non-medical removals	18.5	17.1	13.2	13.8
Woman-years of use	2153	2104	3163	3214

Adapted from Newton J. IUD safety and acceptability recent advances. *Curr Obstet Gynaecol* 1993;3:28–36.

emergency contraceptive. Only eight documented failures have been reported after more than 8400 postcoital insertions [11]. This gives a failure rate of at most 0.1 pregnancies per 100 women treated per cycle, i.e. 15 times more effective than the Yuzpe hormonal regimen. When efficacy is essential, the IUD is the emergency contraceptive of choice. There are no data to support the use of the levonorgestrel IUS as an emergency contraceptive.

Medical removals

The average menstrual blood loss is 30–40 ml per cycle. Inert devices increase this to around 70–80 ml. Copper-bearing devices increase it to 50–60 ml. Removals for bleeding and/or pain are the most common reasons for discontinuation. Bleeding problems and uterine cramping tend to settle after a few months of use. Antiprostaglandins such as ibruprofen or mefenamic acid may help. For copper devices, the removal rates for pain and bleeding are approximately 5 per 100 woman-years.

Life span

Inert devices have an indefinite life span and women with devices *in situ* can keep them as long as they wish. First-generation copper devices showed an increase in pregnancy rates after the second year. WHO studies on the Nova T device showed an increasing pregnancy rate after 3 years [12]. Third-generation copper devices with a surface area of copper of over 300 mm² have life spans that exceed 5 years (Table 8.3), and so save women frequent reinsertions and reduce the chance of adverse events. The TCu 380A was approved for 10 years use by the US Food and Drug Administration in 1993. To date, the longest follow-up of copper-bearing devices is for 12 years of

use [13]. No pregnancies were reported with the TCu 380A between 8 and 12 years of use.

Expulsion

Cumulative expulsion rates at 5 years are less than 10 per 100 women for copper-bearing devices. No consistent patterns have been detected in expulsion rates by device type [9]. Claims of lower expulsion rates for the 'fundal-seeking' Multiload devices have not been borne out. Initial experience with GyneFix® was disappointing [4]; large studies of the modified version are awaited. Variation in expulsion rates is thought to reflect differences in insertion technique, and inserter skill and training, rather than inherent differences in the devices.

Expulsion may occur at any time after insertion, but is most common in the early cycles, usually during menstruation, with the highest risk at the time of the first postinsertion menses. Thereafter the frequency of expulsion decreases. Patients who are older, are of higher parity or who have used a device for longer have lower expulsion rates.

Expulsion may be complete or partial. Partial expulsion may be

Table 8.3 Life span of IUDs/IUSs

Device	Licensed use (years)[a]	Duration of effectiveness demonstrated in clinical trials
TCu 200/200B	3	6
TCu 220C	3	12
Nova T 200	5	5
Nova T 380	5	3 to date
Multiload 250	3	8
Multiload 375	5	8
TCu 380 series	10	12
GyneFix®	5	5
Levonorgestrel IUS	5	7

[a]UK licence; licences vary between countries.

detected by the woman by feeling the tip of the stem or noticing the thread becoming longer; the physician may make these observations at follow-up or may elicit the presence of the stem of the device in the endocervical canal by exploring the canal with a sterile Q-tip. It is important to recognize that protection against pregnancy is reduced.

Women who expel an IUD have a threefold increased risk of expelling the same or another device. However, almost half of women requesting reinsertion following expulsion will retain their second device [14].

Return of fertility

Both cohort and case-control studies show no harmful effects on fertility of previous IUD use, even if the IUD was removed for suspected complications [9]. No difference has been shown in the rate of return of fertility between users of copper-bearing IUDs and the levonorgestrel IUS.

Contraindications to the use of copper IUDs

Absolute contraindications

These are:

- pregnancy

- unexplained genital tract bleeding

- PID – current or within the last 3 months

- STI with purulent cervicitis – current or within the last 3 months

- distortion of the uterine cavity, e.g. congenital malformation, submucous fibroids[a]

- copper allergy

- Wilson's disease

- cavity length less than 5.5 cm (does not apply to frameless devices)

- benign or malignant gestational trophoblastic disease

- known pelvic tuberculosis

- cervical cancer.

Relative contraindications

These are:

- menorrhagia

- anaemia: haemoglobin less than 9 g/dl

- increased risk of STIs – multiple sexual partners or partner who has multiple partners

- age less than 20 years – as a surrogate of STI risk

- Acquired Immune Deficiency Syndrome/Human Immunodeficiency Virus positivity/high risk of HIV

- previous ectopic pregnancy – not for TCu 380

- nulliparity (weak relative contraindication related to increased risk of expulsion)

- risk of bacteraemia:

  - valvular heart disease and septal defects – antibiotic cover at insertion

- renal disease/ dialysis/transplant

- immunosuppressive therapy (not steroids)

- severe dysmenorrhoea.

Assessment of risks and benefits

Intrauterine pregnancy

Failure of an IUD to prevent pregnancy, resulting in an intrauterine pregnancy, leads to an increased risk of both second trimester abortion and premature labour. The risk of abortion is reduced from about 50% to the background rate of about 13%, if the device is gently removed before the threads disappear out of reach [2].

Ectopic pregnancy

Medicated devices have low rates of ectopic pregnancy: indeed, they have a protective effect. Copper-bearing devices with a surface area of more than 350 mm^2 have a lower ectopic pregnancy rate than those with less copper. While the progesterone and microdose levonorgestrel IUSs had unacceptably high ectopic pregnancy rates, the levonorgestrel 20 µg per day IUS has a very low ectopic pregnancy rate. Figure 8.4 shows ectopic pregnancy rates for non-medicated, medicated and hormone-releasing devices.

IUDs provide more protection against intrauterine than extrauterine pregnancies. If a pregnancy occurs in an IUD user, the chance of it being ectopic is 1 in 25 [15] compared with about 1

---

[a]Not necessarily for GyneFix®.

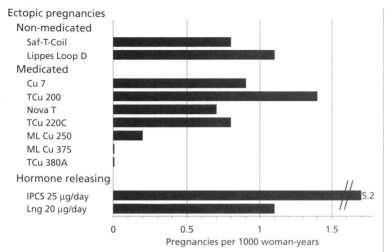

Ectopic pregnancies

- Non-medicated
  - Saf-T-Coil
  - Lippes Loop D
- Medicated
  - Cu 7
  - TCu 200
  - Nova T
  - TCu 220C
  - ML Cu 250
  - ML Cu 375
  - TCu 380A
- Hormone releasing
  - IPCS 25 µg/day — 5.2
  - Lng 20 µg/day

Pregnancies per 1000 woman-years

Fig. 8.4 Ectopic pregnancy rates per 1000 woman-years. Reproduced with permission from *IPPF Med Bull* 1996; 31.

in 250 for non-IUD users; this is the ectopic ratio. The ectopic rate per 1000 woman–years illustrates the protective role of the IUD (Table 8.4).

Pelvic inflammatory disease

Studies in the 1970s and early 1980s that showed an increased risk of PID in IUD users of up to 10-fold had methodological problems. It is now clear that PID is related to lifestyle and sexually transmitted infections (STIs). A landmark WHO paper [16] based on approximately 668 000 cycles of use showed that the risk of PID is increased by a factor of 6.3 in the 3 weeks after insertion; thereafter, the risk is low for up to 8 years (the duration of the study) (Table 8.5). For women in mutually faithful sexual relationships, IUDs pose little ongoing risk of PID.

Clinical suitability criteria

The risk of sexually transmitted infections

Routine microbiological screening

The relevance of testing for *Chlamydia trachomatis*, and possibly other STIs, prior to IUD insertion depends entirely on the local prevalence. In high-prevalence areas, there is a case to be made for making testing routine. At prevalences of less than 6%, it is probably not a reasonable public health measure [17]. At low prevalences, consideration should be given to testing those aged under 25, those with contact bleeding of the cervix, those with a heavy or offensive discharge, and those with a change of partner in the last 6 months. Some of those requesting emergency contraception are more likely to be at risk of STIs.

Previous PID

As long as the episode of PID is longer ago than 3 months and the patient is not assessed on their lifestyle as being at high risk of STIs, previous PID is not a contraindication to the use of an IUD. Some consider it reassuring if the woman has had a pregnancy since the episode of PID.

Antibiotic 'prophylaxis' at insertion

A randomized controlled trial of azithromycin administered immediately prior to IUD insertion had no demonstrable effect on IUD removal within 90 days of insertion, morbidity or use of medical services; the investigators concluded that

Table 8.4 Copper and progestin intrauterine devices: pregnancy and ectopic rates per 1000 woman-years in the first 2 years of randomized non-postpartum trials

Device and surface area (mm²)	Woman-years (1000s)	Pregnancies per 1000 years	Number of ectopic pregnancies	Ectopic ratio per 1000 pregnancies	Ectopic rate/ 1000 years
200 mm²					
Nova T	7.0	13.4 ± 1.4	6	64	0.9 ± 0.2
Cu 7	5.1	25.8 ± 2.3	5	38	1.0 ± 0.4
220–300 mm²					
TCu 220	15.5	9.0 ± 0.8	5	36	0.3 ± 0.1
MLCu 250	4.5	9.4 ± 1.5	2	48	0.4 ± 0.3
350–380 mm²					
MLCu 375	2.5	5.9 ± 1.5	0	0	0
TCu 380	9.9	3.4 ± 0.6	2	59	0.2 ± 0.1
Levonorgestrel					
20	4.1	1.0 ± 0.5	1	250	0.2 ± 0.2

Adapted from Sivin I. Dose and age dependent ectopic pregnancy risks with intrauterine contraception. *Obstet Gynecol* 1991; 78: 291–298.

Table 8.5 Intrauterine devices and pelvic inflammatory disease (PID): subject characteristics and PID rates

Characteristic	No. of insertions	Years of follow-up	PID cases	PID rate/ 1000 woman-years
All women	22 908	51 399	81	1.58
Time after insertion (days)				
≤20	22 908	1243	12	9.66
>21	22 521	50 157	69	1.38
Age (years)				
15–24	5006	9492	33	3.48
25–29	8287	18 292	23	1.26
30–34	6549	15 953	17	1.07
35 +	3066	7663	8	1.04

Adapted from Farley TNM, Rosenberg MJ, Rose PJ, et al. Intrauterine devices and pelvic inflammatory disease: an international perspective. *Lancet* 1992; 339:785–788.

routine antibiotic prophylaxis at IUD insertion is unwarranted [18].

Menstrual history

Menorrhagia is only a relative contraindication to the use of IUDs (see p. 97). The severity of menorrhagia is quite subjective. Menorrhagia is a positive indication for the levonorgestrel (LNG) IUS.

Previous ectopic pregnancy

Such women should be offered a high-load copper device or a LNG IUS in preference to other devices. The impact of a second ectopic pregnancy in a woman who has never had a successful pregnancy may be deemed so devastating that a contraceptive which further reduces the risk of ectopics should be considered, e.g. Depo-Provera.

Age

Age is negatively associated with PID and expulsion, but positively associated with ectopic pregnancy and menorrhagia. As women age and fertility declines, IUDs offer a long-term, low-compliance method. Women over 40 years at IUD insertion may keep their device until their natural menopause.

Parity

Statistically, IUDs are more suitable for parous women. Nulliparity is associated with shorter uterine cavity length (approximately 30 mm compared with 45 mm for those of parity of two or more), pain and bleeding, and expulsion.

Principles of counselling and follow-up

The issues that need to be discussed in counselling once the IUD/IUS has been chosen as a preferred method are as follows:

- advantages/disadvantages of intrauterine contraception – heavier, longer periods with the copper IUD and oligomenorrhoea with the IUS must be included

- a description of the device recommended and its life span

- a description of the insertion (by demonstrating on a model, if possible)

- the timing of insertion and the method to be used in the interim

- the right to have the device removed without undue delay.

Counselling should always be backed up with written material. Some points to consider when making an assessment of STI risk are as follows:

- Is the woman in a stable relationship? If so, for how long?

- Is the relationship monogamous on both sides?

- Does the woman have any of the following symptoms: vaginal discharge, dyspareunia, intermenstrual bleeding?

Follow-up should be 2 weeks after insertion, 3 months later, then annually thereafter; annual visits are probably of little medical benefit, although they provide the opportunity for concerns to be discussed.

Aids to clinical practice for IUD use

Pain relief

Giving mefenamic acid 500 mg orally 1 hour before IUD insertion may be of some benefit in reducing postinsertion uterine cramping. A gel containing 2% lignocaine is now available for uterine use; it is administered through a special quill. Lignocaine gel often provides sufficient anaesthesia to permit dilatation of the cervix; otherwise paracervical or intracervical block will be necessary.

Resuscitation

Manipulation/instrumentation of the internal cervical os can result in 'cervical shock'. The pain experienced by the patient leads to vasovagal attack with bradycardia, nausea and hypotension. If the condition persists, the insertion procedure should be abandoned and the patient monitored for bradycardia, the head should be lowered and the feet elevated, the airway should be maintained, if necessary by elevating the chin. An airway (Brook or Laerdal pocket mask) and atropine must be available. Most cases of 'cervical shock' are mild and self-limiting, and it is important not to overtreat women; a great deal can be done to prevent such reactions by the provision of a calm, relaxed, reassuring environment with 'aural valium' supplied by an assistant.

Very rarely, an epileptic fit may be precipitated by IUD insertion; fainting causes cerebral ischaemia and hypoxia, which trigger a convulsion. The patient should be protected from injuring herself and, if lasting for more than a few seconds, diazepam (10 mg) should be administered per rectum.

Selection of device

The CuT 380 and the Multiload 375 have the lowest failure rates among copper-bearing devices and have long life spans. They are especially suitable where the uterine cavity is of 'standard' dimensions to accommodate the long arms of the T 380. Nulliparous women have a shorter cavity length and the vertical stem of standard devices tends to press down on to the uterine isthmus, causing cramping. If the uterus sounding length is between 5.5 and 6.5 cm, a Multiload 250 short or GyneFix are the devices of choice; if less than 5.5 cm GyneFix is the only suitable device.

Timing of insertion

Insertion may take place either intermenstrually or towards the end of a period. With the latter, one can be sure that the woman is not pregnant and the device may be easier to insert, since the cervix will be softening. However, uterine contractions may compromise placement of the device and increase the risk of expulsion.

The uterus is more relaxed at midcycle. Insertion should be undertaken not later than 5 days after the earliest calculated date of ovulation (day 19 of a 28-day cycle), unless there has been no intercourse that cycle, as beyond day 19, implantation may have occurred.

After childbirth, IUD insertion may be performed by a specifically trained clinician within 48 hours of delivery. Sounding the uterus is best avoided as the uterus is soft. The major disadvantage of postpartum insertion is that the expulsion rate is high. The more usual timing is at least 4 weeks after vaginal delivery or at least 6 weeks after caesarean section. For the IUS, insertion is not recommended earlier than 6 weeks postpartum because of the possibility of prolonged bleeding.

Insertion technique

General points on insertion technique are given in the section on tips for safe practice, and insertion instructions for the Gyne T 380 and Mirena® are provided in Appendix 8.1 and 8.2, respectively. Recognized practical training must be obtained before inserting intrauterine methods of contraception.

Removal

An IUD can be removed at any time providing the woman is wishing to conceive. If pregnancy risk is to be avoided, then the device should only be removed at or beyond midcycle, if there has been no sexual intercourse during the preceding 7 days or if a barrier method has been used carefully since the last period. If an IUD needs removing at midcycle, thought should be given to the provision of emergency contraception.

Women changing to another method of contraception should start it at least from the first day of the cycle during which the device is to be removed. IUDs should be removed 1 year after the last menstrual period for women who have reached the menopause after the age of 50 years, and 2 years after the last period, if this was reached under 50 years of age.

Documentation

It is essential to record discussions with women about their choice of an intrauterine method, why they have selected it, and that efficacy (including ectopic pregnancy risk), mode of action, insertion technique, menstrual pattern, potential side effects, follow-up and symptoms of ectopic pregnancy have been discussed. This verbal information must be backed up by the provision of written information. In the UK it is not considered necessary to ask women to sign a consent form.

It is important to record detailed information about the insertion, including examination findings, the analgesia used and any difficulties encountered. Many services use standard forms to record IUD/IUS insertions (Figure 8.5).

Management of IUD-associated events

Uterine perforation

This is a rare but probably underestimated complication, owing to 'silent' perforations, with rates being estimated at between 0.6 and 1.3 per 1000 insertions [9]. Two studies have suggested that perforation is more likely to occur during lactation; other studies have not supported this and it is now thought that this is not so [9]. Perforation may be a 'silent' phenomenon and the clinician cannot rely on a signal of pain from the patient. An IUD does not 'migrate' through the uterine wall: perforation always occurs at the time of insertion. However, a rare phenomenon is embedding of a poorly placed device in the myometrium with gradual erosion under the influence of uterine muscular activity (partial perforation) [19].

Lost threads

The main reasons for 'lost threads' are:

* the threads are too short or are drawn up into the cervical canal or uterus

* unrecognized expulsion of the device

* a perforation of the uterus resulting in translocation of the device into the peritoneal cavity.

Figure 8.6 shows how to manage the situation. When attempting to locate or remove a device with 'lost threads', pregnancy should be excluded and the woman must be advised that she cannot rely on the IUD (if *in situ*) and she must use other precautions until the problem has been resolved. Instrumentation beyond the internal os should not be carried out in the luteal phase of the cycle. Thread-retrieving devices (Figure 8.7), such as the Emmett, are very useful. As the instrument is swept down the anterior, posterior and lateral aspects of the uterus, the IUD threads become caught on its notches and are brought down on removal.

Copper devices translocated into the peritoneal cavity should be removed as they may cause a sterile inflammatory response and adhesions.

Pelvic infection with IUD *in situ*

The diagnosis is difficult to make with precision without laparoscopy. However, symptoms

---

IUD First Insertion/Subsequent Insertion

Date:	LMP:	
Type removed	....	/ None
Type inserted	....	
OE:	(NB) Tenderness absent	☐
	(IF PRESENT, INSERTION CONTRAINDICATED)	
Vulva/vagina	....	/Normal
Cervix	....	/Normal
Uterus	....	/A/V
	....	/N/S
Sounding depth (centimetres) :..		
Adnexa	....	/Normal
INSERTION DIFFICULTY? Yes ☐ (specify opposite)		None
LA used? ☐	....	/None
SYMPTOMS : Above average ☐ Average ☐		Minimal ☐
Oral Analgesia? ☐	....	/None
Name of Inserting Doctor (capitals) & Signature:		
....		
Supervised by:	....	
(if trainee)		
	Standard letter sent to GP	☐

Fig. 8.5 Standard form for recording IUD/IUS insertion in the UK.

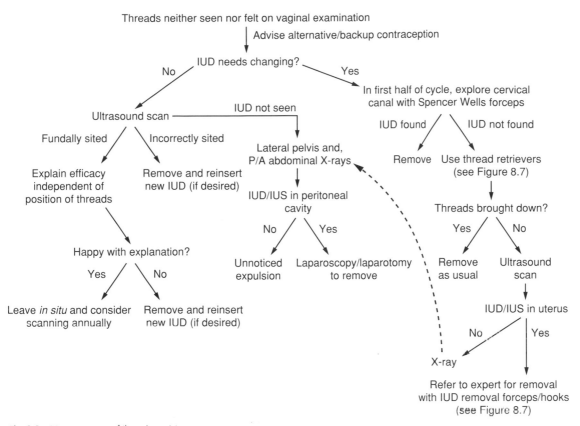

Fig. 8.6 Management of 'lost threads'.

and signs are lower abdominal pain, purulent vaginal discharge and cervical excitation/pain. If all three are present, there is a 50% probability of PID. The probability is increased further by finding a pyrexia greater than 38°C, a palpable adnexal mass, an elevated white cell count or a raised erythrocyte sedimentation rate. Ideally, high vaginal and cervical swabs should be taken. If the diagnosis is in doubt, the woman should be treated rather than waiting. In mild cases, the IUD can be left *in situ*. If there is a lack of response after 48 hours, the device should be removed. More severe cases will need referral.

Actinomyces-like organism (ALO) carriage [20]

These organisms, also known as Gupta bodies (after the person who reported them in 1976), are seen on cervical smears of those with inert and medicated devices *in situ*. There does not appear to be any direct relationship with pelvic actinomycosis, a serious pelvic sepsis that is seen very rarely. There are only a few hundred cases in the literature compared to millions of years of IUD use, although the presence of ALOs on a cervical smear may be a marker for increased risk of developing pelvic actinomycosis. A woman having a smear

showing the presence of ALOs should have an abdominal and pelvic examination, and be asked about the symptoms of pelvic actinomycosis (intermenstrual bleeding, pelvic pain, deep dyspareunia and dysuria). The vast majority of women with ALO carriage are asymptomatic. The management protocol is shown in Figure 8.8.

The levonorgestrel-releasing intrauterine system (LNG IUS)

The levonorgestrel-releasing intrauterine system has many of the properties of an ideal contraceptive: high efficacy, long

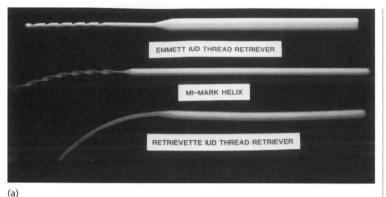

(a)

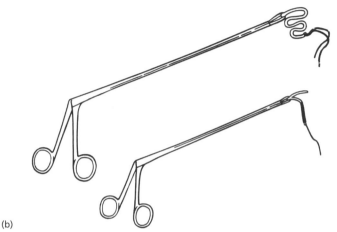

(b)

Fig. 8.7   Thread-retrieving devices. (a) Plastic thread-retrieving devices; (b) IUD retrieving forceps.

duration of action, requirement for minimal compliance, independent of coitus, non-contraceptive benefits, full and immediate reversibility, and largely nuisance-only side effects.

The LNG IUS (Mirena®/Levonova®) consists of a plastic T-shaped frame (32 mm in length and identical to that of the Nova T/Novagard) with a steroid reservoir around its vertical stem (Figure 8.3). This contains 52 mg of levonorgestrel/Silastic mixture surrounded by a highly sophisticated rate-limiting polydimethylsiloxane membrane which regulates the release of levonorgestrel into the uterine cavity to 20 μg per 24 hours.

The LNG IUS is inserted into the uterine cavity by the same technique as the Nova T/Novagard (see Appendix 8.2). The steroid reservoir requires a wider insertion tube (4.8 mm) than Nova T/Novagard and, even though cervical dilatation is rarely required in parous women

Fig. 8.8   Management of *Actinomyces*-like organisms (ALOs) on cervical smear.

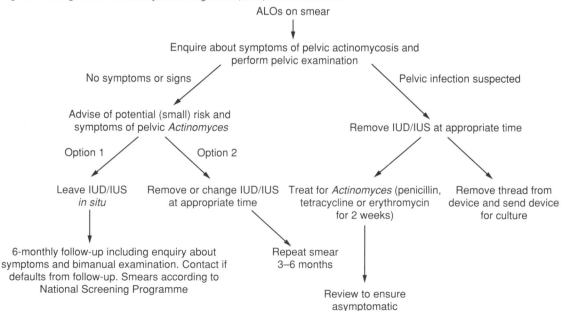

ALOs on smear

Enquire about symptoms of pelvic actinomycosis and perform pelvic examination

No symptoms or signs | Pelvic infection suspected

Advise of potential (small) risk and symptoms of pelvic *Actinomyces* | Remove IUD/IUS at appropriate time

Option 1 | Option 2

Leave IUD/IUS *in situ* | Remove or change IUD/IUS at appropriate time | Treat for *Actinomyces* (penicillin, tetracycline or erythromycin for 2 weeks) | Remove thread from device and send device for culture

6-monthly follow-up including enquiry about symptoms and bimanual examination. Contact if defaults from follow-up. Smears according to National Screening Programme | Repeat smear 3–6 months

Review to ensure asymptomatic

under 45 years, cervical dilators should be available for insertions. If cervical dilatation is needed, this should be performed using a paracervical or intracervical local anaesthetic block with 1% lignocaine. The LNG IUS should be fitted only by those who have received all necessary practical training. Expulsion and perforation rates are similar to those for the Nova T/Novagard.

The LNG IUS releases levonorgestrel into the uterine cavity, where it is absorbed via the capillary network in the basal layer of the endometrium into the systemic circulation. As soon as 15 minutes after insertion of the device, levonorgestrel can be detected in the plasma [21]; maximum concentrations are reached within a few hours. Plasma levonorgestrel concentrations stabilize after the first few weeks at 0.3–0.6 nmol/l and are lower than those seen in users of all other hormonal methods.

The LNG IUS exerts its contraceptive effects by several local and remote mechanisms (Box 8.1). Profound suppression of endometrial growth is seen after only a few months of use but, after removal of the LNG IUS, the endometrium returns to normal and menstruation usually returns within the first month. Fertility also returns promptly, with 79–96% of women having conceived within 12 months [26]. After discontinuation of use of the LNG IUS, there has been no reported increase in congenital abnormality above the background rate. There are no data relating to term pregnancies conceived with an LNG IUS *in situ*.

The LNG IUS has the lowest

Box 8.1 **LNG IUS – Contraceptive mode of action**

- Profound suppression of endometrial growth [22]. Endometrium rendered atrophic and unresponsive to oestrogen
  - Endometrial glands atrophy
  - Stroma becomes swollen and decidual
  - Mucosa thins
  - Epithelium becomes inactive
  - Blood vessels become thick-walled and fibrotic. Thrombosis seen in small capillaries [23]
- 'Foreign body reaction' – inflammatory response with infiltration by leucocytes, plasma cells and macrophages
- Modification of ovarian function in the first 12 months [24]
  - Anovulatory cycles with some inhibition of oestradiol production
  - Anovulation with high follicular activity
  - Ovulation with inadequate luteal phase (after 12 months > 2/3 cycles are ovulatory [25])
- Cervical mucus hostility
- Possible effect on sperm migration in the genital tract

pregnancy rate of any IUD to date (Table 8.6), although there is no statistically significant difference in efficacy between it and the CuT 380 at 7 years. The same is not true of Nova T, and there is a significantly lower rate of both intrauterine and extrauterine pregnancy at 3 years [28]. These studies, against other IUDs and Norplant, lasting for up to 7 years collectively, report more than 12 000 woman-years of use and demonstrate very high effectiveness in preventing unwanted pregnancies – Pearl Index 0–0.3 [29–31] (similar to female sterilization). Unlike copper-bearing devices and all other methods of fertility regulation, which become more effective as users age, the failure rate among women using the LNG IUS is uniformly low.

Because of the very high efficacy of the LNG IUS, ectopic

Table 8.6 Randomized comparative study at 7 years of use (cumulative discontinuation rates per 100) of the LNG IUS and the Cu T 380 Ag

	LNG IUS	Standard error	Cu T 380Ag	Standard error
Pregnancies				
Total	1.1	±0.5	1.4	±0.4
Intrauterine	1.1		1.4	
Ectopic	0		†/*	
Expulsion	11.7	±1.2	8.4	±1.0
Medical removals				
Total	71.9		55.1	
Pain/bleeding	20.4**		30.0**	
Other	23.3		20.4	
Amenorrhoea	24.6***		1.1***	
Pelvic inflammatory disease	3.6		3.6	
Non-medical removals	44.9		48.0	
Woman-years of use	3371		3758	

†There were two cases of ectopic pregnancy, giving a rate of 0.05 per 100.
*$P < 0.05$.
**$P < 0.01$.
***$P < 0.001$.
Adapted from Sivin I, Stern J, Couthino E, et al. Prolonged intrauterine contraception: a seven year randomized study of the levonorgestrel 20 mcg/day (LNg20) and the copper T380Ag IUDs. *Contraception* 1991;44:473–480.

pregnancies are rare, with an incidence of only 0.02 per 100 woman-years [31]; this represents an 80–90% reduction in risk compared with women not using contraception. Approximately 20% of conceptions with the LNG IUS are ectopic [31] and the possibility of ectopic pregnancy should not be ignored in an LNG IUS user, although the device's efficacy makes it possible to offer the LNG IUS to some women with a history of ectopic pregnancy.

Users of the LNG IUS have low rates of pelvic inflammatory disease, with removal rates of the order of 0.5 per 100 users by 3 years of use [31]. A significant reduction in infection rates, particularly among young women, has been seen in some comparative studies, although these findings have not been repeated in other blinded studies.

Although the daily progestogen dose is low, and there are no peaks in plasma levonorgestrel concentrations, some women clearly feel the effect of the progestogen. Reported hormonal side effects include headache, breast tenderness, nausea, acne, hirsutism and mood changes [31]. Most of these symptoms are rare, peak 3 months after insertion and reduce over time. Cumulative discontinuation rates for hormonal side effects are low at 12.1 per 100 LNG IUS users at 5 years [31]. A recent Finnish study has shown continuation rates at 1, 2, 3, 4 and 5 years of use of 94%, 87%, 82%, 76% and 65% of women, respectively. Counselling prior to LNG IUS insertion should always include a discussion about its potential hormonal side effects.

Menstrual irregularity, mostly prolonged spotting, is common in the first few months after LNG IUS insertion. From the fourth month onwards, however, a profound reduction in menstrual blood loss is typical, with up to 20% of women being amenorrhoeic by 12 months of use [32]. Dysmenorrhoea also improves or resolves completely. The amenorrhoea is the result of potent endometrial suppression; plasma oestradiol levels remain within the range for normal fertile women.

LNG IUS use results in increased haemoglobin and serum ferritin levels, and appears to have no significant effect on carbohydrate metabolism, the coagulation cascade, liver enzymes or serum lipid levels [21]. In addition, there is no effect on blood pressure and no objective evidence of weight gain.

The LNG IUS is suitable for almost all women wanting effective long-term contraception – women dissatisfied with their current method, or women unable or unwilling to use oral contraceptives. It is perhaps particularly suitable for women contemplating sterilization or those with heavy menstrual periods. The LNG IUS is particularly useful for women with relative or absolute contraindications to the combined oral contraceptive pill, such as diabetes, severe migraine, hypertension and smokers over 35 years. It is also often suitable for those with severe learning disorders or physical disabilities needing long-term contraception, as an alternative to sterilization.

The LNG IUS should be inserted during the first 7 days of a menstrual cycle and may be inserted immediately at a suction termination of pregnancy, but insertion is usually delayed for 6 weeks after term pregnancy to reduce the risk of prolonged bleeding. No problems have been reported in the infants of breastfeeding women.

The LNG IUS is being increasingly used in the treatment of menorrhagia. In women with menorrhagia, quantitative menstrual blood loss studies have shown a reduction in bleeding of up to 86% after 3 months and 97% after 12 months of LNG IUS use [32, 33]. These results are better than most other pharmacological treatments: whilst danazol and gonadotrophin-releasing hormone agonists are as effective as the LNG IUS in inducing oligomenorrhoea, they induce hypo-oestrogenism and their distressing and potentially serious side effects preclude prolonged use. The LNG IUS represents a simple, effective and cheap treatment for menorrhagia, providing an alternative to both hysterectomy and endometrial ablation/resection with the advantage that it preserves fertility.

A very promising future indication for the LNG IUS is endometrial protection during oestrogen replacement in both perimenopausal and postmenopausal women. Used with oral, transdermal or implanted oestrogen, climacteric symptoms are effectively relieved by the oestrogen, the endometrium is protected from proliferation, women experience few progestogen-related symptoms and many women achieve amenorrhoea, with others having a bleeding pattern typical of continuous combined preparations (period-free but not bleed-free). Other potential applications include the treatment of endometrial hyperplasia, the prevention of tamoxifen-induced endometrial hyperplasia and the management of severe premenstrual syndrome in conjunction with oestradiol implants or continuous high-dose oestradiol skin patches.

Tips for safe practice

IUD insertion should always be carried out in a calm, relaxed, unhurried atmosphere with a gentle reassuring approach to the patient at all times. With patients in whom one might anticipate adverse reactions, oral diazepam 2 mg and/or mefenamic acid 500 mg 1 hour beforehand may help. In such patients, the clinician should also have a low threshold for administering local anaesthetic.

It is essential to know the position of the uterus prior to insertion of an IUD, to sound the uterus to determine the direction of the uterine cavity and to stabilize the cervix with a tenaculum during insertion. The application of traction to the cervix is important in order to straighten the cervicouterine angle and ease the device placement; there is no evidence that it reduces the risk of perforation [19]. If the fundus is not felt with the end of the introducer as the stop arrives at the external os, the introducer and device should be removed and the situation reassessed.

Procedures that minimize the chance of pelvic infection are:

- taking a careful sexual history relating to STIs and performing a pelvic examination

- screening as indicated by the risk profile

- using a meticulous aseptic no-touch technique

- using devices with a long life span to reduce the number of reinsertions.

The future

Intrauterine delivery of various medicinal/contraceptive products using IUDs is a real possibility following the success of the hormone-releasing systems. Enhancing safety through adoption of protocols for intrauterine instrumentation should restore confidence in current devices. The recognition that the efficacy of modern devices is comparable to sterilization should push intrauterine contraception to the top of the 'best–buy' contraceptive league.

Resource list

- Intrauterine devices. Technical and managerial guidelines for services. World Health Organization (WHO), 1997.

- Improving access to quality care in family planning. Medical eligibility criteria for contraceptive use. WHO, 1996.

- McIntosh N, Kinzie B, Blouse A (eds). IUD guidelines for family planning service providers: a problem solving reference manual. Baltimore: Johns Hopkins Program for International Education in Reproductive Health (JHPIEGO), 1993.

Appendix 1

Insertion technique for Gyne T 380 (TCu 380S) (see Figure 8.A1)

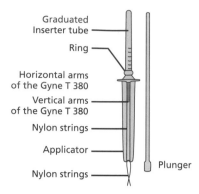

Graduated
Inserter tube

Ring

Horizontal arms
of the Gyne T 380

Vertical arms
of the Gyne T 380

Nylon strings

Applicator

Plunger

Nylon strings

1. Place Gyne T 380 device in introducer.

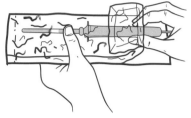

2. The sterile package should be opened on a flat surface to expose the bottom of the plunger and the bottom of the applicator. The plunger should be inserted carefully into the applicator tube until it is in contact with the lower part of the device. From outside the packaging, the ring is moved forward with one hand whilst pulling the applicator back with the other hand. The upper part of the ring should be positioned at the sounding distance.

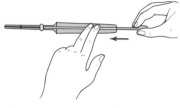

3. The package should be opened completely and the plunger pressed on gently to introduce the Gyne T 380 into the inserter tube. The upper part of the Gyne T 380 must emerge approximately 2 mm from the inserter tube. The arms of the 'T' should not be bent more than 5 minutes before it is to be introduced into the uterus.

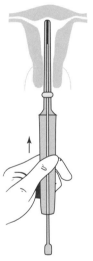

4. The inserter tube should be introduced gently through the cervical canal into the uterine cavity until the Gyne T 380 is in contact with the uterine fundus. (The ring of the inserter tube allows verification of the correct position of the IUD at the fundus.)

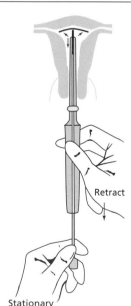

Retract

Stationary

5. The Gyne T 380 is released by retracting the applicator 2 cm while holding the plunger stationary. (This releases the horizontal arms without further upward movement of the device.)

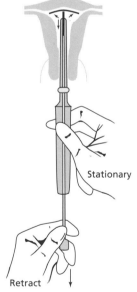

Stationary

Retract

Retract

6. The plunger and then the applicator should be retracted gently and the threads then cut to a length appropriate for checking the presence of the IUD.

7.

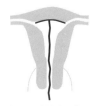

Gyne T 380 in place

Fig. 8.A1 Insertion technique for Gyne T 380 (see text).

Appendix 2

Insertion technique for levonorgestrel-releasing intrauterine system (Mirena®/Levonova®) (Figures 8.A2 and 8.A3)

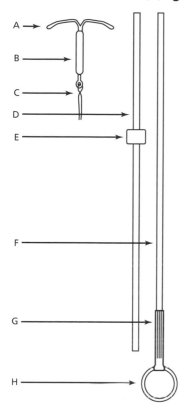

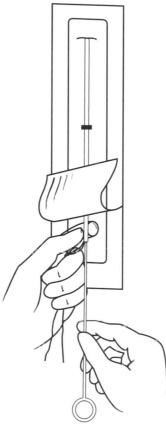

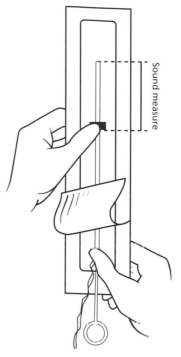

Fig. 8.A2   Instruments. A = horizontal arms; B = hormone cylinder; C = removal threads; D = insertion tube; E = flange; F = plunger; G = grooved part of the plunger; H = ring part of the plunger.

1. Open the plastic covering far enough to reveal the insertion tube. While keeping the removal threads stretched, place the plunger in the insertion tube.
2. Grasp the threads and pull the system *slowly and steadily* into the insertion tube until the knobs at the ends of the horizontal arms of the system cover the distal opening of the tube.

3. Steadying the flange with one hand, move the insertion tube until the distance between the tip of the loaded inserter and the edge of the flange nearest to the physician corresponds to the sound measure. Ensure that the flange is in the same plane as the arms will be when horizontal.

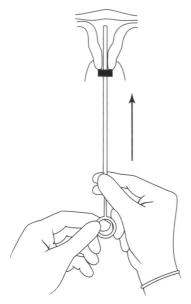
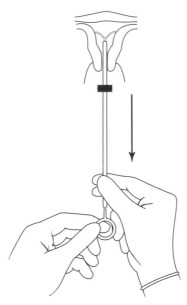
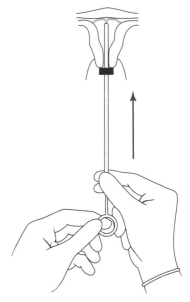

4. Remove the loaded system from the plastic cover and introduce the insertion tube gently into the cervical canal until the flange touches the cervix. The flange must be horizontal to ensure subsequent correct unfolding of the arms.

5. Note the grooved part on the plunger. Hold the plunger still and release the horizontal arms of the system by pulling the insertion tube only until the edge of the insertion tube reaches the grooved part.

6. Observe that the distance between the flange and external cervical os is now about 1.5 cm.

7. Holding the tube and plunger together, gently push the system until the flange again touches the cervix.

8. Release the system completely from the insertion tube by holding the plunger still and then pulling the tube until it touches the ring part of the plunger.

9. Remove the plunger by keeping the tube stationary and then carefully remove the tube. Make sure that the removal threads run freely through the tube and do not draw the system from its fundal position in the uterine cavity.

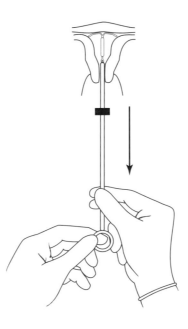

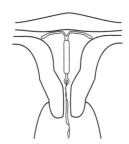

10. Cut the removal threads so that 2 cm remain visible outside the cervix.

Fig. 8.A2 Insertion technique for levonorgestrel-releasing intrauterine system (see text).

References

1. Tatum JH, Connell EB. Intrauterine contraceptive devices. In: Filshie M, Guillebaud J (eds) Contraception: science and practice. London: Butterworths, 1989;144–71.

2. Treiman K, Liskin L, Kols A, Rinehart W. IUDs – an update. *Pop Rep* 1995;Ser B, no. 6:1–35.

3. van Kets HE, Van der Pas H, Delbarge W, Thiery M. A randomised comparative study of the TCu380A and Cu-Safe 300 IUDs. *Adv Contracep* 1995; 11:123–9.

4. UNDP, UNFPA, World Health Organisation (WHO) Special Programmes of Research, World Bank: IUD Research Group. The TCu 380A IUD and the frameless IUD 'the FlexiGard': interim three-year data from an international multicenter trial. *Contraception* 1995;52:77–83.

5. Riphagen FE, Ketting E. Comparative overview of results from eight surveys on contraceptive behaviour. In:Ketting E (ed) Contraception in Western Europe. Carnforth, UK: Parthenon, 1990;77–110.

6. Rowlands O, Singleton N, Maher J, Higgins V. Contraception. In: Living in Britain. Results from the 1995 General Household Survey. London: Office for National Statistics, 1997:144 67.

7. WHO Scientific Group. Mechanisms of action, safety and efficacy of intrauterine devices. Tech Rep Ser 753. Geneva: World Health Organisation, 1987.

8. Alvarez F, Brache E, Fernandez E, et al. New insights on the mode of action of intrauterine contraceptive devices in women. *Fertil Steril* 1988;49:768–73.

9. Chi I. What we have learned from recent IUD studies: a researcher's perspective. *Contraception* 1993;48:81–108.

10. Newton J. IUD safety and acceptability: recent advances. *Curr Obstet Gynaecol* 1993; 3:28–36.

11. Trussell J, Ellerton C. Efficacy of emergency contraception. *Fertil Control Rev* 1995;4:8–11.

12. WHO Special Programme of Research. The Cu380A, T220C, Multiload 250 and Nova T IUDs at 3,5 and 7 years of use – results from three randomized multicentre trials. *Contraception* 1990;42:141–158.

13. United Nations Development Programme/United Nations Population Fund/WHO/World Bank. Long-term reversible contraception: twelve years of experience with the TCu380A and T220C. *Contraception* 1997;56:341–352.

14. Tietze C, Lewit S. Evaluation of intrauterine devices; ninth progress report of the cooperative statistical program. *Stud Fam Plann* 1970;55:1–40.

15. Sivin I. Dose and age dependent ectopic pregnancy risks with intrauterine contraception. *Obstet Gynecol* 1991;78:291–298.

16. Farley TNM, Rosenberg MJ, Rose PJ, et al. Intrauterine devices and pelvic inflammatory disease: an international perspective. *Lancet* 1992; 339:785–788.

17. Genc M, Mardh P-A. A cost-effectiveness analysis of screening and treatment for Chlamydia trachomatis infection in asymptomatic women. *Ann Intern Med* 1996;124:1–7.

18. Walsh T, Grimes D, Frezieres R, et al. Randomised controlled trial of prophylactic antibiotics before insertion of intrauterine devices. *Lancet* 1998;351:1005–1008.

19. Bromham DR. Intrauterine contraceptive devices – a reappraisal. In:Drife JO, Baird DT(eds) Contraception. Edinburgh: Churchill Livingstone, 1993;100–123.

20. Clinical and Scientific Committee Faculty of Family Planning & Reproductive Healthcare of the RCOG. Recommendations for clinical practice: *Actinomyces* like organisms and intrauterine contraceptives. *Br J Fam Plann* 1998;23:137–138.

21. Luukkainen T. Levonorgestrel-releasing intra-uterine device. *Ann NY Acad Sci* 1991; 626:43–9.

22. Silverberg S, Haukkamaa M, Arko H, et al. Endometrial morphology during long-term use of levonorgestrel-releasing devices. *Int J Gynecol Pathol* 1986;5:235–41.

23. Nilsson C, Pertti L, Lahteenmaki A, et al. Ovarian function in amenorrhoeic and menstruating users of a levonorgestrel-releasing device. *Fertil Steril* 1984;41:52–55

24. Nilsson CG, Lahteenmaki P, Luukkainen T. Levonorgestrel plasma concentrations and hormone profiles after insertion and after one year of treatment with a levonorgestrel-IUD. *Contraception* 1980;21:225–33

25. Xiao B, Zeng T, Shanchun W, et al. Effect of levonorgestrel releasing intrauterine device on hormonal profile and menstrual pattern after long-term use. *Contraception* 1995;51:359 365.

26. Andersson K, Batar I, Rybo G. Return to fertility after removal of a levonorgestrel-releasing intra-uterine device and Nova T. *Contraception* 1992;46:575–584.

27. Sivin I, Stern J, Couthino E, et al. Prolonged intrauterine contraception: a seven year randomized study of the levonorgestrel 20 mcg/day (LNg20) and the copper T380Ag IUDs. *Contraception* 1991;44:473–480.

28. Toivonen J, Luukkainen T, Allonen H. Protective effect of intrauterine release of levonorgestrel on pelvic infection: three years' comparative experience of levonorgestrel and copper releasing intrauterine devices. *Obstet Gynecol* 1991;77:261–4.

29. Sivin I, El-Mahgoub S, McCarthy T, et al. Long-term contraception with the levonorgestrel 20 μg/day (LNG

20) and the copper T380Ag
intra-uterine devices: a five year
randomised study. *Contraception*
1990;42:361–78.

30. Luukkainen T, Allonen H,
Haukkamaa M, et al. Five years'
experience with levonorgestrel
IUDs. *Contraception* 1986;
33:139–148.

31. Andersson K, Odlind V, Rybo
G. Levonorgestrel-releasing and
copper-releasing (Nova T) IUDs
during five years of use: a
randomised comparative trial.
Contraception 1994;49:56–72.

32. Scholten P, van Eykeren M,
Chrisiaens G, et al. Menstrual
blood loss with levonorgestrel,

Nova T and Multiload Cu 250
intrauterine devices. Thesis,
Utrecht University Hospital,
1989;35–45.

33. Andersson JK, Rybo G.
Levonorgestrel-releasing
intrauterine device in the
treatment of menorrhagia. *Br J
Obstet Gynaecol* 1990;97:690–4.

Male and female barriers

Jill L Schwartz MD
Mitchell D Creinin MD

Introduction

Throughout the history of contraception, methods have emerged into widespread use only to later be abandoned for newer methods. The common use of the condom in the USA declined in the early 1960s and 1970s as a result of the availability of oral contraception. A resurgence in interest in the condom occurred in the late 1980s owing to increased awareness of sexually transmitted diseases (STDs), driven by human immunodeficiency virus (HIV). Ironically, in our highly technologically advanced society, the oldest and simplest method, the condom, has come back into vogue. The need for a contraceptive that provides protection from STDs has brought both a renewed fervor and remarkable innovations to barrier contraceptive methods.

Not surprisingly, it is projected that the new millennium will witness the manufacture of 20 billion condoms a year of various types (including latex, lamb's intestine and polyurethane), different colors and textures (smooth and ribbed), and with and without lubricants. New forms of barrier methods include the female condom, which is manufactured in the UK, where it is known as Femidom®, and available in the United States as Reality® since 1993. New cervical caps under development include Lea®, available in Canada, Australia and Germany, and the Femcap™. Research is being conducted to develop better spermicides and microbicides, affording more options for protection against pregnancies and STDs. Nonetheless, there continue to be many unanswered questions about the ability of barrier methods to protect against pregnancy and STDs.

Usage of barrier methods

A 1990 worldwide estimate indicates that 5% (45 million) of all married couples, with a female spouse of reproductive age, use condoms as contraception [1]. In contrast, female-controlled barrier methods, such as spermicides and diaphragms, are used by 1% of married women of reproductive age. Direct estimates of how many condoms are used in the world, outside marriage, cannot be made because survey data are inadequate. However, the total number of condoms produced and estimated use by married couples produces a rough calculation that two-thirds of the six billion condoms produced in 1989 were used by unmarried couples.

Barrier methods are used by about 24% of contraceptors in the USA at risk for unintended pregnancy (Table 9.1). According to the 1995 National Survey of Family Growth (NSFG), the total number of condom users in the USA increased between 1988 and 1995 from 5 to 8 million [2]. The simultaneous decline in oral contraceptive use with the increased use of condoms suggest that HIV and other STDs have contributed to the changing patterns of method use among unmarried women. Young women and men concerned about STD transmission are dependent on barrier methods, but have lower efficacy rates than experienced married couples [1,3]. While increased frequency of intercourse and higher fecundity rates are possible explanations for lower efficacy of barrier methods among younger adults, incorrect use is equally suspect. Therefore, education remains an essential component to improve the efficacy of barrier methods.

Most barrier contraceptive methods such as the condom work by acting as a mechanical barrier and preventing sperm

Table 9.1 Percentage distribution and number of contraceptive users aged 15–44, by current method (USA)

Method	1988		1995	
	%	n(000)	%	n(000)
Widely used methods				
Sterilization (male and female)	39.2	13 686	38.6	14 942
OCPs	30.7	10 734	26.9	10 410
Total	69.9	24 420	65.5	25 352
Barrier methods				
Diaphragm	5.7	2000	1.9	720
Male condom[a]	14.6	5093	20.4	7889
Foam	1.1	371	0.4	161
Other[b]	2.1	733	1.3	508
Total	23.5	8197	24	9278
Total[c]	93.4	32 617	89.5	34 663

[a]If 'any' condom use at all is substituted for condom used as the 'primary' method of birth control, the proportion of condom users would rise from 20% to 23% (8 to 9 million).
[b]Includes douche, sponge, jelly or cream alone, and other methods.
[c]Excludes implants, injectable, IUD and withdrawal.
Adapted from Piccinino LJ, Mosher WD. Trends in contraceptive use in the United States: 1982–1995. *Fam Plann Perspect* 1998; 30: 4–10, 46.

from entering the uterus. The diaphragm and cervical cap are used with chemical barriers known as spermicides. Alternatively, spermicidal preparations can be used alone.

Barrier methods have several advantages. Condoms are easily accessible and available over the counter. Most barrier contraceptive devices are free of systemic effects and require use only at the time of intercourse. Other barrier methods such as the diaphragm and the cervical cap require clinician visits, and give varying protection against pregnancy and HIV but provide protection against cervical pathogens (Table 9.2). Women who have used barrier methods, including the condom, the diaphragm, the cervical cap, the sponge, and spermicide used alone or in conjunction with a barrier method, are half as likely to develop cervical cancer [4]. Similarly, women using condoms, spermicides or a diaphragms are at a reduced risk of high-grade cervical dysplasia [5].

The following will review the barrier methods currently available and highlight promising future methods under evaluation.

Efficacy and continuation rates of barrier methods

Contraceptive failure rates are most commonly reported as first-year failure rates, reflecting potential inexperience with a method in a general population of users. This group includes women and men who are both inexperienced and experienced with the method, who have varying incentives for preventing pregnancy, and who have different frequencies of intercourse and baseline rates of fecundity. The failure rate during perfect use is a measure of the inherent efficacy of the actual method with correct use, whereas typical-use failures will include the reality that these methods are sometimes incorrectly or inconsistently used.

In general, the large gap in failure rates between the typical use and the perfect use of barrier methods indicates that user failures are high (Table 9.3). Most failures appear to be associated with poor compliance or incorrect use [6]. The effectiveness of vaginal barrier contraceptives is dependent on user motivation and compliance in addition to the device effectiveness. The one-year continuation rates for barrier contraception for women in the USA range from 40 to 60% (Table 9.3). Contraceptive discontinuation rate in developing countries is high for condoms and vaginal methods. A component of

Table 9.2 Barriers and infection/neoplasia

Condition	Female-controlled barrier	Male condom
Chlamydial cervicitis	? reduced	Reduced
Gonococcal cervicitis	? reduced	Reduced
Trichomonas infection	? reduced	Reduced
Cervical cancer	Reduced (70%)	Reduced (50%)
Cervical intraepithelial neoplasia	Reduced	Reduced
Pelvic inflammatory disease	Reduced	Reduced
Urinary tract infection	Increased	No effect
Candidiasis	? increased	No effect
Bacterial vaginosis	? increased	No effect
Toxic shock syndrome	Increased	No effect
HIV	?? increased[a]	Reduced
HPV	No effect	? reduced
HSV	No effect	? reduced

HIV = human immunodeficiency virus; HPV = human papilloma virus; HSV = Herpes simplex virus.
[a]The female condom probably protective.

Table 9.3 First-year probability of failure for perfect-and typical-use life-table probability and continuation rates

	Perfect-use failure rate	Typical-use failure rate	One year continuation rates[a]
Latex male condoms[a] (non-spermicidal)	2%	12%	64%
Female condom[b]	5.1%	21.1%	
Diaphragm[c]	4–8%	13–17%	57%
Cervical cap[c]	10–13%	18%	63%
Today sponge[c]	11–12%	17%	53–60%
Spermicides[a] (foam and suppositories)	3%	21%	43%

[a]Trussell J, Hatcher RA, Cates W, Stewart FH, Kost K. Contraceptive failure in the United States: an update. *Stud Fam Plann* 1990;21:51–4.
[b]Trussell J, Sturgen K, Strickler J, Dominik R. Comparative contraceptive efficacy of the female condom and other barrier methods. *Fam Plann Perspect* 1994;26:66–72..
[c]Trussell J, Strickler J, Vaughan B. Contraceptive efficacy of the diaphragm, the sponge and the cervical cap. *Fam Plann Perspect* 1993;25:100–5.

the discontinuation rate in developing countries is due to method failure and subsequent pregnancy (Table 9.4).

Male barrier methods

Male condoms

The condom (Figure 9.1) is the only method of male contraception marketed around the world. When used consistently and correctly, latex condoms decrease the risk of STDs and unplanned pregnancy. Studies of serodiscordant couples indicate that using latex condoms substantially reduces the risk for male to female HIV transmission [7]. Although not failproof, male latex condoms are the gold

standard in barrier protection against gonorrhea, chlamydia and HIV infection.

Condoms, however, are often used inconsistently and incorrectly. In addition, some people have allergies to latex that in rare cases can be life-threatening. Lambskin condoms (natural skin) can be used in the setting of latex allergy; although these provide some protection against pregnancy, they have not been proven to provide an acceptable barrier against STDs. Two condoms made of polyurethane are available for people with allergies to latex who desire some protection against STDs: the female condom, Reality®, and a male condom, Avanti®.

The perfect-use failure rate of

the latex male condom is reported to be 2% and the typical use failure rate is closer to 12% [6]. Slippage and breakage rates of condoms are measures of condom performance that vary widely across studies (Figure 9.2). Latex condom performance in a controlled clinical trial indicated a total breakage rate of 0.28% (0.15–0.48%) and a complete condom slippage rate of 0.63% (0.42–0.90%) [8]. These rates are lower than other prospective studies, with clinical breakage rates between 0.5% and 3.7%, and complete slippage rates from 0.6% to 5.4%, but are consistent with a prospective study of sex workers in Nevada which indicated that condoms can provide excellent performance to motivated users [9]. Total breakage and slippage rates quoted have ranged widely from <1% to 14.6% [10].

The efficacy of condom used along with a separate spermicide has not been established in clinical trials. However, estimates of the probability of contraceptive efficacy of the simultaneous perfect use of condoms and spermicide using empirical information of independent efficacies have been calculated [11]. Based on these calculations, perfect use of condoms along with a separate spermicide yields a probability of failure of 0.05% per year, which would provide contraceptive protection at least as efficacious as combination oral contraceptives.

Tips for safe practice
Incorrect placement, such as unrolling before placement, stretching, or trying to unroll condoms with the rim held toward the body can tear

Table 9.4 Cumulative percentage discontinuing a method by 12 months, average for 11 developing countries

	Total	Due to contraceptive failure	Due to side effects
Vaginal methods (jelly, douche, and foam tablets)	68%	29.8%	9.4%
Condoms	64%	12.5%	3.2%

Adapted from The market for new contraceptives: translating unmet need into market demand. In: Harrison PF, Rosenfield A (eds) Contraceptive research and development: looking to the future. New York: Institute of Medicine, National Academy Press, 1996.

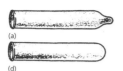 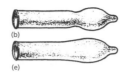 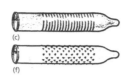

Fig. 9.1a Condom shapes and surfaces.
(a) Straight; (b) contoured; (c) ribbed;
(d) plain ended (no teat); (e) flared;
(f) dotted.

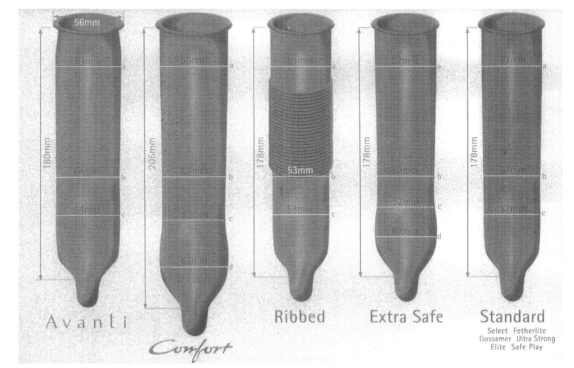

Fig. 9.1b Durex condoms. Size and shape chart. Published with permission of London International Group.

condoms [1]. The most frequently used techniques to prevent breakage include:

- careful handling of the condom;

- placing the condom on the penis after erection and before any genital contact;

- monitoring the condom throughout intercourse, immediate withdrawal post-ejaculation and holding on to the rim of the condom during withdrawal;

- ensuring proper condom use by using additional water-based lubricants as needed. In a case–control study of 525 university students presenting for postcoital contraception and 481 controls, the use of water-based lubricants was associated with a significant reduction in condom 'failure' with no increase in slippage rates [13].

- avoiding expired, dry or brittle condoms;

- leaving space at condom tips [1,9,12].

Principles of counseling

- Discuss the relative effectiveness of condoms in the context of the patient's own risk of failure, taking into account frequency of intercourse, age and other personal factors.

- See that users get an adequate supply of condoms and know where to get more.

- Help users make correct condom use a comfortable, routine part of sexual intercourse.

- Teach the physical skills of condom use by practicing on models.

- Teach the social skills to negotiate male partner usage [14].

- Accurately answer questions and dispel myths and rumors.

- Make sure that the condom users are aware of emergency

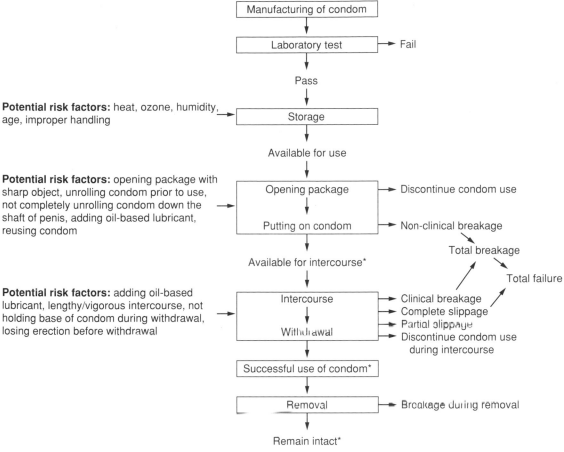

Fig. 9.2 Condom breakage and slippage flow chart. *A small proportion of these may actually be unreported or undetected breaks.

contraception and know how to obtain it if the condom slips, breaks or is not used.

Remember that latex rubber is weakened by ozone, oil-based lubricants (Box 9.1), high temperature, excessive moisture and sunlight.

Male polyurethane condoms

Condoms made of synthetic materials other than latex have been developed. Polyurethane is odorless and transparent, and withstands oil-based lubricants and storage better than latex.

Since it is stronger than latex, the condom can be thinner, allowing for potentially greater sensitivity and comfort. Data assessing polyurethane condom protection against STDs and HIV *in vivo* are lacking, although laboratory studies indicate that polyurethane blocks microbes [15]. A randomized, controlled, cross-over trial comparing Avanti® to latex condoms found a clinical breakage rate of the polyurethane condom of 7.2% compared to 1.1% for the latex condom (RR = 6.6, CI 3.5–12.3) [16]. The complete slippage rate of the polyurethane condom was 3.6% compared with 0.6% for the latex condom (RR = 6, CI 2.6–14.2)

Box 9.1 Commonly used medicinal and non-medicinal preparations that damage latex barriers

- Baby oil/bath oil/body oil/Vaseline
- Cold cream/suntan oil/massage oil
- Cream/ice cream/salad cream
- Lipstick/hair conditioner
- Premarin cream/Dienestrol/Estriol pessaries
- Nystatin cream
- Many anticandidal preparations
- Clindamycin cream
- Progesterone pessaries

However, male users preferred the sensitivity provided by the polyurethane condom to the latex condom [16,17]. Although the clinical breakage and slippage rate is significantly higher compared to latex condoms, polyurethane condoms provide an alternative for couples who have an allergy to latex products or find traditional condoms unsuitable.

Female-controlled barrier methods

Female-controlled methods that are available include the female condom, diaphragm, cervical cap, contraceptive sponge and spermicides. In the UK, latex vimule and vault caps are also available. 'Female-controlled' refers to methods intended primarily for vaginal use potentially without a partner's knowledge. The data available on the relative efficacy of the sponge, cervical cap and diaphragm during typical use are comparative and useful because they are derived from two clinical trials conducted in the USA in which women were randomly assigned to use either the sponge versus the diaphragm or the cervical cap versus the diaphragm (Table 9.3) [18]. The clinical trial of the Reality® female condom did not include comparisons with other barrier methods. However, comparing studies of the contraceptive efficacy of other barrier methods, the efficacy of the female condom during typical use is similar to that of the diaphragm, the sponge or the cervical cap in the USA [19]. Spermicides alone are considered less effective than other barrier methods but have not been studied adequately.

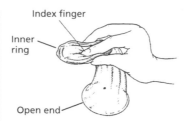

Fig. 9.3 Female condom (Reality®/Femidom®): mode of insertion and structure.

Female condoms

The female condom (Figures 9.3 and 9.4), Reality®/Femidom®, consists of a soft, prelubricated and loose-fitting, 17 cm-long polyurethane sheath with two flexible polyurethane rings. The free ring inside the closed end is used for introduction into the vagina similar to the diaphragm. The attached outer ring rests on the labia covering the external genitalia, potentially reducing genital contact between partners. Many participants in clinical trials reported that they liked the female condom and would recommend it to others [20]. Complaints included dislike of the inner ring, a 'rustling noise' during use, inconvenience and messiness. Non-compliance was due mostly to partner objection, occasional negligence and discomfort using the device. There are no data available to

Fig. 9.4 Female condom (Reality®/Femidom®) *in situ.*

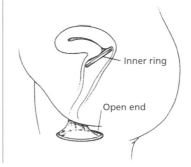

document STD protection *in vivo*. Additionally, the female condom costs approximately 3–4 times more than the male latex condom.

Since the female condom can be inserted in advance of sexual activity, it enables uninterrupted intercourse and allows for intercourse before full erection of the penis. It is a more extensive physical barrier than male condoms, since it covers both the internal and external genitalia of the female, and the base of the penis, theoretically offering more protection against STDs. Leakage studies suggest that Reality® is less prone to leakage than latex male condoms [21].

A female condom not yet available, the Bikini Condom, is made of latex, worn like a panty, and a lubricated rolled portion is pushed into the vagina at the time of intercourse, forming a loose-fitting vaginal liner which is twice as thick as a male condom [22,23]. Another product called Women's Choice, a latex sheath that has an outer ring at the open end and a pleated tip at the inner end that expands when the device is in place, is also in the development stages [22,23].

Principles of counseling

- Discuss the relative effectiveness of female condom use in the context of the patient's own risk of failure, taking into account frequency of intercourse, age and other personal factors.

- Insert inner ring high in the vagina, against the cervix with the outer ring properly outside the vagina.

- During intercourse, be sure that the penis is placed inside the female condom.

- They can be used by a woman who is pregnant or menstruating, but not by a woman who has a tampon inserted.

- They should not be used simultaneously with male condoms because they may stick together.

- The noise during use can be reduced by applying additional lubricant.

- Possibly less effective than latex male condoms against STDs.

- Make sure that the condom user is aware of emergency contraception and knows how to obtain it if the female condom slips, breaks or is not used.

Diaphragm

The diaphragm is a dome-shaped latex contraceptive device used in conjunction with spermicides, with a rim made of flexible metal. It is available in a wide range of sizes, the most common being 65–80 mm in rim diameter. The three types of rims (flat spring, coil spring and arcing spring) are suitable for different women (Figure 9.5). The arcing-spring diaphragm assumes an arch shape when folded in half and it is easier for women to insert because the curve helps guide the diaphragm behind the symphysis and over the cervix. Its ease of insertion allows for successful use even by women with relaxed vaginal muscle tone, with cytoceles and

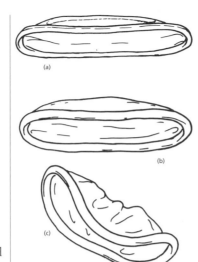

Fig. 9.5 Diaphragms: (a) Flat spring; (b) coil spring; (c) arcing spring.

rectoceles, and with retroverted uteri. The coil spring folds in one plane and is more suitable for women with average vaginal muscle tone and an average pubic arch. The flat spring has a gentle spring which is well suited for nulliparous women with strong vaginal muscle tone or a shallow pubic arch.

Women may choose a diaphragm because it is non-systemic and non-invasive, used only when required but, unlike male condoms, does not interrupt intercourse. It allows intercourse during menstruation. It may reduce the risk of pelvic infection and cervical neoplasia.

The typical-use one-year efficacy rate of the diaphragm ranges from 83% to 87% (Table 9.3). In a retrospective study conducted in Brazil, adjuvant spermicide use with the diaphragm did not significantly improve effectiveness compared to diaphragm use alone [24]. A fit-free diaphragm used without spermicide was developed in London with a high continuation rate but a typical-use failure rate of 24% [25]. Since spermicides may also act as microbicides, and until better data conclusively refute traditional recommendations, the use of spermicides with the diaphragm should not be abandoned. A diaphragm made of silicone has been developed that is worn continuously, removed for washing and available in different colors [22]. Robust documentation of the efficacy of this method is lacking.

Side effects

The risk of toxic shock syndrome is increased with female barrier methods such as the diaphragm and sponge [26]. Because the actual incidence is so rare, only women who have had toxic shock syndrome should be advised to avoid barrier methods. Urinary tract infections (UTIs) are almost twice as common among diaphragm users compared to oral contraception users [27]. While in the past this was attributed solely to pressure of the diaphragm on the urethra, there is recent evidence that spermicides used alone may also affect this risk by changing the normal vaginal flora and increasing the ability of uropathogens to adhere to vaginal epithelial cells [28,29].

Tips for safe practice

Successful use of the conventional diaphragm is dependent upon proper fitting by the clinician, and the ability of the patient to insert and remove the diaphragm correctly. The diaphragm should fit between the pubic symphysis and the posterior fornix. The largest size that is comfortable, does not cause pelvic pressure for the patient and does not come out with bearing down should be chosen. A size that is too small may not cover the cervix during intercourse and a size that is too large may cause discomfort. The patient needs to demonstrate that she can insert and remove the diaphragm, and verify that it is covering her cervix to assure proper placement.

Principles of counseling

- Discuss the relative effectiveness of the diaphragm in the context of the patient's own risk of failure, taking into account the frequency of intercourse, age and other personal factors.

- Place the device all the way against the cervix with the cavity containing the spermicidal cream or jelly covering the cervical opening, and make certain the cervix is completely covered.

- Leave in place at least 6 h after the last act of intercourse, but no more than 24 h in total.

- Additional spermicide should be placed in the vagina before each additional episode of intercourse while the diaphragm is in place.

- Instructing patients to void prior to and after sexual intercourse may be helpful in avoiding urinary discomfort.

- Contrary to popular belief, refitting is not necessary following a weight change or pregnancy, unless the patient recognizes a change in fit or experiences a pregnancy with correct diaphragm usage.

- The diaphragm may be used during menses but must be removed 6 h after intercourse in this case.

- Since the diaphragm might not protect against HIV, it may not be an appropriate method for at-risk women.

- Make sure that the diaphragm user is aware of emergency contraception and knows how to obtain it if the diaphragm malfunctions, is used incorrectly or is not used.

- Remember that latex rubber is weakened by ozone, oil-based lubricants (Box 9.1), high temperature, excessive moisture and sunlight.

Cervical cap

The Prentif™ cavity rim cervical cap was approved for use in the USA in 1988. It is made of latex and is designed to fit snugly over the cervix. It only comes in four sizes with diameters of 22, 25, 28 and 31 mm. Protection against STDs has not been studied. The typical use efficacy is 82%, which is similar to the diaphragm (Table 9.3). There is a higher pregnancy rate for parous compared to nulliparous women [18]. In addition, the cap is more difficult to fit and to situate over the cervix than the diaphragm. If the cervix is very posterior, there is a risk of dislodgement of the cap during intercourse. In a large clinical trial, 10% of subjects could not be fitted [30].

Other caps

The vault (Dumas) is a semicircular, shallow-domed cap

that fits over a 'short' cervix with 'suction' by the vaginal vault. The vimule cap has a thinner rim and therefore greater suction and can accommodate a 'longer' cervix. Both, as well as the cervical cap, may be used in women with poor pelvic muscles or a lax vagina. The Ovis cervical cap is a silicone-rubber, disposable, cervical cap that can be left *in situ* for up to 48 h. It comes in three sizes only (26, 28 and 30 mm). It is not to be used during menstruation. The dome is designed to allow the cervix to be unrestricted. A loop at the rim facilitates removal. Efficacy data are limited.

Figure 9.6 shows a variety of cervical barriers.

Side effects

UTIs occurred with similar frequency in users of both the cervical cap and the diaphragm [31]. Since the cap does not compress the urethra, and both the cervical cap and the diaphragm are used with spermicides, this further implicates spermicides in the pathogenesis of bacteriuria. An increased frequency of abnormal cervical cytology in users of the Prentif™ cavity rim cervical cap compared to the diaphragm has been documented [32]. The difference in abnormal cytology rates is more likely to reflect risk factors which are well known to be difficult to control for. No study has demonstrated that this observation translates to an increase in significant cervical dysplasia or progression to cancer.

Tips for safe practice

Since a common problem associated with failure of the

Fig. 9.6   Cervical barriers: (a) diaphragm; (b) cervical cap; (c) vimule; (d) vault cap (Dumas).

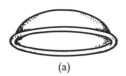

(a)

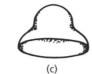

(c)

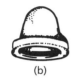

(b)

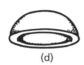

(d)

cervical cap is dislodgement, correct fitting of the cervical cap is essential. The cervix must be symmetrical, uniformly shaped and long enough to secure the cervical cap. Insertion is achieved by squeezing the cap dome, sliding the cap into the vagina and pressing the rim around the cervix. The unfolding dome creates a suction between the cap rim and the cervix. The circumference of the cap should be swept with one finger to be certain that there are no gaps between the cap rim and the cervix. The cap should be pinched gently for evidence of an adequate suction and probed with a finger tip to assess if it is too easily dislodged. To remove the cap, press on the rim until the seal is broken and tilt the cap to hook index fingers under the rim and pull sideways out of the vagina.

Principles of counseling

- Discuss the relative effectiveness of the cervical cap in the context of the patient's own risk of failure, taking into account the frequency of intercourse, age, parity and other personal factors.

- Before inserting, the cervical cap should be filled one-third full with spermicidal cream or jelly.

- The cervical cap must be left in place for 8 h after the last act of intercourse and can be left in place for up to 48 h.

- Although it can stay in place for 48 h this may lead to a bad odor in some women.

- The US FDA currently recommends a follow-up visit at 3 months of cap use for a Pap smear.

- Refitting may be necessary following childbirth, miscarriage or pregnancy termination, owing to a change in the cervical architecture.

- Since the cervical cap might not protect against HIV, it may not be an appropriate method for at-risk women.

- Make sure that the diaphragm user is aware of emergency contraception and knows how to obtain it if the diaphragm malfunctions, is used incorrectly or is not used.

- Remember that latex rubber is weakened by ozone, oil-based lubricants (Box 9.1), high temperature, excessive moisture and sunlight.

Contraceptive sponge

The Protectaid® sponge (Figure 9.7) is available over the counter in Canada and Hong Kong. It is made of polyurethane foam, and theoretically acts as a mechanical barrier both blocking and absorbing semen. In addition, its innovation lies in its role as a chemical barrier through the combination of three active spermicides rather than one, which enables lower concentrations of each compound to be used. It contains F-5 gel®, a combination of sodium cholate (supposed to have antiviral properties), nonoxynol-9 (N-9) and benzalkonium chloride, and a dispersing agent, polydimethyl siloxane, that helps diffuse the gel and forms a protective coating over the entire vaginal mucosa. The sponge comes ready to use with two finger slots in the sponge's matrix to facilitate insertion and removal. In a small study of 20 women, the sponge was 100% effective during 12 months of use

Fig. 9.7   Protectaid® sponge. With permission from Axcan Ltd, Canada.

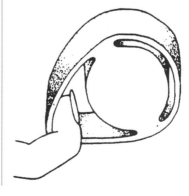

[33]. There is some controversy as to whether the sponge acts independently as a barrier method or is solely a reservoir for holding spermicide over the cervical os. Studies comparing the efficacy of sponges with and without spermicides have not been conducted. The Pharmatex® sponge containing a cream with 60 mg of benzalkonium chloride is available in Europe [34].

Side effects

The three spermicides combined used in low concentrations minimize the risk of cervico-vaginal irritation. In contrast to the Today® sponge, which was available in the USA until 1995 and contained 1000 mg of N-9 (releasing 150 mg of N-9), there is 25 mg of N-9 spermicide in Protectaid®, a substantially lower dosage. In a study evaluating the association between spermicide use and HIV infection, 138 Nairobi sex workers were randomized to use sponges containing 1000 mg of N-9 versus a placebo and were encouraged to use condoms. Despite equivalent condom usage, contraceptive sponge users had a higher rate of HIV infection (45%) compared to placebo users (36%), although this difference was not statistically significant (hazard ratio = 1.7, 95% CI 0.9–3.0) [35]. In studies, women who used the new Protectaid® sponge for up to 1 year had no signs of cervico-vaginal irritation [15].

Principles of counseling

- Discuss the relative effectiveness of the sponge in the context of the patient's own risk of failure, taking into account the frequency of intercourse, age, parity and other personal factors.

- To insert the sponge, the patient should be instructed to place the index finger into the slots and push the sponge into place as deeply as possible inside the vagina.

- The sponge should not be left in place for more than 12 h (these time limits depend on the licence conditions of the product and vary in different countries). Intercourse may be repeated during a 12-h period without changing or removing the sponge, which must be left in place at least 6 h after the last act of intercourse.

- In the unlikely case that the sponge starts to fall out, the patient should insert her finger into the vagina and push it back inside. If it falls out entirely, then immediately insert a new sponge.

- Make sure that the sponge user is aware of emergency contraception and knows how to obtain it if the sponge malfunctions, is used incorrectly or is not used.

Spermicides

Modern spermicides are produced in a variety of formulations, including gels, foams, creams, suppositories, foaming tablets and films. Spermicides are relatively inexpensive and available over the counter. All of the currently available preparations contain a chemical agent or detergent (nonoxynol-9, octoxynol, benzalkonium chloride) which disrupts the sperm cell membrane, and a vehicle or base compound that carries the spermicide. Most spermicides marketed in the USA and Europe contain N-9 at concentrations ranging from 2% to 28% and dosage from 70 mg to 150 mg [36]. Spermicides are locally applied and have no known systemic effects. An extensive review indicates that the use of vaginal spermicides during pregnancy is not associated with congenital anomalies [37]. Vaginal contraceptive film (VCF[USA] or C-Film [Europe]) is perceived as a less 'messy' spermicide. It must be placed high in the vagina at least 5 and preferably 10 min before intercourse. It remains effective for 1 h and the user should not 'douche' for 6 h after intercourse. Its appearance (like a thin plastic membrane) may be an advantage or disadvantage depending on the user. Accurate placement of the film is an issue difficult to monitor and account for in trials.

Many studies have suggested that spermicides containing N-9 provide some protection against gonorrhea and *Chlamydia* cervical infections in women [38,39]. These studies are fraught with serious methodological problems, and do not sufficiently answer the question of whether or not spermicides provide a reasonable amount of protection from STDs [40]. In a double-blind placebo-controlled study of 1292 women, N-9 vaginal film did not reduce the rate of new HIV, gonorrhea or *Chlamydia* infections [41]. Moreover, N-9, the most commonly used spermicide, is a detergent; in addition to killing sperm and micro-organisms, it can irritate the cervico-vaginal epithelium possibly leading to more STD transmission [42,43].

A notable disadvantage of spermicides is that they are less effective in preventing pregnancy compared to other contraceptive methods (Tables 9.3 and 9.4). In addition, a wide variability of efficacy can be attributed to different doses and formulations of spermicides studied, and difference in the study population with respect to fecundity and compliance. Moreover, there have been no clinical trials of spermicide efficacy that meet modern standards of design, execution and analysis. There are neither comparative studies nor reliable estimates of the effectiveness of spermicides. To address this deficiency, a multicenter study to determine the effectiveness, safety and acceptability of five marketed spermicide products is currently under way.

Reformulation of proven spermicidal agents into new products that are less irritating to the vaginal mucosa, provide a more extensive coating of the cervix and vagina, and have a longer duration of action, is being explored. New substances that hold promise as new base compounds include hydrogels or substances with bioadhesive capabilities [44].

Principles of counseling

- Discuss the relative effectiveness of spermicides in the context of the patient's own risk of failure, taking into account the frequency of intercourse, age and other personal factors.

- If used as the primary method of contraception, the spermicidal preparation must be used with each and every act of intercourse to be effective.

- There are many spermicide preparations available. It is important to stress that spermicides used with barrier methods can be different from those that are effective when used alone.

- The spermicide must be placed high in the vagina covering the cervix. Foams, jellies and creams used with an applicator must also be inserted far into the vagina.

- Foams, jellies and creams are effective as soon as inserted and can be inserted up to 1 h prior to intercourse. Suppositories, tablets and films require 5–15 min to dissolve before intercourse. Most are effective for 1–2 h.

- Until proven efficacious, spermicides should optimally be used with another barrier method.

- Make sure that the spermicide user is aware of emergency contraception and knows how to obtain it if the spermicide is used incorrectly or is not used.

Future prospects and developments in barrier contraceptives

Female-controlled barrier contraceptive methods all have characteristics which may reduce their acceptability to women. Several promising innovations are under evaluation. Both Lea® and

FemCap™ are newly tested cervical caps which are unlikely to provide complete protection against viral infections, such as HIV, but may provide protection against cervical pathogens, such as gonorrhea and *Chlamydia*, as the diaphragm does. Both are designed to conform better to female anatomy and to lessen the pressure on the urethra. Additionally, a wide variety of microbicides promise protection against STDs.

Lea®

Lea® is a cervical cap (Figure 9.8) made of silicone rubber, a material more durable than latex that is tolerant of heat, light, chemicals, oil-based lubricants and cleaning procedures [45]. It comes in one size that covers the cervix of most women, is intended for use with spermicide and can be worn for up to 48 h. Two novel features include a one-way valve that prevents the trapping of air and cervical secretions between the cervix and the device, and creates a suction that holds the device in place, and an anterior loop for ease of insertion and removal. In addition, a thicker posterior section is designed to fill the posterior vaginal fornix and hold the device in place, by its volume not its diameter. The valve can also act as an egress for menstrual flow; yet, because of the theoretical risk of toxic shock syndrome, it is not currently recommended for use during menstruation.

Lea® is available in a single size, potentially making it suitable for over-the-counter use. In a multicenter clinical trial, the

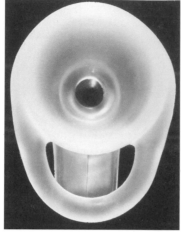

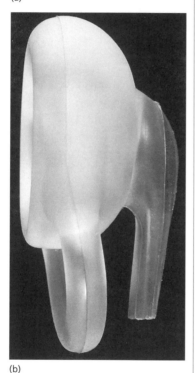

(a)

(b)

Fig. 9.8 Lea® cap/shield. (a) front view;
(b) side view.

6-month life-table pregnancy rate
was 8.7% when used with
spermicides [46]. Those who used
the device without spermicide
experienced almost twice as many
pregnancies. This study, although
not a direct comparison, indicates
that the contraceptive efficacy of
Lea® is comparable with other
barrier methods. Lea® did not
adversely affect cervical cytology,
there were no serious adverse
experiences, and the device was
very acceptable to women and
men.

FemCap™

The FemCap™ (Figure 9.9), is
also made of silicone rubber, has
the shape of a sailor's hat with a
dome that covers the cervix, a
rim that fits snugly into the
fornices, and a brim that adheres
and conforms to the vaginal
walls. The device is manufactured
in three sizes based on obstetrical
history: 24 mm for nulliparous
women, 28 mm for women who
have not had a full-term vaginal
delivery, and 32 mm for parous
women. A spermicide is applied
to the cap and it is positioned
over the cervix. The device can
be left in place up to 48 h and

Fig. 9.9 FemCap™ (second generation).
With permission from Femcap
Incorporated.

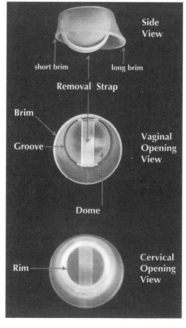

should remain in place at least 8 h
after intercourse.

In a small clinical trial of 121
subjects, the 1 year life-table
pregnancy rate of the FemCap™
was 4.8% with standard error of
2.1% [47]. However, in a larger
multi-center clinical trial, the 6-
month pregnancy rate was 13.5%
among FemCap™ users
compared to 7.9% among
diaphragm users. In general,
study participants reported higher
satisfaction with the FemCap™
than with their previous
contraceptive methods, including
women who had previous
experience with the diaphragm
or Prentif cervical cap [48].
Although difficulty in inserting
and removing the device was
reported as the aspect least liked
about the FemCap™, a new
model with the addition of a
removal strap may prove easier to
use.

Microbicides

A new area of barrier method
research is the development of
novel microbicides, which are
substances that can inhibit or
destroy bacteria, viruses and
protozoa. While male latex
condoms are currently the gold
standard against which other
barriers must be tested, many
women are unable to negotiate
condom use even if their partners
are at risk or infected.
Development of an effective
female-controlled microbicide
would provide an alternative way
to protect women against sexually
transmitted diseases (STDs) that is
invisible to a partner, eliminating
the need to negotiate for safe sex.
Another challenge is the
development of a microbicide

that prevents diseases but does not act as a spermicide.

While studies demonstrate that N-9 rapidly inactivates HIV *in vitro*, *in vivo* studies have been less conclusive [1]. A non-randomized cohort study among 273 sex workers in Cameroon found a protective effect of spermicide use against HIV [49,50]. Other data on female sex workers in Kenya found that sponges containing higher dosages did not protect against HIV [35]. Assessing genital irritation by colposcopy following N-9 use indicates that frequent doses of N-9 increase epithelial disruption on the vaginal and cervix [42,43]. The detergent effect of N-9 may act to disrupt vaginal epithelium, possibly increasing the risk of HIV transmission.

Determining whether existing spermicidal products reliably protect against STDs and HIV, and at what dosages they are most effective, are important research priorities of the turn of the 21st century. Potential new chemical

Table 9.5 Conventional and novel spermicides and microbicides

Agent	Mode of action	Characteristics	Potential microbicide	Spermicide
Nonoxynol-9, menfegol, octoxynol (non-ionic detergent)	Surfactant that disrupts cellular membranes	At high doses can cause cervico-vaginal irritation	Yes	Yes
Benzalkonium chloride (cationic disinfectant)	Surfactant that disrupts cellular membranes	At high doses can cause cervico-vaginal irritation	Yes	Yes
Cholic acid	Natural biodetergent	Found in human uterine fluid	Yes	Yes
Chlorhexidine (antiseptic)	Surface active leading to altered permeability; disrupts envelope	Diffuses into cervical mucus, allowing more time for action	Yes Viricidal (enveloped)	Yes
C31G (amphoteric surfactant)	Similar to other detergents; less irritating to epithelium	Substance in mouth wash; diffuses into cervical mucus	Yes	Yes
Buffer gels	Lowers pH in vagina. Acidity inactivates HIV, HIV-infected leukocytes and sperm	Odorless, colorless and inexpensive; affects acid-intolerant bacteria not lactobacilli	Yes	Yes
Lactobacilli	Secrete lactic acid or hydrogen peroxide; maintain low pH	Maintains normal vaginal ecology	Yes	No
Natural antimicrobial peptides (Squalamine)	Inhibits the sodium hydrogen exchange on cell surface – stops cell growth	Prolonged duration of activity and well tolerated	Yes	Yes
Plant extracts (Praneem)	Membrane active; immunomodulatory activity	Unacceptable odor and difficulty dissolving in the vagina	Yes Viricidal (enveloped)	Yes
Sulfated polysaccharides	Coats epithelial surface of vagina with a film that repels HIV, HIV-infected cells and *Chlamydia*	Forms natural gel; may produce less irritation than currently available spermicides	Yes	No
N-Docosanol (alcohol)	Inhibits lipid-enveloped viruses	Antiviral activity, possible topical treatment for HSV	Yes Viricidal (enveloped)	Yes
Milk fatty acids	Lipophilic molecules have microbicidal activity	Found in human milk	Yes	Yes
Serine proteinase inhibitors (aryl 4-guanidino-benzoates)	Inhibit sperm penetration through zona pellucida; inhibit HIV replication	Inhibit replication without cytotoxicity	Yes	Yes
Peroxidases	Membrane active	Affects peroxide-intolerant bacteria not lactobacillus	Yes	Yes
Monoclonal antibodies	Can serve as natural protective agents for mucosal surfaces	Expected to be potent, flexible, specific, sturdy and inexpensive	Yes	Yes

HIV = human immunodeficiency virus; HSV = Herpes simplex virus.
Adapted from Zaneveld LJD, Anderson KJ, Whaley KJ. Part I: Barrier Methods. In: Harrison PF, Rosenfield A (eds) Contraceptive Research and Development: Looking for the Future. New York: National Academy Press, and Alexander N. Barriers to sexually transmitted diseases. *Sci Am Sci Med* 1996;3:32–41.

barriers (Table 9.5) include the development of preparations that can maintain vaginal acidity even in the presence of semen and cervical mucus to provide high buffer capacity [51].

Tactylon condoms

Latex allergy is an increasingly serious problem. Like polyurethane, Tactylon is a non-latex synthetic polymer from which hypoallergenic surgical gloves are made. Tactylon is more resistant to heat and ozone, and would be expected to have a longer shelf-life than latex condoms.

Conclusion

The current medical climate has focused the spotlight on barrier contraceptives. New physical and chemical barrier methods are being investigated to meet the needs of contraceptive users. To address unanswered questions, more rigorous studies on old methods and the development of novel methods may help to prevent both unplanned pregnancies and STDs more effectively in the future.

References

1. Liskin L, Wharton C, Blackburn R. Condoms – now more than ever. *Pop Rep* 1990; Ser H(8):1–36.

2. Piccinino LJ, Mosher WD. Trends in contraceptive use in the United States: 1982–1995. *Fam Plann Perspect* 1998;30:4–10, 46.

3. Vessey MP, Villiard-Mackintosh L, McPherson K, Yeates D. Factors Influencing use-effectiveness of the condom. *Br J Fam Plann* 1988;14:40–3.

4. Kost K, Forrest JD, Harlap S. Comparing the health risks and benefits of contraceptive choices. *Fam Plann Perspect* 1991;23:54–61.

5. Coker AL, Hulka BS, McCann MF, Walton LA. Barrier methods of contraception and cervical intraepithelial neoplasia. *Contraception* 1992;45:1–10.

6. Trussell J, Hatcher RA, Cates W, Stewart FH, Kost K. Contraceptive failure in the United States: an update. *Stud Fam Plann* 1990;21:51–4.

7. Saracco A, Musicco M, Nicolosi A, et al. Man-to-women sexual transmission of HIV: longitudinal study of 343 steady partners of infected men. *J Acquired Immune Defic Synd* 1993;6:497–502.

8. Rosenberg MJ, Waugh MS. Latex condom breakage and slippage in a controlled clinical trial. *Contraception* 1997;56:17–21.

9. Albert AA, Warner DL, Hatcher RA, Trussell J, Bennett C. Condom use among female commercial sex workers in Nevada's legal brothels. *Am J Public Health* 1995;85:1514–20.

10. Trussell J, Warner DL, Hatcher RA. Condom slippage and breakage rates. *Fam Plann Perspect* 1992;25:20–23.

11. Kestelman P, Trussell J. Efficacy of the simultaneous use of condoms and spermicides. *Fam Plann Perspect* 1991;23:226–7, 232.

12. Centers for Disease Control Update. Barrier protection against hiv infection and other sexually transmitted diseases. *MMWR* 1993;42:589–91, 597.

13. Gabbay M, Gibbs A. Does additional lubrication reduce condom failure? *Contraception* 1996;53:155–8.

14. Albert AE, Warner DL, Hatcher RA. Facilitating condom use with clients during commercial sex in nevada's legal brothels. *Am J Public Health* 1998;88:643–6.

15. Future barrier methods. *Contracep Rep* 1997;8:9–13.

16. Frezieres RG, Walsh TI, Nelson AI, Clark VA, Coulson AH. Breakage and acceptability of a polyurethane condom: a randomized, controlled study. *Fam Plann Perspect* 1998; 30:73–8.

17. Rosenberg MJ, Waugh MS, Solomon HM, Lyszkowski DL. The male polyurethane condom: a review of current knowledge. *Contraception* 1996;53:141–6.

18. Trussell J, Strickler J, Vaughan B. Contraceptive efficacy of the diaphragm, the sponge and the cervical cap. *Fam Plann Perspect* 1993;25:100–5.

19. Trussell J, Sturgen K, Strickler J, Dominik R. Comparative contraceptive efficacy of the female condom and other barrier methods. *Fam Plann Perspect* 1994;26:66–72.

20. Farr G, Gabelnick H, Sturgen K, Dorflinger L. Contraceptive efficacy and acceptability of the female condom. *Am J Public Health* 1994;84:1960–4.

21. Leeper MA, Conrardy M. Preliminary evaluation of reality, a condom for women to wear. *Adv Contracept* 1989;5:229–35.

22. Family Health International. Barrier methods. *Network* 1996; 16(3).

23. Bounds W. Female condoms. *Eur J Contracept Reprod Health Care* 1997;2:113–6.

24. Ferreira AE, Araujo MJ, Regina CH, et al. Effectiveness of the diaphragm, used continuously without spermicide. *Contraception* 1993;48:29–35.

25. Smith C, Farr G, Feldblum PJ, Spence A. Effectiveness of the non-spermicidal fit-free diaphragm. *Contraception* 1995; 51:289–291.

26. Schwartz B, Gaventa S, Broome CV, et al. Nonmenstrual toxic shock syndrome associated with barrier contraceptives: report of a case-control study. *Rev Infect Dis* 1989; 2:S43–9.

27. Fihn SD, Latham RH, Roberts P, Running K, Stamm WE. Association between diaphragm use and urinary tract infection. *JAMA* 1985; 254:240–5.

28. Hooten TM, Hillier S, Johnson C, Roberts PL, Stamm WE. *Escherichia coli* bacteriuria and contraceptive method. *JAMA* 1991;265:64–9.

29. Hooton TM, Fennell CL, Clark AM, Stamm WE. Nonoxynol-9: differential antibacterial activity and enhancement of bacterial adherence to vaginal epithelial cells. *J Infect Dis* 1991;164:1216–9.

30. Richwald GA, Greenland S, Gerber M, et al. Effectiveness of the cavity-rim cervical cap: results of a large clinical study. *Obstet Gynecol* 1989;74:143–8.

31. Bernstein GS Cervical caps and female condoms. In: Fertility control, 2nd edn.: Goldin Publishers, 1985.

32. Gollub EL, Sivin I. The Prentif cervical cap and pap smear results: a critical appraisal. *Contraception* 1989;40:343–9.

33. Psychoyos A, Creatsas G, Hassan E. Spermicidal and antiviral properties of cholic acid: contraceptive efficacy of a new vaginal sponge (Protectaid®) containing sodium cholate. *Human Reproduct* 1993;8:886–9.

34. Psychoyos A. Protectaid, a new vaginal contracepive sponge with anti-STD properties. In: Barrier contraceptives: current status and future prospects. New York: Wiley-Liss, Inc., 1994.

35. Kriess J, Ngugi E, Holmes K, et al. Efficacy of nonoxynol 9 contraceptive sponge use in preventing heterosexual acquisition of HIV in Nairobi prostitutes. *JAMA* 1992; 268:477–82.

36. Cates W, Raymond EG. Vaginal spermicides. In: Contraceptive technology, 17th edn. New York: Irvington Publishers, 1998.

37. Simpson JL, Phillips OP. Spermicides, hormonal contraception and congenital malformations. *Adv Contracept* 1990;6:141–67.

38. Niruthisard S, Roddy RE, Chutivongse S. Use of nonoxynol-9 and reduction in rate of gonococcal and chlamydial cervical infections. *Lancet* 1992;339:1371–5.

39. Cook RL, Rosenberg MJ. Do spermicides containing nonoxynol-9 prevent sexually transmitted infections? A meta-analysis. *Sexually Trans Dis* 1998; 25:144–50.

40. Roddy RE, Schulz KF, Cates W. Microbicides, meta-analysis, and the N-9 question. Where's the research? *Sexually Trans Dis* 1998;25:151 3.

41. Roddy RE, Zekeng L, Ryan KA, et al. Controlled trial of nonoxynol 9 film to reduce male to female transmission of sexually transmitted diseases. *N Engl J Med* 1998;339:504–10.

42. Roddy RE, Cordero M, Cordero C, Fortney JA. A dosing study of nonoxynol-9 and genital irritation. *Int J STD AIDS* 1993;4:165–70.

43. Niruthisard S, Roddy RE, Chutivongse S. The effects of frequent nonoxynol-9 use on the vaginal and cervical mucosa. *Sexually Trans Dis* 1991;18:176–9.

44. Alexander N. Barriers to sexually transmitted diseases. *Sci Am Sci Med* 1996;3:32–41.

45. Archer DF, Mauck CK, Viniegra-Sibal A, Anderson FD. Leas's shield®: a phase I postcoital study of a new contraceptive barrier device. *Contraception* 1995;52:167–73.

46. Mauck C, Glover LH, Miller E. Lea's Shield®: A study of the safety and efficacy of a new vaginal barrier contraceptive used with and without spermicide. *Contraception* 1996; 53:329–35.

47. Shihata AA, Trussell J. New female intravaginal barrier contraceptive device preliminary clinical trial. *Contraception* 1991;44:11–9.

48. Shihati AA, Gollub E. Acceptability of a new intravaginal barrier contraceptive device (FemCap). *Contraception* 1992;46:511–9.

49. Zekeng L, Feldblum PJ, Oliver RM, Kaptue L. Barrier contraceptive use and HIV infection among high-risk women in Cameroon. *AIDS* 1993;7:725–31.

50. Wittkowski KM, Susser E, Dietz K. The Protective effect of condoms and nonoxynol-9 against HIV infection. *Am J Public Health* 1998;88:590–6.

51. Zaneveld LJD, Anderson KJ, Whaley KJ. Part I: Barrier methods. In: Harrison PF, Rosenfield A (eds) Contraceptive research and development: looking to the future. New York: Institute of Medicine, National Academy Press, 1996.

Male hormonal contraception

Christina Wang MD
Ronald S Swerdloff MD

Background

Methods of contraception generally available for men are limited to 'withdrawal', condoms and vasectomy (see Chapter 11). In the 20th century, contraception has been mostly a female 'burden', especially when a man rejects condoms as 'messy' or 'unnatural', and the couple are unable to accept an irreversible method such as vasectomy. History and psychosocial research suggests that men have, do and will continue to play an active part in the contraceptive decision. Currently, one in four couples rely on the male partner for contraception (Table 10.1). If periodic abstinence (fertility awareness) is added to the list of male-dependent methods, the ratio goes up to nearly one in three. What hampers the advent of the 'contracepted' male is the failure of science and technology to understand and conquer the biological challenges of male reproductive physiology (Box 10.1). These challenges are gradually being conquered with molecular and cellular biology advances in the understanding of the male reproductive system.

Although the condom has the advantage of preventing sexually transmitted disease, the contraceptive failure rate of condom use is as high as 12% [1]. To improve compliance and efficacy, non-latex-based condoms are being developed. The prevalence of vasectomy varies between countries and regions. Vasectomy is widely adopted as a contraceptive method by couples in the USA, the UK, Australia and the Netherlands, as well as in less developed countries, such as China, Korea and Thailand. Vasectomy is a safe, well-established procedure with few long-term side effects. Nevertheless, recent improvements in the procedure include a technique, non-scalpel vasectomy, which has even lower postoperative discomfort and is culturally more acceptable in some regions of the world.

Despite its efficacy, vasectomy is considered a potentially irreversible technique because, even though successful

Table 10.1 Current male methods of contraception

Method	Failure risk range per 100 woman-years	Worldwide usage	Advantages	Disadvantages
Coitus interruptus ('withdrawal')	5–20	56 million	Free Always available	Not under the woman's control Requires high motivation and control Reduces sexual fulfilment
Male condoms	3–15	49 million	Non-systemic Protects against sexually transmitted infections	Coitally related Can break Not under the woman's control
Vasectomy	0.1–0.3	45 million	High contraceptive protection Simple outpatient procedure	Irreversible Surgical procedure Not immediately effective

Box 10.1 Biological differences between male and female reproduction

Males	Females
Produce 50 000 spermatozoa per minute	Produce a single egg each month
Sperm survive up to 7 days	Egg is fertilizable for < 24 hours
Fertility maintained to old age	Fertility limited to around 40 years

reanastomosis can be expected in skilled hands in over 90% of corrective surgery, pregnancy occurs in less than 50% of vasectomy reversals. This low pregnancy rate in the partners of vasovasotimized, previously vasectomized men is related to the development of antibodies to spermatozoa after vasectomy. Current developments in this field include using intravasal devices to prevent sperm transport or percutaneous introduction of intravasal cure-in-place occlusive agents, e.g. medical grade silicone or polyurethane [2], similar to the development of tubal occlusion methods in the female (Chapter 11).

Non-hormonal approaches to systemic male contraception have been disappointing (Table 10.2. Agents directly affecting the testis (e.g. gossypol) have been used in some countries but it is generally believed that agents acting on spermatogenesis may induce irreversible effects [3]. The search for agents acting specifically on the epididymis has led to testing of compounds such as α-chlorhydrin, imidazoles and chlorinated glucose. Most of these compounds have other unacceptable toxic effects [4]. Recently, derivatives from the Chinese herb *Tripterygium wilfordii*, have been studied for their effect on male infertility [5]. Studies in men and rats showed that, when the multiglycosides of extracts from the root of *Tripterygium* were administered, sperm motility was markedly reduced while the effect on sperm count was less pronounced. This observation suggested that *Tripterygium* might have an effect on spermiogenesis or maturation of the spermatid. The pure compounds with antifertility effect isolated from these crude extracts have not been tested in man.

In this chapter, the focus will be on hormonal methods of male contraceptive development. Many of the hormonal methods have been tested in clinical trials and represent the most promising method that may be available to men in the near future [6–9].

Hormonal regulation of spermatogenesis: the basis of male hormonal contraception

Spermatogenesis in man is a highly organized process which involves cell proliferation, maturation and death. This orderly process begins with the spermatogonia undergoing multiplication (both mitosis and meiosis) to form spermatocytes and spermatids. The spermatids progress through defined steps to become spermatozoa with flagella (tails) by a process called spermiogenesis. Developing germ cells are embedded in Sertoli cells which provide the necessary environment for development. The intercellular communication between Sertoli cells and germ cells is critical for germ cell development. In the seminiferous tubules, the germ cells are arranged in defined association or stages. The stages follow one another in succession, leading to a wave of germ cell maturation along the seminiferous tubules. In the human this process takes about 73 days. The mature spermatozoa are then released to the tubule lumen where they are transported to the epididymis. In

Table 10.2 Non-hormonal approaches to male contraception

Agent	Advantages/mechanism of action	Disadvantages	Where are we with it?
Gossypol (cotton seed oil extract)	Effective suppressant of spermatogenesis	Slow recovery of sperm numbers; 10% irreversible	Dose finding and toxicity work
Trypterygium wilfordii extract	Reduces motility, not density	Side effects to be ascertained	Toxicity work
Imidazole derivatives	Spermicidal action; active orally	To be ascertained	Phase 1

the epididymis the spermatozoa acquire membrane proteins, forward motility and fertilizing capacity, thereby attaining functional capacity. From the epididymis, the spermatozoa traverse the vas deferens and then through the ejaculatory ducts. The passage through the accessory organs takes about 14 days in man. The normal sperm density is over 20 million per milliliter of ejaculate. Thus, for agents affecting spermatogenesis in the human, it will take about 3 months before their maximum effect will be manifested in the ejaculate.

Spermatogenesis in man is regulated by testosterone (T), produced by the adjacent Leydig cells situated in the interstitium between the seminiferous tubules, aided also by the pituitary follicle stimulating hormone (FSH). Thus, testicular spermatogenesis and androgen production are interlinked functionally by endocrine and paracrine mechanisms. Both testicular functions are driven by the pituitary gonadotrophins through the hypothalamic–pituitary testicular axis. Testosterone exerts a negative feedback on the hypothalamic–pituitary unit, thereby regulating its own levels. The testicular concentration of testosterone is 100 times higher than in peripheral blood. Exogenous administration of testosterone decreases luteinizing hormone (LH) and FSH secretion and endogenous intratesticular T levels, resulting in suppression of spermatogenesis.

The pituitary gland secretes two gonadotropins, LH and FSH, under the influence of the hypothalamic peptide gonadotropin-hormone releasing hormone (GnRH). LH affects spermatogenesis by stimulating the secretion of testosterone within the testis. Testosterone acts through the Sertoli cells, although there is some evidence to show direct actions of testosterone on germ cells. FSH also stimulates Sertoli cell secretory function and promotes spermatogenesis. In man, it is generally accepted that both FSH and testosterone are required for the initiation of spermatogenesis. Testosterone is also required for the maintenance of spermatogenesis. Other endocrine effects include maintenance of male secondary sexual characteristics, libido and sexual potency. Clinical studies have also shown that LH (by increasing endogenous testosterone) alone produces qualitatively normal spermatogenesis but both FSH and testosterone are required to achieve quantitatively normal sperm production. Dysfunction of Leydig cells results in low testosterone production (male hypogonadism). The resultant decreased negative feedback on the hypothalamus–pituitary by low endogenously produced testosterone leads to elevated LH levels. Similarly, seminiferous tubule dysfunction leads to decreased inhibin production by the Sertoli cells. This results in the loss of negative feedback on the hypothalamus–pituitary leading to elevated FSH levels (Figure 10.1).

In addition to the gonadotropins, FSH and LH, a large number of intratesticular factors may affect spermatogenesis. Growth factors, cytokines and other peptides are secreted by the various cell types of the testes, forming a network of cross-communication between germ cells, Sertoli cells, Leydig cells and peritubular myoid cells. The exact role of each of these factors in the regulation of spermatogenesis in vivo is not clear, but together they produce a microenvironment that nurtures the developing spermatozoa.

Hormonal methods of male contraception are based on the suppression of both gonadotropins (LH and FSH) by administration of testosterone alone, or in combination with other gonadotropin suppressors, such as progestogens, estrogens and GnRH analogs (Box 10.2). Testosterone or other sex steroids, when administered exogenously, by virtue of negative feedback mechanisms on LH and FSH secretion, result in marked suppression of spermatogenesis. In principle, the ideal hormonal method should selectively inhibit FSH without lowering LH and serum testosterone levels. Such methods would not require the administration of replacement doses of androgens such as testosterone. Theoretically, this can be achieved by immunization against FSH, development of specific FSH or FSH receptor antagonists or use of inhibin-like substances. In primates, immunization against FSH does not lead to persistent suppression of spermatogenesis. Specific FSH or FSH receptor antagonist and inhibin have not been generally available for testing in vivo. Moreover, a recent report of men with genetic inactivating mutations of FSH receptor suggests that FSH may not be necessary for spermatogenesis. These men with FSH receptor mutations resulting in functionally non-active receptors

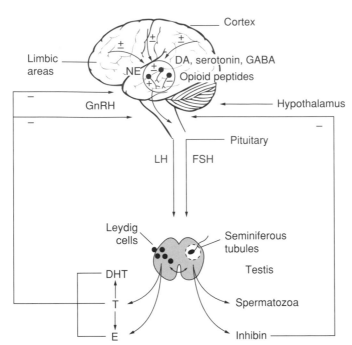

Fig. 10.1 The hypothalamic–pituitary–testicular axis in the male. The hypothalamus is the integrating center for central nervous system (CNS) regulation of gonadotropin-releasing hormone (GnRH). Extrahypothalamic CNS input has both inhibitory and stimulatory influences on GnRH secretion. Neurotransmitters such as norepinephrine (NE), dopamine (DA), opioid peptides, gamma-aminobutyric acid (GABA), serotonin and melatonin serve as regulators of GnRH synthesis and release from the hypothalamus. The human testis is a dual organ with endocrine and reproductive functions. Testicular function is regulated by a series of closed-loop feedback systems involving the higher centers in the CNS, the hypothalamus, the pituitary, and the testicular endocrine and germinal compartments. T = testosterone; DHT = 5α-dihydrotestosterone; E = estradiol. From Wang C, Swerdloff RS. Evaluation of testicular function. In: De Kretser DM (ed.) *Bailliere's Clinical Endocrinology and Metabolism* Vol 6 No 2 London: Bailliere Tindall, 1992.

have a varying phenotype from infertility to proven fertility [10]. This raises doubts as to whether inhibition of FSH secretion or activity alone will be adequate as a male contraceptive.

Box 10.2   Hormonal methods of male contraception

Suppression of both LH and FSH

- Androgen [testosterone esters (TE), modified testosterone such as 19-nortestosterone]
- Androgen + progestogen (injectable progestin such as DMPA or oral progestin such as levonorgestrel or norethisterone)
- Androgen + estrogen
- Androgen + antiandrogens (cyproterone acetate 50 mg per day + TE)
- Androgen + GnRH agonist (such as buserelin)
- Androgen + GnRH antagonist

Suppression of FSH only

- FSH immunization
- FSH antagonists
- FSH receptor antagonists
- Inhibin or related substances

Clinical studies of hormonal methods for men

Androgens alone

In the 1970s, studies were initiated based on the use of testosterone esters alone (testosterone enanthate, TE) as a potential method of male fertility regulation. These short-term (4–6 months) studies showed that TE, when administered at a weekly dose of 200–250 mg, induced oligozoospermia (suppressing the sperm count to less than 5 million/ml) in 90–95% of men and azoospermia (no sperm in ejaculate) in about 40–60% of men. If the TE injections were administered less frequently, then only about 45–65% of the men would reach oligozoospermia [11].

Administration of TE as a weekly injection is not practical. Moreover, the pharmacokinetic profile of serum testosterone after TE administration, with initial high levels followed by progressive decrease to pretreatment levels, is not ideal. The high initial levels of testosterone may lead to side effects such as acne, seborrhea and mood fluctuations. Other modalities of androgen delivery are currently being developed which might be suitable for male fertility regulation purposes (Table 10.3).

Long-acting testosterone preparations, such as testosterone undecanoate (monthly injections), testosterone buciclate (2–3-monthly injections), testosterone-loaded biodegradable microspheres (2–3-monthly injections) and testosterone implants (implants

Table 10.3 Androgen preparations with a potential as hormonal male contraceptive agents

Preparations currently available	Features
Injectables	
Testosterone enanthate	The prototype formulation tested by WHO for many years
Testosterone undecanoate (China, Europe)	
19-Nortestosterone (nandralone) (modified testosterone)	Has some progestogenic effects, may be used alone or in combination
Transdermal systems	
Scrotal (Testoderm®)	See Table 10.4
Non-scrotal (Androderm®)	See Table 10.4
Testosterone implants	Subcutaneous pellets; last 4–6 months

Preparations under development	Features
Injections (long acting)	
Testosterone buciclate	In higher doses can produce azoospermia
Testosterone microspheres	A depot injection, 3 monthly, zero-order release
Transdermal systems	
Non-scrotal patches without enhancers	To be ascertained
Creams/gels	
Implants	
7α Methyl-19-nortestosterone (MENT)	Subdermal implant for androgen replacement; lasts 1 year; highly potent
Oral	
Testosterone undecanoate	To be ascertained

lasting for 4–6 months) might be more acceptable as male contraceptive agents because of their prolonged action and their ability to provide more steady physiological levels of testosterone after administration compared with TE [12,13]. Testosterone pellets, when inserted subcutaneously at a dose of 1200 mg into normal volunteers, led to suppression of spermatogenesis to a degree similar to that achieved by weekly TE injections and with fewer side effects. A major advantage is their low production costs. However, the insertion of pellets required a minor surgical procedure and a trained provider. Testosterone buciclate (1200 mg, single injection) was studied in eight volunteers and found to induce azoospermia in only three men. The other preparations are in various stages of development for use as replacement therapy for hypogonadal men and have not been tested in male contraceptive trials.

Recently available transdermal systems (Table 10.4) have not been studied in androgen-alone regimens. Some of the gel preparations (testosterone or dihydrotestosterone; DHT) had been used in conjunction with progestogens in some earlier studies. The transdermal testosterone delivery systems achieve low- to mid-range, adult male serum testosterone levels. The observations from the data derived from previous studies on TE and testosterone pellets suggest that high physiological serum testosterone levels, achieved with exogenous androgens, are required for adequate suppression of spermatogenesis [14–16]. Such high doses of testosterone produced significant but reversible side effects, such as weight gain, acne, gynecomastia, a decrease in high-density lipoprotein (HDL) levels and an increase in hematocrit [17].

The long-term consequences in normal men of maintaining relatively high serum testosterone levels required for

Table 10.4 Transdermal androgen delivery systems

System	Features	Potential as contraceptive
Testoderm®	Scrotal 'patch' in two doses, 2.4 mg/day and 3.6 mg/day. Daily change. Physiological/plasma levels. Matrix patch	Unknown
Andropatch®	Non-scrotal patch. Daily change. Physiological plasma testosterone levels. Reservoir patch	Unknown
T or DHT gel	To be ascertained	To be ascertained

spermatogenesis suppression are not known. It is known that TE injections induce a small but significant decrease in HDL-cholesterol. The long-term effects of slightly decreased HDL-cholesterol and the relationship with coronary heart disease are not clear. The other concern is that long-term administration of testosterone may lead to prostatic dysfunction. There is no clear evidence that androgens will induce benign prostatic hyperplasia or carcinoma of the prostate. However, it is recognized that the presence of androgens is required for the development of prostatic disease. There are no long-term studies of the effects of exogenous androgens on the prostate in normal men. 5α-dihydrotestosterone is the active androgen metabolite in the human prostate. Inhibitors of 5α-reductase enzymes are used to decrease prostatic volume in patients with benign prostatic hyperplasia. Owing to the concern about long-term androgen administration to normal men, androgens which are not reduced to 5α-dihydrotestosterone (thus with less effect on the prostate) are being developed. One such androgen is MENT (7α-methyl-19-nortesterone), which is being studied by the Population Council (New York) as an androgen implant.

The effects of high doses of androgens on sexual function and behavior have been studied when TE was administered at a dose of 200 mg per week. No significant change in sexual or aggressive behavior was found. A double-blind cross-over study with appropriate instruments to assess behavioral changes is currently in progress to answer the specific question of whether exogenous administration of androgens causes behavioral changes, including aggression.

Androgen and progestagen combinations

Concerns about long-term safety of high-dose androgen-alone contraception led to the development of a combined regimen with a non-androgenic spermatogenesis suppressant used with testosterone as an add-back androgen replacement therapy. Progestogens, when administered to men, depress pituitary function and suppress spermatogenesis: they can be used as the main suppressant in the progestogen–androgen combination. Because serum testosterone levels are also suppressed with progestogen administration, supplementary testosterone will be necessary to prevent the symptoms and side effects of androgen withdrawal.

Combinations of progestogens and androgens might allow a reduction in the dose of androgen and greater suppression of gonadotropins than androgen-alone regimens. Many progestogen–androgen combinations were used in single and multicenter clinical trials sponsored by the World Health Organization (WHO) and the Population Council. In these earlier studies, the most widely clinically tested progestogen was depot- medroxyprogesterone acetate (DMPA) given by injection in combination with TE or 19-nortestosterone. Using DMPA 200–250 mg per month together with TE 200–250 mg per month, both by intramuscular injections, azoospermia was achieved in 50–60% of men and severe oligozoospermia in an additional 30–40% [18–20]. When such a regimen was tested in Indonesian men, 97% of the men developed azoospermia and no pregnancies were reported [21]. The cause of this ethnic variability is unknown, but the potential of using lower doses to achieve contraceptive efficacy in some groups is immense. There were relatively few side effects, since libido and potency were retained when progestogens were used in combination with androgen supplementation. Other important side effects include weight gain and occasional gynecomastia. Progestogens also lower HDL levels. The effect of long-term suppression of HDL levels in men and its relationship to risks of atherosclerosis have to be clarified. An acceptable injection routine needs to be developed with a long-acting testosterone.

Recently, in a comparative study of TE (100 mg per week) alone versus TE plus oral levonorgestrel (500 mg per day), Bebb et al.[22] demonstrated that the latter androgen plus progestagen combination was more effective and that it had a more rapid onset of action than TE alone in the suppression of spermatogenesis. Thus it is apparent that combinations of androgens and progestogens may be synergistic in the suppression of gonadotropins, allowing the lowering of the doses of both androgens and/or progestogen to achieve the same goal. This combination of levonorgestrel plus TE suppressed HDL-cholesterol by 24% and total cholesterol by 6%. Development of long-acting progestogens with less impact on lipid profile and testing of the effect of lower doses of progestogens in combination with androgens for suppression of spermatogenesis are currently in progress. Further work needs to be carried out to explore the long-term effects of progestogens in men.

Androgens and estrogens

Combinations of androgens and estrogens have been tested in experimental animals. The advantage would be that estrogens neutralize the effects of androgens on lipids and may have a neutral effect on behavior, but the effect of the combination on the prostate is not known. Clinical studies on combinations of androgen plus estrogen are in progress.

Androgens and antiandrogens

The antiandrogen cyproterone acetate was studied as a potential male contraceptive agent. Cyproterone acetate has both antiandrogenic and progestational properties. Administration of cyproterone acetate alone leads to decreases in sperm production and serum testosterone levels. It also interferes with sperm maturation. Studies in India have suggested that the combination of cyproterone acetate with testosterone resulted in much more marked suppression of sperm production. These studies have been confirmed recently with a combination of

cyproterone acetate and TE. However, cyproterone acetate is not approved for use in the USA. The advantage of cyproterone acetate plus TE regimens over progestogen and androgen combinations is that cyproterone acetate does not lead to changes in lipid profile, and has the theoretical benefit of lesser effects on prostate growth [23]. Other new antiandrogens have not been tested for efficacy in suppression of spermatogenesis.

GnRH analogs and testosterone

GnRH analogs are classified as either agonists or antagonists based on their acute effect on LH and FSH secretion. The agonists were initially developed as therapeutic agents to stimulate LH and FSH, and therefore treat GnRH deficiency (hypogonadotropic hypo-gonadism). Early experimental studies demonstrated that GnRH agonists, when given in repeated doses, had interesting paradoxical effects on gonadotropin secretion and even more striking inhibition of testosterone secretion and intratesticular content. The mechanisms by which GnRH agonists downregulate the reproductive system are complex but, for the purpose of this discussion, can be thought of as initially stimulative, and later inhibiting the pituitary's secretion of biologically active gonadotropins. This results in testosterone deficiency and decreased spermatogenesis.

GnRH agonist preparations have been tested by at least 12 investigators studying the effects

on 106 volunteer subjects. The overall results were summarized recently [8]. They indicated that about 20% of men became azoospermic, an additional third developed severe oligo-zoospermia (less than 5 million/ml) and the remainder had lesser degrees of sperm suppression. Several explanations exist for the limited success of GnRH agonist and androgen combinations. These include inadequate dose, suboptimal route and frequency of administration, and interference of analog effect by combined androgen therapy. The most likely reason for incomplete suppression of spermatogenesis in clinical trials with GnRH agonists and testosterone combinations is their inability to inhibit LH and FSH secretion completely.

Ongoing studies are examining whether administering higher doses of GnRH agonist (5–10 times the dose previously studied) in combination with physiological replacement doses of testosterone will be more efficacious in complete suppression of gonadotropins and consequently of spermatogenesis. The advantage of pursuing studies with GnRH agonists is the lack of side effects of these groups of agents and the relative lower costs compared with GnRH antagonists.

GnRH antagonists are analogs of GnRH, which inhibit the action of the endogenous hormone via competitive binding with pituitary receptor sites. Through this action, LH and FSH secretion are prevented (without the transient simulatory phase seen with GnRH agonist treatment), resulting in a decrease in endogenous testosterone and a reduction in spermatogenesis. Because of these actions, GnRH antagonists have been studied as potential agents for fertility control. In several short-term studies, these compounds have been shown to suppress testosterone production and inhibin levels, while longer term studies have demonstrated their ability to inhibit spermatogenesis. There is as yet no prototype product.

Since it is known that both GnRH antagonists and testosterone inhibit gonadotropin secretion, the combination of these two drugs has been investigated as a potential male contraceptive agent. The results of several studies have shown the combination regimen to be more effective at suppressing spermatogenesis (60–80%) than testosterone alone (50–70%) [24,25]. Several different replacement doses of testosterone have been studied in these trials, ranging from 25 mg/week to 200 mg/week. In addition, many studies have delayed the initiation of androgen replacement until 2–3 weeks after commencing GnRH antagonist administration to avoid counteracting the suppressive effects of the antagonist on the testes.

Like GnRH agonists, GnRH antagonists are administered as daily subcutaneous injections. In contrast to GnRH agonists, some GnRH antagonists produce local reactions at the site of injection, such as redness, itchiness and painful wheals which might last for 7 days. GnRH antagonists are also more expensive to synthesize and the doses used were higher than GnRH agonists. The advantages of the GnRH antagonist include complete

suppression of FSH and LH without an initial flare. Recent studies suggest that azoospermia induced by GnRH antagonists plus testosterone can be maintained by testosterone alone. The long-term goal of these studies with GnRH analogs is to develop non-peptide analogs that may be potent, safe, easier to administer (e.g. orally) and less expensive to synthesize than the peptide analogs.

Are hormonally based male contraceptive methods efficacious?

In 1985, the WHO embarked on a multicenter study to investigate whether hormonally induced azoospermia could be maintained to provide effective contraception for 12 months. Testosterone enanthate (200 mg/week administered by intramuscular injection) was selected for this purpose as a prototype of a hormonally based male contraceptive based on its known safety, reversibility and efficacy in humans. This study included 271 couples in 10 centers in seven countries. During the suppression phase, TE injections were administered weekly until azoospermia was achieved in three consecutive semen samples. A total of 157 couples then entered the efficacy phase, where all other methods of contraception were withdrawn and the weekly TE injections were the sole method of fertility regulation. This efficacy phase lasted for 12 months. At the end of the suppression phase, the cumulative azoospermia rate was 64.5%. There was one pregnancy in the 1486 months of efficacy

exposure, giving a Pearl rate of 0.8 (95% CI 0.02–4.5) per 100 person-years. Complete recovery occurred in all subjects [14]. The study established TE as a reversible suppressant of spermatogenesis as effective as female injectables.

The second multicenter study sponsored by WHO began in 1989 to examine whether men rendered severely oligo-zoospermic (less than 3 million/ml) by hormonally based agents would be infertile. Again the prototype treatment was TE 200 mg once every week. The protocol was similar to that described above. If consistent oligozoospermia was attained, then the couple entered an efficacy phase of 12 months. A total of 399 men from 15 centers in nine countries participated in the study. Of these subjects, 98% achieved azoospermia or severe oligozoospermia to allow them to enter the efficacy phase. There were four pregnancies in the 49.5 person-years of the oligo-spermic group (sperm count between 0.1 and 3.0 million/ml) and none in the 230.4 person-years in the azoospermic group. The combined method failure for azoospermia and oligo-zoospermia was 1.4 (95% CI 0.4–3.7) per 100 person-years. The pregnancy rate was directly related to the sperm concentration in the ejaculate, with 3–5 million sperm being the threshold for acceptable efficacy. Once azoospermia or oligozoospermia was achieved, escape from suppression of spermatogenesis was very unusual [15]. These studies showed for the first time that, if azoospermia was achieved in most men and oligozoospermia in the remainder, a hormonally based contraceptive agent would be efficacious. Moreover, in these studies, complete recovery of sperm counts after withdrawal of TE injection occurred in all subjects; the acceptability of the injection routine remains the main drawback.

Future development

The development of hormonally based contraceptive methods has progressed steadily in the past 20 years. Firstly, it has been shown that suppression of spermatogenesis to azoospermia or sperm concentration less than 3 million/ml by exogenous hormone administration can achieve contraceptive efficacy comparable to that of the female reversible methods (Chapter 3, 5 and 7). Secondly, it has also been demonstrated that addition of a gonadotropin suppressive agent such as a progestogen or GnRH antagonist to androgen will lead to more complete and faster

inhibition of spermatogenesis. Thirdly, through an active synthesis program jointly sponsored by international (WHO) and national organizations (National Institute of Health), a number of new steroid compounds have been synthesized, toxicology studies performed and preliminary clinical studies completed. These compounds include testosterone buciclate (a long-acting androgen) and levonorgestrel butanoate (a long-acting progestogen).

Plans for future developments in male contraception for the next decade include the following:

- New preparations and new androgen delivery systems to yield a more stable level of testosterone.

- 'Designer' androgens, which can maintain sexual function, bone and muscle mass, but without adverse actions on the prostate and lipid profile.

- New long-acting progestogens with favorable pharmacokinetics to be used in conjunction with androgens. The progestogens should have minimal effects on lipid profile.

- Non-peptide GnRH agonists or antagonists, which will be highly potent, without side effects and can be administered orally or as long-acting injectables.

- Determination of the minimum dose of androgens, progestogens or GnRH analogs required to achieve complete suppression of spermatogenesis.

- Home monitoring kits or 'dipsticks' to determine when sperm concentration falls below a threshold, e.g. 3 million/ml or near zero.

- Assess when these potential methods will be acceptable to men from different cultural, ethnic and geographical backgrounds.

References

1. Trussel J, Kost K. Contraceptive failure in the United States: a critical review of literature. *Stud Fam Plann* 1987; 18:237–83.

2. Liu X, Li S. Vasal sterilization in China. *Contraception* 1993; 48:255–65.

3. Meng GD, Zhu JC, Chen ZW, et al. Recovery to normal sperm production following cessation of gossypol treatment: a two center study in China. *Int J Androl* 1988;11:1–11.

4. Ford WCL, Waites GMH. A reversible contraceptive action of some 6-chloro-6-deoxy sugars in the male rat. *J Reprod Fertil* 1978; 52:152–7.

5. Qian SZ. *Tripterygium Wilfordii*: a Chinese herb effective in male fertility regulation. *Contraception* 1987; 36:247–63.

6. Swerdloff RS, Wang C, Bhasin S. Male contraception: 1988 and beyond. In:Burger H, de Kretser D (eds) The testis, 2nd edn. *New York: Raven Press* 1989; 547–68.

7. Waites GMH. Male fertility regulation: the challenges for the year 2000. *Br Med Bull* 1993;49:210–21.

8. Cummings DE, Bremner WJ. Prospects for new hormonal male contraceptives. *Endocrinol Metabol Clin North Am* 1994;22:893–922.

9. Wang C, Swerdloff RS, Waites GMH. Male contraception: 1993 and beyond. In: Van Look PFA, Perez-Palacio (eds) Contraceptive research and development 1984 to 1994. Delhi: Oxford University Press, 1994:121–34.

10. Tapanainen JA, Ailtomaki K, Min J, Vaskivuo T, Huhtaniemi IT. Men homozygous for an inactivating mutation of the follicle-stimulating hormone (FSH) receptor gene present variable suppression of spermatogenesis and fertility. *Nature Genet* 1997;15:205–6.

11. Patanelli DJ (ed). Hormonal control of male fertility. Bethesda: US DHEW, 1978, Publication no. (NIH) 78–1097.

12. Nieschlag E, Behre HM. (eds) Testosterone: action, deficiency, substitution. Berlin: Springer-Verlag, 1990.

13. Bhasin S, Gabelnick HL, Spieler JM, Swerdloff RS, Wang C. (eds) Pharmacology, biology and clinical applications of androgens. New York: Wiley-Liss, 1996.

14. World Health Organization Task Force on Methods for the Regulation of Male Fertility. Contraceptive efficacy of testosterone-induced azoospermia in normal men. *Lancet* 1990; 336:955–9.

15. World Health Organization Task Force on Methods for the Regulation of Male Fertility. Contraceptive efficacy of testosterone-induced azoospermia and oligo-zoospermia in normal men. *Fertil Steril* 1996;65:821–9.

16. Handelsman DJ, Conway AJ, Boylan LM. Suppression of human spermatogenesis by testosterone implants in man. *J Clin Endocrinol Metab* 1992;75:1326–32.

17. Wu FCW, Farely TMM, Peregoudov A, Waites GMH, World Health Organisation Task Force on Methods for the Regulation of Male Fertility. Effects of testosterone enanthate in normal men: experience from a multicenter contraceptive efficacy study. *Fertil Steril* 1996;65:626–36.

18. Paulsen CA, Bremner WJ, Leonard JM. Male contraception: clinical trials. In: Mishell DR Jr (ed) Advances in Fertility Research New York: Raven Press, 1982:157–70.

19. Knuth UA, Nieschlag E. Endocrine approaches to male fertility control. *Clin Endocrinol Metab J* 1987;1:113–131.

20. Schearer SB, Alvarez-Sanchez F, Anselmo J, et al. Hormonal contraception for men. *Int J Androl* 1978; Suppl 2:680–712.

21. World Health Organization Task Force on Methods for the Regulation of Male Fertility. Comparison of two androgens plus depo-medroxyprogesterone acetate for suppression to azoospermia in Indonesian men. *Fertil Steril* 1993;60:1062–8.

22. Bebb RA, Anawalt BD, Christiansen RB, Paulsen CA, Bremner WJ, Matsumoto AM. Combined administration of levonorgestrel and testosterone induces more rapid and effective suppression of spermatogenesis than testosterone alone: a promising male contraceptive approach. *J Clin Endocrinol Metab* 1996;81:757–62.

23. Merigiolla MC, Bremner WJ, Paulsen CA, et al. A combined regimen of cyproterone acetate and testosterone enanthate as a potentially highly effective male contraceptive. *J Clin Endocrinol Metab* 1996;81:3018–23.

24. Tom L, Bhasin S, Salameh W, et al. Induction of azoospermia in normal men with combined Nal-Glu gonadotropin-releasing hormone antagonist and testosterone enanthate. *J Clin Endocrinol Metab* 1992;75:476–483.

25. Bagatell CJ, Matsumoto AM, Christiansen RB, Rivier JG, Bremner WJ. Comparison of a gonadotropin-releasing hormone antagonist plus testosterone (T) versus T alone as potential male contraceptive regimens. *J Clin Endocrinol Metab* 1993;77:427–432.

Female and male sterilization

G Marcus Filshie DM FRCOG MFFP

Female sterilization

Historical overview

The first reported case of female sterilization appeared in a textbook over 160 years ago by James Blundell who recommended tubectomy at the time of caesarean section in patients with a contracted pelvis. Fifty years later, in Ohio, USA, in 1880 Lungren ligated the fallopian tube, also at caesarean section, in a woman with a similar problem. Since then a multitude of different methods of occlusion of the fallopian tubes have been developed, the most notable being the Madlener procedure of 1910 and techniques of Irving (1924), Pomeroy (1930), Aldridge (1934), Kroener (1935) and Uchida (1946). These have been ably reviewed by Rioux [1]. In 1965, Sir Dugald Baird delivered his famous lecture – The Fifth Freedom (from the fear of unwanted pregnancy) – and highlighted the role of sterilization.

The main indications were for medical reasons or for grand multiparity. The procedures were performed at the time of caesarean section or immediately postpartum. Female sterilization was not performed frequently until the advent of laparoscopy, which enabled the patient to have the procedure performed safely on a daycare basis. Although crude laparoscopy was originally performed in 1910 by Kelling, in dogs, Jacobeus from Sweden first introduced a laparoscope into humans in 1911 and it was he who coined the phrase 'laparoscopy'. The use of the laparoscope to perform female sterilization was first recorded by Ruddock in 1934.

Anderson from the USA first designed a purpose-built electrode for tubal fulguration in 1937, and Powers and Barnes in 1941 wrote an article on laparoscopic tubal fulguration techniques. However, it was not until 20 years later when Palmer of France in 1960 gave a huge impetus to laparoscopic tubal fulguration and popularized the method in France. Later, in Germany in 1964 and the UK in 1965, Frangenheim and Steptoe popularized these methods in their respective countries.

The laparoscope was substantially improved by the addition of the Hopkins Rod Lens system together with the advent of the cold light source, and laparoscopic tubal ligation was later adopted by Cohen and Wheeless in the USA. This technique became so popular that it was used for sterilizing women for social as well as medical reasons. As the operation was performed on large numbers of patients, so complications and fatalities relating to bowel burns from unipolar diathermy came to light; these burns were often at a site distant from the operating field. Bipolar cautery was introduced by Rioux (in Canada), Kleppinger (in the USA) and Hirsch (in Germany) in an attempt to reduce these complications. Despite bipolar cautery, thermal injuries still continued, which led to the emergence of a number of mechanical methods of tubal occlusion (Figure 11.1). These included the Falope ring in 1973 [2], the Hulka clip in 1973 [3] and the Filshie clip in 1981 [4]. Tupler and Bleier plastic clips also emerged, but today only the Falope ring, Hulka and Filshie clips are used on a regular basis.

Prevalence

It is estimated that over 160 million women throughout the world are protected from pregnancy by female sterilization. In the UK it has been estimated that over 70 000 procedures are

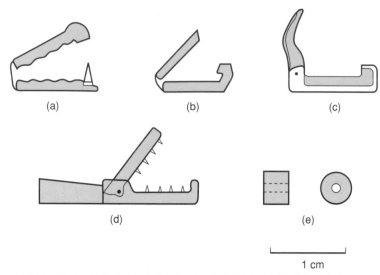

Fig. 11.1 Methods of tubal occlusion (mechanical): (a) Tupla; (b) Bleier; (c) Filshie;
(d) Hulka Clemens; (e) Falope ring.

performed each year, with a similar number of vasectomies. Of couples over 40 years approximately 50% rely on male or female sterilization; over the age of 35, over 30% of women in the UK have been sterilized. In the USA, the figures are similar. By the end of the century it is estimated that over 328 million women [5] will have been sterilized throughout the world. In the USA, approximately half the number of sterilizations are performed in the postpartum period or at the time of caesarean section – mainly for economic reasons. In the Developing World, postpartum sterilization is very popular as it is more convenient to perform an immediate postpartum sterilization than to arrange for the patient to have the procedure 6–8 weeks later. This is particularly so if the patient has to travel a long distance to the hospital.

Surgical approaches

- laparoscopy

- mini-laparotomy – suitable for early puerperal sterilization

- transvaginal – higher complication and failure to complete rates

- transcervical – remains experimental.

Laparoscopies

The laparoscopic technique is widely used and preferred. Its use is popular both in developed and developing countries. The procedure may be performed under local [6] or general anaesthesia. The patient is placed on the operating table, usually in the lithotomy position, and following catheterization a pneumoperitoneum is created by instilling, through a Veress needle just below the umbilicus, 2–3 litres of carbon dioxide or nitrous oxide if local anaesthetic is employed. A trocar and cannula is inserted just below the umbilicus to allow the insertion of a standard laparoscope. The patient

is placed in the Trendelenburg position and the pelvic organs, including the fallopian tubes, are visualized. Using a suprapubic second puncture, a further trocar and cannula is inserted to allow the introduction of the appropriate operating instrument, e.g. a clip applicator, a ring applicator or cautery forceps. The tubes may be anaesthetized by dropping local anaesthetic, e.g. 2 ml 4% lignocaine or 10 ml 0.5% marcaine to reduce the peroperative and postoperative discomfort, whether the procedure is performed using local or general anaesthesia. There are single puncture techniques for all these methods and their use depends on the surgeon's preference. As a rule, a single puncture technique is more difficult to perform but may be more acceptable for certain patients.

Mini-laparotomy

In countries or locations where laparoscopy is not available, then mini-laparotomy, performed either under local or general anaesthetic, is available. This method is perfectly acceptable and has minimal extra morbidity when performed by skilled surgeons. It is especially suitable for puerperal sterilization. A transverse incision 2–3 cm above the pubic symphysis allows access to the tubes provided the uterine fundus is elevated using vaginal manipulation. For puerperal sterilization a subumbilical incision is best.

Culdoscopy or culdotomy

This route is feasible and well utilized, but its reputation for increasing pelvic infection has made it less popular.

Methods and efficacy

Although female sterilization has been adopted by over 140 million women throughout the world, there have been remarkably few pivotal comparative studies comparing the most popular methods of tubal occlusion. Most studies are single and not comparative. The results therefore demonstrate a wide scatter of effectiveness, making comparisons difficult. Pivotal studies are when patients are randomized to methods where the surgeon is competent at each method and follow-up data are obtained without the knowledge of the method employed. The popular methods to consider are:

- partial salpingectomy (Pomeroy or Parkland)
- electrocautery
- Falope rings
- Filshie clips
- Hulka clips.

Partial salpingectomy

This method [7] is commonly performed in the postpartum period or at the time of caesarean section. It is also employed for interval tubal occlusion in the developing world when laparoscopic facilities are not available. The principles are division of the tube, ligation with an absorbable suture and separation of the ligated ends. The Pomeroy technique is popular and has a failure rate of 3.3 per thousand. The Parkland technique involves the excision of a portion of the fallopian tube and each end is then ligated separately. This involves slightly more surgery, but has a low failure rate [8].

Unipolar cautery

This is of interest from an historic point of view as it is considered to have a complication rate which is unacceptable by today's standards (e.g. sparking and thermal injury to viscera).

Bipolar cautery

This is usually performed laparoscopically. Unipolar cautery, which is very efficient, has largely been replaced by bipolar cautery because of the rare, but serious, consequences, of inappropriate bowel burns. When cautery is used, the tube is desiccated in two or three places which usually involves a substantial portion of the fallopian tube. The temperature at the point of contact may reach over 300°C. Cutting the tube following the procedure has been used, but has been associated with a higher failure rate. The short-term failure rate is reportedly below 2 per thousand [9] but long-term failures are much higher [8].

Cold coagulation

A low-voltage low-temperature technique has been developed to decrease further complications of heat. The temperature between the jaws of the forceps reaches approximately 120–140°C. When the forceps have become heated to the peroperative temperature, they are kept in place for 20 s at each place of burning.

The Falope ring

This is the most commonly used mechanical device throughout the developing world. It is an ingenious technique and the ring can be made relatively cheaply. The ring is made of silicone rubber 1 × 2.2. × 3.6 mm, which is expanded on to the end of a cannula. The forceps grasp the isthmic portion of the fallopian tube and pull the tube into the lumen of the operating cannula. The expanded ring is then pushed off the cannula to contract around a knuckle of approximately 3 cm of the fallopian tube. The failure rate is less than 4 per thousand [10,11]. This method is not recommended for postpartum use as the tubes are hypertrophied. Postoperative pain is more likely as the mesosalpinx tends to be 'tensed'.

Hulka Clemens clip

This is a spring-loaded clip first described in 1972. The clip is made of lexan plastic and has interdigitating teeth on the jaws to prevent expulsion of the tube during closure of the clip. The clip is kept closed by a spring made of gold-plated stainless steel to minimize peritoneal reaction. This clip maintains pressure between its jaws, holding the enclosed tube so that a vascular necrosis occurs within the jaws. The clip is 3 mm wide and 15 mm long. The short-term failure rate is less than 5 per thousand but is higher for sterilizations associated with pregnancy [10,11]. Reversal is feasible.

Filshie clip

This clip is made of titanium with an inner cushion lining of silicone rubber. It has a front-locking mechanism (the upper jaw flattens on closure and slides under the hook-shaped end of the lower jaw) to reduce the chance of the tube slipping out of the jaws when correctly applied. The silicone rubber 'expands' as the tube shrinks, thus maintaining complete occlusion. It is the most widely used method in the UK [12], Canada and Australia and has been available in the USA since September 1996. The clip is 4 mm wide and 13 mm long. The failure rate is less than 3 per thousand, but is higher in the postpartum period [13].

Operative risk

All operations have risks, particularly of sepsis and haemorrhage. The laparoscopic approach, when performed, correctly, has remarkably few immediate complications, particularly of sepsis. In one of the largest mortality survey series published involving 29 deaths [14], 38% were related to anaesthetic problems and 24% due to sepsis – most of which related to bowel injury including bowel burns. Haemorrhage was associated with 14% of cases. The remainder were due to miscellaneous causes including myocardial infarction, pulmonary embolus and gas embolus. The present estimated mortality from female sterilization is 3.6 per 100 000 [15], which is considerably lower than the mortality of childbearing which is 5.5 per 100 000 [16]. This benefit is particularly important in developing countries where the maternal mortality can be in excess of 100 per 100 000.

Long-term effects of tubal ligation

These include long-term failures, ectopic pregnancies and menstrual effects.

Long-term failures (8–14 years) [8]

The quoted failure rate of female sterilization is 2–3 per 1000 woman-years; 50% of failures can be due to technical errors. Failures in women under 35 are three times higher than in women over 35. The notion that most failures occur within 2 years of the operation has been challenged recently by the CREST Study [8], which showed the risk to continue for years with a 10-year cumulative pregnancy rate of 1.8% for female sterilization versus 2% for a copper T intrauterine device (IUD). Young age seems to increase the risk of regret and pregnancy. This should be considered when counselling, especially since some reversible contraceptives now approach the efficacy of sterilization.

The CREST Study, a long-term follow-up study of female sterilization, was conducted by the Center for Disease Control [8]. As this is an American study, the Filshie clip data were not included. However, a long-term study is presently being conducted. Long-term follow-up data for unipolar coagulation, bipolar coagulation, Falope rings and Hulka clips are now available. In the CREST collaborative study, 10 863 patients were enrolled and 10 685 were followed up. Data were collected at 1, 3, 5, 8 and 14 years following the procedure. Cumulative 10-year morbidity was highest in the Hulka clip method (36.5 per 1000 cases) and was lowest in the unipolar coagulation (7.5 per 100 000). Young women have the highest failure rate and this included 53.3 per 1000 with bipolar coagulation and 51.2 per 1000 with Hulka clip application.

Pregnancies occurred fairly evenly throughout the successive years following the operation.

Common causes of failed sterilization are:

- tubal fistula/recanalization
- luteal sterilization with existing pregnancy
- incorrect application of clip or ring
- application of ring or clip to round ligament
- 'puerperal' sterilization is more likely to fail.

Ectopic pregnancy following sterilization

Ectopic pregnancies are potentially life-threatening complications, particularly in less developed countries where access to surgery may be limited. There are three types of fistulae leading to ectopic pregnancies:

- a direct tubo-peritoneal fistula derived from the stump of the tube following any method of tubal ligation
- as a result of endosalpingeosis following tubal ligation
- a tubo-tubal fistula causing an ectopic pregnancy to lodge in the site of the fistulous connection.

Electrocoagulation methods have the highest rate of ectopic pregnancy in relation to failures, whereas mechanical failures have the lowest. A recent review has quantified the ectopic risk post sterilization [13] (Table 11.1).

Menstrual problems

Evidence about the long-term effect of sterilization on menstrual

Table 11.1 Risk of ectopic pregnancy following female sterilization

Sterilization technique	Ectopic pregnancies (as % of total failures)
Filshie clip	4%
Hulka clip	0%
Falope ring	20%
Electrocautery	67%

function has been conflicting. Increased loss and spotting has been reported, as has the instance of pelvic pain [17]. Some studies have involved over 10 000 subjects. In a prospective study of 5000 patients followed up for 5 years, it was found that an increased number of menstrual disturbances occurred, including pain, bleeding and spotting [18]. These problems were not related to the degree of tissue destruction at the time of the original operation. The disturbances increase with time since the procedure and may be due to age-related hormonal dysfunction or the consequence of discontinuation of menstrual regulating systemic contraception.

Hysterectomy has been reported to involve an increased number of women following sterilization but no causality is established. It has also been concluded that women who have been sterilized are more likely to be offered, and more readily accept, a hysterectomy in the future.

Several studies show an unexplained reduction in ovarian cancer in sterilized women; the largest study [19] showed 30% less risk.

Pelvic abscesses have been recorded with the Filshie clips in one patient [20]. Expulsion of Hulka clips has also been reported [21]: in a study of 6000 Filshie clip patients [13], three patients had a clip pass per urethram, per rectum and per vaginam. All three patients were subsequently examined and no cause or morbidity was found. Migration is a common problem of clips but it is only rarely associated with morbidity.

Counselling

Counselling is a process of information gathering by the couple so that they can understand the nature of the operation and its consequences sufficiently well to be able to give an informed consent. The principle of counselling is the same for both female and male sterilization. A medical history of both partners is important and concomitant pathology should be noted in either partner, e.g. menstrual problems relating to fibroids or the presence of ovarian cysts may make gynaecological surgery imminent or, as far as the man is concerned, he may have a hernia or scrotal tumour. If related surgical procedures are contemplated, then the sterilization could be performed at that time. If both clients are fit and well, then either may be sterilized. There are a number of special circumstances which need extra time when formulating a decision.

Age
When a client is under 25 years of age, a couple should understand fully that regret is more likely as there is longer time to have a change in terms of life events, e.g. marital breakdown or death of a child or spouse.

Low parity
As with younger clients, low parity patients should be certain that they understand the permanency of the procedure and accept the consequences, even in the face of loss of a child or spouse.

Performing a sterilization in association with pregnancy
Regret of the procedure following birth, termination of pregnancy or miscarriage is higher. This fact must be clearly understood by the client and accepted. There is some evidence that there is a higher failure rate with some methods at this time. If the method is associated with a higher failure rate, then the client should be made aware of this.

Financial considerations
Poor financial circumstances can be highly motivating towards sterilization. Clients should be aware of the potential for improved financial circumstances in the future.

Illness of a spouse or child
These circumstances are difficult to respond to as the condition could be genetically transmitted, familial or sporadic. On balance it would be preferred if the ill spouse be sterilized, provided that it would not compromise his/her health. Ultimately, however, it is the couple's decision as to who should be sterilized.

Marital disharmony or psychosexual problems
A sterilization only rarely improves a marital relationship

or psychosexual problems. If such problems are identified, then the issue should be addressed by marital guidance or psychosexual counselling prior to sterilization.

Proximity to the menopause

The cost effectiveness of a sterilization operation is much less as menopause is approached, particularly as fertility declines substantially at this time. However, there are some couples who would not accept an abortion under any circumstances and would prefer to have a method with the highest efficacy.

Reversibility of sterilization

This should not be a serious consideration. Although methods with minimal tissue destruction, e.g. clips, have a higher success rate when reversed, most UK Health Authorities have virtually excluded the operation from their service contracts. The permanency of the operation should be emphasized and accepted.

Cycle changes

If a woman is to come off the combined oral contraceptive pill after many years, then her periods are likely to become heavier, whereas if she has a copper IUD prior to the sterilization, her periods may become lighter.

Postoperative period

Both laparoscopy and mini-laparotomy cause postoperative discomfort which can last for several days; the woman may need to take several days off work.

Medico-legal considerations

A failure of a sterilization procedure is the most common cause of medico-legal complaints. The UK Medical Protection Society reports that this is responsible for 29% of claims in obstetrics and gynaecology [22]. The three areas of litigation involve:

1. failure to warn patients that there is a failure or complication rate
2. negligence in performing the sterilization
3. inadvertent injury during the course of the procedure.

Careful and meticulous attention to surgical techniques should reduce (2) and (3). To reduce (1), careful counselling should be adopted by the general practitioner, the counsellor and also the surgeon. It is helpful if full documentation can be made of the counselling. This should include the following:

1. The client should be aware of other methods of family planning available, including vasectomy.
2. The client should be aware of the main complications of a sterilization procedure. This should include the failure rate, which is usually given as 2–3 per 1000 (anything less than 1% should be acceptable).
3. The patient should accept the responsibility of not becoming pregnant at the time of tubal ligation and continue with family planning methods until the next menstrual period has arrived. Ideally, the operation should be performed in the follicular phase of the cycle. If the operation is performed in the luteal phase, then it is possible that a sperm could have already entered the reproductive tract and this could result in an intrauterine pregnancy, or indeed an ectopic pregnancy. If an IUD is to be removed at operation, the client should be advised not to depend on it for the 7 days prior to the operation.
4. The client should accept the permanency of the operation.
5. If the patient is obese or has medical problems, then this could increase the risk. This fact should be discussed and documented.

A dedicated consent form for sterilization should be signed. Although a spouse is often requested to sign, this is not a legal necessity.

New methods being evaluated

Most new methods of tubal occlusion are mainly related to the transcervical route as this would be less intrusive than the abdominal route. These are detailed below.

Transcervical thermal obliteration of the interstitial portion of the fallopian tube

Cryocautery, diathermy and ND:YAG lasers have all been used to destroy the interstitial portion of the fallopian tube. The power of regeneration of the endosalpinx is substantial and patency has been reported in up to 50% of cases.

Transcervical insertion of tubal blocking devices

There have been a number of intrauterine plugs of titanium and silicone rubber, ceramics and nylon plus hydrogel. The latter is called P-block, which is designed by Brundin [23] and has undergone a number of studies. Recent studies have demonstrated a Pearl index of 0.3.

Both transcervical thermal obliteration of the interstitial portion of the fallopian tube and transcervical insertion of tubal blocking devices require hysteroscopic expertise in identifying tubal ostia.

Transcervical application of chemical agents

The use of caustic chemicals (silver nitrate, zinc chloride, copper sulphate), formaldehyde, phenol paste, methyl cyanoacrilate, which flow down the fallopian tubes, and quinacrine pellets has been described. Methyl cyanoacrilate is a powerful tissue adhesive which results in 89% occlusion after two instillations. The most promising of these, however, has been the development of quinacrine pellets. This technique involves the introduction of 7×36 mg pellets through a modified copper T IUD introduced into the uterine cavity. A single application, or two applications separated by a month, is satisfactory. In one study [5] of over 31 000 subjects, there were no deaths and the pregnancy rate varied between 2.63 in 1 year to 4.3 at 2 years [5]. The method is promoted as a safe and effective procedure. In developing countries, blind canalization of the tubes is likely to be superior to blind instillation of chemical agents. The anxiety about quinacrine relates to the paucity of systemic toxicological appraisal.

Vasectomy

Historical background

Vasectomy was only rarely performed prior to 1970. However, following a publication from the Margaret Pyke Centre, London, of 1000 vasectomies followed up for 1 year after the operation, it gained widespread support [24]. When family planning services became freely available in 1974, many local authorities included vasectomy amongst their services. This was further enhanced when vasectomy became an item of service for family planning.

Prevalence

Vasectomy is becoming increasingly popular. A total of 42 million couples worldwide rely on vasectomy. Whereas it was estimated that some 50 000 procedures were performed annually in the UK in 1975, some 100 000 procedures are now thought to take place annually in the UK. In the developed world there are approximately equal numbers of vasectomies and female sterilizations. However, vasectomy is less popular, may be culturally unacceptable or is illegal in some developing countries.

Methods

A vasectomy may be performed under general or local anaesthesia. At present, most patients have a local anaesthetic procedure as it is quicker and safer. Traditionally the local anaesthetic is administered to the skin and vas either in the midline or in preparation for a lateral incision. An incision (1–2 cm long) is made in the skin down to the spermatic sheath. The sheath and vas are then grasped through the incision by special forceps, e.g. Soonawalla, and the sheath is incised until the vas is encountered. The vas is picked out from the sheath (a No. 1 needle is helpful here) and freed from the surrounding tissue. A portion of the vas is removed and both ends are ligated. Ideally, a needle point diathermy is then inserted down each vas to cauterize the lumen. The testicular end is sometimes tied back on itself. This helps to keep one end out of the sheath whilst the other end falls into the sheath. Bleeding points are cauterized and the procedure is repeated on the other side. A dissolvable skin suture is usually placed in the skin incision.

The no-scalpel technique

This procedure was developed in China by Dr Shungiang Li [25] and involves the use of two special instruments (Figure 11.2). These are ring-grasping forceps and a sharp pair of pointed dissecting forceps. A local anaesthetic is injected into the skin and to the vas 2–3 cm away from the testicular end to effect a proximal block. Both vasa are anaesthetized. The oedema generated by the local anaesthetic is therefore 2–3 cm away from the operating site so that the vas can be easily palpated. The vas, and the anaesthetized overlying

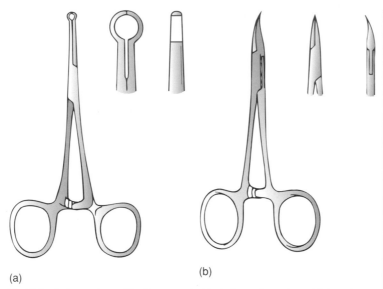

Fig. 11.2 Instruments used for the no-scalpel technique of vasectomy (a) ringed clamp; (b) dissecting forceps. Adapted from *No-scalpel Vasectomy: an Illustrated Guide for Surgeons*. New York: AVSC 1992.

skin, is grasped in the ring forceps. The skin is punctured by one blade of the sharp dissecting forceps and, through this puncture site, both blades are inserted down to the vas. The forceps blades are then opened to spread the tissue. The vas can therefore be seen immediately and exteriorized by the dissecting forceps. The vas is stripped clear of any tissue and ligated as before. The placing of fascia between the two ends has been advocated to reduce the failure rate, although this stage has been regarded as optional. No suture is usually required.

In a study from Bangkok, Thailand, at the King's Birthday Festival on 5 December 1987, 1203 patients were operated on [26], and a comparison was made between a standard vasectomy technique and the no-scalpel technique. The following results were recorded. Twenty-eight physicians operated on 1203 patients. Twelve physicians utilized the no-scalpel technique, whereas 16 physicians used a standard technique. The mean number of procedures was 57 (SD = 12) for the no-scalpel technique compared with 33 (SD = 13) for the standard procedure. Nineteen complications were reported during the 2 weeks following the operations. Sixteen occurred in the standard technique (3.1 per 100 procedures) and three occurred following the no-scalpel technique (0.4 per 100 procedures). Haemorrhage was the most common complication and two patients required surgical drainage. Nine of 11 haemorrhages (including those requiring drainage) resulted from the standard procedure. Eight patients had an infection diagnosed and seven of those resulted from the standard technique and one occurred following the no-scalpel technique.

The advantages of the no scalpel technique are as follows:

• shorter time required

• less pain and oedema (0.09%)

• lower risk of infection (0.9%)

• more acceptable to men

• vasal nerve block ensures painless procedure

• quicker resumption of sexual intercourse.

Morbidity

Vasectomy has a very low mortality [27], but has a relatively high morbidity. Approximately 4–5% of cases will develop a small haematoma or experience sepsis. Large haematomas may need evacuation, as would an abscess. However, such interventions are required only one or two times per 1000 cases. Long-term problems are rare: sperm granulomas and neuromas have been noted. There is no evidence that either testicular cancer or cardiovascular disease is increased with vasectomy. However, there may be a very small increase in prostatic cancers, but it is regarded to be so small as to be insignificant relative to the advantages of a vasectomy [28].

Counselling

The principles of counselling are the same as those adopted for female sterilization. However, there are extra facts to be understood and accepted by the patient. There is a short-term failure rate of 3–5 per 1000. These can be identified by performing two sperm counts following the procedure. This may take between 10 and 20 weeks postoperatively and is said to require an average of 20 ejaculations. Patients are therefore advised to continue other forms of contraception until these two counts have proved negative. There is evidence of long-term intermittent presence of sperm in the ejaculate, which could, very rarely, result in a pregnancy [29,30]. Complications of the procedure should be mentioned and also accepted by the patient. It is wise to ensure that the client seeks immediate advice should any complications occur. A leaflet describing the procedure and its complications should be available for the couple to read.

New methods

Intravasal chemicals and silicone plugs are being evaluated. The object would be to have a simple, reversible method. The techniques are more cumbersome and prolonged than existing methods, and the results of the efficacy and reversibility are being evaluated. Percutaneous diathermy of the vas has also been investigated. The procedure appears simple and safe, but the efficacy appears to be less than optimal. However, should the operation fail, a repeat procedure is easy to perform.

References

1. Rioux JE. Female sterilisation. In: Filshie GM, Guillebaud J (eds). Contraception, science and practice. London: Butterworths, 1991.

2. Yoon I, King TM. A preliminary and immediate report on a new laparoscopic tubal ring procedure. *J Reprod Med* 1975;15:54–7.

3. Hulka JF, Fishbourne J, Mercer JP, et al. Laparoscopic sterilisation with a spring clip. A report of the first fifty cases. *Am J Obstet Gynecol* 1973;116:715–8.

4. Filshie GM, Casey D, Pogmore JR, et al. The titanium/silicone rubber clip for female sterilisation. *Br J Obstet Gynaecol* 1981;88:655–62.

5. Mumford SD, Kessel E. Sterilisation needs in the 1990s: the case for quinacrine nonsurgical female sterilisation. *Am J Obstet Gynecol* 1992;167:1203–7.

6. Mackenzie IZ, Turner E, O'Sullivan GM, Guillebaud J. Two hundred outpatient laparoscopic clip sterilisations using local anaesthesia. *Br J Obstet Gynaecol* 1981;94:449–53.

7. Population Reports. Female sterilisation. 1990; C (10), page 11. Population Information Program, Johns Hopkins University. Baltimore, Maryland, USA.

8. Peterson HB, Zhisen X, Hughes JM, et al. The risk of pregnancy after tubal sterilisation: findings from the US Collaborative Review of Sterilisation. *Am J Obstet Gynecol* 1996; 174:1161–70.

9. Hirsch HA, Nesser E. Bipolar high frequency coagulation. In: van Lith DAF, Keith LG, van Hall EV (eds) New trends in female sterilisation. Chicago, London: Year Book Medical, 1983:83–90.

10. Chi I-C, Lauffe LE, Gardner SD, et al. An epidemiological study of risk factors associated with pregnancy following female sterilisation. *Am J Obstet Gynecol* 1980;136:768–71.

11. Chick PH, Frances M, Paterson PJ. A comprehensive review of female sterilisation – tubal occlusion methods. *Reprod Fertil* 1985;3:81–7.

12. Penney GC, Souter V, Glasier A, Templeton AA. Laparoscopic sterilisation: opinion and practice among gynaecologists in Scotland. *Br J Obstet Gynaecol* 1997;104:71–7.

13. FDA Advisory Panel Meeting, 26 February 1996.

14. Peterson HB, De Stefano F, Rubin GL, et al. Deaths attributable to tubal sterilisation in the United States: 1977–1981. *Am J Obstet Gynecol* 1983;164: 131–6.

15. Kawachi I, Colditz GA, Hankinson S. Long term benefits and risks of alternative methods of fertility control in the United States. *Contraception* 1994;50:1–16.

16. Report on Confidential Enquiries into Maternal Deaths in the United Kingdom, 1991–1993. London: HMSO.

17. Bhiwandiwala PP, Mumford SD, Feldblum PJ. A comparison of different laparsocopic sterilisation occlusion techniques in 24,439 procedures. *Am J Obstet Gynecol* 1982;144:3.

18. Wilcox L, Martinez-Schnell B, Peterson HB, et al. Menstrual function after sterilisation. *Am J Epidemiol* 1992;135:1368–81.

19. Miracle-McMahill HL, Calle EE, Kosinski AS, et al. Tubal ligation and fatal ovarian cancer in a large prospective cohort study. *Am J Epidemiol* 1997; 145:349–57.

20. Robson S, Kerin J. Recurrence of pelvic abscess associated with a detached Filshie clip. *Aust NZ J Obstet Gynaecol* 1993;33:446.

21. Gooden MD, Jaroslav F, Hulka MD, Cristman GM. Spontaneous vaginal expulsion of Hulka clips. *Obstet Gynecol* 1993;81:884–6.

22. Orr CJB. Female sterilisation – the medico–legal aspects. In: Chamberlain GVP, Orr CJB, Sharp F (eds) Litigation and obstetrics and gynecology, Vol. 163. London: Royal College of Obstetrics and Gynaecology, 1985:76.

23. Brundin J. Hysteroscopy for sterilisation. In: Hafez ESE, Os WAA van (eds) Contraceptive delivery systems, Vol. 3.

Amsterdam: Elsevier, 1982:
63–74.

24. Margaret Pyke Centre. One
thousand vasectomies. *Br Med J*
1973;4:216–21.

25. Li S, Goldstein M, Zhu J, et al.
The no-scalpel vasectomy. *J Urol*
1991;145:341–4.

26. Niraphpongporn A, Huber D,
Krieger JN. No scalpel vasectomy
at the King's birthday vasectomy
festival. *Lancet* 1990;335:894–5.

27. Giovannucci E, Tosteson TD,
Speizer FE, et al. A long-term
study of mortality in men who
have undergone vasectomy. *N
Engl J Med* 1992;326:1392–8.

28. Schwingl PJ, Guess HA.
Vasectomy and cancer: an update.
Gynaecol Forum 1996;1:24–8.

29. Philip T, Guillebaud J, Budd D.
Late failure of vasectomy after
two documented analysis
showing asoospermic semen. *Br
Med J* 1984;289:77–9.

30. Thomson JA, Lincoln PJ,
Mortimer P. Paternity by a
seemingly infertile vasecomised
man. *Br Med J* 1993;307:
299–300.

Emergency contraception

Ali Kubba MBChB MFFP FRCOG
John Guillebaud MA FRCSE FRCOG

Introduction

Emergency contraception has been described as the best kept secret in family planning. Worldwide, there is poor awareness of this important emergency method, and its provision remains extremely patchy and passive. This fact sits uncomfortably against a background of a clear need. The impulsive liberating nature of sexual activity means that it can never be rationally controlled and planned on every occasion. It is therefore not surprising that, in 1994, up to 49% of pregnancies in the USA were unintended. The figure for teenagers was 79% [1]. All reversible contraceptives in current use are imperfect and many are user dependent. Discontinuation is the extreme expression of unacceptability of particular methods to their users. A more prevalent trend is for users occasionally to 'opt out' of the use of the method, putting themselves at risk of pregnancy. The more user dependent the method, the more this is likely to happen. Users of such methods as coitus interruptus, condoms and fertility awareness would recognize any risk-taking events. Emergency contraception should complement their chosen method, enhancing its efficacy.

In one survey, 70% of those requesting an abortion would have prevented an unplanned pregnancy if they had accessed emergency contraception [2]. Indeed, emergency contraception was preferred by 90% of a group of women requesting termination of pregnancy. Their access to this method was hindered by lack of awareness [3]. Box 12.1 summarizes the indications for emergency contraception.

Emergency contraception methods

There are two broad categories – hormonal methods and copper intrauterine devices (IUDs). The use of vaginal douches or postcoital spermicides is unlikely to be effective because spermatozoa are 'too quick' for such methods, accessing endocervical mucus within 90 s of ejaculation, and are retrievable from tubal washings within 5 min of deposition in the vagina. Of the hormonal methods, the combined oestrogen–progestogen method, popularized by Albert Yuzpe [4,5], has been the dominant postcoital contraceptive in the Western world. Progestogen-only emergency contraceptives have been widely used in eastern Europe, China and some developing countries. Among the many progestogen-only regimens, the one emerging as the most effective is the levonorgestrel regimen popularized by Ho and Kwan [6]. Table 12.1 lists the hormonal methods and their dosing regimens.

The antiprogesterone, mifepristone, proved a highly effective postcoital contraceptive in two World Health Organization (WHO)-sponsored trials [7,8]. It was given as a single dose of 600 mg within 72 h of unprotected intercourse. It exhibited a low risk of gastrointestinal side effects but tended to delay the onset of subsequent menses owing to a delay of ovulation. The prolonged treatment to menses period is seen as a disadvantage as couples may run further risks of contraceptive accidents or unprotected intercourse. Recurrent/regular use of mifepristone is likely to lead to menstrual chaos.

Copper-containing IUDs are the most effective postcoital contraceptives, with a failure rate of under 1%. While hormonal

Box 12.1 Indications for emergency contraception

1. Unprotected intercourse
   - No method – especially first-time intercourse, well known to be unprotected
   - Coitus interruptus/failed coitus interruptus
   - Ejaculation on external genitalia
   - Miscalculation of the rhythm method (fertility awareness method/periodic abstinence)
   - Spermicide use alone in women at high risk of pregnancy

2. Potential barrier method failures
   - Condom rupture, dislodgement or misuse
   - Diaphragm or cap inserted incorrectly, dislodged during intercourse, found to be torn or removed too early

3. Potential pill failures
   - Missed pills

4. Potential IUD failures
   - Complete or partial expulsion of an IUD
   - Midcycle IUD removal considered absolutely necessary

5. Sexual assault
   Sexual assault of whatever nature is an important indication for emergency contraception. The provision of emergency contraception should not be affected by the probability of legal proceedings in such cases. Providers must be aware of the possibility of sexually transmitted infections. The question of police involvement in order that forensic tests may be conducted should also be raised. Any woman experiencing sexual assault may require long-term emotional support

6. Recent use of suspected teratogens
   - Drugs, e.g. cytotoxics
   - Live vaccines such as yellow fever

Reproduced with permission of the Faculty of Family Planning and Reproductive Health Care of the Royal College of Obstetricians and Gynaecologists from Kubba A, Wilkinson C. Recommendation for Clinical practice: Emergency Contraception. London: Faculty of Family Planning and Reproductive Healthcare, 1998.

methods are effective when given up to 72 h from unprotected intercourse, the IUD can be used up to 5 days. Emergency IUDs prevent pregnancies at least partly through inhibition of implantation of a fertilized ovum. They therefore remain highly effective when used up to 5 days from the earliest calculated date of ovulation [9]. Table 12.2 compares the characteristics of different methods of emergency contraception.

Worldwide, the use of emergency contraception is mainly 'off licence'. IUD licences do not cover emergency use. The combined hormonal method is licensed in six western European countries, South Africa, Australia, New Zealand and,

recently, the USA. A licensed product was introduced in the UK in 1983 (Schering PC4®) and in the USA in 1998 (Preven™). Progestogen-only emergency contraceptives are licensed in at least ten countries. These include Hungary (where Postinor® was licensed in 1981), China, Singapore, Uruguay, Pakistan, Switzerland and Egypt.

The conditions that should be satisfied by the doctor when a licensed product is used for an indication outside its licence are [9]:

- The doctor ensures that he or she is adopting a practice that would be endorsed by a responsible body of professional opinion;

- the doctor has explained clearly to the woman that this is an unlicensed prescription;

- the doctor has explained clearly the perceived risks and benefits, so that informed consent can be obtained and recorded;

- the doctor keeps a record of the woman's details and prescription.

Hormonal methods

Combined hormonal emergency contraception (combined emergency pills)

Oestrogen–progestogen combined pills are administered in two doses. Each dose is 100 μg ethinyloestradiol plus 1000 μg norgestrel equivalent to 500 μg levonorgestrel. The first dose should be initiated within 72 h of intercourse, followed by the second dose 12 h later (Figure 12.1). The method is effective throughout the 72-h window but recent work by the WHO shows higher efficacy of earlier administration. The failure rate, when given within 12 h of intercourse, was 0.5% versus 4.1% when given in the last 12 h of the 72-h window [10]. For every 12-h delay of treatment the failure rate increased 50%.

Contraindications to hormonal emergency contraception are few. None, apart from pregnancy, is absolute (Table 12.3). The WHO has designated this method as safe, with no contraindications, apart from pregnancy.

The main side effects of the combined method are

Table 12.1 Hormonal emergency contraception methods

(a) Combined methods:

1. Licensed products

Single dose	Initiated	Repeated	Brand name
100 µg EE + 1000 µg NG	Within 72 h	12 h later	*Schering PC4®* E-Gen-C® SA, Neo Primovlar 4® Finland, Tetragynon® Denmark, Germany, Norway, Sweden, Switzerland
100 µg EE + 500 µg LNG + pregnancy test	Within 72 h	12 h later	Preven®

2. 'Home-made' preparations (unlicensed)[a]

Tablet composition in micrograms	Number of tablets to make a single dose	Brand name
EE 50 + LNG 250	2	*Ovran*
EE 50 + LNG 250	2	Ovral
EE 30 + LNG 150	4	*Microgynon 30 Ovranette Levlen/Levora* Nordette *Rigevidon*
EE 30 + NG 300	4	Lo/Ovral/Femenal
EE 20 + LNG 100	5	Alesse/Levlite
Phasic	4 *ochre*	*Logynon/Trinordial*
EE 30 + LNG 125	4 yellow	Triphasil/Tri-levlen
	4 pink	Trivora

(b) Levonorgestrel-alone home-made preparations (unlicensed)[a]

Tablet composition	Number of tablets to make a single dose	Brand name
0.03 mg LNG	25	*Microval/Norgeston/Microlut*
0.075 mg NG	20	Ovrette *Neogest*
0.75 mg LNG	1	Postinor-2

[a]The treatment course is of two doses, the first initiated within 72 h and repeated 12 h later
Italics are used for products available in the UK, otherwise the products are US products unless otherwise indicated.
EE = ethinyloestradiol; LNG = levonorgestrel; NG = norgestrel.
NB Danazol has been used in a number of trials; efficacy is not proven.

gastrointestinal: nausea has been reported in up to 66% of users and vomiting in up to 24% of users. Other minor side effects include mastalgia and headaches.

Emergency contraception may cause a change in the timing of the post-treatment menses. Menstruation occurs early in 15–20% of users, is late in 20% and is on time in over 50%. A total of 98% of users would have had a period within 3 weeks of the treatment [4,5].

Amenorrhoea beyond 3 weeks should be investigated to exclude a pregnancy. A sensitive pregnancy test, done at that time, would be positive if pregnancy was the result of treatment failure.

There is currently no evidence of an adverse effect on pregnancy outcome in cases where emergency hormonal contraception fails and pregnancy continues to term. A register of pregnancies continuing to term after failed emergency hormonal contraception is kept by the Faculty of Family Planning and Reproductive Healthcare of the Royal College of Obstetricians and Gynaecologists in the UK, and shows no excess congenital abnormalities [11]. However, counselling patients requesting emergency contraception must emphasize that a normal outcome to a pregnancy cannot be guaranteed.

The following counselling points on the outcome of pregnancy after failed hormonal emergency contraception should be considered.

- The impact of the postcoital hormones is limited to the peri–implantation embryo phase. Noxious agents acting at such a time have an 'all or nothing' effect.

- Evidence from the literature shows no excess risk of congenital abnormalities.

- A normal outcome to any pregnancy cannot be guaranteed. There is a background risk of a major congenital abnormality of 2%.

- The woman has to be positive enough about the unplanned pregnancy to continue to term without undue anxiety.

- Failed hormonal emergency contraception is not an indication for a therapeutic termination of pregnancy.

The mechanism of action of hormonal emergency contraception, be it combined or progestogen–only, is likely to be multifocal at ovarian, endometrial and tubal levels. The endometrium is 'desynchronized' through an effect on endometrial enzymes and endometrial progesterone receptors, which are significantly downregulated [12]. The endometrium is therefore rendered unreceptive to a

Table 12.2 Comparison of hormonal emergency contraception (progestogen-only and combined) and intrauterine emergency contraception

	Emergency hormonal contraceptive	IUD
Efficacy	High	Very high
Contraindications	Few	Fewer
Method provides contraceptive cover for the rest of the cycle	No (condoms may be used)	Yes (and long term, if appropriate)
Requires medical intervention (procedure or examination)	Infrequently	Always
Suitable for multiple exposures over 72 h from presentation	No data on efficacy yet	Suitable, as long as within 5 days of earliest ovulation
Breastfeeding[a]	Not contraindicated unless lactation is already poor or not well established Warn the mother that a female infant may get a withdrawal bleed Give the option of stopping breast feeding for 24 h to minimize exposure of baby	Acceptable but beware placement problems in early postpartum period

[a]NB The lactational amenorrhoea method (LAM) confers substantial contraceptive cover.
Reproduced with permission of the Faculty of Family Planning and Reproductive Health Care of the Royal College of Obstetricians and Gynaecologists.

fertilized ovum. These are the only consistently reported 'effects'. Many authorities in the field believe that transient disruption of ovarian activity is the most important action of the combined method. When given preovulation, hormonal methods tend to delay ovulation by approximately 7 days and would prolong the cycle in question [13]. Given at or after ovulation, the ovarian effect is variable but predominantly disruptive to corpus luteum function [14]. Both oestrogens and progestogens affect tubal motility, and this action may interfere with sperm and ovum transport and fertilization.

Progestogen-only emergency contraception

There is a long history of postcoital use of progestogens alone. They were originally introduced for repeated use timed to follow coitus as a simple, easy to teach method that promotes compliance in the less motivated.

In such cases, coital frequency defines the exposure to hormones, with a likely reduction in the total dose if coital frequency is restricted by protocol or the lifestyle of the user (e.g. the levonorgestrel product Postinor has a use limit of 4× per cycle). Efficacy of progestogen-only emergency methods is quoted as being high and is likely to be higher with higher frequency of use.

The Chinese home visiting/ vacation pills were used to provide planned contraceptive hormone cover for a period of 2 weeks a year, when couples working apart during the rest of the year were united and likely to have a high level of sexual activity [15] (Table 12.4). The treatment is started 2 days before the 'vacation'. Providers of such methods claim acceptable efficacy but evidence from controlled trials was lacking.

Several progestogen-only regimens have been used as emergency contraceptives. Efficacy was perceived to be inferior to the combined regimen

until the publication of the Ho and Kwan comparative study confirming comparable efficacy to the Yuzpe method. In 1998, a large, well-conducted, WHO trial, comparing levonorgestrel–alone and the combined 'Yuzpe' regimens, revealed an efficacy of the levonorgestrel regimen which was higher than earlier studies and which surpassed the highest efficacy stated for the Yuzpe regimen [16].

Other advantages of progestogen-only emergency contraception are the absence of oestrogen, the lower risk of gastrointestinal side effects and possibly that it is especially suitable for lactating women. There is a variable effect of progestogens on ovarian function. They can inhibit ovulation if used in frequent high doses.

Emergency intrauterine contraception

Postcoital use of copper-bearing IUDs started in the late 1960s. They were found to be effective if

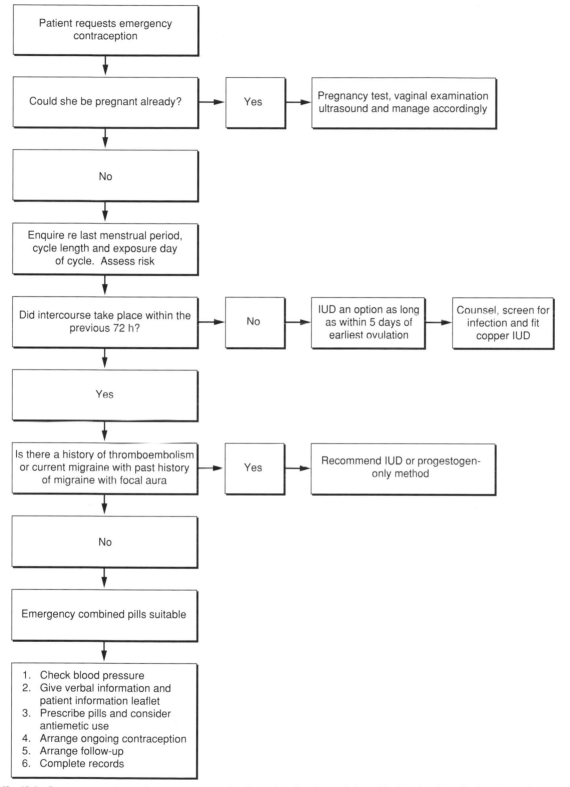

Fig. 12.1 Emergency contraception management plan. Reproduced with permission of the Faculty of Family Planning and Reproductive Health Care of the Royal College of Obstetricians and Gynaecologists.

Table 12.3 Contraindications to emergency contraception

Condition	Combined hormonal method	Progestogen-only hormonal method	Copper IUD
Suspected pregnancy	Contraindicated	Contraindicated	Contraindicated
Past history of ectopic pregnancy	Not contraindicated	Not contraindicated	Relative contraindication[a]
Past history of thromboembolism	Relative contraindication[b]	Not contraindicated	Not contraindicated
Migraine at presentation	Contraindicated only if previous history of migraine with focal aura	Not contraindicated	Not contraindicated

[a]Can be removed at next menses.
[b]Progestogen-only method preferable.
Reproduced with permission of the Faculty of Family Planning and Reproductive Health Care of the Royal College of Obstetricians and Gynaecologists.

used up to 5 days from unprotected intercourse. When efficacy is calculated per cycle of treatment, the emergency IUD has the lowest failure rate of all postcoital agents. Only half a dozen failures have been reported in a literature comprising over 8000 woman–cycles. The mechanism of action is hypothesized to be through prevention of implantation and the spermicidal/blastocidal action of copper. Studies seeking

evidence of implantation in emergency IUD users by detection of beta-human chorionic gonadotrophin have failed to find such evidence. This refutes the notion that postcoital IUDs are abortifacient. The emergency IUD is versatile, in that it can be used up to 5 days from the earliest calculated date of ovulation (up to day 19 of a 28-day cycle, assuming that ovulation occurred on day 14) [9]. This also means that an IUD

can cover multiple exposures, as long as they have occurred within this time window. The use of the IUD up to 7 days from unprotected intercourse was investigated in a couple of studies. No conclusions on efficacy can be drawn owing to small numbers.

The usual precautions that underpin IUD-use protocols apply to postcoital use. It is especially important to screen and/or administer prophylactic

Table 12.4 Chinese home visiting or vacation pills

Name	Dosage (mg)	Efficacy (% of cycles)[a]	Mode of administration
Simple progestogens			
Norethisterone	5	99.5	In case of vacation, one pill in the evening, then one pill each day for 10–14 days; change to pill no. 1 (norethisterone-ethinyloestradiol combination pill – various doses) or no. 2 (megestrol + ethinyloestradiol combination pill – various doses) if vacation longer than 2 weeks
Megestrol	2	99.6	One pill at midday before vacation and then in the evening. Afterwards, one pill each day until the next day after vacation
Quingestanol	80	98.8	One pill daily for 2 weeks
Norgestrel	3	99.9	One pill 1–2 days before vacation, then one pill every day. Change to pill no. 1 or no. 2, if vacation longer than 2 weeks
R-2323	2.5	99.5	Similar to norgestrel
Norethisterone acetate-3-oxime	1	99.3	Similar to norgestrel
Progestogen combinations			
Mequingestanol	Megestrol 0.55 Quingestanol 0.88	98.2	One pill at midday before vacation, then one pill postcoitally
Chlorquingestanol	Chlormadinone 0.25 Quingestanol 0.85	99.5	One pill at midday before vacation, then one pill every evening
Non-progestogen			
Anordrin	7.5	99.5	Was used as a postcoital agent. Results were equivocal

[a]Woman-cycles, not woman-years.
Reproduced with permission of Butterworth from Yuzpe A, Kubba A. Postcoital contraception. In: Filshie M, Guilleband J (eds) Contraception: science and practice. London: Butterworths, 1989:126–43.

antibiotics in situations where there is a risk of sexually transmitted infections, such as when unprotected intercourse has taken place with a new partner, was the result of a casual encounter or in cases of sexual assault.

The classic contraindications to the use of the IUD, such as menorrhagia or a past history of ectopic pregnancy, do not apply to the use of the IUD postcoitally as the device is only required in the latter half of the cycle of treatment and, indeed, may be removed with the next menses. However, an advantage of the IUD is that it will serve as a contraceptive for the rest of the cycle of treatment and may be kept *in situ* for ongoing contraception if that is the woman's wish.

Table 12.2 compares the attributes of emergency intrauterine contraception with those of hormonal methods.

When used in young nulliparous women, consideration should be given to use of local anaesthesia. Choice of devices with a small insertion diameter, such as the recently introduced GyneFix®.

Hormone-releasing intrauterine systems are not suitable for emergency contraception, as copper, through its instantaneous effect on endometrial environment, seems to be important for the antifertilization–implantation effect of the emergency IUD [9].

Efficacy of emergency contraception

The variables that influence efficacy include the couple's fertility, the use of 'dubious' contraceptives, such as douching, the patient's recall of the timing of exposure(s) and the lack of a control group in all studies owing to ethical considerations.

Failure of emergency contraception can be expressed in two ways. Crude failure rates are based on the percentage of treatment failures per cycle (woman–month). A more accurate assessment of failure is to calculate the ratio of the pregnancies observed to those which would have otherwise been expected if a postcoital agent was not given (17).

The IUD is the most effective emergency contraceptive with a failure rate of under 1%.

The probability of conception on each day of the menstrual cycle was calculated from previous studies and formed the basis for calculating the ratio of observed to expected pregnancies [17–19]. A review of the efficacy of the Yuzpe regimen looked at seven studies in which the number of women treated and the outcome of treatment by cycle day of unprotected intercourse were identified [20]. The range of efficacy of the Yuzpe regimen was estimated to be between 44.2% and 88.7% (i.e. it prevented at least two out of three pregnancies, and may prevent as many as four out of five). In everyday practice, efficacy–failure rates are expressed as number of failures per 100 women-months. The failure rate of the Yuzpe regimen in this model ranges from under 1% to 5%, with the higher rate applying to unprotected intercourse in midcycle. Efficacy tends to be higher in well-conducted studies, where users had a single unprotected intercourse and gave accurate menstrual histories. One of the postulated reasons for apparent lower efficacy of the method is poor recall or reporting of previous coital exposures and/or menstrual dates (i.e. some women are already pregnant when treated). This may explain the observation in some studies that women treated in the latter third of their menstrual cycles, supposed to be the least 'fertile' phase, seem to experience higher failure rates than expected for that particular phase of the cycle. Some women may have unprotected intercourse following treatment, contributing further to the apparent failures.

The WHO's randomized controlled trial comparing the Yuzpe regimen with the progestogen-only regimen confirmed the efficacy of the Yuzpe regimen, but showed it to be lower than earlier studies. Although the WHO trial has the advantage of large numbers (nearly 1000 in each group) and fairly tight confidence intervals, this finding needs further confirmation. The overall failure rate of the Yuzpe regimen in this study was 3.2%, equivalent to a true efficacy rate of 57%, i.e. at least one in two pregnancies were prevented.

In the same study, the efficacy of the Yuzpe and levonorgestrel regimens in a subset of 1157 women who used the assigned regimens correctly was 76% and 89%, respectively. The fact that, in the whole group, the Yuzpe regimen was less effective makes one suspect that gastrointestinal side effects may have led to violation of the protocol in some users, with this not being reported to the investigators.

The same study found levonorgestrel alone to be highly effective when given up to 72 h from unprotected intercourse. The overall failure rate was 1.1%, with a significant trend of higher efficacy the earlier the treatment is given, with a failure rate of 0.4% in the first 24 h rising to 2.7% in the last 24 h of the 72-h window. Ethnic origin did not affect efficacy.

An ectopic pregnancy has been reported following the Yuzpe regimen but a causal link has not been established [21].

A WHO comparative trial of a three-dosage regimen of 600 mg, 50 mg and 10 mg mifepristone administered as a single dose within 120 h of unprotected intercourse showed the 10 mg dose to be as effective as the 600 mg [22]. However, failures did occur, which is a departure from findings from previous research [7,8]. Efficacy was still at the upper end of the efficacy range, with 85% of expected pregnancies prevented by mifepristone.

Recurrent use of emergency contraception

The total dose of the Yuzpe regimen is equivalent to seven low-dose, combined oral contraceptive pills. The levonorgestrel-alone method has 50% more progestogen but the total dose is still relatively low. Even if used repeatedly, the total dose of emergency contraception would be small compared to regular pill taking. There is no evidence to suggest that women resort to the use of emergency

contraception in place of ongoing regular family planning. Those women who may experience recurrent episodes of unprotected intercourse or contraceptive failure may be best served by emergency contraception to avoid an unplanned pregnancy, and should not be denied the treatment.

Antiemetics

In case of vomiting of the tablets within 2 h of ingestion, a repeat dose with an antiemetic is recommended or the use of an IUD should be considered. The optimal antiemetic is domperidone because of its safety profile and the lack of extrapyramidal side effects or sedation. Domperidone acts on the chemoreceptor trigger zone, which is the area that triggers nausea and vomiting in hormonal method users. Antiemetics do reduce the risk of nausea and vomiting. Routine concomitant use of antiemetics has been associated, in one study, with a lower failure rate [23].

Drug interaction

Broad-spectrum antibiotics are unlikely to have an impact on bioavailability of the contraceptive steroids, so no alteration of the dosage is required. Drugs that induce hepatic enzymes may be expected to reduce bioavailability and, thereby, efficacy. It is recommended that the dose of the Yuzpe regimen is increased by 50% (i.e. three tablets used within 72 h and repeated 12 h later, instead of two tablets).

Use in older women

Age is not a contraindication to emergency hormonal or intrauterine contraception.

Ethical objections to the method

As some of the pregnancies prevented by emergency contraception are likely to be prevented through an antinidation effect of the treatment, patients who have a moral objection to methods that may work postfertilization should be counselled accordingly and allowed to make an informed decision. Failure of emergency contraception is not an indication for a termination of pregnancy.

Postpartum use

The IUD or progestogen-only method should not interfere with lactation. It is unlikely that the Yuzpe regimen would have a significant effect where lactation has been established, which would be the case by the time an emergency contraceptive is indicated. The mother should be warned that, if she continues to breastfeed in the immediate post-treatment day or so, enough exposure of a female infant to oestrogen and its subsequent elimination may lead to the baby experiencing a small withdrawal bleed.

Restarting regular contraception

Emergency hormonal contraception does not have a

prospective protective effect and couples must use a barrier method, or abstain, until the next period. Oral contraception can be started on the first day of the subsequent period. The woman should seek advice if she suspects that her post-treatment menses was abnormal in any way.

Figure 12.1 illustrates an emergency contraception management plan.

The future

Mifepristone remains a promising product whose true potential remains untested. It has the attraction of a single, low dose of a non-oestrogenic preparation with high efficacy and low gastrointestinal side effects.

The true potential of emergency contraception in reducing unplanned pregnancies and abortions is still unrealized because of poor awareness and motivation from some health professionals and the public in many parts of the world. The fact that emergency contraception remains a prescription medication is a barrier against wider use, although one also has to address the pharmaceutical houses' anxiety about uncontrolled use and the potential for litigation. A compromise solution may be the provision of emergency hormonal contraception through pharmacists working with a local, regional or national protocol and liaising with local healthcare providers.

Self-administration/'take home' emergency contraception can be a fail safe option and should encourage responsible use of ongoing contraception. The largest study so far in this area confirms that making emergency contraception available for self-administration does not reduce the use of other mainstream methods of contraception [24]. In the study, the relative risk of unintended pregnancies was 0.7 in the self-adminstering group compared to controls. Although this was not statistically significant, it points to a potential advantage when emergency contraception is made more accessible.

The concept of a 'once a month' hormonal contraceptive is unlikely to be practical because of the need to time the treatment accurately for midcycle when ovulation suppression is the target. Ethical considerations hinder use of a once a month method late in the cycle when implantation may have occurred.

Resource list

USA

- The American College of Obstetricians and Gynecologists produce a patient education leaflet on emergency contraception (August 1997). Contact: ACOG, 409, 17th Street SW, PO Box 96920, Washington DC, 20090-6920.

- ACOG Practice Patterns – Emergency Oral Contraception 1996, no. 3

- Emergency contraception hotline 1–888–NOT–2–LATE 1–888–668–2528

- Program for Appropriate Technology in Health (PATH) produce information for professionals and the public. Contact: PATH, 4 Nicherson Street, Seattle, WA 98109

- Websites
  - www.PREVEN.com
  - www.path.org info@path.org
  - http://opr.Princeton.edu/ec/ (in English and Spanish)

UK and Europe

- The UK Family Planning Association produce leaflets on all aspects of contraception including emergency contraception. Contact: UKFPA, 2–12 Pentonville Road, London N1 9FP

- UK Health Education Authority run emergency contraception campaigns. Contact: UK HEA, 30 Great Peter Street, London SW1P 2HW

- ADMCU (Association pour le Développement des Méthodes de Contraception d' Urgence), Hôpital Broussais, 96 rue Didot, 75014 Paris, France (Tel. 01 43 95 90 60)

Worldwide

- Emergency Contraception. A guide for service delivery. WHO 1998. WHO/FRH/FPP/98.19

- Emergency Contraceptive Pills. A Resource Packet for Health Care Providers and

Programme Managers –
Consortium for Emergency
Contraception 1998

References

1. Henshaw SK. Unintended pregnancy in the United States *Fam Plann Perspect* 1998; 30:24–9, 46.

2. Duncan G, Harper C, Ashwell E, et al. Termination of pregnancy: lessons for prevention. *Br J Fam Plann* 1990;15:112–7.

3. Bromham DR, Cartmill RS. Knowledge and use of emergency contraception among patients requesting termination of pregnancy. *Br Med J* 1993;306:556–7.

4. Yuzpe AA, Lance WJ. Ethinylestradiol and DL-norgestrel as a post-coital contraceptive. *Fertil Steril* 1977;28:932–36.

5. Yuzpe AA, Percival Smith R, Rademaker AW. A multi-center clinical investigation employing ethinylestradiol combined with DL-norgestrel as a post-coital contraceptive agent. *Fertil Steril* 1982;37:508–13.

6. Ho PC, Kwan MSW. A prospective, randomised comparison of levonorgestrel with the Yuzpe regimen in post-coital contraception. *Hum Reprod* 1993;8:389–92.

7. Glasier A, Thong KJ, Dewar M, Baird DT. Mifepristone (RU 486) compared with high dose estrogen and progestogen for emergency postcoital contraception. *N Engl J Med* 1992;327:1041–4.

8. Webb AMC, Russell J, Elstein M. Comparison of the Yuzpe regimen, Danazol and mifepristone (RU 486) in oral postcoital contraception. *Br J Med* 1992;305:927–31.

9. Kubba A, Wilkinson C. Recommendation for clinical practice: emergency contraception. London: Faculty of Family Planning and Reproductive Health Care, 1998.

10. Piaggio G, von Hertzen H, Grimes DA, Van Look PFA, on behalf of the Task Force on Postovulatory Methods of Fertility Regulation. Timing of emergency contraception with levonorgestrel or the Yuzpe regimen. *Lancet* 1999;353:721.

11. Cardy GC. Outcome of pregnancies after failed hormonal postcoital contraception: an interim report. *Br J Fam Plann* 1995;21:112–15.

12. Kubba AA, White JO, Guillebaud J, et al. The biochemistry of human endometrium after two regimens of postcoital contraception: a dl-norgestrel/ethinylestradiol combination or Danazol. *Fertil Steril* 1986;45:512–16.

13. Ling WY, Wrixon W, Acorn T, et al. Mode of action of dl-norgestrel and ethinyl estradiol combination in postcoital contraception. III. Effect of preovulatory administration following luteinizing hormone surge on ovarian steroidogenesis. *Fertil Steril* 1983;40:631–6.

14. Ling WY, Wrixon W, Zayid I, et al. Mode of action of DL-norgestrel and ethinylestradiol combination in post-coital contraception. II. Effect of postovulatory administration on ovarian function and endometrium. *Fertil Steril* 1983;39:292–7.

15. Yuzpe A, Kubba A. Postcoital contraception. In: Filshie M, Guillebaud J (eds) Contraception, science and practice. London: Butterworth, 1989:126–43.

16. Task Force on Postovulatory Methods of Fertility Regulation. Randomised, controlled trial of levonorgestrel versus the Yuzpe regimen of combined oral contraceptives for emergency contraception. *Lancet* 1998;352:428–33.

17. Kubba A. The efficacy of emergency hormonal contraception. In: Paintin D (ed) The provision of emergency hormonal contraception. London: RCOG Press 1995.

18. Dixon GW, Schlesselman JJ, Ory HW, et al. Ethinylestradiol and conjugated estrogens on post-coital contraceptives. *JAMA* 1980;244:1336–9.

19. Trussell J, Steward F. The effectiveness of postcoital hormonal contraception. *Fam Plann Perspect* 1992;24:262–4.

20. Trussell J, Rodriguez G, Ellertson C. New estimates of the effectiveness of the Yuzpe regimen of emergency contraception. *Contraception* 1998;57:363–9.

21. Kubba AA, Guillebaud J. Case of ectopic pregnancy after postcoital contraception with ethinyloestradiol-levonorgestrel. *Br Med J* 1983;287:1343–4.

22. Taskforce on Postovulatory Methods of Fertility Regulation. Comparison of three single doses of Mifepristone as emergency contraception: a randomised trial. *Lancet* 1999;353:697–702.

23. Baghshaw SN, Edwards D, Tucker AK. Ethinyl oestradiol and dl-norgestrel is an effective emergency postcoital contraceptive: a report of its use in 1,200 patients in a family planning clinic. *Aust NZ J Obstet Gynaecol* 1988;28:137–40.

24. Glasier A, Baird D. The effects of self-administering emergency contraception. *N Engl J Med* 1998;339:1–4.

The contraceptive decision: information and counselling

Toni Belfield BSC FRSH

'The methods of fertility regulation from which most couples choose represent a choice among unpleasant alternatives. The choice is not so much a positive discrimination but a negative one, in that the methods not chosen are even more disliked than the method that is chosen. The contraceptive methods most people use are therefore the least unpleasant of an unpleasant set of alternatives. However, it is most important that this realistic summary is set against the other reality that consumers greatly prefer the available range of methods to no methods at all.'[1]

The last 30 years has seen a huge change in the availability and provision of contraceptive methods. Research shows that people are knowledgeable about contraception, yet a substantial body of research throughout the world consistently demonstrates that women and men using contraception lack knowledge about how methods work, how to use methods and what to do if a contraceptive method's effectiveness is compromised. As a result, unintended pregnancies and requests for abortion remain high. Contraception enables people to choose whether and/or when to have children. It is by its very nature inextricably linked with emotional and sexual well-being, and it is impossible to talk about contraception without addressing sexuality – the two are inseparable.

Obtaining harmonized, objective information on reproduction and fertility is not only a need, it is a right. Such knowledge provides an understanding of *how* health, emotions and behaviours relate to fertility, it *enables* an unravelling of the myths, misconceptions and misinformation that exist, and can *minimize* the embarrassment and anxieties that surround this often taboo subject. Knowledge and choice on contraception provide empowerment and confidence, which in turn enable improved reproductive decisions and choices to be made.

Women's and men's contraceptive needs, expectations and choices are influenced by many factors: knowledge, information, lifestyle need, age, religion, ethnicity, perceptions (their own and others), anxieties and embarrassment [2–4]. Provider preference and service delivery contribute to limiting or improving acceptability and choice [5,6]. The ability to control fertility has been shown to be in direct proportion to the amount of information an individual has, how they feel about their sexuality and sexual identity as well as feelings of personal self-worth and determination. An extensive literature review of research in the area of users' perspectives on fertility regulation is discussed and summarized in a WHO report entitled 'Beyond acceptability: users' perspectives on contraception' [4].

The main findings from that review include the following.

- Contraceptive users lack complete information about both methods and services.

- Women's and men's needs and preferences for contraception change over time, and vary with the person's stage of life.

- Universally, women and men would like a method that is safe and effective, but it is not clear what these concepts mean. Side effects and health concerns (particularly with respect to hormonal methods) and method failure (particularly with respect to barrier methods and periodic abstinence) are the major reasons why women discontinue or do not use contraception.

- Individual perspectives and preferences vary widely and defy generalization.

- The limited range of methods available in many developing countries necessarily limits people's perceptions and preferences.

- Research on people's reactions to a hypothetical method does not usually yield information predictive of subsequent use or behaviour with the method.

- There is a particular lack of information about the perspectives of men, adolescents, women having an abortion, especially repeat abortion, and women in the postpartum period.

Research continues to confirm Snowden's findings that women for the most part still perceive contraceptive choices as a matter of finding the 'least-worst' option, balancing effectiveness and ease of use with perceptions and expectations of side effects and health risks [3,6].

Increasing knowledge and confidence depend on identifying and countering misinformation on promoting the benefits of use through accurate, complete, consistent and memorable information about the method of choice [7]. The motive for providing information is to help patients/clients understand their clinical situation and help them make the best choices [8]. Patient choices and behaviour depend not simply on the provision of information, but on the context in which people are involved in making decisions and on how that information is understood – 'its not *what* you say, it is also *how* you say it'. For patients to participate fully in decision making, they need first of all to be authorized to ask questions, to make demands, to make informed decisions and be able to consent.

Providing good contraception and sexual health services today requires training, knowledge, skill and sensitivity. The facilities offered and the way in which they are offered are important factors in determining where people want to go to receive their contraception. Yet there is little information on the way in which professionals inform or advise their clients, and so affect consumer decisions to start, continue or stop a contraceptive method. Communication skills have a major influence on the adequacy of the contraceptive consultation: questioning, listening, non-verbal communication and care given during physical examinations. It relates to patient/client satisfaction: lack of friendliness, poor communication and use of appropriate or suitable language. It affects patient compliance: failure to understand or remember what has been said. Many professionals make assumptions, often underestimating a person's degree of motivation, ability or needs, and 'censor' or limit information. Many also adopt a variety of ways to pressure a woman to use certain methods. Because of this, women (quite rightly) express feelings of anger, frustration and powerlessness because they feel they are not listened to, not spoken to on equal terms, and not given time or permission to voice fears or anxieties. These findings are backed up daily by the enquiries to the UK Family Planning Association's (FPA) national Contraceptive Telephone Helpline, which handles over 100 000 enquiries a year on all aspects of contraception, sexual and reproductive health, including service provision. Research shows women and men want *more* information not less. This is in direct contrast to the opinion of a number of professionals who feel that the public cannot deal with 'too much' information. Clearly, there is information which people have a *right* to know – advantages, disadvantages and the uncertain areas about risk and benefit, and the information that people *need* to know in order to use their chosen method safely and effectively. Professionals need to be aware of how far they ought to go in determining choice rather than influencing it.

Hatcher et al. [9] discuss the importance of informed consent in family planning and reproductive health as having three bases:

- pragmatic
- ethical
- legal.

Pragmatically, a person who thoroughly understands their contraceptive method or medical procedure will be more likely to use it safely and effectively. Ethically, every person has a right to information about methods or procedures that can affect their health. Legally, the doctor must provide information that enables patients to make an informed decision. If patients are not given sufficient information, they may sue for negligence. The general standard for medical negligence is the Bolam test. As long as a 'responsible body of medical opinion' would support the doctor's action, then the action is not negligent. The focus of patient choice is therefore not simply the provision of information, but the context in which patients are involved in making decisions in a voluntary and non-coerced way.

The US Department of Health and Human Services regulations – informed consent – is comprised of seven basic elements. Hatcher et al. [9] provides a useful mnemonic for these: BRAIDED:

- **B**enefits of the method;

- **R**isks of the method (both major risks and all common minor ones), including the consequences of method failure;

- **A**lternatives to the method (including abstinence and no method);

- **I**nquiries about the method are the patient's right and responsibility;

- **D**ecision to withdraw from using the method without penalty is the patient's right;

- **E**xplanation of the method is owed to the patient – including uncertainties in medical knowledge and opinion;

- **D**ocumentation that the clinician has covered each of the previous six points by providing good case notes or consent forms.

Ensuring a positive partnership between patients and professionals is vital and can be achieved by recognizing the need to improve patient information and counselling, understanding the issues surrounding the doctor–patient interaction, and considering the influences of power, knowledge and different expectations of both doctor and patient. Baraitser [10] identifies six different types of 'knowledge' which may influence a contraceptive consultation:

- doctors' knowledge from formal training;

- doctors' knowledge from their observations of patients' experience with different contraceptives;

- contraceptive users' knowledge from their own experience;

- doctors' knowledge of contraception from their own or their partners' personal experience;

- contraceptive users' knowledge from the experience of friends and relatives;

- various kinds of knowledge more or less in the public domain, for example from the media.

Baraitser then argues that many types of knowledge must be legitimized within the consultation because:

- if health professionals impose a medical frame of reference on contraceptive consultations which undervalues women's experience of their own

bodies, it will, for example, discourage women reporting side effects because they do not expect to be taken seriously;

- legitimizing many types of knowledge leads to better understanding of client choices and actions – if a client presents with an unplanned pregnancy having stopped using a particular contraceptive method, her reasons need to be understood to help her plan contraception in the future.

Recognizing the complexities in contraceptive choices, a number of strategies can be introduced to address and improve contraceptive services and the contraceptive decision process.

Contraceptive service provision

- Provide accessible and flexible clinical services that address the diversity of sexual and reproductive health care needs within the community.

- Provide a full range of contraceptive methods or accessible referral to other services that do.

- Ensure all staff (medical and non-medical) are appropriately trained, updated and properly resourced – use the different skill mix to the best advantage.

- Provide information about services so people *know* about them.

- Ensure confidentiality in visits, communications and record keeping. This is vital for all age groups but especially teenagers, where aspects of confidentiality outweigh any anxieties about the consequences of unprotected sex [11–13]. Arrange for staff to sign a confidentiality clause.

- Practice an ethos of equality regarding age, gender, race, sexual orientation and disability.

- Ensure an established rapport and mutual respect with clients.

- Ensure consulting rooms are pleasant and do not have barriers (i.e. desks) between the professional and client.

- Provide sufficient *time* for contraceptive consultations, especially the first visit.

- Provide, where appropriate, a choice of male or female doctors, advocacy workers and interpreters.

- Provide effective services that are designed, developed and delivered on the basis of local needs assessment, which include the views of users, past users and non-users of services.

- Provide efficient and good-quality audited services.

- Know about other sexual and reproductive health services for referral.

Contraceptive information and counselling

- Recognize that contraception and sex are inextricably linked.

- Always provide accurate, complete, consistent and objective information.

- Use suitable, appropriate language that both enables and informs.

- Be aware and note non-verbal cues, such as body language, tone of voice and speed of talking.

- Always discuss risks *and* benefits *and* uncertainties. All information and advice should be explicitly supported by the best available evidence.

- Be a catalyst and facilitator not an 'educator' who tends to tell what needs to be done. *Check out* information needs and concerns by asking questions.

- Recognize people are not always comfortable and need 'permission' to ask questions. Listen to the client and respond.

- Spend more time on compliance-related issues at the initial consultation.

- Provide verbal information and 'back-up' written information about methods, recognizing that client's questions and choices are based on the following:

(a) Effectiveness, i.e. will the method work? There is no perfect method and giving information about contraceptive efficacy is complex. Research by the FPA [14] illustrates the need to present this information in both percentages and numbers with definitions. This must also recognize the need to discuss the difference between 'user' and 'method' failure rates.

(b) Suitability, i.e. will it harm me?

(c) Risks and benefits – known and unknown.

(d) How to use, i.e. when to start a method, when it becomes effective, when to stop it (e.g. a planned pregnancy), how long it can be used for.

(e) What to do if it fails, if it is not used consistently, and if there is concomitant use of drugs or illness.

(f) How the method works, i.e. does the method's primary or secondary actions prevent ovulation, or work before or after ovulation? This has important considerations for those who believe that life begins at fertilization, rather than the general medical and legal opinion defining life beginning at implantation.

- Increase motivation – be prepared to offer solutions to practical difficulties which the client experiences in using methods correctly *and* consistently (such as provision of written information or telephone support).

- Be aware of clients not attending follow-up or not collecting repeat prescriptions.

- Recognize that a compliant attitude does not necessarily reflect compliant behaviour.

- Recognize that non-compliance may result from feelings of loss of status and/or control.

- Pay attention to discussed side effects (whether real or perceived).

- Discuss the transient nature of side effects that relate to hormonal methods when first starting (e.g. unpredictable bleeding).

Patient information

One of the forces driving the concept of evidence-based patient choice is the wish to provide patients with information [8]. The value of patient information is enormous and research has demonstrated consistently that giving information does have beneficial effects as well as enabling people to make choices [6,15]. The growth and wider availability of the Internet means more information is available; however, much of it is inaccurate and misleading [16], providing a continued role for professionals to check fact from fiction for their clients (and themselves!). Various checklists reviewed by Entwistle [17] have been proposed to enhance the quality of health information. 'DISCERN' has been developed as new guidelines to provide quality criteria for the content of written consumer health information [18].

Criteria addressed include:

- accessibility;
- acceptability;
- readability;
- comprehensibility;
- style, layout and attractiveness of presentation;
- accuracy and reliability of content;
- review for updating;
- references to source and strength of evidence;
- credibility of authors, organizations, publishers, etc.

There is an absolute need to research patients' information needs and involve them in developing and testing materials. Information produced and given needs to ensure that *all* groups have the same access and ability to information and care. Failure to pay attention to the quality of information obtained by patients can have serious consequences. Providing good information will enhance the quality and appropriateness of healthcare.

Conclusion

Korsch and Harding [19] discuss why patients and doctors often have different interpretations of their encounters and look to provide solutions for patients. 'Barriers to communication can be avoided by greater understanding, trying harder, increasing sensitivity and more imagination'. Patient satisfaction is not based on whether a medicine, product or method is obtained, but on whether they think their doctors understand their needs and concerns.

Contraception, sexual and reproductive health, more than any other branch of medicine, are areas where a partnership between the professionals and public is vital. Ensuring access, quality and continuity of care in contraception services, recognizing the dynamics between professionals and patients/clients, and providing full, accurate and objective information contribute to that partnership. Through this, truly informed choices and decisions can be made which recognize the complexity of peoples' lives and the multiplicity of psychosocial factors which influence sexual relationships and reproductive choices.

References

1. Snowden R. Consumer choices in family planning. London: FPA, 1985.

2. Belfield T. Consumer perceptions of family planning. *Br J Fam Plann* 1988;13:46–53.

3. Oddens BJ. Determinants of contraceptive use – national population-based studies in various Western European countries. International Health Foundation. London: Eburon Publishers, 1996.

4. Ravindran Sundari TK, Berer M, Cottingham J. Beyond acceptability: users' perspectives on contraception. Reproductive Health Matters for World Health Organisation. Geneva: WHO, 1997.

5. Belfield T. Problems of compliance in contraception. *Br J Sex Med* 1992;19:76–8.

6. Walsh J, Lythgoe H, Peckham S. Contraceptive choices – supporting effective use of methods. London: FPA, 1996.

7. Belfield T. A standardised patient information leaflet on oral contraception for Europe: just around the corner or never-ending circles? In: Hannaford PC, Webb AMC (eds) Evidence-guided prescribing of the pill. London: Parthenon, 1996.

8. Hope T. Evidence-based patient choice – promoting patient choice. London: Kings Fund Publishing, 1996.

9. Hatcher RA, Trussell J, Stewart F, et al. Contraceptive technology.

New York: Irvington Publishers Inc., 1994.

10. Baraitser P. Power and knowledge in family planning consultations: can a reanalysis of doctor–patient interaction improve client satisfaction? *Br J Fam Plann* 1995;21:18–19.

11. Hadley A. Private and confidential. Women's Health 1997;2:20–2.

12. Brook Advisory Centres. Someone with a smile would be your best bet – what young people want from sex advice services. London: Brook Advisory Centres, 1998.

13. Kishen M. Adolescent contraception. *The Diplomate* 1997;4:207–13.

14. Godwin K. Consumers' understanding of contraceptive efficacy. *Br J Fam Plann* 1997;23:45–6.

15. Coulter A. Evidence based patient information – is important, so there needs to be a national strategy to ensure it. *Br Med J* 1998;317:225–6.

16. Wyatt JC. Measuring quality and impact of the world wide web. *Br Med J* 1997; 314:79–81.

17. Entwistle VA, Sheldon TA, Sowden A, et al. Evidence-informed patient choice – practical issues of involving patients in decisions about health care technologies. *Int J Technol Assess Health Care* 1998;14:212–25.

18. Charnock D. The DISCERN handbook – quality criteria for consumer health information. Oxford: Radcliffe Medical Press Ltd, 1998.

19. Korsch B, Harding C. The intelligent patient's guide to the doctor–patient relationship. Oxford: Oxford University Press, 1998.

Section 3:
Special groups

The postpartum period

Pramilla Senanayake MBBS DTPH PhD FRCOG
Roni Liyanage MA

Introduction

There are many different definitions of the postpartum period. The time period varies according to definition from a few hours, to describe the length of time in the delivery room after expulsion of the placenta, to several months, to describe the time interval to the resumption of menses after birth [1]. The postpartum period is often confused with the puerperium, which is defined physiologically as the time to involution of the uterus (around 42 days postpartum). The postpartum period has typically been divided into three distinct phases:

1. immediate postpartum, which is the time immediately after delivery of the placenta;
2. time through to 6 weeks postpartum;
3. 6 weeks to 6 months postpartum.

This definition considers the postpartum period only in terms of its physiology. However, the postpartum period is a psychosocial state with physiological, cultural and psychological components in which a woman recuperates from pregnancy whilst meeting the physiological requirements of her child. As such, postpartum programmes must consider not just the needs and desires of a woman as an individual, but also the needs of the mother–child dyad and the infant itself (S Diaz, personal communication, 1996). Defined accordingly, the postpartum period very much depends on the individual and her circumstances. In essence, it is the mother who should define her postpartum period rather than the service provider. The duration of her postpartum period is influenced by a number of factors, including the psychological condition of the mother, the cultural significance of the postpartum period, and the duration of amenorrhoea and lactation. This may vary from a few weeks in the absence of breastfeeding to several months where breastfeeding is prolonged.

Psychological significance of the postpartum period

The period immediately following parturition is a time of extreme physiological and psychological change. Many women suffer from postpartum blues, a mild depressive condition, with symptoms including insomnia, restlessness, fatigue, instability, sadness, headaches and lability of mood. In the USA, 50–70% of women experience postpartum blues. It should not be confused with postpartum depression, which is a true depressive state affecting only one or two per 1000 [2]. In many non-Western societies, the postpartum period is culturally recognized with measures to protect the new mother, social seclusion, mandated rest and assistance with tasks. In these societies, postpartum blues are absent, indicating a strong role for culture [3].

Postpartum sexuality

Childbirth can have a significant effect on sexuality. Diminished vaginal lubrication, tenderness in the perineum and heavy lochial discharge may interfere with a woman's sexual desire and make intercourse painful. Breastfeeding and the formation of the maternal–child bond may also decrease sexual drive. Conversely, the emotional high of the childbirth experience may promote an increase in sexual intimacy. In a survey of American couples, 66% of lactating women were sexually active in the first month postpartum and 88% in the second month [4].

The situation is very different in many developing countries, particularly in sub-Saharan Africa, where postpartum abstinence is observed lasting up to 3 years following the birth of a child. In many societies, such as contemporary Java, people believe that the man's semen contaminates the mother's milk [5]. Moreover, infant diseases are frequently attributed by the community to the resumption of intercourse. Postpartum sexual abstinence is seen as a rational means of ensuring the preservation of the health of the mother and the baby.

Postpartum fertility

During pregnancy, increased levels of progesterone and oestrogen, essential for the maintenance of the implanted embryo, suppress pituitary secretion of follicle stimulating hormone (FSH) and luteinizing hormone (LH). After placental delivery, there is a rapid decline in circulating levels of progesterone and oestrogen, allowing the resumption of the pulsatile release of FSH and LH from the pituitary [6]. In non-lactating women, plasma levels of FSH and LH gradually rise and, by 4 weeks postpartum, levels of FSH are typically within the normal menstrual range, while LH levels reach the lower limit of normal [7]. Non-lactating women resume menses within 4–6 weeks of parturition, although about one-third of first cycles are anovulatory and a high

proportion have luteal-phase defects.

Breastfeeding

Advantages to the infant

Breast milk provides nutrition and protection against disease for the infant. Studies have shown that breastfed infants are less likely to contract respiratory and gastrointestinal diseases, including neonatal necrotizing enterocolitis. This applies to babies in developing as well as developed countries. Colostrum, the breast milk in the immediate postpartum period, contains essential nutrients and host humoral and allergy prophylaxis factors. As a result, breastfed infants are less susceptible to allergies such as eczema, cows' milk allergy and allergic rhinitis [8–11]. Furthermore, breast milk continues to provide calories, essential proteins and immunological protection for toddlers up to 2 years and beyond. Lactation prolongs the interval between births, enhancing child survival by increasing parental attention and decreasing competition between siblings where resources are scarce. Breastfeeding also plays an important role in mother–infant bonding. Breast milk may have specific nutrients required for postnatal brain development and may influence intelligence later in life.

Advantages to the mother

Women who breastfeed tend to return to their normal weight

soon after childbirth, owing to the considerable caloric demand of lactation. Well-nourished women typically lose 0.5–1 kg/month while nursing. In addition, suckling induces the release of pituitary oxytocin, which promotes the return of uterine tone [12]. The birth-spacing effect of lactation is also of benefit to the mother, allowing her more time to recuperate from the physiological demands of childbirth. Breastfeeding reduces a woman's lifetime risk of breast cancer by as much as 50% in some studies. Whilst the benefits of breastfeeding, to both the infant and the mother, are well known, no woman should be forced into breastfeeding. If the mother chooses not to breastfeed, her decision should be respected.

Breastfeeding and HIV

The human immunodeficiency virus (HIV), which causes the acquired immunodeficiency syndrome (AIDS), can be transmitted from mother to infant during pregnancy and childbirth, and through breastfeeding. According to the World Health Organization (WHO) and the United Nations Children's Fund (UNICEF), roughly one-third of the babies born worldwide of HIV-infected women become infected themselves [13]. Much of this transmission occurs *in utero* or during childbirth. The risk of HIV transmission through breastfeeding is much greater among women who become infected during the postpartum period than among women infected prenatally [14]. The

WHO and UNICEF advise HIV-infected women to continue breastfeeding in regions where the primary causes of infant deaths are infectious diseases and malnutrition, because the immunological and nutritional benefits of breast milk outweigh the risk of HIV infection. In populations where infectious diseases make a less significant contribution to infant mortality, HIV-infected mothers are advised not to breastfeed but to use a safe feeding alternative for their babies.

Lactational infertility

Breastfeeding prolongs the period of postpartum infertility. In developing countries, particularly in Africa and South Asia, the anovulation associated with breastfeeding continues to be a major determinant of fertility control. In the absence of breastfeeding or contraception, a woman might have 13–15 children during her reproductive life, yet in Africa, women have an average of seven children, and in Asia, five. Breastfeeding and contraception are the two most important proximate factors in determining the realized fertility of a woman. Although lactational amenorrhoea provides natural contraceptive protection, family planning programmes, until recently, have paid little attention to the role of breastfeeding in pregnancy spacing.

Physiological basis of lactational infertility

The physiological mechanism of lactational infertility appears to be related to patterns of suckling. Infant suckling induces a suppression of the pulsatile release of gonadotropin releasing hormone (GnRH) from the hypothalamus which, in turn, suppresses the pulsatile release of LH. An inadequate LH pulse frequency is associated with failure or inadequacy of follicular development. In addition, if follicle growth does occur during lactational amenorrhoea, the resulting increase in oestrogen inhibits sustained GnRH release from the hypothalamus by a suckling-induced negative feedback mechanism, preventing ovulation. As a result, a lactating woman is less likely to ovulate and more likely to have an anovulatory first bleeding episode [7]. The exact mechanism by which suckling suppresses GnRH release is not yet known, but it is believed to be related to increased hypothalamic secretion of β-endorphin in response to suckling, hence the association of intensive breastfeeding with amenorrhoea. Suckling also stimulates prolactin release which is essential for milk production. However, the role of prolactin in lactational amenorrhoea, if any, is unclear.

Lactational amenorrhoea

There is considerable variation in the duration of postpartum amenorrhoea between populations, ranging from a mean length of 1.8 months in Taiwan among women who did not lactate to 14–15 months in Bangladesh and Guatemala where breastfeeding is prolonged [15]. The length of amenorrhoea is influenced by many factors, most significantly by breastfeeding patterns and the introduction of infant food supplements. Full or nearly full breastfeeding is associated with longer periods of lactational amenorrhoea and infertility than partial breastfeeding. The critical factors which prolong the period of infertility appear to be high suckling frequency and the avoidance of long intervals between feeds. The contraceptive effect of lactation can be maximized by delaying the introduction of infant food supplements for as long as possible without jeopardizing infant growth and development. Food supplementation reduces the suckling stimulus, increasing the possibility of earlier resumption of ovarian activity. Maximal suckling stimulus is maintained by giving the infant supplements after a breastfeed. Strictly exclusive breastfeeding is difficult to achieve. Often, demands on a woman's time, such as responsibilities at work and family care, can limit the suckling frequency and duration.

A number of studies have been carried out to evaluate the relationship between lactation and the resumption of ovulation and pregnancy. A longitudinal study in Durango, Mexico, found that the rate of ovulation for exclusively breastfeeding amenorrhoeic mothers was 4% at 6 months postpartum [16]. A study of fully nursing Chilean women revealed that the cumulative rate of pregnancy at 180 days postpartum for women who were still amenorrhoeic was under 2% [17].

Return of fertility during lactation

The return of fertility can be predicted, with reasonable accuracy, from the time of return of menses, the breastfeeding pattern and the time postpartum. Menses is defined as the first vaginal bleed after 56 days postpartum in order to exclude the bleeding episode experienced by some women around 40 days postpartum. Lactational infertility decreases with time. After 6 months, full breastfeeding is less likely to be practised and food supplements are more likely to have been introduced. Moreover, the likelihood that ovulation precedes the return of menses increases later in lactation.

Bellagio consensus

The Bellagio consensus statement on lactational amenorrhoea as a family planning method concluded that the maximum birth-spacing effect of breastfeeding is achieved when a mother:

1. 'fully' or nearly fully breastfeeds; and
2. remains amenorrhoeic [18].

If both conditions are satisfied, lactation provides more than 98% protection from pregnancy in the first 6 months postpartum, an efficacy comparable to other available contraceptive methods. At the end of 6 months, or if breastfeeding ceases to be full or nearly full, or if menses return, the risk of pregnancy increases.

Contraceptive methods

Ideally, contraceptive counselling should begin in the prenatal period. The choices available to women in the postpartum period depend on whether the mother chooses to breastfeed her child (Table 14.1).

Timing of contraceptive use

The timing of postpartum contraceptive use is a critical

Table 14.1   When to initiate contraception post partum

Contraceptive	Lactating	Non-lactating	Considerations
Male and female condoms	Immediately	Immediately	Protects against STDs and HIV
Spermicides	Immediately	Immediately	May alleviate dryness
Diaphragm, cervical cap	Delay 6 weeks	Delay 6 weeks	Elevated risk of toxic shock syndrome Increased failure rate for women who have given birth
IUD	Delay for 4–8 weeks	Delay for 4–6 weeks	High risk of expulsion for IPPI-IUDs Lactating women experience less discomfort during insertion
Female sterilization	Immediate or delay 6 weeks	Immediate or delay 6 weeks	Lactation disrupted during mother/child separation
Male sterilization (vasectomy)			Can be performed during the antenatal period Relieves the woman of contraceptive burden
POCs			
Depo-Provera	Delay 6 weeks	Delay 6 weeks	Effect on lactation and infant not yet clarified
POPs	Start beginning of week 4	Start beginning of week 4 or earlier if practical	WHO advises 6 weeks delay
Norplant	Delay 6 weeks	Start beginning of week 4	
Combined pills	Delay 6 months May be allowed if lactation well established	Delay 3 weeks	Oestrogen may decrease milk supply Increased risk of thromboembolism in immediate puerperium
Lactational amenorrhoea method	Immediately	N/A	Requires full or nearly full breastfeeding Pregnancy risk increases after 6 months
Rhythm, ovulation and symptothermal methods	Delay until menstrual cycle has resumed	Delay until menstrual cycle has resumed	Rhythm method requires prediction of ovulation by use of calendar, date of menstruation and symptothermal methods Mucus changes difficult to interpret during lactational amenorrhoea

IUD = intrauterine device; IPPI = immediate post-placental insertion; POCs = progestin-only contraception; POPs progestin-only pills; STDs = sexually transmitted disease.

component in the development of postpartum programmes responsive to the needs and desires of women who use the services. Since services are maternity-based with shared administrative and medical facilities, start-up costs for immediate postpartum programmes are low. However, given that worldwide the majority of women do not deliver in health facilities, access to services poses problems. The Sfax Postpartum Programme in Tunisia, where postpartum health care for mother and child is integrated with family planning services, had an 83% return rate for postpartum visits in 1987 [19].

Contraceptive choices for non-lactating women

A non-lactating woman may choose to initiate contraceptive use immediately postpartum or at least by the first postpartum check-up (3–6 weeks postpartum). The guidelines for contraceptive use in non-lactating women are less restrictive than those for lactating women. Diaphragms and cervical caps cannot be inserted until the uterus has involuted, usually 6 weeks postpartum. Although progestin-only contraceptives can be used immediately postpartum, some clinicians recommend that initiation is delayed until 3 weeks postpartum to avoid an increased risk of puerperal bleeding. Similarly, women are cautioned not to use combined oral contraceptives until 3 weeks postpartum to avoid an increased risk of postpartum thromboembolism, which is

greatest immediately after delivery. Although the risk of pregnancy in the first 3–6 weeks postpartum (i.e. before the postpartum check-up) is very low, women are advised to practice sexual abstinence or use condoms if sexual relations are resumed, until a more reliable contraceptive method is employed. Contraceptive cover is assured as long as a systemic method is initiated before the fourth postpartum week.

The lactational amenorrhoea method

The lactational amenorrhoea method (LAM) formalizes breastfeeding into a structured method of natural family planning (Figure 14.1). In order for the method to be effective, three conditions must prevail:

1. the woman is amenorrhoeic;
2. she is fully or nearly fully breastfeeding;
3. her baby is less than 6 months old.

If satisfied, LAM predicts at least 98% protection from pregnancy. If any of these conditions are no longer met, the mother is advised to use a complementary method of family planning. Women using LAM are advised to maintain a high breastfeeding frequency with short intervals between feeds. If supplements are introduced, at least 85% of feeds must be breastfeeds [20].

In the clinical trial of the LAM in Santiago, Chile, it proved highly efficacious with 99.5% protection after 6 months [21].

LAM is an inexpensive, efficacious postpartum method of

contraception which introduces new users to family planning services. The positive effects of LAM are enhanced breastfeeding practices resulting in improvements in child survival, maternal health and infant nutrition. All postpartum women have the right to receive information on breast feeding, lactational infertility and LAM.

However, women should not be made to feel guilty or inadequate if, for whatever reason, they choose not to breastfeed.

Integrating the LAM into family planning programmes

LAM proved to be attractive to first-time family planning users at the Centro Medico de Orientacion y Planificacion Familiar (CEMOPLAF) in Ecuador. A total of 73% of LAM acceptors had no prior experience of family planning services. Around 90% used the method correctly and initiated the timely use of a complementary contraceptive after only one follow-up visit [22]. In some regions where lactational amenorrhoea typically continues beyond 6 months, extended LAM programmes have been introduced. In Rwanda, a LAM-9 programme was introduced following LAM guidelines for the first 6 months and then breastfeeding before supplemental feeds up to 9 months. Efficacy was high with no pregnancies among the acceptors who returned to follow-up (419 out of 445) [23]. The increased risk of pregnancy in the additional LAM months

Ask the mother, or advise her to ask herself these three questions:

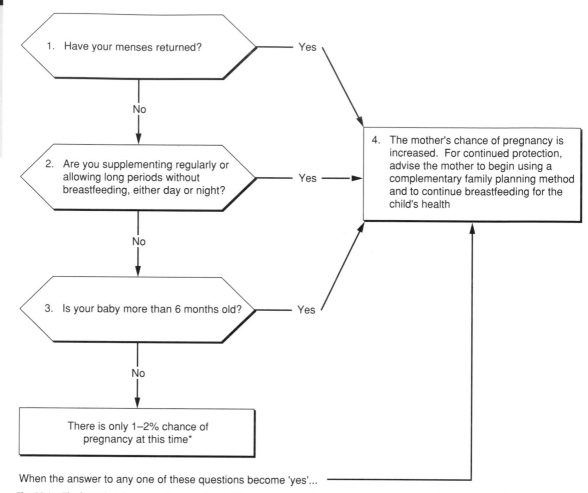

1. Have your menses returned? ——— Yes

No

2. Are you supplementing regularly or allowing long periods without breastfeeding, either day or night? ——— Yes

No

3. Is your baby more than 6 months old? ——— Yes

No

4. The mother's chance of pregnancy is increased. For continued protection, advise the mother to begin using a complementary family planning method and to continue breastfeeding for the child's health

There is only 1–2% chance of pregnancy at this time*

When the answer to any one of these questions become 'yes'...

Fig. 14.1 The lactational amenorrhoea method. *However, the mother may choose to use a complementary method at any time.

may be acceptable in some settings where access to family planning services is limited.

In most developed countries, breastfeeding is encouraged, but in practice many women breastfeed for shorter periods (usually 3 months) and introduce supplementary foods earlier. It is therefore more reliable for the postpartum contraceptive plan to be based on a reliable contraceptive started at 3 weeks postpartum for lactating women not practising LAM and 3 months postpartum for lactating women who choose to depend on LAM in the first 3 postpartum months.

Non-hormonal intrauterine devices

Postpartum intrauterine device (IUD) insertions are defined by the WHO according to the timing of insertion. *Immediate post-placental insertion* (IPPI) should be carried out within 10 min of placental delivery, *postpartum insertion* within the first 48 h postpartum, and *interval insertion* at least 4 weeks after delivery and preferably 6–8 weeks in breastfeeding women. A lower segment caesarean section scar should have healed and involuted by the sixth postpartum week and should allow safe IUD insertion. Delayed insertion, 2 days to 4 weeks after delivery, is not recommended owing to the increased risk of uterine perforation.

Contraindications to postpartum IUD use include recent molar pregnancy (because of the confusing effect of any irregular bleeding), postpartum sepsis and continuing bleeding or the presence of pain (suggesting retained placental tissue).

IUDs need to be inserted by experienced health care workers. The IUD expulsion rate for IPPIs is estimated to be just over 10 per 100 users per year, whilst the expulsion rate for interval insertions is about 3 per 100 users [24]. Although expulsion rates are higher in postpartum IUD fittings, lactation does not seem to increase the risk.

At the time of IUD insertion, sexually transmitted micro-organisms can be introduced into the uterine cavity, leading to pelvic inflammatory disease (PID). Moreover, where aseptic technique cannot be ensured, insertion of IUDs may be unsuitable owing to the increased risk of infection.

IUDs are a very convenient method of postpartum contraception. The use of the Copper T 380 among lactating women is both widespread and effective. It is the device of choice in parous women. The copper does not affect the quantity or quality of breast milk nor does it affect infant health. Lactating women have less painful IUD insertions and fewer bleeding problems during IUD use than non-lactating women; the belief that uterine perforation is more common in lactating women needs further confirmation. IUDs are highly efficacious and cost effective. If inserted properly, the 'new-generation' copper IUDs are 99.4–99.9% effective [25].

Barrier methods

Male and female condoms and spermicides are coitus dependent,

making them attractive contraceptive methods in populations where postpartum intercourse is infrequent. Moreover, the lubricative effect of spermicides can alleviate vaginal dryness owing to oestrogen deficiency, which is common in lactating women. However, diaphragms and cervical caps are not advisable for immediate postpartum use. They usually cannot be fitted until 6 weeks postpartum when the uterus and vagina have returned to normal. The cervical cap has a higher failure rate for women who have recently given birth, even with perfect use [26].

The main advantage of condoms is the protection they confer against STDs and postpartum endometritis. Barrier methods are particularly effective as part of a broad postpartum family planning strategy, either as a temporary method employed by women (especially those who are not breastfeeding) who will later use oral contraceptives or an IUD, or as a complementary method for women using the LAM.

Hormonal methods

Progestin-only contraceptives
Progestin-only contraceptives (POCs) such as Norplant, Depo-Provera (DMPA) and progestin-only pills (POPs) are safe and appropriate methods for breastfeeding women throughout the period of lactation. The WHO investigated the effect of POCs used during lactation on infant growth and development, and found no significant differences between acceptors of

progestin-only methods and non-hormonal methods [27, 28] and no adverse effect on growth and development to age 4 years [29]. Moreover, POCs have no adverse effects on breast milk volume (some studies suggest they may even enhance milk production) or duration of breastfeeding.

The timing for initiating progestin-only contraception in breastfeeding women is still subject to debate. According to the WHO, the theoretical or proven risks of using POCs in the first 6 weeks postpartum usually outweigh the advantages, and the WHO recommends that the initiation of POCs should be delayed until at least 6 weeks postpartum [30]. The risk of ovulation in fully lactating women up to the fourth postpartum week is negligible, making it prudent to delay the initiation of hormonal contraception until then to allow establishment of lactation. Such an approach avoids exposing the infant to exogenous steroids during the time when the infant's liver enzymes are still maturing. Where it is deemed more practical, POP or Norplant use can be initiated at the beginning of the fourth postpartum week.

In circumstances in which a breastfeeding woman is unlikely to return for a postpartum visit, the contraceptive benefit of immediate postpartum Norplant insertion should exceed the theoretical risks. Women who have difficulty complying with the strict pill-taking schedule for POP use may wish to switch to combined oral contraceptives, which are acceptable for use whilst breastfeeding after 6 months postpartum.

Levonogestrel releasing intrauterine system

Similar guidelines apply to the use of progestin-releasing IUDs such as LNG-IUS (Levonova®, Mirena®). Interval insertions are advised, given the need to avoid infant progestin ingestion before the establishment of lactation and the high rate of expulsions for IPPIs. In the long term, the LNG-IUS may prove to be an excellent postpartum contraceptive method, offering health benefits such as reduction of blood loss and anaemia.

Combined oral contraceptives

Combined oral contraceptives (COCs) should be avoided during the early (absolute contraindication) and perhaps the entire period of lactation (relative contraindication). The lowest effective hormonal combination should be used. There is considerable evidence that the oestrogen component in combined pills has a detrimental effect on breastfeeding by reducing breast milk volume [31,32]. The dose of ethinyl-oestradiol transferred to the infant in breast milk (about 10 ng per day) is very low and is comparable to the dose of naturally occurring oestradiol (6–12 ng per day) in the breast milk of ovulatory mothers not taking COCs [33]. Most studies have focused on high-dose COCs. With low-dose COCs, the effect of oestrogen on lactation may be minimal. However, it may be prudent to caution women against the use of

COCs early in breastfeeding and instead advise the use of an alternative contraceptive method until 6 months postpartum or until the child is weaned. Where compliance is a potential problem, COCs have an advantage over POPs; they also provide better cycle control.

Emergency contraception

Lactation is not a contraindication to hormonal or intrauterine emergency contraception. Postpartum women who have unprotected intercourse should be informed about and offered emergency contraception (see Chapter 12). Once lactation is established, it is unlikely that the short course of high oestrogen/progestin combination would inhibit lactation. Oestrogen would pass in breast milk to a breastfed infant: a withdrawal bleed might therefore follow; the mother must be alerted to this. She may choose to discard her breast milk over the 24 h of the emergency contraception treatment. Another option is to choose an IUD, if appropriate, or to use the progestin-only emergency contraceptive (see Chapter 12).

Female sterilization

Postpartum women must also consider whether female sterilization is an appropriate course of action for their needs. Female sterilization is a single surgical procedure providing permanent contraception for

couples who wish to limit the size of their family before the end of their reproductive life span. A considerable number of sterilizations are performed during the immediate postpartum period while women are still in the hospital after delivery. In the USA, 33% of female sterilizations are performed within 48 h of delivery. Interval sterilizations are performed when the uterus is fully involuted at 4 or more weeks postpartum. The timing of sterilization is important in determining the surgical technique and method of occlusion.

Tubal occlusions are permanent and difficult to reverse. Therefore, where immediate postpartum sterilizations are planned, comprehensive counselling should take place during the prenatal period. The physical and emotional stress of childbirth may unduly influence the decision to have surgical sterilization. Postpartum sterilizations are associated with an increased incidence of regret [34,35] Moreover, potential clients should be informed of the availability of long-term contraceptive methods, such as IUDs and Norplant. If a woman has been fully counselled and has had time to reflect on her decision to be sterilized, then an immediate postpartum procedure can be performed. Conversely, if the woman has had insufficient time to reflect on her decision and if acceptance of sterilization is contingent on the survival of the child, it may be prudent to advise the delay of sterilization until 6 weeks postpartum, despite the economic and practical advantages of immediate postpartum procedures.

In the future, non-surgical methods of female sterilization, such as quinacrine pellets, may become viable options for postpartum women [36]. However, quinacrine has yet to be approved by the WHO, International Planned Parenthood Federation (IPPF) or the drug regulatory authority in any country, since current data on efficacy and toxicology are insufficient.

Male sterilization

In certain circumstances, a couple may choose male sterilization in the postpartum period. Vasectomies are highly effective, safer and less expensive than female sterilizations. Vasectomies are not immediately effective, but LAM can provide sufficient contraceptive protection for lactating women in the meantime. Vasectomy can be performed during the antenatal period as long as the couple are determined to have no more children, irrespective of the outcome of the current pregnancy. Vasectomy is especially suitable for the postpartum period, since there is no physiological and negligible psychosocial impact on the postpartum mother and the newborn infant. However, the mother is still at risk of pregnancy, making vasectomy a suitable choice for couples in stable relationships and where the woman has no other sexual partners. Where infant mortality is high, as in developing countries, the health of the newborn may need to be taken

into consideration prior to deciding on a male or female sterilization.

Recent developments in contraceptive technology

Newer methods of contraception, such as cyclofem (monthly injections), the oestrogen/progestin vaginal rings and the progestin/progesterone-only vaginal rings, will have their place in postpartum family planning programmes when they become widely available.

Double protection

In certain circumstances, the immediate postpartum contraception strategy may not be the best approach to produce the longest birth intervals. This is especially apparent in populations where breastfeeding is prevalent and prolonged, and continuation rates of contraceptives are low. In a study of pill use in rural Bangladesh, women who initiated use of oral contraceptives during lactational amenorrhoea had shorter intervals to the next pregnancy as continuation rates were very poor, with an average duration of contraceptive use of less than 7 months [37,38]. A demographic analysis from Zimbabwe revealed that the total fertility rate was high (5.7 in 1988) despite a contraceptive prevalence rate of 43% amongst women aged 15–49. Given this rate of contraceptive prevalence, the expected fertility rate would be 4.3 [39]. The discrepancy between the observed and

expected fertility rates can be accounted for by the overlap between contraceptive use and lactational amenorrhoea. During this period of lactational infertility, contraception has no effect on fertility. Overall, 29% of the potential birth-spacing effect of contraception is wasted owing to this period of double protection. Double protection is a problem in populations where discontinuation rates are high. In Zimbabwe, where the average duration of amenorrhoea is 12.5 months and the average duration of contraceptive use is less than 2 years, later initiation of contraception when protection from lactational amenorrhoea diminishes would result in lower fertility than early initiation.

Postpartum programmes

In developing programmes for postpartum women, due consideration should be given to the location of such programmes (Table 14.2).

Postpartum reproductive care

Maternal health care during the postpartum period is an important element of women's health. Postpartum advice should cover the areas of:

1. breastfeeding, including the encouragement of feeding on demand;
2. nutrition for the mother after delivery;
3. general maternal health and infant health;
4. resumption of sexual activity;
5. contraception.

Table 14.2 Postpartum programmes

Place of delivery	Location of postpartum programme	Personnel
Hospital or maternity units	Hospital maternity units or community facility	Midwives supported by doctors
Home	Domiciliary	Outreach (community) midwives and health visitors
Hospital or maternity units or home	Primary health care facility or community clinic	Designated member of primary health care team supported by community reproductive health team

Immediate puerperium

Irrespective of LAM use, breastfeeding should begin immediately after birth, promoted by rooming-in practices and close contact between the mother and the child. Non-lactating women, in particular, must receive family planning advice and contraceptive supplies before leaving the hospital after delivery because the resumption of ovarian activity may precede the postnatal check-up.

Counselling and support must be provided for mothers following a neonatal death. It is important to provide support for women who may experience feelings of isolation intensified by guilt and failure, and to address the anxieties a woman may have about when to embark on another pregnancy.

Postnatal depression affects 10–15% of mothers. Up to 50% of cases may go undetected. Women at risk include those with a personal or family history, primiparae, those lacking partner support or those with a history of childhood abuse. Interventions include offering support at home and recognizing the signs of serious depression; liaison with psychiatrists and psychologists should facilitate access to cognitive behavioural therapy and psychotherapy, if required. Access to a mother and baby unit allows multidisciplinary team work. Antidepressants may be required in 30% of cases. The tricyclic antidepressants imipramine and amitriptyline are still deemed safe in breastfeeding women [40]. Lofepramine, however, is safer in overdose, has a shorter half life, and is less likely to accumulate in the infant [41].

The postnatal check-up and beyond

The timing of the postnatal visit has been the subject of recent debate. Typically, the postnatal check-up is scheduled for 6 weeks (in some countries it is earlier). However, many couples have resumed intercourse by then and, since ovulation may occur as early as the fourth week postpartum, the postnatal visit may be too late at 6 weeks with respect to discussion on and initiation of contraceptive use. At the postnatal check-up, the mother should receive a physical examination to ensure the correct involution of the uterus, and her blood pressure and weight should be checked.

The infant must also receive a thorough check-up at this time. Interval IUD insertions and female sterilizations are often performed at the same time as the postnatal check-up. In populations where breastfeeding is infrequently used as a method of contraception, the postnatal check-up is typically the time of the initiation of contraceptive use and the prescription of POCs (this argues for timing the visit at 2–3 weeks rather than 6 weeks). In populations where the mean duration of lactational amenorrhoea is several months, a delayed initiation of backup contraception may be warranted, although contraceptive counselling should be accessible throughout the postpartum period. After the postnatal check-up, subsequent visits may be arranged to monitor the progress of the chosen method of contraception and/or the lactational status of the mother.

Components of postpartum counselling and reproductive health care

Breastfeeding

The principles of counselling have been discussed earlier. A mother should be encouraged to maintain a high frequency of suckling, ideally on demand or at intervals of no more than 4 hours. Women who return to work must be instructed on how to adapt their breastfeeding patterns to increased mother–child separation and informed of the advantages of giving expressed breast milk before other food supplements. When supplements

Table 14.3 Drugs affecting lactation

Drug group	Effect	Mechanism of interaction
Oestrogens	Milk volume and content reduced	Direct action on breast
Alcohol and nicotine	Milk volume reduced	Oxytocin suppression
Dopamine, dopamine agonists	Milk volume reduced	Inhibit prolactin
Diuretics	Milk volume reduced	Disrupt fluid balance

are introduced (from 3 months postpartum), women must be advised of methods to maintain high suckling frequency if they wish to prolong the contraceptive effect of lactation. Drugs that may affect lactation are listed in Table 14.3.

Suppression of lactation

High-dose oestrogen therapy is not recommended. Avoiding breast stimulation, ensuring adequate breast support and analgesia are usually sufficient; engorgement with or without mild pyrexia resolves within a few days. To suppress established lactation, bromocriptine (2.5 mg b.d.) is given for 14 days. Mastitis present after the first week is usually staphylococcal and responds to penicillin.

Maternal nutrition

Lactation places significant nutritional demands on the mother, which are accentuated by the combination of puerperal blood loss and possible anaemia. Not only must the caloric requirements for lactation be met through nutrition but there must also be an adequate supply of micronutrients, such as iron and calcium. In some cases, it may be necessary to introduce iron supplements for anaemic women. Nutritional advice is particularly important where cultural taboos place limitations on a postpartum woman's diet. Although there is evidence that maternal physiology adapts to ensure that lactational performance is relatively unhindered by maternal malnutrition, this is achieved at the expense of the mother's own health.

The health of the parturient mother

Most maternal deaths occur during the puerperium. A study in Bangladesh showed that six out of ten maternal deaths took place during the puerperium, most of them due to infection or haemorrhage [42]. Maternal health care is often overlooked since the focus is switched to the care of the new-born infant.

Maternal blood loss at delivery can be fatal. A study in Australia showed that 17% of new mothers suffered postpartum haemorrhage, making them vulnerable to anaemia and maternal death. Anaemic women suffer from fatigue and have reduced resistance to infection. The latter, unless treated promptly with antibiotics, can lead to death in both the mother and/or the baby. In some regions, infections account for a third of maternal deaths. Infections, and their sequelae of PID and tubal damage, can be prevented by the use of aseptic technique during delivery and prompt antibiotic treatment of such conditions as premature rupture of membranes and uterine trauma. Hypertension and the risk of thromboembolism continues from pregnancy into the immediate puerperium. Although maternal risk from both conditions is low, it could be increased by the use of oestrogen-containing COCs. In any case, these are an 'overkill' in the immediate puerperal phase even for non-lactating women and can be safely (from the maternal health and contraceptive viewpoints) initiated when the baby is 21 days old.

Sexuality after childbirth

The demands of the new baby, the physical 'trauma' to the lower genital tract, and the anxiety about resumption of sexual activity and risk of pregnancy may all contribute to lack of libido in the early postpartum phase. However, couples should be supported and reassured in expressing sexual feeling, touching and non-penetrative sex, progressing to full intercourse whenever they are ready. Pelvic floor exercises reduce perineal pain and are confidence building; instruction should be given without undue pressure or encouraging unrealistic expectations.

Dyspareunia

Dyspareunia tends to be associated with perineal tears/stitching accentuated by a lack of lubrication, a hypo-oestrogenized vagina and anxiety.

References

1. Winikoff B, Mensch B. Rethinking postpartum family planning. *Stud Fam Plann* 1991;22:294–307.

2. Campbell SB, Cohn JF. Prevalence and correlates of postpartum depression in first time mothers. *J Ab Psych* 1991;100:594–9.

3. Harkness S. The cultural mediation of postpartum depression. *Med Anthropol Q* 1987;1:194–209.

4. Ford K, Labbok M. Contraceptive usage during lactation in the United States: an update. *Am J Public Health* 1987;77:79–81.

5. van de Walle E, van de Walle F. Postpartum sexual abstinence in tropical Africa. In: Gray R, Leridon H, Spira A (eds) Biomedical and demographic determinants of reproduction. Oxford: Clarendon Press, 1993:446–60.

6. Hodgen GD, Itskovitz J. Recognition and maintenance of pregnancy. In: Knobil E, Neill JD, Ewing LL, Greenwald GS, Markert CL, Pfaff DW (eds) The physiology of reproduction. New York: Raven Press, 1988:1995–2021.

7. McNeilly A. Breastfeeding and fertility. In: Gray R, Leridon H, Spira A (eds) Biomedical and demographic determinants of reproduction. Oxford: Clarendon Press, 1993:391–412.

8. Howie PW, Forsyth JS, Ogston SA, Clark A, du V Florey C. Protective effect of breastfeeding against infection. *Br Med J* 1990;300:11–16.

9. Kovar MG, Serdula MK, Marks JS, Fraser DW. Review of the epidemiological evidence for an association between infant feeding and infant health. *Pediatrics* 1984;74(Suppl 4):615–38.

10. McCann MF, Liskin LS, Piotrow PT, Rinehart W, Fox G. Breastfeeding, fertility and family planning. *Pop Rep* 1984;12(2):Ser J(24).

11. Lucas A, Cole TJ. Breastmilk and neonatal necrotising enterocolitis. *Lancet* 1990;336:1519–23.

12. Hatcher R, et al. In: Contraceptive technology, 16th edn. New York: Contraceptive Technology Communications, Inc., 1994:433–52.

13. World Health Organisation. Consensus statement from the WHO/UNICEF consultation on HIV transmission and breastfeeding. Global Programme on AIDS. Geneva: WHO, April–May 1992.

14. Hira S, Mangrola U, Mwale C, et al. Breastfeeding and HIV-1 transmission (Abstract). Montreal conference, 51.

15. Ford K, Kim YJ. Demographic research on lactational amenorrhea. In: Gray R, Leridon H, Spira A (eds) Biomedical and demographic determinants of reproduction. Oxford: Clarendon Press, 1993:359–71.

16. Rivera R, Kennedy K, Ortiz E, et al. Breastfeeding and the return to ovulation in Durango, Mexico. *J Biosoc Sci* 1985; Suppl 9:127–36.

17. Diaz S, Rodriguez D, Peralta O, et al. Lactational amenorrhea and the recovery of ovulation and fertility in fully nursing Chilean women. *Contraception* 1988;38:53–67.

18. Kennedy K, Rivera R, McNeilly A, et al. Consensus statement on the use of breastfeeding as a family planning method. *Contraception* 1989;39:477–96.

19. Coeytaux F. Celebrating mother and child on the fortieth day: the Sfax, Tunisia postpartum program. *Wuality/Calidad/Qualite* 1989, The Population Council, NY.

20. Labbok M, Perez A, Valdes V, et al. The lactational amenorrhea method (LAM): a postpartum introductory family planning method with policy and program implications. *Adv Contracept* 1994;10:93–109.

21. Perez A, Labbok M, Queenan J. Clinical study of the lactational amenorrhea method in family planning. *Lancet* 1992; 339:968–70.

22. Wade K, Sevilla F, Labbok M. Integrating the lactational amenorrhea method into family planning program in Ecuador. *Stud Fam Plann* 1994;25:162–75.

23. Cooney K, Hoser H, Labbok M. Assessment of the nine month LAM method experience in Rwanda (Presentation and Abstract). American Public Health Annual Meeting, October 1993.

24. Thiery M. Contraception for postpartum use: non-hormonal methods intrauterine devices. Postpartum Conference, 1991.

25. Farley TMM. Evolution of IUD performance. *IPPF Med Bull* 1997;31:4.

26. Trussell J, Sturgen K, Strickler J, et al. Comparative contraceptive efficacy of the female condom and other barrier methods. *Fam Plann Perspect* 1994;26:66–72.

27. World Health Organisation, Task Force for Epidemiological Research on Reproductive Health. Progestin-only contraceptives during lactation: 1. Infant growth. *Contraception* 1994;50:35–53.

28. World Health Organisation, Task Force for Epidemiological Research on Reproductive Health. Progestin-only contraceptives during lactation: 1. Infant development. *Contraception* 1994;50:55–68.

29. Anonymous. Progestin-only methods safe during lactation. *Network* 1993;14:32–3.

30. World Health Organisation. Improving access to quality care in family planning: medical eligibility criteria for contraceptive use. Geneva: WHO, 1996.

31. Tankeyoon M, Dusitin N, Chalapati S, et al. Effects of hormonal contraceptives on milk volume and infant growth. *Contraception* 1984;30:505–22.

32. Wharton C, Blackburn R. Lower-dose pills. *Pop Rep* 1988;16: Ser A(7).

33. McGregor JA. Lactation and Contraception. In: Neville MC, Neifert MR (eds) Lactation: physiology, nutrition and breastfeeding. New York: Plenum Press, 1983:405–21.

34. Wilcox LS, Chu SY, Peterson HB. Characteristics of women who considered or obtained tubal reanastomosis: results from a prospective study of tubal sterilization. *Obstet Gynecol* 1990;75:661–5.

35. Wilcox LS, Chu SY, Eaker ED, Zeger SL, Peterson HB. Risk factors for regret after tubal sterilization: 5 years of follow-up in a prospective study. *Fertil Steril* 1991;55:927–33.

36. El Kady AA, Nagib HS, Kessel E. Efficacy and safety of repeated transcervical quinacrine pellet insertions for female sterilization. *Fertil Steril* 1993;59:301–4.

37. Bhatia S, Becker S, Kim YJ. The effect of fecundity on pill acceptance during postpartum amenorrhea in rural Bangladesh. *Stud Fam Plann* 1992;13:200–7.

38. Bhatia S, Becker S, Kim YJ. The effect of oral contraception acceptance on fertility in the postpartum period. *Int J Gynecol Obstet* 1987:25(Suppl):1–14.

39. Adamchak DJ, Mbizvo MT. The relationship between fertility and contraceptive prevalence in Zimbabwe. *Int Planned Parenthood Perspect*, 1990;16:103–6.

40. Duncan D, Taylor D. Which antidepressants are safe for use in breast-feeding mothers? *Psych Bull* 1995;19:551–552.

41. Nicholls KR, Cox JL. Lofepramine and breast feeding. *Psych Bull* 1996;20:309.

42. Anonymous. Postpartum care is crucial for health and survival. Safe *Motherhood Newslett* 1994;13:4–6.

Contraception and disability

Raymond E Goodman MSc MRCS LRCP DRCOG CBiol MIBiol

Background

Sexuality and disability

Throughout history, the pendulum has swung towards and away from sexual permissiveness, but it was the Victorian attitudes to morality that shaped much of Western beliefs, at least for the earlier part of this century. This was to continue until the sexual liberation movements of the 1960s and 1970s relaxed the sexual mores of many people. One of the good things to arise out of this was the recognition that sexuality is an essential part of being human, and the belief that no one should be denied such a basic right. This has particular relevance when one considers people who have disabilities.

Physical problems

Stewart [1] reported on a study of 212 people who suffered from a physical disability. He found 250 separate physical disorders, which affected to varying degrees aspects of mobility, manual dexterity, or the ability of the individual to care for himself or herself or to communicate with others. Stewart pointed out that as up to between 20% and 40% of

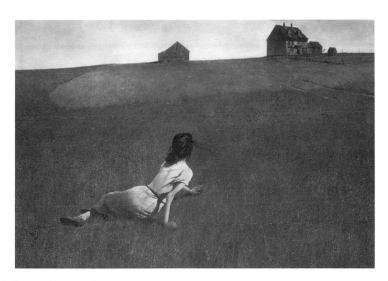

Christina's World (1948) by Andrew Wyeth
Andrew Wyeth was a post-war American painter. In 1939 he came to know a brother and sister on a remote farm in Maine. This troubling painting shows that Christina Olson, who many assumed to be an attractive young girl, sprawled in youthful abandon on the grass, was actually a mature woman, so severely crippled that she had to crawl on her arms in order to progress at all.

The unusual perspective of the painting, which was prompted by a sight of her from a window in the house, shows the tragedy and the effort involved with vivid poignancy. The house seems so far away, the effort so great, yet the determination to overcome highlights human endurance.

Tempera on gessoed panel, 32¼ × 47¾ in (81.9 × 121.3 cm). The Museum of Modern Art, New York. Purchase © 1998 The Museum of Modern Art, New York.

non-disabled people have sexual difficulties at some time in their lives, it was not surprising that the disabled, considering all the extra problems they have to cope with, were found to have a sexual difficulty incidence of 72%. Of these difficulties, 45% were caused by physical factors, 15% psychological and 36% were of mixed aetiology. Some people described their sexual difficulties as starting before the onset of disability, but most felt the problems had resulted from the illness. More men than women reported problems, perhaps partly because it was easier for men to talk about sex during that period, but also because of the fragility of the erectile mechanism. In women, however, providing the disability itself was not preventing penetration, coitus was usually possible.

Psychological problems

The timing of acquiring a disability may be important. Carcinomas or leukaemias, for instance, are particularly devastating in adolescence. This is just the time when the individual is breaking away from parental care and having to deal with the transition to adulthood, and the illness now makes him or her more dependent than ever upon parental help, and so interferes with normal development. Peer-group interaction, an essential aspect of growing up, may also be affected as the young person has to cope with the general malaise and other stigmata of the illness. 'Looks' are very important, particularly in this age group, and hair loss due to chemotherapy may damage self-esteem further.

Procedures such as mastectomy and hysterectomy in women can

invoke powerful feelings of deformity and loss, which may be compounded by a sense of loneliness and isolation if the illness coincides with the time that adolescent children are leaving home. Women who have had families before becoming ill and who require surgery may already have a sense of fulfilment, so that the surgery may be less devastating to them than to their younger counterparts who are at the start of reproductive life. A woman who has had a good sex life and to whom sex was important may experience a more profound sense of loss at any interference with her reproductive life than would a woman to whom sex was not so important.

Amputations and facial disfigurements can invoke in the individual feelings of repugnance and hatred towards themselves, and these feelings can prevent attempts to form a loving relationship. Furthermore, the sexual partners may find it difficult to adopt a double role, i.e. that of carer and lover.

Grief reactions, with the resultant feelings of anger, guilt and depression and the lowering of sense of worth, may surface after the diagnosis of serious pathology. Very real fears about the impending surgery, such as the anticipated discomfort, the loss of control under anaesthesia and the possibility of death, may all take their toll on the patient's psychological well-being [2].

Societal attitudes

Educational, health and social services tend to discourage expression of sexuality and sexual development in children and adults with learning or physical

disabilities. To some, the idea of people who are less than physically whole and beautiful having sex is disturbing. The disabled are either seen as forever innocent/childlike, or unable to control sexual impulses and therefore a threat. Perhaps some people harbour unconscious sexual anxieties and even feelings of jealousy, especially if they themselves are having or have had sexual difficulties. The anxieties felt by society and professional carers about who will care for possible offspring of such unions, and fears that the disabilities may be inherited, put a further burden on the sexual relationships of the disabled. Perhaps too many people see the handicap rather than the person first.

The individual's particular background, social class, education, religious and sexual beliefs may engender attitudes that preclude dealing with people who are somehow felt to be different. Carers such as parents, social workers, district nurses and health visitors, and particularly those who work in residential homes for the disabled, have much to cope with. Many feel great ambiguity and confusion about the sexuality of their charges. Help with sexual matters, however, is often discreetly given. This may mean the carers lifting a paralysed couple into bed together to facilitate sex, or supplying a vibrator to a patient to help him or her masturbate. Perhaps more problematic for some would be to help gay men and women with disabilities in the same way. The carers' anxieties in these matters are numerous and include such problems as worry about damage to the reputation of the home, their own jobs, the feelings of parents and legal consideration (see later). Simple concepts like privacy may be difficult to envisage in a communal setting.

Contraception

Historical

Early references to birth control are mentioned in the Ebers Papyrus of Egypt around 1500 BC, where pessaries of acacia leaves and crocodile dung are described. Hebrew writings describe a 'cup of roots' drunk by women to ensure sterility, and an early reference to a diaphragm appears in Greek mythology when the goddess Athene protects herself against Hephaestos' advances by inserting a spider's web into her vagina to prevent conception [3].

In modern times, the first advocates of birth control were Thomas Malthus and Francis Page at the beginning of the 19th century and, by the end of that century, contraception was widely in use by the upper middle classes. In the early part of the 20th century, two organizations forwarded progress in this area in the UK, namely the Malthusian League and the Society for Constructive Birth Control and Racial Progress, formed by Marie Stopes. The former concentrated on overpopulation arguments, the latter on the quality of family life. Some members of the church and medical profession hindered progress, but Lord Dawson, Physician in Ordinary to the King, argued that family planning was a necessity and he helped to sway opinion in favour. The National Birth Control Council

formed in 1930 gave way to the Family Planning Association in 1939. It was not until 1967, however, that the Family Planning Act involved the government in family planning. In the USA, Mrs Margaret Sanger established the first birth control clinic in 1916 in Brooklyn and also invoked the help of individual doctors. Dr Abraham Stone founded the *Journal of Contraception* in 1935 and by 1948 the International Planned Parenthood Federation was formed [4].

General nature of debilities and contraceptive choice

Box 15.1, based on Hakim-Elahi's work [5], presents a functional review of disability; it aims to describe major problem areas only. Some of the disabilities could be placed in more than one section. A brief description follows. The factors that should be considered when choosing a contraceptive are as follows [6]:

- the general level of understanding;
- the medical history, particularly of medical conditions that contraindicate combined oral contraceptives e.g. thromboembolism, hepatitis and carcinoma;
- psychiatric illness, e.g. depression, schizophrenia;
- current medication;
- the degree of mobility and manual dexterity;
- the quality of the circulation, especially in the limbs;
- whether or not there is sensory loss;
- problems with menstrual or genital hygiene, especially relevant to the use of a diaphragm or intrauterine device.

Mobility impairment

This may result from one or a combination of causes. The most

---

Box 15.1 Classification of disability – a functional approach

Mobility impairment
- Arthritis
- Spinal cord injury
- Amputations
- Poliomyelitis
- Multiple sclerosis

Major chronic illness
- Cardiac debility
- Strokes
- Carcinomas
- Rheumatic disease

Ostomies and catheters
- Ileostomy, colostomy and ureterostomy
- Catheters

Special senses
- Blindness
- Deafness

Mental handicap
- General
- Legal problems

Specific genetic syndromes and congenital disorders
- Down's syndrome
- Haemophilia
- Cystic fibrosis
- Spina bifida
- Cerebral palsy

Miscellaneous
- Burns
- Drugs
  - effects on sexual function
  - interactions between COCs and drugs

common of these are considered
below.

Arthritis

Rheumatic disease affects both
men and women, all ethnic
groups and people of all ages from
children to the elderly. It is the
most common debilitating illness,
affecting some 30 million
Americans outside of institutions.
In the UK, 5 million people suffer
from osteoarthritis, half a million
from rheumatoid arthritis and
12 000 from the juvenile form.

The timing of medication may
be important to facilitate sexual
function. Analgesics given 30
min to 1 h before coitus often
dull the pain and increase the
potential for sexual arousal.
Orgasm itself tends to give the
patient some relief from pain,
perhaps because of the release of
endorphins. Pain relief may last
for several hours or more [7].

Menstruation and fertility are
not affected, but delivery may
require a caesarean section if
there are pelvic deformities.

A condom or a diaphragm may
be too difficult to use if the hands
are badly affected, although the
unaffected partner may be able to
assist. Combined oral
contraceptive pills (COCs) may
be contraindicated owing to the
risk of thrombosis in patients
who are in a wheelchair or
generally immobile. The
coexistent use of other drugs may
also forbid the use of COCs.
Progestogen-only contraceptives,
particularly the long-acting depot
modalities, should be considered.
In some cases, sterilization may
be appropriate. The couple
should be supported in exploring
non-coital sexual techniques that
involve touching/masturbation
or oral stimulation.

Spinal cord injury (SCI)

Traumatic injury to the brain and
spinal cord involves some
200 000 children in the USA
each year. The resulting loss of
function depends on the location
and severity of the lesion. Some
degree of motor and sensory loss
is not uncommon. Voluntary
movement, bowel and bladder
control, and sexual function may
all be affected. In lesions above
the sixth thoracic vertebra,
respiratory function may be
compromised. Prolonged
inactivity may result in
circulatory problems, spasticity,
decubitus ulcers and general
susceptibility to infection.
Urinary incontinence may cause
difficulties, and only certain coital
positions may be possible or
comfortable.

To allow heterosexual or
homosexual relations, the couple
need permission to try. Practical
suggestions include the use of
pillows to keep legs up or open,
having sex in a wheelchair with
the sides removed or trying the
'spoons' position which provides
support for both partners and
allows penetration. Impotent
men can be offered
intracavernous alprostadil or a
penile prosthesis secured with a
harness if necessary. Vibrators can
be used as 'hand extensions' to
stimulate a partner or can be used
as an aid to masturbation.

In SCI men, 80–90% can still
have erections but only 10–20%
can ejaculate, 3–5% of whom are
fertile. Spastic paraplegics usually
retain more erectile function than
do flaccid paraplegics. In SCI
women, menstruation and
fertility are usually unaffected so
that contraception must be
considered. Immobility and
COCs are both risks for

thrombosis. Injectable
progestogens seem safer and may
be the method of choice for
many such women. Barrier
methods such as a diaphragm may
be too difficult for the patient to
fit. Sterilization should always be
discussed; for a review, see
Yarkony and Chen [8].

As mentioned earlier,
amputations may cause
psychological problems to do
with body image and sense of
wholeness, but physical problems
such as loss of balance, difficulties
in masturbation and problems
with phantom limb pain may also
occur. Prosthetic devices may be
helpful [9].

Poliomyelitis

This was a leading non-traumatic
cause of paraplegia. Menstruation
and fertility are not affected. As
recently as the 1950s, UK couples
who wished to marry were often
frowned upon, and such unions
were called tut-tut marriages (P.
Mohr, personal communication,
1996). '(Tut-tut' is an English
expression which indicates mild
disapproval and distaste. It was
used by some misguided
individuals to show their
disapproval of marriage between
those who had polio, or indeed
between anyone who suffered
from physical handicap. Hence
the name given to these unions.
It was taken up by those involved
as a symbol of defiance.)

Multiple sclerosis (MS)

This is a chronic debilitating
disease that affects primarily
young people between the ages of
20 and 40. Symptoms include
slurred speech, visual disorders,
problems with vertigo and
transient attacks of paralysis, as
well as difficulty in micturition

and erectile dysfunction in men. Psychological factors include periods of euphoria often mixed with depression and feelings of extreme fatigue. Unreasonable jealousy projected at the partner is not uncommon.

The manual dexterity required to fit a diaphragm for contraceptive purposes may be too difficult for affected women. The use of a COC has no contraindications. Pregnancy seems to be beneficial to the course of the illness but relapses may occur postpartum [10].

Major chronic illness

Anyone recovering from major illness, say a myocardial infarction (MI) or a stroke, or who is living with a chronic debilitating illness such as carcinoma, rheumatoid arthritis or MS, is obviously concerned about survival. Krop et al. [11] explored the anxieties of 100 men who had suffered an MI, and found worries about chest pain and the possibility of a reinfarction during coitus, as well as anxieties about potency. Men with quadriplegias and paraplegias reported that their main concern was to regain control of their limbs, bowel and bladder, while sexual function, although important, perhaps understandably came lower in order of priority [12].

Patients who survive a stroke and who are left with hemiplegias or other stigmata understandably feel extremely anxious about both future survival prospects and their loss of function. The latter may affect sexual life and they may need advice on how to cope with specific difficulties. Numbness,

which may occur in parts of the body, means the spouse or sexual partner should learn to caress other still-sensitive areas. If there is a hemianopia, he or she should approach from the visually intact side, and speech-loss may necessitate the couple learning to communicate by non-verbal clues. Feelings of hopelessness and guilt in either the patient or partner should alert the doctor to the onset of a depressive illness, which is amenable to treatment [13].

Hellerstein and Friedman [14] showed that sex need not necessarily be a high-energy activity, especially in older men and women. Moreover, following an illness or surgery, after a suitable period of convalescence, sexual activity is often beneficial and speeds recovery. Common-sense suggestions include having sex with a caring and familiar partner if possible, and sex need not imply full coitus if this is too difficult. The patient should wait for 3 or so hours after a bath or a meal, and timing medication may be important. Sublingual glyceryl trinitrate taken just before coitus may prevent angina or occipital cephalgia, which may occur in some patients, while the timing of analgesics may ease pain in many conditions and facilitate arousal [15].

Contraception is limited by both the illness and concomitant drug treatment. After an MI or a stroke in women, COCs are contraindicated, and barrier methods may be appropriate. Although chemotherapy for carcinoma may affect spermatogenesis and ovarian function, young sexually active adolescents should not rely on this and will still need to take

precautions. Patients with bleeding diseases or who are on long-term steroid or immunosuppressive drugs may be unable to use either COCs or the IUD, and barrier methods or sterilization may be appropriate.

Ostomies and catheters

Ostomies
In the USA and Canada, there are close to 1 000 000 ostomates. In the UK, there are about 100 000 patients with a colostomy and 10 000 with an ileostomy, 5000 of whom have carcinoma. Ostomies are also used to manage incontinence, both urinary and faecal, in people with various congenital abnormalities such as spina bifida. Burnham et al. [16] found that ileostomy without rectal excision caused no sexual dysfunction in either sex, although 30% of patients did report feelings of embarrassment. Colectomy with rectal excision, however, did cause impotence in 70% of the men. In women, orgasm remained intact, but 30% reported dyspareunia.

Psychological problems involve having to deal with the presence of urine or faeces, with the associated smell and unpleasantness, loss of control if the device slips off, and the effects on the partner. General advice consists firstly in giving the patient permission to have sex. Other suggestions include avoiding foods that may cause problems in the few hours before intercourse is anticipated, and judicial emptying of any device prior to coitus. Finding a comfortable position and wearing sexy underwear helps, as does a sense of humour [16]. Contraception will depend on the primary condition and any drug treatment. Resection of the small bowel may interfere with absorption of the COC steroids and affect efficacy [5].

Catheters

Many disabilities in both men and women necessitate the need for catheterization. It is not necessary, however, to remove the catheter in either sex before attempting coitus. In men it should be left to slide freely as the penis erects, then it can be bent and folded down the shaft of the penis, so that insertion into the vagina is facilitated. If extra lubrication is needed, use of a water-soluble rather than an oil-based lubricant is advised. Sexual intercourse should be comfortable for both parties. In women a catheter *in situ* can be pushed out of the way and, if necessary, taped on to the lower abdomen before penetration [17]. Contraception will depend on the primary condition and relevant medication.

Special senses

Blindness and visual impairment

Nearly half a million people in the USA are registered blind. There are differing degrees of blindness that range from some loss of vision to total loss. Senile changes and glaucoma account for two-thirds of blindness in the UK, while diabetes causes some 7–10%, mainly due to vitreous haemorrhage and cataract. Trachoma is the commonest worldwide cause. Psychological factors may be involved in

hysterical blindness, but physical causes should be excluded before the diagnosis is made.

Non-verbal body language from visual cues is an important part of mother/child bonding, psychosexual development and adult interaction between the sexes. The child with severe visual impairment is obviously at an extreme disadvantage in these matters. Body parts, particularly sexual organs of the opposite sex, remain mysterious. The use of dolls in order to learn about anatomy is usually of limited help. Boys' usual use of erotic material for masturbation fantasies is unavailable to the blind. Inappropriate behaviours, such as masturbating in public, have to be redirected. Meeting potential sexual partners is difficult without sight and eye-to-eye contact, and the mere ability to walk over to someone is fraught with difficulty.

Coexistent pathology, such as diabetes, MS or depressive illness, may cause further problems, which include loss of libido and erectile dysfunction. Menstruation, fertility and pregnancy are unaffected if there is no coexistent illness, but if there is, care must be taken over contraceptive choice [5,18].

Deafness

This is the most common cause of chronic physical debility in the USA today and it remains the most invisible of handicaps. Over 90% of deaf children are born to hearing parents, and nearly this figure of hearing children are born to deaf parents. It is helpful to distinguish between those born deaf (congenital deafness) and those who become deaf

(adventitious deafness). The latter are further divided into those who lose hearing early on before speech and language are acquired (prelingual deafness) and those who lose it after this time (postlingual deafness). The developmental and social effects of deafness are obviously more severe with the congenital and prelingual types. Although IQ is not generally affected, comprehension and reading ability are lowered. Lip reading is often difficult for the deaf and sign language is preferable.

The main causes of congenital deafness are maternal rubella and genetic disorders, while acquired deafness may result either from conductive impairment as a sequel to otitis media and otosclerosis, or from damage to the eighth cranial nerve by infection or trauma.

Psychosexual development depends on verbal cues which help the child to appreciate the 'do's' and 'don'ts' of sexuality. Deaf people, particularly the congenital and prelingual groups, have problems with understanding abstract concepts, such as aspects of relationships, pregnancy and the role of parents, as such ideas are difficult to pick up from sign language. Sexual delinquency is not an infrequent problem among deaf adolescents and may occur as a result of the isolation of the sexes that is enforced in certain residential facilities. Unfortunately, misinformation and the acceptance of sexual myths, which result from a lack of teaching of sexual matters, are sadly all too common [19]. Contraception needs the same consideration as for the blind, as described above.

Mental handicap

General

In the USA alone there are nearly three million young people with learning difficulty. Now that care has moved towards the community, emphasis has been put on enabling people, specifically those with a mental disability, to lead as full and normal a life as possible. This means, among other things, allowing them opportunities to form relationships in which they are able to express physical and emotional needs, and to form sexual relationships. Marriages between people with different degrees of handicap are becoming increasingly common and studies point to the overall success of such liaisons [20]. The apparent low fecundity of couples with mental handicap may have been due in the past to their limited opportunity to have a sexual relationship and partly to their low fertility. Children resulting from such unions do have a greater risk of mental handicap and of congenital abnormalities. If both parents are mentally handicapped, their offspring have a 40% risk of being affected, whereas if one parent only is handicapped, the risk falls to 15%.

Contraception should be considered on the one hand, if there is evidence of casual sexual behaviour and, on the other, if there is the possibility of a more stable relationship. Some form of special counselling should be offered and special training for the professional to meet the needs of such patients may be required. Parents or those caring may ask for contraception on behalf of the mentally handicapped person,

but for the systemic methods (e.g. COC, depot progestogen) or the intrauterine device (IUD) the person's consent is required. Simple explanation should be offered, but if there are problems, more expert help and opinion should be sought.

Severely mentally handicapped people rarely require contraception, but if a liaison has developed, for example, between such an individual and a less severely affected partner, contraception may be appropriate. As such, individuals cannot give consent; the doctor should consult widely with the relatives, those providing care and others concerned and act in the best interests of the patient. Special care must be taken at all times to ensure there is no danger of exploitation.

Sterilization of either partner with appropriate consent is sometimes the method of choice. However, it is final and other methods should be considered first. It should never be done without full agreement, where possible, with the individual concerned: there are reports of mentally handicapped individuals who feel bitterness and regret that this was done to them without previous discussion. Sometimes parents erroneously believe that the operation will take away all sexual interest [21].

Legal problems

The UK has no written constitution but has instead a common law system derived from statute law, from Acts of Parliament, and case law derived from individual cases heard in the higher courts. The law is divided into civil and criminal and it is

the latter that is usually concerned with sexual behaviour. The Crown Prosecution Service decides if prosecution should go ahead.

In general, there are laws which apply to everyone, including people with a disability, and laws which make particular reference to this group. There are eight Acts which deal specifically with the disabled and cover matters such as age of consent, sexual intercourse with a mentally handicapped person, marriage, indecent assault and rape. Other acts deal with homosexuality, sex education and the role of those providing care.

Those professionals who deal with the handicapped in institutions often have anxieties about their role in helping with such matters. Sex education may involve instruction in the use of a condom or the fitting of a diaphragm, intimate procedures in themselves, but teaching masturbation may be even more problematic, although necessary when indirect methods such as books or videos fail to instruct. The role of the professional in instruction may not be clearly defined.

Staff must not have a sexual relationship, specifically sexual intercourse, with a patient. If a woman carer does so, she could be charged with assault and/or failure to exercise proper care, while a male who has sex with a female patient risks a charge of rape if the latter is deemed unable to give consent. In theory, staff who helped a couple to have intercourse could be considered to have aided and abetted the behaviour.

In general, the law seeks to

protect such patients from exploitation or abuse, but if from the circumstances it is apparent that none has taken place, and furthermore that the staff have acted in good faith, then prosecution is highly unlikely. Consultation with the individual in charge of the institution, the relevant medical personnel, such as the psychiatrist and the general practitioner, as well as a discussion with the immediate family and perhaps legal advice, will minimize risk of prosecution. Careful notes as to what was done and who was present should be kept in the patient's records. At the end of the day, however, prosecution is a possible risk that all professionals providing care have to take [22].

In the USA, as in many other countries, there is a written constitution, which consists of laws passed by the Congress and interpreted by the Federal Judiciary by means of the Supreme Court. Each state may also pass local legislation through its judiciary. The education for All Handicapped Children Act of 1974 governs the various debilities and ensures that each individual will receive appropriate education, tailored to his/her specific needs. Section 504 of the Rehabilitation Act of 1973 is somewhat wider in scope and applies to all handicapped people, not just to children, and covers many areas of discrimination. It includes measures such as the providing of appropriate transport and the modifying of buildings to cater for the disabled, and it covers such issues as their right to participate in sports. Other legislation covers sex discrimination and child abuse [23].

Specific genetic syndromes and congenital disorders

Those involving some degree of mental and physical debility affect 5% of all children. Conditions include Down's syndrome, spina bifida, cerebral palsy and neuromuscular disease. Cystic fibrosis, an autosomal recessive condition, occurs in Caucasians from one in 1500 to one in 15 000 live births.

Down's syndrome

Men with Down's syndrome may have libido and may be able to obtain an erection, but they are usually sterile. Women so affected, however, are usually fertile and the chance of their having a Down's syndrome child is significant. Most methods of contraception are acceptable, but care and supervision is needed.

Cystic fibrosis

Sexual intercourse is usually possible in men and women so affected, but problems do occur. In women, inadequate lubrication, which results in vaginal dryness and dyspareunia, is not uncommon, but can be overcome with appropriate lubricants. In men, potency is good but 85% are usually sterile owing to anomalies in spermatogenesis. Sexual activity may precipitate bouts of coughing and respiratory distress.

Turner's syndrome

Owing to the presence of dysgenic ovaries, these women are infertile, but use of the pill regulates the cycle and is a form of hormone replacement therapy.

Klinefelter's syndrome

Men with this disorder are infertile unless they are mosaics who have cells with normal karyotypes present. Most have a diminished libido because of low testosterone levels, although this may be replaced artificially.

Spina bifida (SB)

This condition, i.e. defective closure of the vertebral column during development, varies from the occult type to the clinical type, where the meninges, the spinal cord itself or both meninges and cord protrude, the so-called myelomeningocoele. Various associated anomalies, such as hydrocephalus and club foot, often occur as well as problems with bladder and anal sphincters. Most men so affected have erections, although these are often unpredictable and of limited use for coitus. Fertility is decreased but some affected patients have fathered children. The risk of SB in the general population is 0.1%, rising to 3% if one parent is affected.

Cerebral palsy (CP)

Cerebral palsy is a general term that refers to a broad spectrum of disabilities affecting between 0.1% and 0.2% of children. Trauma *in utero* or at birth and jaundice are among the precipitating factors. CP is loosely classified into spastic, athetoid, ataxic or mixed forms.

CP does not affect genital sensation, menstruation or fertility. The presence of contractures, however, may make certain coital positions impossible or masturbation difficult, and sexual arousal may increase spasticity or athetoid movements.

Contractures and spasticity of joints in spina bifida and the abnormal movements in cerebral palsy may cause problems with the fitting a diaphragm or an IUD. COCs are contraindicated if circulatory problems are present (Table 15.1).

Miscellaneous

Burns

The skin is the largest organ of the body and is intimately involved in psychosexual development, both between mother and child, and later between sexual partners. Damage by lesions such as psoriasis or by burn injury leaves the patient with feelings of being impure or dirty. Lesions on the face, breasts or genital regions have more symbolic sexual meaning, and injuries sustained under the age of 11 years do more to lower self-esteem. Therapies should involve the partner and the use of soothing oils, and touching is the keystone to treatment. There are no special restraints on contraception [24,25].

Drugs
Effects on sexual function

Sexual arousal and performance involve a host of systems which include the cerebral cortex, the limbic system, hypothalamus, the autonomic nervous system, neurotransmitters, relevant arteries and veins, hormones and volatile substances called pheromones. Illness and drugs may affect these mechanism at any level, often acting at more than one site. More research has been carried out on male sexuality than female sexuality (Table 15.2).

Disabled people specifically are often required to take various medications and these may have sexual side effects. For example, analgesics taken for pain by patients with chronic rheumatic disorders may cause sedation and so prevent sexual arousal or response.

Interactions between oral contraception and drugs

In general, drugs which induce liver enzymes and those which prevent reabsorption from the gut reduce the effectiveness of COCs (see Chapter 6).

The future

Progress does seem to depend at first on the ideas and work of individuals. As society evolves to accept some of these views, medicine and the law follow. The International Year of the Disabled in 1981 brought to the general public through the media various issues that concern people with disabilities, which included sexual matters. Organizations have arisen, such as SPOD (Sexual and Personal Problems of the Disabled), which have worked with other organizations in this field to enhance the quality of life for people with disability.

Table 15.1 Contraception and disability

Method	Attributes	Disadvantages
COC	Reduces menstrual loss and dysmenorrhoea Eliminating the PFI ensures amenorrhoea Reduces frequency of cyclical symptoms (PMS, epilepsy)	Risk of VTE Poor compliance Drug interaction
Injectables	Minimal compliance Amenorrhoea may be an advantage PMS, epilepsy and seizures reduced	Issues of consent Long-term amenorrhoea may be a disadvantage
Subdermal implants	No compliance required	Irregular bleeding May be distressing if palpable Insertion may be problematic if patient is uncooperative
IUD/IUS/IUI	No compliance required	Heavier menses with IUD/IUI Insertion difficult sometimes; may need anaesthesia Reactive hypertension in SCI
Barriers	Protect against STIs Condom use can be taught	Difficult to use for some and need motivation
Sterilization	Permanent	Legal and ethical dilemmas

COC = combined oral contraceptive; PFI = pill-free interval; VTE = venous thromboembolism; PMS = premenstrual syndrome; IUD = intrauterine device; IUS = intrauterine system; IUI = intrauterine implant; SCI = spinal cord injury; STI = sexually transmitted infection.

Table 15.2 Sexual side effects of some commonly used drugs

Drug[a]	Mode of action	Sexual effects
Analgesics	Sedative	Loss of libido
Cardiovascular		
Digoxin	Oestrogenic effect	Impotence
Bendrofluazide	?	Impotence
Propranolol	Lowers testosterone production and has a vascular effect	Impotence (dose related)
Calcium channel blockers and ACE inhibitors		Minimal or nil
Methyldopa		Erectile failure/ reduced vaginal lubrication and anorgasmia
Psychotropic		
Hypnotics and anxiolytics, e.g. benzodiazepines and opiates	GABA system	Diminish libido in both sexes Impotence in men
Antidepressants, e.g. tricyclics, SSRIs and MAOIs	Neurotransmitters	Interfere with libido, erection and ejaculation/orgasm
Antipsychotics, e.g. thioridazines	Central and peripheral neurotransmitters	Depress libido in men and women Retrograde ejaculation
Anti-epileptics		
Phenobarbitone	Induce liver enzymes, increase SHBG and lower free testosterone	Impotence, orgasmic problems in women
Carbamazepine	No effects	Nil
Antipeptics		
Cimetidine	Vascular	Erectile dysfunction/ poor lubrication
Drugs of abuse		
Alcohol	Affects liver enzymes, steal syndrome[b]	Impotence
Heroin	Steal syndrome	Impotence
Cigarette smoking	Testosterone binding, arterial effects	? impotence

[a]Only a few drugs in each class have been considered. Sexual side effects are relatively rare.
[b]Steal syndrome – blood is diverted away from the penis to the limbs during arousal.
GABA = gamma aminobutyric acid; SSRIs = selective serotonin reuptake inhibitors; MAOIs = monoamine oxidase inhibitors; SHBG = sex hormone binding globulin.

Today, every family doctor should make use of available information on where he or she can obtain advice on the management of sexual problems of the disabled. Postgraduate courses should have this topic in the syllabus as a basic part of medicine or nursing.

Tips for safe practice

- Each patient has sexual needs: choose your language carefully.

- Discuss choices with the patient, relevant family and staff. Remember that the patient often needs practical help but may be embarrassed to ask. Be explicit.

- Spend extra time with the patient and use simple diagrams when necessary.

- Write clearly in the patient's medical records what is done and why.

- Inform the general practitioner, psychiatrist, superintendent and relevant personnel.

- Ensure that usual check-ups, i.e. blood pressure monitoring, cervical smears, are made.

- Keep abreast of developments: attend lectures and read journals on these topics.

Resources

- Local general practitioner and primary care team.

- Local geriatric/psychiatric services.

- Family Planning Clinics, Brook Advisory Centres.

- Organizations to provide help, information, leaflets, books, videos, etc.:

- Sexual and Personal Relationships of People with a Disability (SPOD), 186 Camden Road, London, N7 0BJ (Tel. 0207–607–8851).
- UK Disabled Living Foundation, 380–384 Harrow Road, London W9 2HU.
- UK Royal Society for Mentally Handicapped Children and Adults, 123 Golden Lane, London EC1Y ORT.
- For 'sexual toys' in the USA:
  - Townsend Institute, PO Box 8855, Chapel Hill, NC 27515 (Tel. 1-800-888-1900).
  - Good vibrations, 938 Howard Street, San Francisco, CA 94103 (Tel. 1-800-289-84123).

References

1. Stewart WFR. Sex and the physically handicapped. Horsham: The National Fund for Research into Crippling Diseases, 1975.

2. Goodman RE. Psychosexual effects of carcinoma. *Psychiatr Practice* 1987;6:6–10.

3. Green S. The curious history of contraception. London: Ebury Press, 1971.

4. Peel J, Potts M. Textbook of contraceptive practice. Cambridge: Cambridge University Press, 1969.

5. Hakim-Elahi E. Contraceptive choice for the disabled (handicapped) person. *N Y State J Med* 1982:1601–8.

6. Leavesley G, Porter J. Sexuality, fertility and contraception in disability. *Contraception* 1982;26:417–41.

7. Lim PAC. Sexuality in patients with musculoskeletal disease. In: Monga TN (ed.) Sex and disability Philadelphia: Hanley & Belfus, Inc., 1995;401–15.

8. Yarkony GM, Chen D. Sexuality in patients with spinal cord injury. In: Monga TN (ed.) Sex and disability. Philadelphia: Hanley & Belfus, Inc., 1995;325–44.

9. Comfort A. Miscellaneous medical and surgical conditions. In: Comfort A (ed.) Sexual consequences of disability. Philadelphia: George F Stickley Co., 1978.

10. Burnfield A, Burnfield P. Common psychological problems in multiple sclerosis. *Br Med J* 1978;1:1193–4.

11. Krop H, Hall D, Mehta J. Sexual concerns after myocardial infarction. *Sex Dis* 1979;2:91–7.

12. Hanson RW, Franklin MR. Sexual loss in relation to other functional losses for spinal cord injured males. *Arch Phys Med Rehab* 1976;57:291–3.

13. Renshaw DC. Stroke and sex. In: Comfort A (ed.) Sexual consequences of disability. Philadelphia: George F Stickley Co., 1978.

14. Hellestein HK, Friedman EH. Sexual activity and the post-coronary patient. *Arch Intern Med* 1970;125:987–99.

15. Goodman RE. Sex counselling for the post-coronary patient. *Br J Sex Med* 1989;16:25–8.

16. Burnham WR, Lennard-Jones JE, Brooke BN. Sexual problems among married ileostomists. *Gut* 1977;18:673–7.

17. Mooney TO, Cole TM, Chilgren RA. Sexual options for paraplegics and quadiplegics. Boston: Little Brown & Co., 1975.

18. Hicks S. Relationship and sexual problems of the visually handicapped. *Sex Dis* 1980;3:165–76.

19. Fitzgerald D, Fitzgerald M. Sexual implications of deafness. *Sex Dis* 1987;1:57–69.

20. Craft A, Craft M. Sexuality and mental handicap: a review. *Br J Psychiatr* 1981;139:494–505.

21. Edgerton RB, Dingman HF. Good reasons for bad supervision: dating in a hospital for the mentally retarded. *Psychiat Quart Suppl* 1964;38:221–33.

22. Gunn MJ. Sex and the law, 3rd edn. London: Family Planning Association, 1991.

23. Underwood J. Legal protection for at risk children. In: Lakebrink JM (ed.) Children at risk, Vol. 7 Springfield, Illinois: Charles C Thomas, 1989:90–118.

24. Bowden ML, Feller I, Tholen D, Davidson TN, James MH. Self-esteem of severely burned patients. *Arch Phys Med Rehabil* 1980;61:449–52.

25. Bogaerts F. Burns and sexuality. *J Burn Care Rehabil* 1992; 13:39–43.

Further reading

- ARC (Association for Residential Care). It could never happen here – a UK document on sexual abuse.

- Comfort A. Sexual consequences of disability. Philadelphia: GF Stickley Co., 1978.

- Darnbrough A, Kinrade D. Directory for disabled people 1995. Prentice Hall/Harvester Wheatsheaf.

- Gunn MJ. Sex and the law, 3rd edn. London: Family Planning Association, 1991.

- Institute for the Study of Drug Dependence. Drugs, pregnancy and childcare (revised edition). London.

- Monga TN (ed.) Sexuality and disability. Philadelphia: Hanley & Belfus Inc., 1995.

- Mooney TO, Cole TM, Chilgren RA. Sexual options for paraplegics and quadriplegics. Boston: Little Brown & Co., 1975.

- Owens T. The outsiders club: practical suggestions. Integration Trust, 1986.

Contraception and medical disorders

Barbara A Hollingworth MBChB DRCOG MFFP

Introduction

There is a wide range of contraceptive methods that are currently available. The choice of any particular method over any other is, therefore, often a complex decision for the healthy individual or couple, and is based on a number of considerations. The final decision, however, usually rests with the user.

The factors involved in the choice of contraceptive method are as follows (see also Chapter 13 on 'The contraceptive decision'):

- acceptability;
- ease of obtaining supply;
- ease of use;
- efficacy;
- frequency of attendance for follow-up;
- health risks of the contraceptive method;
- health risks of a pregnancy;
- mode of action;
- need for medical intervention to initiate the method;
- possible long-term effects;
- reversibility;
- side effects.

The choice of a contraceptive method for a woman with a coexistent medical disorder is complicated by the need to take the disorder itself into consideration. A balance needs to be struck between any risk of a pregnancy and the suitability and/or acceptability of the contraceptive:

- Will the medical disorder be affected by use of the contraceptive; if so in what way?

- What will the effect of pregnancy be on this medical disorder, or what will the effect of this medical disorder and/or its drug treatment be on a pregnancy?

Counselling in this situation must be sympathetic and thorough, as the client's preferred methods may be medically unacceptable. A good rapport between the user and the provider as well as ongoing support for the user is essential to encourage adherence [1]. It is important that a full range of options is available for the couple to try and for them to have the final decision as to which to use. Liaison with any others who care for the couple is also important.

Barrier methods

Male and female condoms, diaphragms and caps would appear to be ideal choices. They are easy to use, require little or no medical intervention, have no side effects and no interaction with coexistent medical disorders. Unfortunately, their efficacy is comparatively low and a more secure option is likely to be desirable for a woman in whom a pregnancy would constitute a significant risk to her health.

Barriers prevent sexually transmitted infections and their use should be encouraged; however, a woman with a history of or susceptibility to urinary tract infections is not a good candidate for a diaphragm.

It should be stressed that oil-based vaginal preparations may not be used with latex barriers as they affect the integrity of latex rubber.

Sterilization

If pregnancy is a severe threat to health and/or the family is complete, sterilization could be offered. Vasectomy may be an option if female sterilization is perceived as too great a medical risk but would only be appropriate in a stable relationship without there being any undue pressure on the male partner to make this choice. If the woman's medical condition carries a significant risk of mortality, this also must be taken into consideration before sterilizing her partner.

Combined oral contraceptives (COCs)

Low-dose COCs contain ethinyl oestradiol (EE) less than 50 μg together with a progestogen; this section relates to the use of low-dose COCs unless otherwise stated. COCs containing ≥ 50 μg EE are not recommended for use other than in certain specific situations where bioavailability is compromised by the medical disorder or concurrent medication.

COCs provide very effective contraception: method failure is low with good compliance. Serious, but uncommon, adverse effects are due to the synthetic oestrogen, which promotes an increase in blood coagulability, leading to a higher risk of thromboembolic events among users. Venous thromboembolic events are more common than arterial ones, which are almost exclusively seen in women with underlying arterial disease or marked risk factors for arterial disease. Existing cardiovascular disease and the risk factors which predispose to it are a major deciding factor in prescribing the COC; they may constitute absolute contraindications (Box 16.1a–c) or relative contraindications (Box 16.2a,b). Two or more coexisting relative

Box 16.1 Combined oral contraceptives (COCs): absolute contraindications

(a) Cardiovascular
- Blood pressure 160/95 mmHg or greater
- Body mass index (BMI) >39
- Cardiomyopathy
- Cigarette smoking >40 per day
- Cigarette smoking and over the age of 35 years
- Combined risk factors for arterial or venous disease
- Complicated diabetes mellitus
- Existing arterial disease, e.g. angina, ischaemic heart disease
- Focal or classical migraine, migraine with aura, treatment of migraine with ergotamine; severe or prolonged migraine
- History of arterial or venous thrombosis
- History of cerebral haemorrhage secondary to cerebral thrombosis
- Lipid disorder predisposing towards atherogenesis
- Predisposition towards arterial or venous thrombosis, e.g. the thrombophilias[a]
- Prolonged immobility; major elective surgery or leg surgery, 4 weeks before and 2 weeks after full mobilization
- Pulmonary hypertension
- Valvular heart disease and most types of structural heart disease

(b) Liver Disease
- Abnormal liver function tests/current active liver disease
- Cholestatic jaundice, either recurrent or in a previous pregnancy
- Dubin–Johnson and Rotor syndromes
- Gallstones (COCs acceptable after cholecystectomy)
- Liver adenoma or carcinoma
- Porphyria

(c) History of a medical condition known to be affected by sex steroids, precipitated by or exacerbated by previous use of COCs
- Chorea
- COC-induced hypertension
- Haemolytic uraemic syndrome
- Otosclerosis
- Pancreatitis due to hypertriglyceridaemia
- Pemphigoid gestationis
- SLE with antiphospholipid antibodies
- Stevens–Johnson syndrome
- Trophoblastic disease until blood levels of hCG are undetectable.

(d) Oestrogen-dependent neoplasia
- Biopsy-proven premalignant epithelial atypia of the breast
- Breast cancer (COC becoming more acceptable in selected women in discussion with their oncologists)

(e) Pregnancy

(f) Undiagnosed genital tract bleeding

[a] The thrombophilias:
- Factor V Leiden Mutation;
- Activated protein C deficiency;
- Protein C deficiency;
- Protein S deficiency;
- Antithrombin III deficiency;
- Acquired antiphospholipid antibodies:
  - Lupus anticoagulant
  - Anticardiolipin antibodies;
- Prothrombin 20/20A.

contraindications are usually considered to be an absolute contraindication [2].

COCs are absorbed through the intestinal wall and both oestrogen and progestogen are metabolized in the liver where they are conjugated and excreted with the bile back into the intestine. Any degree of hepatic malfunction or disease may

Box 16.2   Combined oral contraceptives (COCs): relative contraindications

(a) Risk factors for arterial disease
- Age 35–50 years without any other risk factors
- BMI = 30–39
- Blood pressure: systolic 135–165 mmHg, diastolic 85–95 mmHg
- Family history of arterial disease in a first-degree relative aged below 45 years
- Hyperlipidaemia
- Insulin-dependent diabetes with no complications
- Migraine without focal signs/aura (common migraine)
- Sickle cell disease
- Smoking less than 40 cigarettes per day

(b) Risk factors for venous thromboembolism
- Active inflammatory bowel disease
- BMI = 30–39
- Family history of venous thromboembolic disease in a first-degree relative under 45 years, clotting factors normal
- Long-term immobility such as being confined to a wheelchair
- Severe varicose veins, episode of thrombophlebitis in varicose veins
- Sickle cell disease

(c) Drug treatments which may interfere with the efficacy of COCs
- Hepatic enzyme-inducing drugs
  - Barbiturates
  - Carbamazepine
  - Griseofulvin
  - Rifampicin/Rifabutin
  - Phenytoin
  - Primidone
  - Ritonovir/Melfinavir
  - Topiramate
  - Spironolactone
  - Modafinil
- Broad-spectrum antibiotics, particularly:
  - Amoxycillin
  - Ampicillin and related penicillins
  - Broad-spectrum cephalosporins
  - Tetracyclines

interfere with COC efficacy or be affected by its use (Box 16.1b). Some of the oestrogen conjugates are hydrolysed by the gut flora, allowing free oestrogen to be reabsorbed and so recycled: the so-called enterohepatic circulation. How important this secondary absorption of oestrogen is to the efficacy of the COC is uncertain: owing to the high interindividual variability of oestrogen, the recycled oestradiol may be important for some women [3]. Factors interfering with the enterohepatic circulation, such as the effect of broad-spectrum antibiotics on the gut flora, may reduce COC efficacy (Box 16.2c).

Microsomal enzymes in the hepatic endoplasmic reticulum and, to a lesser extent, in the gut wall inactivate COC steroids; drugs which induce these enzymes will increase the rate of inactivation of the COC, decreasing its efficacy [4] (Box 16.2).

Major surgery and COCs

Women taking a COC should discontinue use 4 weeks before any major elective surgery and resume with the first period at least 2 weeks after full mobilization. Most day-case procedures do not require this precaution but any surgery to legs such as stripping of varicose veins is included. Following surgery where the legs are bandaged, COCs cannot be resumed until after the bandages have been removed and a further 2 weeks after full mobilization [5].

Progestogen-only pills (POPs)

POPs have not been as widely used as COCs and there are limited data available concerning their potential adverse effects. However, based on available information, POPs would seem to be a good choice where synthetic oestrogens are contraindicated but an oral contraceptive is preferred. Efficacy is high, although there is some small variation between studies: Vessey found the failure rate to be between 0.3 and 3.1 per 100 woman–years and to decrease with age [6]. Adherence to pill-taking regimen is important: the POP should be taken daily at a regular time and no more than 3 h late to maximize the progestogenic effect of thickening cervical mucus.

Coagulation factors are not adversely affected by POPs, which may be used by women with a personal history of thrombosis or at high risk of thrombosis. Studies have not shown any significant changes in lipid metabolism, although some have shown very small reductions in high-density lipoprotein (HDL) and HDL_2 cholesterol. Total cholesterol, HDL_3 low-density lipoprotein (LDL) and very low-density lipoprotein (VLDL) are unaltered.

The POP is a good choice for diabetics. It does not seem to affect insulin requirement or diabetic retinopathy. Carbohydrate metabolism shows only small changes of doubtful clinical significance.

Studies of POPs have not shown them to increase blood pressure, therefore, progestogen-only methods of contraception may be used by women with hypertension. POPs would also seem to have little or no effect on hepatic function, but should not be used in the presence of acute disease until liver function tests have returned to normal. There is no evidence to suggest POPs cause hepatic tumours or liver disease. However, steroid hormones are metabolized by the liver and, in the presence of severe disease, the increased steroid load of the POP is best avoided [7].

Hepatic enzyme-inducing drugs will diminish the efficacy of the POP and, although the dose may be increased to two or more pills per day to try and overcome this interaction, it is impossible to gauge how effective it will be. An alternative method of contraception is recommended.

Antibiotics (other than those which induce hepatic enzymes) do not interact with the POP as progestins are not 'recycled' in the enterohepatic circulation.

Contraindications to the use of POPs are:

- acute liver disease;
- benign and malignant liver tumours;
- hepatic enzyme-inducing drugs;
- malignancies of the breast, ovary or genital tract (but may be allowed after discussion with the oncologist);
- pregnancy;

- severe arterial disease;
- severe chronic liver disease;
- trophoblastic disease until human chorionic gonadotrophin has returned to normal (partly due to the confusing effect of any irregular bleeding);
- unexplained abnormal vaginal bleeding.

Injectable progestogens and implants

These methods have the advantage over oral contraceptives of being independent of the user for their efficacy but the disadvantage that they cannot be discontinued immediately. Medical considerations are similar to those of the POP and these methods may be used by women who should avoid synthetic oestrogens.

Enzyme-inducing drugs may have a small theoretical effect on the efficacy of injectables, although data either way are very sparse. It is suggested that women on such drugs should reduce the interval between injections, e.g. depot medroxyprogesterone acetate (DMPA) from 12 to 10 weeks.

The effect of liver enzyme-inducing drugs on the efficacy of implants is uncertain and, as there is no way to compensate for any effect, another method would be preferable.

Injectables and warfarin

There is no known drug interaction but there is a concern about haematoma formation at

the injection site. This should be seen in relation to the need for contraception and the suitability of other methods.

Intrauterine devices (IUDs)

The new generation copper-containing IUDs have a high efficacy, the Copper T 380 Slimline (T-380 S) giving a failure rate of 0.3 per 100 woman-years in the first 3 years, falling to 0.1 thereafter. This is comparable to or better than all other methods of contraception.

Contraindications in respect of coexisting medical disorders are few but include the following:

- current immunosuppressive therapy (other than with oral corticosteroids);
- heart valve prosthesis;
- history of bacterial endocarditis;
- human immunodeficiency virus (HIV) infection (relative contraindication);
- true copper allergy (rare);
- Wilson's disease.

The following conditions should be taken into consideration before using the IUD:

- iron deficiency anaemia and/or menorrhagia (there is the potential for increased blood loss with an IUD);
- a history of pelvic
- infection/lifestyle at risk of sexually transmitted infection, leading to tubal disease and compromise of future fertility;

- structural heart disease or prosthesis which needs to be protected from blood-borne infection.

Management of patients at risk of bacterial endocarditis

An IUD should only be fitted in such women under antibiotic cover. The antibiotic regimen would be similar to that recommended for any minor surgical procedure in these circumstances, such as dental treatment, and the current regimen may be confirmed by the cardiologist caring for the patient. An example of such prophylaxis is to give an oral dose of 3 g amoxicillin 4 h before and another 8 h after the procedure.

Patients with a prosthetic valve or who have had endocarditis should receive intramuscular (im) or intravenous (iv) amoxycillin 1 g plus im or iv gentamicin 120 mg before the procedure and oral amoxycillin 500 mg 6 h later.

Removal of an IUD does not require antibiotic cover unless it is complicated, needing instrumentation of the uterine cavity.

Intrauterine system (IUS)

The levonorgestrel-releasing intrauterine system releases levonorgestrel (LNG) at a rate of 20 µg per 24 h into the endometrial cavity over a 5-year period. This causes atrophic change in the endometrium as a local effect. Once this endometrial change is complete, after approximately 3–4 months, blood levels are about one-

quarter the levels of POP users. The menstrual loss is dramatically reduced and the woman may become oligomenorrhoeic or amenorrhoeic.

Medical contraindications to IUS use are slightly different from those for the IUD:

- allergy to LNG;
- current severe active arterial disease;*
- current active hepatic disease;*
- current immunosuppressive therapy (other than with oral corticosteroids);
- current trophoblastic disease;
- heart valve prosthesis;
- history of bacterial endocarditis;
- liver tumour.*

In women at particularly high risk, the disease process can be closely monitored and the device removed if there is any sign of deterioration. Insertion of an IUS in a woman with structural heart disease or with a prosthesis who is at risk of blood-borne infection should include antibiotic prophylaxis at insertion as described in the IUD section above.

Contraceptive management of various medical disorders

There is very little information regarding contraceptive usage in

---

*In view of the low blood levels of LNG, these may be considered cautions rather than absolute contraindications, taking into consideration the high efficacy of the method.

the presence of specific medical disorders – most studies have been conducted among healthy users. In the World Health Organization (WHO) document 'Medical eligibility criteria for contraceptive use' [2], the suitability of contraceptives for use in any medical condition have been assessed in the light of the most recent available clinical and epidemiological data, and these medical conditions are classified as follows:

1. A condition for which there is no restriction for the use of the contraceptive method.
2. A condition where the advantages of using the method generally outweigh the theoretical or proven risks.
3. A condition where the theoretical or proven risks usually outweigh the advantages of using the method.
4. A condition which represents an unacceptable health risk if the contraceptive method is used.

There is a further subdivision:

- Initiation of the contraceptive method in the circumstances; and
- Continuation of the method should the condition develop or progress.

Table 16.1 Summarizes the suitability of different contraceptives for use in various medical disorders, using this system of classification.

For any given medical disorder, a good medical history must be obtained and an examination performed as necessary in order

Table 16.1 Eligibility criteria for systemic and intrauterine contraception in women with medical disorders. See also Tables 6.8 and 6.9.

Medical disorder	COC	POP	DMPA	IUS	IUD
Age					
<35	1	1	1	1	1
>35			1	1	1
>35 with no other risk factor for CVD	2	1			
>35 with one other CVD risk factor	4	1			
AIDS	1	1	1	2	3 Concern about increased blood loss, susceptibility to STDs and PID
Alopecia	1	1	1	1	1
Arterial disease					
Pre-existing, e.g. MI, CVA, angina	4 (see Box 16.1a)	3/4 depending on severity	3/4	2/3 Theoretical risk of adverse effect on lipids; amount absorbed small and insufficient data	1
With risk factors	I = 2 (see Box 16.2a) C = 2, 3 or 4 (subject to regular review)	1			
		1/2	2	2	1
Asthma	1	1	1	1	1
Body mass Index (BMI)					
Any value	1	1	1	1	1
BMI < 30	1	1			
BMI 30–39		1			
With no other risk factor	2				
With one other risk factor	4	1			
BMI >39	4	1			
Breast disease					
Benign breast disease	1	1	1	1	1
Epithelial atypia (proven)	4	2	4	2/3	1
Carcinoma	4 (3 after discussion with oncologist)	4 (3 after discussion with oncologist)	4	2/3	1
Breastfeeding	3 May reduce quantity of milk	1			
<6 weeks postpartum			3 Concern about steroid load on fetal liver	3 Concern about steroid load on fetal liver and increased risk of uterine perforation	2 Concern about increased risk of uterine perforation
>6 weeks postpartum			1	1	1
Cervical intraepithelial neoplasia	2	2	1	1	1
Cholestasis					
In pregnancy	4	2	1	1	1
Past COC use	3/4	2/3	2	2	1
Cigarette smoking					
<40 per day	I = 2 provided age ≤ 35 years I &C = 4 at age ≥ 35	1 1	1	1	1
≥ 40 per day	I & C at any age = 4	1	1	1	1
Cystic fibrosis	2 (see Boxes 16.2c and 16.2 text for management of long-term prophylactic antibiotics)	1	1	1	1

Table 16.1 *continued*

Medical disorder	COC	POP	DMPA	IUS	IUD
Diabetes Mellitus					
With diabetic complications	4	2	1	1	1
Without diabetic complications	2	1	1	1	1
History of gestational diabetes	1	1	1	1	1
Drug interactions					
Liver enzyme-inducers (long- or short-term use)	2 Efficacy may be significantly compromised (see Box 16.2c and text) Another method may be preferable	2/3 Efficacy may be significantly compromised (see Box 16.2c text) Another method may be preferable	1 Decrease injection interval to 10 weeks	2 Some concern about reduced efficacy; however, no data	1
Broad-spectrum antibiotics (long- or short-term use)	1 Efficacy may be compromised (see Box 16.2c and text)	1 No interaction	1	1	1
Cyclosporin	2/3 COC may delay clearance of cyclosporin and lead to toxicity. Levels should be monitored regularly	1	1	1	1
Ectopic pregnancy in past	1	2/3 Lower risk than no method but other methods preferred	1	1[a]	1
Endometriosis	1	1	1	2[b]	1
Epilepsy	1 Beware of drug interactions with enzyme inducers (see Box 16.2c and text)	2/3 Beware of drug interactions with enzyme inducers Other methods preferable	1 Beware of drug interactions with enzyme inducers see Box 16.2c and text)	2 Some concern about reduced efficacy; however, no data	1
Fibroids	1	1	1	1 Unless uterine cavity is distorted preventing correct fundal placement of the device	1 Unless uterine cavity is distorted preventing correct fundal placement of the device
Gallbladder disease					
Current	4	1	1	1	1
Medical treatment	4	1	1	1	1
Cholecystectomy	1	1	1	1	1
Gilbert's disease	1	1	1	1	1
Glandular fever	LFTs normal: I & C = 1 LFTs abnormal: I & C = 4	1 4	1 1	1 1	1 1
Glycogen storage disease	1	1	1	1	1
Hereditary lymphoedema	1	1	1	1	1
Hodgkin's disease	1	1	1	1	1
Hyperprolactinaemia	1/2 after assessment and initiation of treatment	1	1	1	1

[a]Risk of ectopic very low with T380 or LNG-IUS. Increasing with other types of copper IUDs due to the slightly lower effectiveness of these devices.
[b]Copper IUD use may worsen pain.

Table 16.1 *continued*

Medical disorder	COC	POP	DMPA	IUS	IUD
Hypertension					
≥160/95	I =4, C=4	I=1, C=1	1	1	1
≤160/95	I = 2/3, C=2/3 with regular monitoring.	I = 1, C=1	1	1	1
≤160/95 on antihypertensives	I & C = 2/3, if no other risk factors for CVD	I = 1, C=1	1	1	1
Inflammatory bowel disease					
Crohn's disease	I & C quiescent = 2/3 I & C during exacerbations = 4	1	1	1	1
Non-granulomatous Crohn's disease	I & C = 4	1	1	1	1
Ulcerative colitis	I & C quiescent = 2/3. I & C during exacerbations = 4	1	1	1	1
Lipid disorders					
Total cholesterol ≥ 7.5 mmol/l	4	1	3	2	1
Total cholesterol 6.0–7.5 mmol/l	2/3 (in absence of any other risk factor for arterial disease)	1	2	2	1
Hypertriglyceridaemia	4	1	2	2	1
Liver disease					
Acute	I & C = 4 until LFTs return to normal, then 2	I & C = 2/3 until LFTs return to normal, then 1	3	2/3	1
Chronic	I & C 3/4 depending on degree of liver function	I & C = 2/3 depending on degree of liver function	2	2	1
Cholestatic jaundice, either recurrent or In a previous pregnancy	4	I = 1/2 C = 4, if condition occurs when taking POP	2	1/2	1
Dubin–Johnson and Rotor syndromes	4	1	1	1	1
Porphyria	4	4	4	4	1
Liver Tumours					
Benign	4	4	4	3/4 Very low levels of hormone absorbed but data lacking	1
Malignant	4	4	4	3/4	1
Migraine					
With aura and with focal neurological signs preceding headache	4	1	1	1	1
Without aura but with a history of more than one additional risk factor for stroke	4	1			
Use of ergot derivatives	4	1			
Without aura but with a history of one additional risk factor for stroke	3	1			
Without aura and with no additional risk factors for stroke	2	1			
'Triptan' treatment (naratriptan, sumatriptan, zolmitriptan)	2	1			
Multiple sclerosis	1	1	1	1	1
Myaesthenia gravis	1	1	1	1	1

Table 16.1 *continued*

Medical disorder	COC	POP	DMPA	IUS	IUD
Otosclerosis	3/4	1	1	1	1
Ovarian cysts	1	3 Increased incidence of functional ovarian cysts	1	2 Functional ovarian cysts may occur and be a source of pelvic pain; usually disperse spontaneously	1
Pancreatitis	4 Unless due to gallbladder disease, now treated by cholecystectomy	1	1	1	1
Pelvic inflammatory disease					
Past	1	1	1	2	2/3
Current or within past 3 months	1	1	1	4	4
Postpartum					
non-lactating					
<21 days	3/4	1 (although unnecessary)			
>21 days	1	1			
<6 weeks			2 Possibility of heavier and prolonged bleeding	2/3 Increased risk of uterine perforation	2/3 Increased risk uterine of perforation
> 6 weeks			1	1	1
Post-abortion (1st or 2nd trimester)	1	1	1	1	1
Pre-eclampsia in previous pregnancy	1	1	1	1	1
Pregnancy	4 No known deterimental outcome to mother or fetus if taken accidentally in early pregnancy	4 No known detrimental outcome to mother or fetus if taken accidentally in early pregnancy	4	4	4
Pulmonary hypertension	4	2	2	2	1
Raynaud's disease	1	1	1	1	1
Renal dialysis (without lipid abnormalities or hypertension)	2	1	2	1	1
Retinitis pigmentosa	1	1	1	1	1
Rheumatoid arthritis	1	1	1	1	1
Sarcoidosis	1	1	1	1	1
Sickle Cell					
Trait	1	1	1	1	1
Disease	2–3	1	1	1	1
Spherocytosis	1	1	1	1	1
After splenectomy	I & C platelet count $< 500 \times 10^7/l = 1$ I & C platelet count $< 500 \times 10^9/l = 4$				
Structural heart disease (including those abnormalities predisposing to atrial fibrillation)	4	1	1	2 Antibiotic prophylaxis at insertion to prevent bacterial endocarditis (see text)	2 Antibiotic prophylaxis at insertion to prevent bacterial endocarditis (see text)
Mild asymptomatic valvular abnormalities	I = 2 C = subject to regular review	1 1	1	1 (as above)	1 (as above)

Table 16.1 *continued*

Medical disorder	COC	POP	DMPA	IUS	IUD
Systemic lupus erythematosus (SLE)					
With antiphospholipid syndrome	4	2	1	1	1
Mild SLE	2/3	1	1	1	1
Thalassaemia major	1	1	1	1	1
Thrombocytopenic purpura	See spherocytosis	See spherocytosis	1	1	1
Thyroid disease	1	1	1	1	1
Tuberculosis	1 Beware drug interaction with enzyme inducers	1 Beware drug interaction with enzyme inducers	1	1	1
Venous thromboembolic disease (VTE)	4	1	1	1	1
Past history VTE	4	1	1	1	1
Thrombophilia	I & C = 2/3 if only one factor present	1	1	1	1
Risk factors for VTE (see Box 16.2b)	I & C = 4 if more than one VTE risk factor or in presence of any other risk factor	1	1	1	1
Wolff–Parkinson–White syndrome	1	1	1	1	1
Warfarin use	3 Possible justification to control heavy bleeding Other methods preferred	2	2 Possible haematoma formation at injection site	2	2 Possibility of longer, heavier menstruation and inter-menstrual bleeding

COC = combined oral contraceptive; POP = progestogen-only pill; DMPA = depot medroxypregesterone acetate;
IUS = intrauterine system; IUD = intrauterine device; CVD = cardiovascular disease;
MI = myocardial infarction; CVA = cerebrovascular accident; STDs = sexually transmitted diseases; PID = pelvic inf lammatory disease; LFTs = liver function tests.
1 = a condition for which there is no restriction for the use of the contraceptive method.
2 = a condition where the advantages of using the method generally outweigh the theoretical or proven risks.
3 = a condition which represents an unacceptable health risk if the contraceptive method is used.
4 = a condition which represents an unacceptable health risk if the contraceptive method is used.
I = initiation of the contraceptive method in the circumstances.
C = continuation of the method should the condition develop or progress.

Table 16.1 *continued*

to detect the presence of any recognized absolute and/or relative contraindications to the available contraceptive methods. An assessment of the disorder itself should be made to decide whether or not it could lead to contraindications over time, exacerbate any existing contraindications or require treatment which would affect or be affected by a contraceptive method in some way. For example, before prescribing the COC, consideration of the following questions will indicate the potential for summation of the effects of the medical disorder with the known adverse effects of the COC:

- Does this medical disorder increase the risk of venous thromboembolism?

- Does this medical disorder increase the risk of arterial wall damage?

- Has the woman already got one or more risk factors for cardiovascular disease independent of the medical disorder?

- Does this medical disorder interfere with hepatic function?

- Does this medical disorder display hormone dependency which could be exacerbated by the use of the COC?

- Is medication being used which may interfere with or be interfered by the COC?

- AIDS
- Alopecia
- Asthma
- Gilbert's disease
- Glandular fever provided LFTs are normal
- Glycogen storage diseases
- Hereditary lymphoedema
- Multiple sclerosis
- Myaesthenia gravis
- Non-hormone-dependent cancers under treatment, provided no
  increased risk of thrombosis
- Otosclerosis
- Raynaud's disease
- Renal dialysis (beware of hypertension and/or lipid abnormalities)
- Retinitis pigmentosa
- Rheumatoid arthritis
- Sarcoidosis
- Spherocytosis ⎫ unless splenectomy with platelet
- Thrombocytogenic purpura ⎭ count > 500 ×10⁹/l
- Thalassaemia major
- Thyrotoxicosis
- Treated Hodgkin's disease
- Wolff–Parkinson–White syndrome

Certain conditions that are not known to be adversely affected by the use of steroid hormones are listed in Box 16.3.

Epilepsy

Women with epilepsy need effective contraception. They have an increased risk of complications in pregnancy, such as stillbirth, and some anticonvulsants are teratogenic. No method of contraception is contraindicated.

Seizures are usually less frequent among COC users, although rarely they may increase. Seizures may rarely be provoked at IUD insertion also; suitable resuscitation measures must be available at all IUD and IUS insertions. DMPA may decrease the frequency of seizures.

Common anticonvulsant drugs are hepatic microsomal enzyme-inducers (Box 16.2c) and can lower the efficacy of hormonal methods.

Management of common drug interactions

Enzyme-inducers (Box 16.2c)

COCs

These should be given as a 50 µg EE-containing preparation to compensate for this this and the pill-free interval (PFI) reduced from 7 to 4 days. The EE content of the COC can be raised further if breakthrough bleeding occurs, titrating the dose of the pill to ensure good cycle control.

The so-called tricycle regimen, where three packets of pills are taken consecutively without a break followed by a 4-day PFI, may be particularly useful in epilepsy if seizures tend to occur around the PFI, a time of hormonal fluctuations. For the same reasons, a monophasic pill should be used in preference to a phasic preparation.

POP

Although the dose can be raised empirically to two tablets daily there are insufficient data to confirm the efficacy of this regimen. An alternative contraceptive method is recommended.

Norplant

Norplant may have a lowered efficacy; this would be a consideration rather than a contraindication. Additional contraceptive precautions should be used.

LNG IUS

There are no data to suggest a lowered efficacy as the contraceptive effect is mainly at a local level on the endometrium. The manufacturers mention enzyme-inducing drugs as a precaution. Most experts allow its use having informed the user of the lack of data.

DMPA

This is usually given at 10-weekly intervals to compensate for any drug effect, although there is no good evidence that efficacy is lowered if given at the usual 12-week interval.

Enzyme-inducing effects cease between 4 and 8 weeks after stopping the drug; contraceptive precautions/protocols should be continued for 4 weeks after discontinuation of the interacting drug.

Enzyme-inducing antibiotics Rifampicin

This is an antibiotic that is used as a long-term treatment for tuberculosis and as a short course for the protection of those exposed to meningococcal meningitis. As it is a powerful enzyme-inducing drug, neither the COC nor the POP are recommended for use concurrently and for 4 weeks after the end of treatment. If the COC is to be used, then it should contain 50 µg of EE; pills containing Mestranol (a prodrug for EE) should not be used.

Griseofulvin

This is an antifungal drug which induces aneuploidy and is a potential teratogen. Men should avoid fathering children whilst using this drug and for 6 months after cessation of treatment. Women should avoid pregnancy during treatment and for 1 month afterwards. Owing to the enzyme-inducing nature of this drug, the advice concerning contraception is the same as that given in the section on epilepsy.

Broad-spectrum antibiotics (other than enzyme-inducers) COCs

These may show reduced efficacy in a small but as yet unidentifiable group of users who rely on the EE reabsorbed from the enterohepatic circulation. Short-term users of such antibiotics should be advised to use extra contraceptive precautions for the duration of the course of treatment and for 7 days afterwards. Long-term users should take extra contraceptive precautions for the first 2 weeks of the antibiotic, after which time antibiotic resistance should have developed.

Progestogen-only methods

No effect has been shown on POP, LNG IUS, Norplant or injectable progestogens.

Inflammatory bowel disease

Both ulcerative colitis and Crohn's disease are associated with hypercoagulability during exacerbations, leading to an increased risk of thrombotic episodes.

COCs

COC use is advisable only in mild forms of these conditions and not at all during exacerbations. Colonic non-granulomatous Crohn's disease appears to be more common amongst COC users and improvement has been reported when the COC is discontinued.

Progestogen-only methods and IUDs

There are no known contraindications to their use. Acute abdominal pain may present a clinical dilemma in an IUD user; both the patient and her physician should be aware of this potential confounding factor.

Injectable progestogens

These are ideal in bowel disease where severe diarrhoea is a feature.

Other bowel disorders

Ileostomy, colostomy COCs

There have been reports of successful use of COC among women with both these conditions. The rapid absorption of the contraceptive steroids from the more proximal small bowel would appear to provide satisfactory plasma levels.

Progestogen-only methods and IUDs

There are no known contraindications to their use.

Coeliac disease COCs

Absorption does not seem to be impaired. There are no known contraindications to their use.

Progestogen-only methods and IUDs

There are no known contraindications to their use.

Liver disease

Both oestrogens and progestogens affect hepatic function, but progestogens to a much lesser extent except in porphyria.

COCs

They should not be used in acute or severe chronic liver disorders; a history of cholestasis of pregnancy or cholestasis with previous COC use would be an absolute contraindication. Following an episode of acute liver disease, COCs may be used after liver function tests (LFTs) return to normal.

Progestogen-only methods

Little or no effect has been found on hepatic function with the use of the progestogen-only methods. Neither the POP nor DMPA should be used by women with a history of COC-related cholestatic jaundice as it is uncertain which of the two hormones is implicated.

LNG IUS

There is concern about an increased load on the liver, although the amount of LNG involved is very small and would have to be seen in the context of prognosis of disease and the suitability of alternative contraceptive methods.

Copper-containing IUDs

These are preferable to a LNG IUS.

All hormonal methods should be avoided in acute liver disease until LFTs return to normal; steroid hormones may be imperfectly metabolized if liver function is compromised.

Chronic liver disease, if mild or compensated, would be compatible with a progestogen-only method but, if the disease is severe or decompensated, hormones should be avoided as they represent an extra load on the damaged liver.

Hepatic tumours

There is an increased incidence of both benign and malignant liver tumours among COC users. No association has been shown between any of the progestogen-only methods and the incidence of hepatocellular tumours.

COCs

These are contraindicated in the presence of hepatic tumours.

POP, Norplant and DMPA

These are also contraindicated.

Gallbladder disease

There is no evidence to suggest an increase in the incidence of gallbladder disease among COC users but COCs may accelerate its presentation in those who are predisposed, probably owing to altered bile composition.

COCs

Their use should be avoided in those with known gallbladder disease. They can be used after cholecystectomy but not after medical treatment for gallstones.

Progestogen-only hormonal contraceptives

There is no known effect and they may be used.

Lipid disorders

COCs

Hypercholesterolaemia is a risk factor for atherosclerosis. Levels of total cholesterol above 7.5 mmol/l are a contraindication. Lower levels may allow the use of COCs in the absence of any other risk factor for arterial disease.

COCs can cause adverse changes in lipids which vary according to the formulation used; some more modern COCs have a negligible effect on lipid profile and are to be preferred (desogestrel, norgestimate or gestodene) where lipid abnormality exists. Hypertriglyceridaemia precludes COC use because of the increased risk of pancreatitis.

POPs and Norplant

These do not cause significant change in lipid metabolism; however, in the presence of severe arterial disease, another contraceptive would be preferred.

DMPA

Changes in HDL cholesterol have been reported in some studies. Another method is recommended in the presence of severe arterial disease or in women with several predisposing factors for arterial disease.

Connective tissue disorders

Systemic lupus erythematosus (SLE)

This may deteriorate or be precipitated by oestrogens. The presence of lupus anticoagulant or antiphospholipid antibody increases the risk of thrombosis.

COCs

These are only acceptable in very mild cases; the antiphospholipid syndrome (Hughes syndrome) is an absolute contraindication to COCs.

Progestogen-only methods

These have not been shown to affect SLE adversely and are to be preferred to COCs.

Rheumatoid arthritis

Any method of contraception may be used. Female barriers may be difficult to insert and remove if there is severe arthritis of the fingers.

Immune system disorders

COCs

These are contraindicated in Behçet's syndrome and erythema nodosum.

Drug interactions

Oestrogens and progestogens are mild enzyme inhibitors: the activity of certain other drugs may be enhanced in oral contraceptive users.

Corticosteroids

No clinically significant effects have been shown.

Warfarin

Concurrent COC use is unlikely in the presence of increased thrombogenicity, although its use to control menorrhagia may be justified. If the combination occurs, coagulation screening and warfarin dosage would need to be monitored closely.

Cyclosporin

Cyclosporin levels may be raised with the risk of hepatotoxicity.

Mucolytics

These are used in cystic fibrosis and do not adversely affect the POP's effect on cervical mucus.

Venous thromboembolic disease (VTE)

For women who have a past history of VTE or who have a known thrombophilia.

COCs

These are absolutely contraindicated (see Boxes 16.1a and 16.2b).

Progestogen-only methods

They are all suitable.

Cardiovascular disease

Cardiovascular disease encompasses a wide variety of conditions each having a spectrum of severity.

Arterial disease

Whether or not this is associated with an underlying disease process, the use of synthetic oestrogens is contraindicated because of the increased risk of thrombosis, cerebrovascular accident (CVA) and myocardial infarction (MI) (Boxes 16.1a, 16.2a and 16.3).

Progestogens may adversely affect lipid metabolism and there is a theoretical possibility of exacerbating severe arterial disease; however, there is no direct evidence for this and a pregnancy may be a far greater health threat.

Structural heart disorders
COCs

Marked structural abnormalities carry an increased risk of thromboembolic phenomena, thus precluding the use of COCs. Associated arterial problems such as pulmonary hypertension also contraindicate COCs, as does atrial fibrillation with its thromboembolic risk.

Women with mild, asymptomatic, valvular abnormalities without history of thromboembolism or other risk factors for arterial disease may use COCs with supervision.

Progestogen-only pills and injectables

These may be used.

IUDs and LNG IUS

These may be used but may require antibiotic cover at insertion.

Diabetes mellitus (DM)
Pregnancy

The pregnancy outcome is related to diabetic control; there is an increased risk of fetal loss (of up to 44% with poor control), congenital abnormality, prematurity, stillbirth and neonatal morbibity.

Maternal diabetic complications may be exacerbated and maternal mortality is 50 times higher. Pregnancy should be planned and unwanted pregnancy avoided.

COCs

Low-dose COCs have been shown to have only very minor effects on carbohydrate metabolism; there is a small increase in insulin secretion, and an insignificant or no change in glucose tolerance or glycosylated haemoglobin levels.

DM carries an increased risk of arterial disease, so COCs should be used only by fit young diabetics who have no signs of any diabetic complications and who are without any other, non-DM-related risk factors for arterial disease.

Progestogen-only methods

These have not been shown to affect DM adversely. However, there is concern that the small adverse changes in HDL cholesterol seen in DMPA users may worsen diabetic arteriopathy and it should be used with caution.

POPs

These are seen as highly appropriate for women with DM.

IUDs

These are a good option; there is no reduction in efficacy.

Barrier methods

These should be encouraged to reduce the risk of pelvic inflammatory disease.

Sterilization

This is a good option once the family is considered complete.

Haemoglobinopathies

Sickle cell trait

Carriers may use any method.

Sickle cell disease

Those with either SS or SC types may be at increased risk of thrombosis.

COC

Pregnancy is known to precipitate crises, although studies have not shown COCs to do so; another method would be preferable.

Progestogen-only methods

These avoid the theoretical concerns about thrombotic risk.

Injectable progestogens

These reduce the incidence of sickling crises and improve the haematocrit. Progestogens stablize the red cell membrane.

Thalassaemia

This is not a contraindication to COC use.

Migraine

Cerebral thrombosis is rarely associated with migraine (Table 16.2).

COCs

Women who have a history of migraine without aura (previously known as 'simple' or 'common' migraine) may use the COC provided they have none of the other risk factors for stroke (see Box 16.2a). They should be monitored regularly for the development of new risk factors and advised to report changes in either the frequency or symptoms of their migraine without delay.

In the presence of one risk factor for arterial disease, COCs should be used with great caution. COCs should be stopped immediately with any adverse change in either the migraine or the risk factor. Another method of contraception should be encouraged.

The following symptoms, which suggest transient ischaemia in a migraine attack, should preclude the use of the COC:

- loss of a part of the visual field;

- unilateral fortification spectra;

- any unilateral neurological symptoms such as weakness or paraesthesiae;

- disturbance of speech;

- first-ever migraine attack after starting the COC;

- severe migraine, 'status migrainosus' (formerly known as crescendo migraine: a migraine lasting for 3 or more days and worsening over that time, with or without focal symptoms and whether or not treatment has been used).

Blurred vision, photophobia, phonophobia and flashing lights affecting the whole visual field are not focal in nature and are included in the category of migraine without aura.

The COC should not be prescribed together with ergotamine because of its vasoconstricting properties; sumatriptan may be used with caution [8].

Progestogen-only methods

These are all acceptable.

Endocrine disorders

Thyroid

Pregnancy

Both hyperthyroidism and hypothyroidism can increase obstetric morbidity; antithyroid drugs can cross the placenta.

Contraception

Any method of contraception may be used.

Hyperprolactinaemia

Pituitary microadenomas and macroadenomas causing hyperprolactinaemia are frequently associated with amenorrhoea and hypo-oestrogenism. After treatment is begun with bromocriptine or equivalent, COCs may be used; this is a way of providing both contraception and oestrogen replacement to help prevent bone loss.

Once thought to be the cause of hyperprolactinaemia, COCs may in fact have been therapeutic but masked the underlying menstrual irregularities or amenorrhoea. Studies have now shown no difference in the rate of growth of pituitary adenomas between COC users and non-users.

Polycystic ovarian syndrome (PCOS)

PCOS is associated with a wide spectrum of symptoms of different degrees of severity.

Hyperandrogenism with acne and hirsutism can be treated with an appropriately antiandrogenic COC as can any irregular menstrual patterns ranging from amenorrhoea to irregular bleeding.

Hypo-oestrogenism and hyperoestrogenism with an

Table 16.2 Association of COC and migraine with thrombotic risk of cerebral thrombosis stroke

		At age 20 per 100 000 women	At age 40 per 100 000 women
No migraine or COC	Background risk	2	20
Migraine only	Absolute risk	5.6	56
COC only	Absolute risk	3.6	36
Migraine and COC	Absolute risk	10	100

COC = combined oral contraceptive.

increased risk of endometrial carcinoma can be features of PCOS. Again the COC is the treatment of choice.

Psychiatric disorders

Pregnancy

Certain psychiatric disorders are exacerbated by pregnancy. Issues to consider include compliance with antenatal care, the future welfare of the child and an increased need for support services.

Depression

There is no good evidence that any of the hormonal contraceptives precipitate or exacerbate depression, although manufacturers' information leaflets frequently mention it to be a consideration before prescribing. This is also mentioned in some patient information leaflets and deters

women from trying these methods. However, an unwanted pregnancy or the trauma of termination arguably has a much more profound influence on mood.

In severe depression, long-acting hormonal methods may be inadvisable because of their lack of immediate reversibility but they should not be denied if requested.

Psychoses

Compliance with contraception is most important and is usually optimal when the method has been chosen by the user herself.

Long-acting methods have advantages in poor compliers; however, obtaining informed consent from some women might pose a problem. Liaison with the psychiatrist might help.

Intrauterine contraception, although highly effective, does not protect against sexually

transmitted infections and sexual behaviour/lifestyle should be taken into consideration.

Drug interactions

Antidepressants

No clinically significant interactions have been reported between antidepressants and hormonal contraceptives.

Phenothiazines and tricyclic antidepressants

These may depress gonadotrophin levels with resultant amenorrhoea and lowered oestrogen levels; this does not reliably indicate infertility and contraception should be used. Any acceptable method is appropriate.

Galactorrhoea is a well-documented side effect of these psychotropic drugs. It need not affect the choice of contraceptive method.

References

1. Sapire KE. Contraception and sexuality in health and disease. London: McGraw-Hill, 1986:3.
2. World Health Organisation (WHO). Improving access to quality care in family planning. Geneva: WHO, 1996.
3. Gillmer MDG. Metabolic effects of combined oral contraceptives. In: Filshie M, Guillebaud J (eds) Contraception, science and practice. London: Butterworths, 1989:16–17.
4. Gillmer MDG. Metabolic effects of combined oral contraceptives. In: Filshie M, Guillebaud J (eds)
5. Contraception, science and practice. London: Butterworths, 1989:31.
6. Guillebaud J. Contraception, your questions answered. Edinburgh: Churchill Livingstone 1993.
7. Vessey MP, Villard-Mackintosh L, Yeates D. Effectiveness of progestogen-only oral contraceptives (letter). *Br J Fam Plann* 1990;16:79.
8. McCann MF, Potter LS. Progestin-only oral contraception. *Contraception* 1994;50: (Suppl 1).
9. MacGregor EA, Guillebaud J. Recommendations for clinical practice-oral contraceptives,

migraine and ischaemic stroke. *Br J Fam Plann* 1998;24:53–60.

Further reading

- Filshie M, Guillebaud J (eds) Contraception, science and practice. London: Butterworths, 1989.
- Sapire KE. Contraception and sexuality in health and disease. London: McGraw-Hill, 1986.
- WHO. Improving access to quality care in family planning. Geneva: WHO, 1996.

Section 4:
Sexual health

Lower genital tract infection

Sebastian Faro MD PhD
Christopher Wilkinson MFFP

Introduction

Lower genital tract infections encompass a variety of diseases caused by bacteria, fungi, viruses and protozoa. These diseases include both sexually and non-sexually transmitted infections. The differentiation can be difficult but is important because infection caused by sexually transmitted organisms have major implications for both the public health and the health of the individual. For example, chlamydial infection, which is both common and readily transmitted through sexual intercourse, may result in damage to the fallopian tubes which could cause ectopic pregnancy or infertility. Both sexually and non-sexually transmitted infections may develop into systemic disease, resulting in significant morbidity.

Bacterial skin infections

There are a variety of bacterial infections that affect the vulvar skin: folliculitis, furuncles and carbuncles are common, whereas pyoderma, erysipelas, impetigo and hidradenitis are less so. Whilst these infections may be caused by exogenous organisms, they are more commonly due to bacteria which are part of the normal skin flora. Infection is usually preceded by trauma such as a scratch. The patient often notes localized pruritus and a small erythematous raised lesion followed by local spread to adjacent tissues and local lymphadenopathy.

Folliculitis

Folliculitis begins when bacteria gain access into the base of the hair follicle causing a localized inflammatory reaction. The tendency to scratch or squeeze the lesion can introduce *Staphylococcus aureus* and an abscess may develop [1,2].

Furuncles and carbuncles

Furuncles are abscesses that occur following folliculitis and are usually due to *Staphylococcus aureus* [3]. If a fistula develops between adjacent furuncles, a carbuncle forms. The infected area becomes erythematous, swollen and painful due to the increasing pressure within the follicle, which eventually results in pointing on the surface of the skin. The area may develop a core, a solid accumulation of purulent material, which is removed surgically if the lesion does not drain spontaneously.

Treatment of folliculitis, furuncles and carbuncles

Bacterial skin infections are commonly caused by Gram-positive bacteria, especially *Staphylococcus aureus*, which, being community acquired, is usually sensitive to first-generation cephalosporins. Cephalexin 250–500 mg orally, four times a day for 7–10 days is recommended. Patients allergic to penicillin and cephalosporins can be treated with a quinolone, such as ciprofloxacin or ofloxacin. Warm compresses should be used to assist drainage. If the lesion drains spontaneously, the area should be cleansed with warm water.

Genital ulcers

Genital ulcers are common. It is important to differentiate between those that are due to trauma, infection or to cancer (Box 17.1) as specific management is required. Traumatic ulcers are usually due to chronic rubbing or localized scratching. Whilst ulcers associated with infectious diseases may appear similar to malignant ulcers (Box 17.2), they usually heal without treatment whereas the latter should be suspected by their failure to heal.

Syphilis

Syphilis is an infection due to *Treponema pallidum*, a spirochete. Transmission is either vertically or by close, predominantly sexual contact. Transmission usually occurs when a lesion comes into contact with a mucosal surface. Syphilis is referred to as being acquired or congenital. It is useful to consider acquired syphilis as being early (which includes primary, secondary and early latent syphilis). If untreated 25–30% of patients develop late syphilis which includes late latent and tertiary syphilis (Table 17.1).

The incidence in the USA is 15 per 100 000. Fifty per cent of congenital syphilis occurs in women receiving no antenatal care.

Primary syphilis

Primary syphilis is characterized by the presence of an ulcer, known as a chancre, that is typically painless and usually solitary. The margins are raised, well defined, the base is usually indurated, erythematous and clean. If the ulcer becomes secondarily infected, its base becomes grey or yellow. A chancre can occur at any site where infection was transmitted, but is most commonly found on the vulva, labia, vaginal walls and cervix. A chancre can easily be missed on clinical examination, especially if it occurs on the cervix, in the oropharynx or anal canal. In association with the ulcer, the patient typically develops bilateral painless rubbery inguinal lymphadenopathy [4].

Secondary syphilis

The initial presentation of secondary syphilis can resemble a flu-like syndrome: malaise, myalgia, headache and sore throat. Characteristic features are a generalized maculo-papular rash which may affect the palms of the hands and the soles of the feet, generalized lymphadenopathy, condylomata lata, hepato-splenomegaly, snail track lesions on mucous membranes and (rarely) patchy alopecia. Condylomata lata are waxy flat lesions involving the vulva and perianal areas. A coexistent persisting chancre may occur.

Tertiary syphilis

Tertiary syphilis includes benign tertiary syphilis, and syphilis with involvement of the cardiovascular and central nervous systems. Although usually only clinically relevant in tertiary syphilis involvement of the central nervous system may occur at any stage of infection.

Syphilis in pregnancy

Syphilis in pregnancy is often diagnosed by routine screening of the asymptomatic woman. Untreated syphilis is associated with a 75–95% risk of vertical transmission and a 40% risk of perinatal death. Vertical transmission of syphilis can occur at any time in pregnancy and has been recorded as early as 9 weeks' gestation. Transplacental transmission is commonest in secondary syphilis and declines during late latent infection [4]. A pregnant woman with syphilis should be treated to reduce the risk of vertical transmission which can lead to intrauterine death, preterm labor and 'congenital' syphilis. All babies born to women with positive syphilis serology will themselves have maternal immunoglobulin

Box 17.2   Characteristics of genital ulcers associated with infection

Syphilis:	base is clean, erythematous, margins raised, painless
Chancroid:	base clean and covered with a grey, necrotic exudate; margins are narrow and ragged; painful
Lymphogranuloma venereum:	base clean, erythematous; painful
Granuloma inguinale:	base appears beefy red; margins are well defined; painless
Herpes simplex:	painful, multiple small erythematous lesions but can coalesce to form large ulceration

Table 17.1 Working classification of acquired syphilis

	Early acquired syphilis			Late acquired syphilis	
	Primary	Secondary	Early latent	Late latent	Tertiary
Time from infection to onset	9–90 days	6 weeks–6 months	<2 years	>2 years	Years
Duration	Weeks	Weeks	<2 years	>2 years	Variable
Clinical features present	Yes	Yes	No	No	Yes
Infectious					
Vertically	Yes	Yes	Yes	Low/nil	Nil

G (IgG) and should be tested for IgM antibodies. Congenital syphilis is a progressive condition that requires treatment.

Diagnosis

The diagnosis of syphilis is aided by clinical suspicion. Specific diagnostic tools available are: microscopy (darkfield and the direct fluorescent antibody test); non-specific serologic tests; and specific serologic tests. Darkfield microscopy is of value in primary and secondary disease and requires that a lesion be present and that the patient is referred to a facility that has the appropriate equipment and expertise. For oral lesions where commensal treponemes are likely, the direct fluorescent antibody test is preferred to darkfield microscopy.

The serologic tests available may vary from one laboratory service to another. The initial tests include non-specific tests such as the *rapid plasma reagin* (RPR), or the *Venereal Disease Research Laboratory* (VDRL) test and the specific *total treponemal antibody* (TTA) test. If positive, then confirmatory specific treponemal tests are usually automatically performed by the laboratory. These include the *fluorescent treponemal antibody absorbed test* (FTA-ABS) or the *microhemagglutination assay* for antibodies to *Treponema pallidum* (MHA-TP or TPHA) [5]. These

tests tend to remain positive for life, and are highly specific for treponemal infection but do not differentiate syphilis from other non-sexually transmitted treponemal infections, such as yaws, pinta or bejel. They are therefore of value in excluding those individuals who have not had syphilis. False-positive serology reactions occur more with non-specific tests (2%) than with specific tests (1%); for this reason, several tests are used to screen for, diagnose and monitor the disease. The titers of non-specific tests in individuals with biological false-positive results are often low (1:2) and the specific test negative (Box 17.3).

The serologic tests become positive at different times after the initial infection; for example, the FTA IgM test becomes positive at about 2 weeks, whereas the VDRL and the TPHA do so at 4 and 6 weeks, respectively. In early primary syphilis, as many as 30% of infected individuals will therefore have a negative non-

specific test at presentation. Repeat tests should then be carried out at 1 week, 1 month and 3 months. Individuals with a negative test at 3 months can be considered non-infected. Individuals with secondary syphilis usually have a titer greater than 1:16. In the absence of clinical features, patients with positive test results who are known to have had a negative test in the previous year should at least be considered to have early latent syphilis. If the results of previous tests are not known, then the patient should be categorized as having late latent syphilis, and be evaluated for involvement of the cardiovascular and central nervous systems. Non-specific tests tend to become negative with time and approximately 20% of patients with latent syphilis will have negative serology when such a test is performed in isolation. If a patient is considered to have late latent syphilis, a spinal tap (lumbar puncture) should be considered,

Box 17.3   Causes of biological false positive non-specific tests

1. Pregnancy
2. Recent infection
   - Bacterial
   - Viral, including early human immunodeficiency virus (HIV) infection
3. Autoimmune disorders
4. Other
   - Recent immunization
   - Narcotic use

especially if there are clinical signs of neurological disease.

Follow-up

The non-specific screening tests are also used to follow the efficacy of treatment. In early syphilis it is suggested that repeat serology (VDRL or RPR) be performed at the end of treatment, monthly for 3 months, at 6 months and 1 year. Patients who are HIV-positive or with late active syphilis (e.g. neurosyphilis) should be reviewed yearly for life.

After treatment for early disease, there should be a decrease in the titers of non-specific tests, which may take 6–12 months. By 3 months there usually is a fourfold decline in titer and an eightfold decline by 10 months. Individuals treated appropriately for primary syphilis will have a negative VDRL or RPR after 1 year. After successful treatment of latent syphilis, there may be no decline in titers, but about 50% will have a lower titer after 2 years. As specific tests remain positive for life, a 2–4-fold rise in titer indicates failed therapy or reinfection.

Treatment

The treatment regimens for early- and late-acquired syphilis are detailed in Table 17.2.

Jarisch–Herxheimer reaction

The Jarisch–Herxheimer reaction is a transient, flu-like reaction consisting of fever, headache and myalgia which may start within 24 h of initiating treatment for syphilis. It occurs in 50% of cases of primary and 70% of secondary syphilis. The exact mechanism is not known. Patients should be warned that it may occur and advised to take paracetamol or

Table 17.2 Treatment of syphilis

	MMWR [6]	UK [7]
Early acquired syphilis		
Not allergic to penicillin	Benzathine penicillin G 2.4 million units intramuscularly in a single dose	Bicillin[a] 3 ml intramuscularly daily for 10–14 days
Allergic to penicillin and not pregnant	Doxycycline 100 mg orally twice daily for 14 days or Tetracycline 500 mg orally four times a day for 14 days	Doxycycline 300 mg as a single dose (or 100 mg three times a day) orally for 21 days
Pregnant and allergic to penicillin	Admit to hospital for penicillin desensitization	Oral erythromycin 500 mg four times a day for 21 days followed by oral doxycycline 300 mg daily after delivery 21 days[b]
Late acquired syphilis (not including cardiovascular or neurosyphilis)		
Not allergic to penicillin	Benzathine penicillin G, 7.2 million units total, as three doses of 2.4 million units intramuscularly each, weekly for 3 weeks	Bicillin 3 ml intramuscularly daily for 21 days
Allergic to penicillin and not pregnant	Doxycycline 100 mg orally twice daily for 28 days or Tetracycline 500 mg orally four times a day for 28 days	Doxycycline 100 mg orally three times a day for 28 days
Pregnant and allergic to penicillin	Admit to hospital for penicillin desensitization	Oral erythromycin 500 mg four times a day for 21 days followed by oral doxycycline 300 mg daily after delivery 21 days[b]

[a]Bicillin (Yamanouchi Pharm) contains 300 mg (300 000 units) procaine penicillin and 60 mg (100 000 units) benzylpenicillin equivalent to total penicillin dose of 0.4 mU/ml.
[b]Retreatment of mother and baby after delivery recommended due to risk of treatment failure.

aspirin if required. Pregnant patients treated for syphilis may need to be observed as premature labour and intrauterine death have rarely been reported following treatment for syphilis and the Jarisch–Herxheimer reaction [8,9].

Treatment of sexual contacts

Sexual partners of patients with primary or secondary syphilis should be screened for syphilis and offered epidemiological treatment or seen at fortnightly intervals for examination and repeat serologic tests at each visit. It may take 90 days for tests to become positive. Contacts of latent or late syphilis should have serologic tests monthly for 3 months. Treatment is not required if tests are negative 3 months after exposure.

Chancroid

Chancroid is caused by the Gram-negative bacillus *Haemophilus ducreyi*. It is usually sexually transmitted by mucosal contact with an ulcerated lesion. Chancroid is probably the most common cause of genital ulcer disease in tropical countries.

Although it is not commonly seen in Europe or the USA, two endemic outbreaks occurred in New Orleans and Dallas in the late 1980s.

Following contact with an infected lesion, there is an incubation period of 7 days or longer. Initially, a papule forms at the point of inoculation and rapidly develops into a pustule. The center of the pustule undergoes spontaneous necrosis and an ulcer forms with undermined and irregular edges. The ulcer can be up to 2 cm in size with an indurated base surrounded by an erythematous halo. In men, the lesion tends to be painful; however, in women, the ulcer may be asymptomatic and therefore easily mistaken for a syphilitic chancre. The patient may develop painful unilateral lymphadenopathy known as a buboe. After 1–2 weeks, the skin overlying the lymph node becomes erythematous, the center undergoes necrosis and the node becomes ulcerated. [10]

Diagnosis

The diagnosis is established by culturing the lesion and isolating the organism. The laboratory should be notified prior to obtaining the specimen in order to prepare to receive and process it properly. A specimen should be obtained from the ulcer for Gram staining. A tentative diagnosis can be made on microscopy because *Haemophilus ducreyi* stains Gram negative and appears in typical (shoal of fish) chains [11]. The diagnosis is confirmed by culture. Other causes of genital ulcer disease, especially syphilis, should be excluded.

Treatment

Antibiotic resistance has been described, but is unusual in developed countries. Recurrences are usually successfully treated with an alternative regimen. Single-dose treatments are not recommended for HIV-positive patients in whom higher failure rates have been observed. The following treatments are recommended:

- azithromycin 1 g orally in a single dose; or

- erythromycin base 500 mg orally four times a day for 7 days; or

- ciprofloxacin 500 mg orally twice a day for 3 days;

- ceftriaxone 250 mg intramuscularly as a single dose.

An alternative therapy is sulfamethoxazole/trimethroprim 800 mg/160 mg orally twice a day for 10 days or ciprofloxacin 1 g orally as a single dose, or spectinomycin 2 g intramuscularly as a single dose.

Treatment of sexual contacts

All sexual contacts in the 2 weeks prior to the onset of the ulcer are likely to have been exposed to infection and should be examined and have appropriate tests. In the absence of clinical disease, epidemiological treatment according to the above regimens should be advised.

Granuloma inguinale

Granuloma inguinale or Donovanosis is caused by the Gram-negative bacterium *Calymmatobacterium granulomatis* [12]. It is thought to be sexually acquired but of low infectivity. The bacterium is endemic to India, Western Australia, tropical regions in Africa, Vietnam, Indonesia, Papua New Guinea and the West Indies. It has also been reported in the southern part of the USA, although it remains rare.

Clinically, multiple ulcerative lesions appear on the external genitalia. The lesions rupture spontaneously and form round, elevated, velvety, granulomatous ulcers. These lesions bleed easily and are infectious. As subsequent lesions develop secondary to autoinoculation, involvement of regional lymph nodes occurs. Indolent masses (pseudobuboe) may develop in the inguinal area, forming granulomatous lesions in the subcutaneous tissue. Subsequent scarring causes lymphatic obstruction resulting in pseudoelephantiasis [13]. Donovanosis has frequently been misdiagnosed as carcinoma or as condylomata acuminata, especially when perianal.

Diagnosis

Donovan bodies can be identified on microscopy using Wright's or Giemsa stains on specimens obtained from an ulcer. An immunofluorescent antibody test using Donovan bodies as the antigen is available.

Treatment

Suitable treatment regimens include:

- trimethoprim–sulfamethoxazole as one double-strength tablet orally twice a day for 3 weeks minimum; or

- doxycycline 100 mg orally twice a day for 3 weeks; or

- ciprofloxacin 750 mg orally twice a day for 3 weeks minimum; or

- erythromycin 500 mg four times a day for a minimum of 3 weeks.

Treatment should be continued until complete resolution of the lesions.

Treatment of sexual contacts

All recent sexual contacts likely to have been exposed to infection should be examined and have appropriate tests. In the absence of clinical disease, epidemiological treatment according to the above regimens should be advised.

Genital herpes simplex

Genital herpes simplex is a common sexually transmitted infection that affects approximately 55 million people in the USA. Genital herpes is caused most commonly herpes simplex type 2 (HSV-2) and to a lesser extent by herpes simplex type 1 (HSV-1). The converse is true of oral (cold sores) and ocular herpetic disease. It is now accepted that that unrecognized, subclinical initial infection is not uncommon. There is immunological cross-reactivity between the two HSV types and their antibodies which affects the clinical picture.

Primary, first and recurrent episodes

Primary genital herpes is the term used to define the clinical episode occurring at the time of initial HSV infection. It occurs in individuals without previous exposure to HSV (1 or 2) and symptoms are usually severe [14]. Some presenting episodes are, however, milder and shorter and are referred to as *first episodes*. In such cases, the initial infection will usually have occurred sometime previously and the patients will have pre-existing antibody from the earlier exposure, usually to HSV-1.

Herpes viruses exhibit latency giving rise to *recurrent episodes*. It is not uncommon to experience more than one recurrence of HSV-2 in the first year after infection, although recurrences of HSV-1 are less common. The lesions of first episodes and recurrences may be very minor and atypical: the diagnosis of HSV may therefore not be considered. This, together with asymptomatic shedding of virus which occurs in about 3% of those infected, is an important factor in the spread of this disease.

Primary genital herpes

In primary genital herpes, the patient initially develops a clinical state that resembles a flu-like syndrome with fever, malaise and myalgia. Aseptic meningitis is not uncommon. After 3–4 days multiple lesions develop at the site of infection, usually the vulva. Other common sites are the peri-anal area, vagina and cervix. The lesions begin as small blisters or vesicles which become unroofed, leaving small and sometimes pinpoint ulcers. Vesicles may arise in close proximity and coalesce to form a large ulcer that may be mistaken for a syphilitic chancre. Individuals with primary genital herpes frequently develop bilateral tender inguinal lymphadenopathy, vulval oedema, vaginal discharge and severe dysuria. Urinary retention can also occur. Complete healing can take up to 3 weeks.

Recurrent genital herpes

Individuals with recurrent genital herpes typically experience a prodrome, e.g. neuralgic-type pain, tingling, itching and hyperasthesia at a localized site where a lesion is to develop. The lesions are few in number and tend to recur at the same site with each outbreak. Recurrences become less severe and less frequent with time.

Pregnancy and genital herpes

In comparison to genital herpes, neonatal herpes is very rare, but is important as the morbidity and mortality is high. Infection of the newborn occurs at the time of delivery. Perinatal maternal primary herpes exposes the neonate to greatest risk. A cesarean section is commonly performed and appears to offer some protection even if herpetic lesions are present during labor, provided the membranes are intact or have been ruptured for less than 4 h. Routine testing for viral shedding during pregnancy has not been demonstrated to be of value.

Herpes and immunocompromised patients

In the presence of HIV infection, HSV infection tends to be severe and chronic, and worsens as the HIV infection progresses. Lesions are often large and secondary infection is common. Antiviral prophylaxis is commonly required to prevent pain and systemic infection.

Diagnosis

The diagnosis is frequently made on clinical examination. However, like any other sexually transmitted infection, the diagnosis should be confirmed, preferably by isolating the virus in tissue culture. Electron microscopy or immuno-fluorescence can be useful if available especially for rapid diagnosis. Enzyme-linked immunosorbent assays (ELISA) are sometimes available. Other less sensitive methods include Tanzck, Giemsa, Wright–Giemsa and Papanicolaou stains [15–17]. HSV serology can be difficult to interpret as it does not indicate the time or site of infection, and caution should be exercised in interpreting the results.

Viral culture is best performed on vesicular fluid taken from an unroofed blister. If an ulcer is present, the base of the ulcer should be blotted with a sterile cotton or Dacron-tipped applicator, and inoculated in tissue culture vials. Lesions that are crusted over are less likely to yield virions for culture.

Management

It is vital that patients diagnosed as having genital herpes are given clear factual information and time for discussion. Psychological or psychosexual complications are common. Primary and severe clinical episodes should be treated with oral antiviral agents in addition to symptomatic treatment with simple analgesics and lignocaine gel. Recurrences are often best managed with symptomatic treatment alone.

Suppressive antiviral therapy is used for patients with frequent documented recurrences. This reduces symptoms but is not guaranteed to stop viral shedding.

Treatment

The treatment regimens for herpetic infections are detailed in Box 17.4.

Lymphogranuloma venereum (LGV)

LGV is caused by *Chlamydia trachomatis*, serovars L1, L2 and L3. This disease is sexually transmitted and is seen predominantly in tropical and sub-tropical areas and is rarely found in the USA or Europe. It is primarily a disease of the lymphatics and, if untreated, is characterized by abscess formation. Healing is by scarring which can rarely lead to a frozen pelvis, rectal stenosis or vulval elephantiasis.

Diagnosis

The diagnosis of LGV can be established by clinical signs, combined with specific laboratory tests, such as complement fixation, microimmunofluorescence (a titer greater than 1:512 is usually associated with active disease) and the isolation of the organism in tissue culture [18].

Clinically LGV presents in one of three stages of disease: primary, secondary or late. Primary disease is characterized by the development of an ulcer or chancre 1–3 weeks after inoculation. It is commonly a small papular or herpetiform lesion which, although it is painful and lasts only a few days [19], may be confused with syphilis and herpes.

Secondary LGV typically presents as unilateral inguinal tender lymphadenopathy. The femoral lymph nodes may also be involved. The inguinal and femoral lymph nodes are

---

Box 17.4 Treatment of herpetic infections

Primary herpetic infection
- Aciclovir: 200 mg orally five times a day for 5 or 10 days or
- Aciclovir: 400 mg orally three times a day for 7–10 days or
- Valaciclovir: 1 g orally twice daily for 10 days or
- Famciclovir 250 mg orally three times a day for 7–10 days

Recurrent herpetic infection
- Aciclovir:
  - 200 mg orally five times a day for 5 days or
  - 400 mg orally three times a day for 5 days or
  - 800 mg orally twice a day for 5 days or
- Valaciclovir: 500 mg orally twice daily for 7 days or
- Famciclovir: 125 mg orally twice a day for 5 days

Severe or disseminated herpetic infection
- Aciclovir: 5–10 mg/kg of body weight administered intravenously every 8 h until clinical resolution of signs and symptoms of the infection is achieved

Suppressive therapy
- Aciclovir: 400 mg orally twice a day or
- Famciclovir: 250 mg orally twice a day or
- Valaciclovir:
  - 250 mg orally twice a day or
  - 500 mg orally once a day or
  - 1000 mg orally once a day

separated by Poupart's ligament which gives rise to the characteristic 'groove' sign. The nodes eventually become soft and are referred to as 'buboes', which can frequently rupture spontaneously producing a thick purulent exudate and fistulae [18]. Anorectal syndrome comprises acute proctocolitis with involvement of the perianal lymphatics. In addition to proctitus, such patients typically have pruritus, rectal pain and tenesmus. The rectal mucosa is edematous, friable and bleeds easily. Multiple rectal lesions can lead to the development of rectal and perianal abscesses and rectal fissures. The perianal lymphatics become obstructed, enlarged and dilated and resemble hemorrhoids. Progression of the disease leads to the formation of rectovaginal fistulae and the development of granulomatous tissue and fibrosis. This leads to the formation of rectal strictures approximately 3–5 cm above the anocutaneous junction which narrows the rectum, producing thin 'pencil stools' [20]. The disease may progress outside the rectum infiltrating the adjacent pelvic tissues with the development of granulation tissue producing a frozen pelvis.

The patient can develop extragenital lesions with bubo formation and disseminated disease characterized by fever, malaise, pneumonitis, hepatitis or meningoencephalitis or other complications. Rarely, erythema multiforme or erythema nodosum may develop. Tertiary LGV is characterized by vulvar elephantiasis due to obstruction of the vulval lymphatics, producing edema. Painful sclerosing ulcerations can also develop.

Treatment

Doxycycline 100 mg orally twice a day for 21 days

Alternative regimens are erythromycin 500 mg orally four times a day for 21 days or sulfoxazole 500 mg orally four times a day for 21 days.

Treatment of sexual contacts

(As for granuloma inguinale.)

Diseases causing cervicitis

Gonorrhoea

The incidence of gonorrhea in the USA is 323 per 100 000 with the highest prevalence in 20–24-year-olds.

The etiologic agent is the Gram-negative diplococcus, *Neisseria gonorrhoeae*. The prevalence of gonorrhea in a population is dependent upon many factors, in particular behavioral and social. It is seen predominately in inner cities where it is often endemic. In other communities, outbreaks occur sporadically. The incubation period for gonorrhea is about 7 days but may be longer.

Gonorrhea is usually contracted through sexual intercourse or mucosal contact with an infected site. The sites of infection in women are: cervix, urethra, rectum, oropharynx, Skene's glands and Bartholin's glands. The main complication is pelvic inflammatory disease, occurring in 10–20% of cases (see Chapter 18). Vertical transmission leads to neonatal ophthalmic infection which can cause blindness.

As genital gonococcal infection is typically asymptomatic in women, a high index of suspicion should prevail. Infection may be suspected if the patient reports relevant symptoms, has clinical signs of infection or has had sexual contact with an infected individual. Taking a history of sexual contacts is useful in assessing risk. When present, symptoms include postcoital or intermenstrual bleeding and dyspareunia [21]. Signs include endocervical mucopus, hypertrophy of the endocervical epithelium, contact bleeding and the signs of pelvic inflammatory disease. Coexistent urethral infection is common but is rarely symptomatic. Bartholin's abscesses have been associated with genital gonococcal infection. Rectal infection can occur as a result of contamination with vaginal discharge or by anal intercourse. Disseminated infection with skin lesions and arthritis is rare.

Diagnosis

If gonorrhea is suspected, specimens should be taken from the endocervix (Stuart's medium) and preferably also the urethra, rectum and, if indicated, the oropharynx. A presumptive diagnosis can be made in about 50% of women by microscopy of endocervical discharge demonstrating the typical appearance of Gram-negative intracellular diplococci within polymorphonucleocytes. Culture is, however, the mainstay of diagnosis and confirmation, and provides important information about antibiotic sensitivity. If gonorrhea is strongly suspected and test results are negative, it is often recommended that they are repeated prior to treatment. Gonococcal cervicitis is commonly associated with *Chlamydia trachomatis* and appropriate tests for this should also be taken. A bimanual examination should be performed for signs of pelvic inflammatory disease.

Treatment

Worldwide resistance to penicillin is not uncommon and, as resistance to other antibiotics also occurs, a knowledge of local sensitivity to antibiotics is important in planning treatment. Penicillin should only be used as a first-line treatment if the incidence of resistance is known to be low.

The following treatment regimens may be used for uncomplicated genital gonorrhea:

- ceftriaxone 125 mg intramuscularly as a single dose; or

- cefixime 400 mg orally in a single dose; or

- ofloxacin 400 mg orally in a single dose; or

- spectinomycin 2 g intramuscularly in a single dose; or

- ciprofloxacin 500 mg orally in a single dose (contraindicated in pregnancy and children); or

- ampicillin 2 g with 1 g probenecid orally in a single dose.*

As chlamydial infection frequently occurs concurrently with gonococcal infection [22], it is common practice to treat it with a combination of antibiotics effective against both organisms.

All patients with gonorrhea should be advised to abstain from sexual intercourse until treatment is completed, sexual contacts have been tested and treated as appropriate and at least one test of cure has been carried out and is negative.

Infection of Bartholin's glands can lead to abscess formation. This is associated with a cellulitis and pain. Initially, the tissue overlying the abscess is indurated and thick. Some clinicians perform surgical drainage immediately, whilst others initiate therapy with antibiotics such as amoxicillin/clavulanic acid 500 mg orally three times a day for 10 days, or ofloxacin 300 mg orally twice a day for 10 days. The patient should be re-examined in 48 h to determine if the outer abscess wall has thinned out. If so, needle aspiration should be performed followed by a suitable procedure to allow communication to be formed between the gland and the skin such as incision, drainage and marsupialization or insertion of a balloon catheter. Any aspirate obtained should be cultured for gonorrhea.

Treatment of sexual contacts

Sexual contacts within the previous 3 months should be screened for gonorrhea and other sexually transmitted infections. If the risk of gonorrhea is high, they should be offered epidemiological treatment whilst awaiting results.

Chlamydia trachomatis

Urogenital chlamydial infection is the most common sexually transmitted infection (STI) in the USA, with a prevalence of 3% in asymptomatic women and 25% in those attending STI clinics. In the UK, the prevalence varies between 4% in low-risk populations to 10% in attendees of STI clinics and 20% in teenagers seeking a therapeutic abortion.

Serovars D to K are obligate intracellular bacteria that cause a genital infection with similar clinical presentation to gonococcal infection. The main sites of infection are the urethra and cervix. It is a rare cause of conjunctivitis, proctitis and perihepatitis. When transmitted vertically, it is also a cause of ophthalmia neonatorum and neonatal pneumonia. Chlamydia is more prevalent than gonorrhea and is less confined to inner city areas. Chlamydia is responsible for the majority of cases of pelvic inflammatory disease due to sexually transmitted infection. Tubal damage due to chlamydial infection can occur without the development of classical clinical PID.

Less than 10% of women and about 25% of men with *C. trachomatis* have symptoms, thus long-standing asymptomatic genital infection is not uncommon. When they occur, the symptoms in women include intermenstrual and postcoital bleeding, mild dysuria, lower abdominal pain with dyspareunia and vaginal discharge.

Diagnosis

A sexual history identifies women who are at risk of chlamydial infection. Risk factors include being under 25 years old and having a change of partner within

*This regimen should only be used where local resistance to penicillins is known to be low.

the previous 12 months. As a public health measure, routine or selective screening protocols have been developed by some health providers

Until recently, *Chlamydia* culture was regarded as the gold standard test, although ELISA tests were commonly used as they are more robust. However, the development of DNA amplification tests such as the ligase chain reaction (LCR) and polymerase chain reaction (PCR) have revealed that culture and ELISA have sensitivities well below those attainable with PCR or LCR [23]. The latter also have the advantage that they can often be carried out on urine specimens, thus avoiding the need for a vaginal examination and facilitating their use as screening tests. The full potential of these tests is being evaluated.

Treatment

The recommended treatments for uncomplicated chlamydial infection in non-pregnant women are doxycycline 100 mg orally twice daily for 7 days or azithromycin 1 g orally as a single dose.★ For women who are pregnant or who do not tolerate these regimens, the following may be used: erythromycin 500 mg orally two times a daily for 10 days.† The rate of failed treatment with the preparations recommended for use in pregnancy is high relative to other regimen. Retesting 3 weeks after completing therapy is recommended.

★The safety of azithromycin in pregnancy has not been established.
† Erythromycin estolate is contraindicated in pregnancy, unlike the stearate.

Treatment of sexual contacts

Sexual contacts within the previous 3 months should be screened for *Chlamydia* and other sexually transmitted infections. If the risk of *Chlamydia* is high, they should be offered epidemiological treatment whilst awaiting results.

Diseases causing vaginal infection

Trichomoniasis

Trichomoniasis is caused by the flagellated protozoan *Trichomonas vaginalis* (TV). It is almost always sexually transmitted. Clinical features range from no symptoms or minor discomfort and pruritus to a severe vulvovaginitis with profuse vaginal discharge. Classically the vaginal mucosa is markedly erythematous and a frothy grey/green malodorous discharge is noted. Long-term complications do not occur.

Diagnosis

The clinical features and a vaginal pH above 5 suggest TV: the diagnosis is confirmed by the presence of trichomonads on microscopy of a wet saline mount of vaginal discharge. Culture in Diamond's medium is sometimes deployed but offers only slightly higher sensitivity than microscopy in good hands. The organisms can also be identified with high vaginal swab, Gram stain, pap smear or with DNA testing.

The presence of *T. vaginalis* should alert the physician to the possible presence of other

sexually transmitted infections and bacterial vaginosis. Typically, when trichomoniasis is present, the patient's endogenous vaginal microflora is disrupted and is dominated by anerobic bacteria.

Treatment

Metronidazole is the only effective treatment available in the USA. It can be administered in the following dosages: 2 g in a single dose or 250 mg three times daily for 7 days, or 375 mg twice daily for 7 days, or 500 mg twice a day for 7 days, or 400 mg twice a day for 5 days.

Successful treatment is dependent upon patient compliance and the simultaneous treatment of her partner(s). In men, microscopy and culture for TV are lacking in sensitivity and often not routinely carried out; however, other STIs should be excluded and the partner offered epidemiological treatment. The patient should abstain from sexual intercourse until it has been confirmed that the trichomonads have been eradicated. Metronidazole gel is not effective in treating trichomoniasis because trichmonads migrate to extragenital sites.

Bacterial vaginosis

Bacterial vaginosis (BV), previously known as anerobic vaginosis, is a disturbance in the normal vaginal ecosystem. BV is the most commonly identified cause of vaginal discharge. The prevalence varies with the population being studied, and can be as high as 20%. Bacterial vaginosis is characterized by an absence of lactobacilli and a preponderance of anerobic bacteria such as *Mobiluncus* spp., *Gardnerella vaginalis*, *Bacteroides* spp. and mycoplasmas. Although the etiology of BV is poorly understood, it is related to sexual activity. However, a sexually transmitted pathogen has not been identified and treatment of the male partners does not affect recurrence rates, which are high. There is an association with vaginal douching and the use of intrauterine contraceptive devices. Recurrences are frequently noticed after intercourse or menstruation.

Bacterial vaginosis presents with a malodorous vaginal discharge, although 50% of women who meet the diagnostic criteria do not report symptoms. Clinically the findings are of a characteristic, grey homogenous (i.e. non-viscous, adherent and free from particulate matter) malodorous (often described as fishy) vaginal discharge. Unlike TV, BV does not cause inflammation of the vagina and vulva, or associated symptoms such as pruritus and soreness.

The significance of BV is that it may predispose the patient to postoperative pelvic infection and, if pregnant, to preterm birth, second trimester loss, chorioamnionitis and postpartum endometritis [24]. It also believed to play a role in the pathogenesis of PID.

Diagnosis

There are three main methods of diagnosing BV: clinical criteria [25], a wet slide saline preparation of vaginal discharge looking for the presence of 'clue' cells (epithelial cells with bacteria obscuring their borders), an absence of lactobacilli and a Gram-stained smear [26]. The

latter has the advantage that it allows an intermediate pattern between normal and BV to be identified and should be used for research. Microbiological culture is not of use in the diagnosis of BV.

The clinical criteria include a vaginal pH of greater than 4.5 (normal pH = 3.5–4.5) and fishy odor on clinical examination or 'whiff test'. This is performed by adding 10% potassium hydroxide to a sample of vaginal discharge and noting the odor of amines, released if BV is present.

Treatment

In the presence of symptoms, BV should always be treated. Those who are asymptomatic and pregnant should be offered treatment as there is evidence that this may reduce the risk of the complications of pregnancy mentioned previously. Many clinicians treat all women diagnosed as having BV irrespective of their disclosed symptoms. Usual treatment options include:

- metronidazole 500 mg (400 mg in the UK) orally twice daily for 7 days; or

- 0.75% metronidazole vaginal gel (5 g) intravaginally twice daily for 5 days; or

- clindamycin 300 mg orally twice daily for 7 days; or

- clindamycin 2% vaginal cream, one applicator full (5 g) intravaginally for 7 days. (This preparation is oil-based and may weaken latex condoms, diaphragms and cervical caps and may lead to contraceptive failure.)

Clindamycin and high-dose metronidazole regimens are not recommended in pregnancy.

Vulvo-vaginal candidiasis

Candidiasis (a yeast infection) is usually caused by *Candida albicans*. It is common: about 60–70% of women will experience at least one episode of *Candida* in their lifetime. Predisposing factors, such as reduced immunity, steroid therapy and undiagnosed diabetes, are occasionally involved in recurrent infections. The condition is not sexually transmitted, although some male partners of women with candidiasis develop a mild, pruritic balanitis which usually resolves on abstention from unprotected vaginal intercourse until the vaginal infection is treated.

Diagnosis

The most notable symptom is vulval pruritus. Soreness and dysuria due to broken skin may also be present and a white vaginal discharge may be noted. The clinical findings may vary from appearing almost normal to a severe vulvo-vaginitis and a typical white curdy vaginal discharge. The vulval erythema usually has a marked edge with adjacent satellite lesions. The diagnosis of vulvo-vaginal candidiasis is made by detecting yeast and pseudohyphae on microscopy of vaginal discharge either by a wet preparation using 10% potassium hydroxide or by Gram stain. The pH of vaginal discharge is usually less than 4.5 unless BV or TV are also present. Culture confirms the diagnosis and the causative species.

Treatment

The mainstay of treatment is with the topical azoles, many of which are available over the counter. Typical drugs and doses include: clotrimazole 500 mg vaginal tablet nocte, or clotrimazole 200 mg vaginal tablet nocte for 3 days, or clotrimazole 100 mg vaginal tablet in hs for 7 days. Other topical agents include:

- butoconazole 2% cream for 3 days;
- clotrimazole 1% cream for 7–14 days;
- miconazole 2% cream or vaginal tablet for 7 days;
- nystatin vaginal tablets, ticonazole ointment and terconazole.

The preferred oral treatment, which is available over the counter in some countries, is fluconazole 150 mg orally in a single dose. After treatment no specific follow-up is required.

Other viral infections

Molluscum contagiosum

Molluscum contagiosum (MC) is caused by the virus of the same name. In adults, MC is usually sexually transmitted, especially when it affects the groin, genital area or lower abdomen. MC commonly occurs in children but affects the face, trunk and upper limbs, and is not indicative of sexual activity. Lesions appear about 1–3 months after infection and can last for up to 2 years. Complications are rare and are limited to secondary infection and postinfection dermatitis. The

lesions are usually asymptomatic or associated with mild pruritus. The clinical appearance is of a few papules with shiny umbilicated domes 2–3 mm across. The color varies but may be the same as the surrounding skin. Treatment is by cryotherapy, or curettage and cautery to the exposed base. The latter is carried out with silver nitrate or trichloracetic acid. Contacts should be seen if they have noticed lesions.

Genital warts and human papilloma virus (HPV) infection

Genital HPV infection is the most common viral STI in industrialized countries.

There are in excess of 70 subtypes of HPV of which only a few are implicated in the development of clinical genital infection, with subtypes 6 and 11 being the most frequent. It is likely that at least 60% of sexually active young people will harbor subclinical infection [27]. Although clinical infection is not as frequent as subclinical infection, most diagnoses of genital warts are made in sexually active people between 16 and 25 years. Approximately 50% of those with a partner with genital warts will also develop them. The incubation period for genital warts is typically 3 weeks to 6 months, although longer periods do occur. In time, these benign tumors resolve spontaneously. The clinical findings in genital HPV infection range from lesions only visible at colposcopy to confluent exophytic genital warts (Table 17.3). The factors affecting the clinical presentation are poorly understood, but genital

Table 17.3 Sites of clinical HPV infection in women [28]

Site	% of cases	Range
Vulva	85	77–94
Perianal area	58	13–85
Vagina	42	35–52
Cervix	34	16–64

From Brown DR, Fife KH. Human papillomavirus infections of the genital tract. *Med Clin North Am* 1990;74:1455–85.

warts are more common in pregnancy and in association with HIV infection. Vertical transmission during delivery is rare, but is associated with the development in the neonate of perianal warts and laryngeal papillomatosis.

HPV subtypes 16, 18, 31, 33 and 35, which may not lead to clinical wart infection, are implicated in the etiology of cervical intraepithelial neoplasia (squamous intraepithelial lesions) and squamous cervical cancer. They are also associated with vaginal and vulvar intraepithelial neoplasia. It is recommended that cervical cytology screening should not be performed in women with genital warts more frequently than in women without genital warts unless indicated for another reason [29].

Diagnosis

Genital warts are diagnosed by a careful and thorough clinical examination. Biopsy is only required for cervical lesions and (rarely) for warts occurring at other sites if the diagnosis is uncertain or there is a possibility of malignancy. The differentiation between warts and molluscum contagiosum or condylomata lata of secondary syphilis is not usually difficult. On examination, genital warts are most commonly seen on the posterior fourchette, the labia minora and the vestibule. When vulvar warts are diagnosed, the possibility of vaginal, cervical, perianal and anal warts should be considered.

Treatment

Therapy is usually cytotoxic or destructive with the aim of treating clinically evident lesions rather than subclinical infection. It is increasingly recognized that treatment is a cosmetic procedure that may reduce symptoms if present. The effect of treatment on infectivity or the duration of the infection is unknown.

The preferred method of treatment for genital warts is cryotherapy using a cryoprobe or liquid nitrogen. Other methods of treatment include the topical application of podophyllin or podophyllotoxin, which are cytotoxic agents. Neither should be used when there is a possibility of pregnancy. Podophyllin, usually as a 10% or 25% resin, is applied to the lesion and washed off after 4–6 h. It is irritant to normal skin and should be applied by a healthcare professional. The related product podophyllotoxin 0.5% (Podofilox 0.5%) and Imiquimod 5% cream are available in some countries for self-application. Trichloroacetic acid, electrocautery, scissor excision, surgical removal and intralesional interferon are also occasionally used. When treating intravaginal warts, care should be taken when applying topical agents or when using cryotherapy to avoid damage to adjacent epithelium or deeper structures. The effects of treatment should be assessed and treatment repeated at weekly intervals until the warts have been eradicated. Improvement should be seen within 3 weeks and resolution is usually achieved in 6 weeks.

Appendix 1

Features of common lower genital tract infections

Feature	Candidiasis	TV	BV	Chlamydia[a]	Gonorrhea[a]	Herpes	Other
An STI	No	Yes	No	Yes	Yes	Yes	
Discharge	Cottage cheese	Yellow–green, foul	Thin homogenous Fishy odor	Uncommon	Uncommon Can be mucopurulent	Not a feature	Foreign body can cause profuse and offensive discharge
Vulval pruritis	Yes + erythema	Soreness rather than itching + erythema	No	No	No	Soreness and pain not itching	Consider pubic lice, scabies and dermatoses
Genital ulceration	Skin cracks in severe cases	No	No	No	No	Yes	Consider syphilis and other ulcerative conditions
Pelvic pain	No	No	No	May occur	May occur	No	
Dysuria	In severe cases	No	No	May occur	May occur	Yes	Consider UTI
Risk of PID	No	No	?	Yes	Yes	No	

TV = *Trichomonas vaginalis*; BV = bacterial vaginosis; UTI = urinary tract infection.
[a]Chlamydia and gonorrhea may cause intermenstrual bleeding.

Appendix 2

Common causes of vaginal discharge

Feature	Condition			
	Normal	BV	TV	Candidiasis
Appearance	White/clear	Grey/milky, homogenous Thin, slightly frothy	Yellow–green Frothy May be offensive	Curdy-white
Odor	None	Fishy	Foul	None
pH	<4.5	>5	>5	<5
Polymorphs	None	None/few	+++	++
Amine (whiff) test[a]	Negative	Positive	Weakly positive	Negative
Wet film	Bacilli	'Clue' cells	Flagellates	Pseudohyphae
Gram stain	Normal flora (normal Gram stain)	Mixed flora Gram -ve rods 'Clue cells' Absence of Gram +ve bacilli	Parabasal cells	Spores/pseudohyphae

TV = *Trichomonas vaginalis*; BV = bacterial vaginosis; +++ = high number; ++ = moderately high number.
[a]Amine test: add two drops of 1–5% KOH to vaginal secretion on a slide or swab. Sensitivity = 85%, specificity >90%.

References

1. Ghoneim ATM, McGoldrick J, Blick PWH, et al. Aerobic and anaerobic bacteriology of subcutaneous abscesses. *Br J Surg* 1981;68:498–500.

2. Noble WC. Microbiology of the human skin, 2nd edn. London: Lloyd-Luke. 1981.

3. Gould JC, Cruikshank JD. Staphylococcal infection in general practice. *Lancet* 1957;ii:1157.

4. Csonka GW, Oates JK. Syphilis. In: Csonka GW, Oates JK (eds) Sexually transmitted diseases. Philadelphia: Bailliere Tindall, 1990:227–76.

5. Jaffe HW, Larsen SA, Jones OG, Dans PE. Hemagglutination tests for syphilis antibody. *Am J Clin Pathol* 1971;78:53.

6. Centres for Disease Control and Prevention. 1998 Guidelines for treatment of sexually transmitted diseases *MMWR* 1998; 47L:RR–1.

7. North Thames (East). Guidelines for the management of syphilis. London, 1996.

8. Negussie Y, Remick DG, DeForge LE, et al. Detection of plasma tumor necrosis factor, interleukins 6 and 8 during the Jarisch–Herxheimer reaction of relapsing fever. *J Exp Med* 1992;175:1207–12.

9. Hanlon-Lundberg DM, Ismail MA. Syphilis. In: Pastorek JG (ed.) Obstetric and gynecologic infectious disease. New York: Raven Press, 1994:479–89.

10. Hammond GW, Slutchuk V, Scatliff J, et al. Epidemiology, clinical, laboratory and therapeutic features of an urban outbreak of chancroid in North America. *Rev Infect Dis* 1980;2:867–69.

11. Nsanze H, Plummer FA, Magwa A, et al. Comparison of media for the primary isolation of Haemophilus ducreyi. *Sex Transm Dis* 1984;11:6–9.

12. Kuberski T. Granuloma inguinale (Donovanosis). *Sex Transm Dis* 1980;7:29–36.

13. Rosen T, Tschen JA, Ramsell W, et al. Granuloma inguinale. *J Am Acad Dermatol* 1984;11:433–7

14. Baker DA. Herpes simplex virus infections. *Curr Opin Obstet Gynecol* 1992;4:676–81.

15. Benedetti J, Corey L, Ashley R. Recurrence rates in genital herpes after symptomatic first-episode infection. *Ann Intern Med* 1994;121:847–54.

16. Lipson SM, Salo RJ, Leonardi GP. Evaluation of five monoclonal antibody-based kits, or reagents for the identification and culture confirmation of herpes simplex virus. *J Clin Microbiol* 1991;29:466–9.

17. Zimmerman SJ, Moses E, Sofat N, et al. Evaluation of a visual, rapid, membrane enzyme immunoassay for the detection of herpes simplex virus antigen. *J Clin Microbiol* 1991;29:842–5.

18. Abrams AJ. Lymphogranuloma venereum. *JAMA* 1968;205:199–202.

19. Coutts WE. Lymphogranuloma venereum. A general review. *WHO Bull* 1950;2:545.

20. Dan M, Rotmench HH, Eylan E, et al. A case of lymphogranuloma venereum of 20 years duration. Isolation of *Chlamydia trachomatis* from perianal tissue. *Br J Vener Dis* 1980;56:344–6.

21. Alary M, Laga M, Vuylsteke B, et al. Signs and symptoms of prevalent and incident cases of gonorrhoea and genital Chlamydia infection among female prostitutes in Kinshasa, Zaire. *Clin Infect Dis* 1996; 22:477–84.

22. Braddick MR, Ndinya-Achola JO, Mirza NB, et al. Towards developing a diagnostic algorithm for *Chlamydia trachomatis* and *Neisseria gonorrhoeae* cervicitis in pregnancy. *Genitourinary Med* 1990;66:62–5.

23. Taylor-Robinson D. Tests for infection with *Chlamydia trachomatis*. *Int J STD AIDS* 1996;7:19–26.

24. McGregor JA, French JI. Pregnancy Introduction. In: Ison CA, Taylor-Robinson D (eds) Bacterial vaginosis. *Int J STD AIDS* 1997;8 (Suppl 1):26–7.

25. Amsel R, Totten PA, Spiegal CA, et al. Non-specific vaginitis. Diagnostic criteria and microbial and epidemiologic associations. *Am J Med* 1983;74:14–22.

26. Nugent RP, Krohn MA, Hillier SL. Reliability of diagnosing bacterial vaginosis is improved by a standardized method of Gram stain interpretation. *J Clin Microbiol* 1991;29:297–301.

27. Ho GYF, Bierman R, Beardsley L, et al. Natural history of cervico-vaginal papillomavirus infection in your women. *N Engl J Med* 1998;338:423–7.

28. Brown DR, Fife KH. Human papillomavirus infections of the genital tract. *Med Clin North Am* 1990;74:1455–85.

29. Duncan ID (ed.) Guidelines for Clinical Practice and Programme Management, 2nd edn. NHSCSP Publication no. 8, 1997.

Further reading

- Holmes KK, et al. (eds) Sexually transmitted diseases, 2nd edn. New York: McGraw-Hill, 1990.

- Adler M. ABC of STDs. London: British Medical Journal, 1995.

- Csonka GW, Oates JK (eds) Sexually transmitted diseases. Philadelphia: Bailliere Tindall, 1990.

- Barlow D, Ison CA. Neisseria gonorrhoeae. In: Weatherall, Ledingham, Warrell (eds) Oxford textbook of medicine, 3rd edn. Oxford: Oxford University Press, 1996:544–50.

- Center for Disease Control and Prevention. 1998 guidelines for treatment of sexually transmitted diseases. *MMWR* 1998;47L:RR–1.

Pelvic inflammatory disease and other infections

Tommaso Falcone MD
Jeffrey M Goldberg MD

Epidemiology

Pelvic inflammatory disease (PID) refers to infections of the upper female reproductive tract: endometritis, salpingitis and oophoritis. It is a disease of a woman's reproductive years. The incidence of acute PID is not precisely known, although it is estimated that 1–2% of women aged 15–35 are affected each year [1]. Estimates were based on patient self-reporting to national surveys, reported visits to physician offices and hospital discharge diagnoses. Data from emergency rooms, hospital outpatient clinics and sexually transmitted disease (STD) clinics were not included. The true incidence may also be underestimated due to asymptomatic patients with 'silent PID'. Also, PID may be difficult to diagnose as the clinical criteria are vague and the site of infection is not accessible for culture. Laparoscopy performed for presumed PID may reveal other etiologies, such as appendicitis, ectopic pregnancy and adnexal torsion. In a number of series, as many as 50% of laparoscopies in patients with a presumptive diagnosis of PID were negative [1].

Currently, it is estimated that one million women annually in the USA will be diagnosed with acute PID. About a third of those will require hospitalization and approximately 150 000 will undergo surgery for complications of PID. There has been a reduction in the incidence of hospitalization for PID since 1983, while the annual number of private physician visits for PID has been increasing, suggesting a greater proportion of patients are being diagnosed earlier with milder disease [2]. At least 25% of patients with laparoscopically verified PID will develop long-term consequences such as infertility, ectopic pregnancy, tubo-ovarian abscess (TOA), pelvic adhesions and chronic pelvic pain. The direct and indirect costs of PID and its sequelae were estimated to exceed $4 billion in 1990 and were projected to approach $10 billion a year by 2000 [3].

Several demographic variables have been determined to influence the risk of acquiring PID. There is an inverse relationship between patient age and the incidence of PID. Younger women may be predisposed due to a larger zone of cervical ectopy for the attachment of *Chlamydia trachomatis* and *Neisseria gonorrhoeae*. This population also tends to have anovulatory cycles with unopposed estrogen effect on the cervical mucus, facilitating access of micro-organisms to the upper genital tract. In addition, the adolescent population tends to have multiple sexual partners and not use contraceptives effectively, and thus has a higher prevalence of STDs. For these same reasons, women of lower socioeconomic status also have a increased risk. These women are less likely to seek medical care in a timely fashion. Married women have a lower rate of PID [4].

Women who have had an episode of PID are at high risk for recurrences secondary to damage of local host defenses and/or to continued exposure to the risk factors which predisposed them to the initial infection. Vaginal douching increases the risk of PID by impairing natural protective mechanisms due to altering the vaginal environment and/or by flushing cervico-vaginal organisms into the uterus and fallopian tubes. Coitus during menses may also increase the risk of developing PID. Other risk-taking behaviours, such as cigarette smoking and substance abuse, have been associated with a greater risk of PID. In all probability, this is because they are markers for other risk behaviors such as multiple partners and non-use of barriers.

Contraceptive practices can affect the risk for PID (Table 18.1) [5]. Barrier methods, such as condoms and to a lesser extent the diaphragm, reduce the risk of PID by helping to prevent the antecedent STDs. These barriers prevent access of the infecting organisms to the cervical glands and mucosa, as well as by eliminating sperm as a vehicle for ascending infection. Data are lacking regarding the ability of the female condom or cervical cap to protect against PID. Spermicides decrease the risk of STDs and PID. Oral contraceptives have also been shown to reduce the risk of PID. Suggested mechanisms include cervical mucus becoming less penetrable by bacteria, reduced menstrual flow and duration, and altered immune responses. While oral contraceptives may offer a protective effect against PID, patients at risk for STDs should still be strongly encouraged to use condoms to prevent viral STDs. Intrauterine devices (IUDs) carry a higher risk of PID only within the first 20 days, suggesting that insertion introduces cervico-vaginal pathogens into the endometrial cavity. This risk may be reduced with screening and/or prophylactic doxycycline at the time of insertion [6]. Patients at risk for PID would be best advised to consider other contraceptive options.

Pathogenesis

The basic mechanism in the development of PID is an ascending infection. The use of endometrial sampling and laparoscopy has documented that the infectious process progresses sequentially from cervicitis to endometritis, salpingitis, peritonitis and perihepatitis. Access to the upper tract may be facilitated by menstrual blood reflux or attachment to sperm. Factors that may increase the probability of an ascending infection are:

- bacterial vaginosis;

- bacterial attachment to sperm;

- vaginal douching;

- loss of cervical barrier as in
  - menstruation
  - cervicitis;

- uterine instrumentation as in
  - insertion of an IUD
  - induced abortion, and other intrauterine procedures.

The organisms that have been associated with PID are:

- sexually transmitted bacteria
  - *N. gonorrhoeae*
  - *C. trachomatis*;

- bacteria of the vaginal flora
  - anaerobes
  - facultative anaerobes
  - mycoplasmas;

- hematogenous spread
  - tuberculosis;

- *Actinomyces*.

C. trachomatis, N. gonorrhoeae and bacteria of the vaginal flora are responsible for an ascending infection, while tuberculosis is spread hematogenously and *Actinomyces* is associated with the IUD.

The interaction of the classical STDs, *C. trachomatis* and *N. gonorrhoeae*, and the anerobic and facultative anaerobic bacteria in the vaginal flora is controversial. Theories proposed include the initiation of tissue damage by *C. trachomatis* and *N. gonorrhoeae* with subsequent invasion of the vaginal flora, a primary mixed infection, and a primary vaginal flora abnormality followed by the ascent of chlamydia and gonorrhea. The latter has recently received much attention [7]. Bacterial vaginosis is thought to be an important factor that could lead to an ascending infection. Bacterial vaginosis is a common vaginal infection with a significant overgrowth of anerobes and facultative anerobes such as *Bacteroides* (*Prevotella*), *Peptostreptococcus* and *Mobiluncus* species, *Gardnerella vaginalis* and *Mycoplasma hominis*. These organisms are recovered with varying frequencies in patients with PID. The large

Table 18.1 Contraceptive effects on upper and lower female genital tract infection

	Lower genital tract		Upper genital tract	
	GC	Chlamydia	PID	Tubal infertility
Oral contraceptives	−	− −	++	+
Norplant	+	?	+	?
Copper IUD	0	+/0	−/0	0
Male condom	++	++	++	++
Diaphragm	++	++	+	+
Spermicide	++	+	+	?

GC = gonococcus; PID = pelvic inflammatory disease; IUD = intrauterine device.
+/++ = slightly/strongly protective; −/−− = slightly/greatly increased risk; 0 = no effect.
Adapted from Rowe PJ. *Aust NZ J Obstet Gynaecol* 1994;34:299–305 [5].

inoculum size of these bacteria may be important in the pathogenesis of PID. These bacteria are more likely to be isolated with severe forms of PID. Regardless of the relative frequencies with which these organisms appear, PID should be regarded as a polymicrobial disease.

C. trachomatis is the most common sexually transmitted bacterial organism in many countries, including the USA, and is responsible for half the cases of PID. It is an obligate intracellular bacterium with more than 20 serotypes. Strains D to K are associated with STDs. Serological tests that are used to detect past exposure to C. trachomatis may cross-react with strains that are not associated with an STD. Chlamydia has two biological forms: the extracellular elementary body and the intracellular reticulate body. The elementary body attaches itself to an epithelial cell. It enters the cell by endocytosis and remains in there as an identifiable vesicle called an inclusion. Reorganization into a reticulate body results in division. Condensation into elementary bodies and release from the cell of infectious organisms then occurs.

The epithelial cells of the endocervix, upper genital tract, urethra and rectum are the initial site of infection of C. trachomatis. The squamous epithelium of the adult vagina is impervious to C. trachomatis infection but the prepubertal vagina is susceptible. There is an initial polymorphonuclear cell response followed by lymphocytes, macrophages, plasma cells and eosinophils. In a series of experiments in a monkey model,

Patton et al. have shown that the host immune response causes the extensive damage and scarring associated with a chlamydial infection [8,9]. The host inflammatory response which causes the cervical, endometrial and tubal inflammation is elicited by a specific heat-shock protein [10]. Interestingly, in spite of such an inflammatory response, most patients with C. trachomatis infection remain asymptomatic or have minimal symptoms [11]. Infection does not confer immunity to reinfection. The risk of infection of a woman from a symptomatic man with non-gonococcal urethritis is estimated to be approximately 30% [12]. Most patients with cervical chlamydial infections will not develop PID.

N. gonorrhoeae is a Gram-negative coccus that grows in pairs. It infects columnar or cuboidal epithelial cells. As with chlamydia, gonococcal PID is an ascending infection. The urethra is usually infected along with the cervix but is rarely the sole site of infection except in hysterectomized women. The pharynx and the rectum are seldom the only site of infection in women. Most patients with the latter sites of infection are asymptomatic. Rectal infection in women is usually acquired by perineal contamination from a cervical infection. Pharyngeal infection is usually acquired by fellatio and uncommonly by cunnilingus [13].

Gonococcus attaches to epithelial cells via pili or outer membrane proteins. Phagocytosis then occurs with transport across the cell to the subepithelial tissue where cellular destruction occurs. This is accomplished by

production of endotoxins as well as lipases and peptidases. Production of immunoglobulin A (IgA) proteases by the bacteria inhibit the protective effect of host IgA. In addition, the pili can prevent phagocytosis by neutrophils. As with chlamydia, gonorrhea can elicit an immune-mediated epithelial cell destruction. It is proposed that there are different strains of gonorrhea, with some having an inherent ability to cause fallopian tube damage. The risk of infection in women from a symptomatic male infected with gonorrhea is higher than with chlamydia and is estimated to exceed 50%. In contrast to chlamydial infections, most women with gonorrhea develop symptoms. However, many women remain asymptomatic or develop only mild symptoms. PID is estimated to occur in 10–20% of women with gonorrhea of the lower genital tract [14].

Uterine procedures, such as therapeutic abortion and insertion of an IUD, may increase the probability of infection. Legal abortion is not commonly associated with PID if performed by experienced practitioners. Preoperative assessment is key to prevention. High-risk patients, especially adolescents, should be screened for cervical infection. Perioperative antibiotics as described in Appendix 2 should be considered. Contact tracing, if feasible, is an important public health intervention.

The association of the IUD with PID has been the subject of much controversy and recent reviews have shown it has been overestimated [15,16]. The strongest association of PID with the IUD is found immediately after insertion (within the first 4 weeks), related to the introduction of cervical bacteria into the uterine cavity. Apart from the insertion-related infections, most PID occurring with the IUD is related to the acquisition of an STD. Spread of an STD to the upper genital tract may be enhanced by the presence of an IUD.

Actinomyces is a filamentous Gram-positive bacterium that can be identified, usually on a cervical pap smear test, in a minority of patients with an IUD in place. Its overall role in PID is limited. An ascending infection with endometritis followed by TOA and progressive involvement of all pelvic organs can rarely occur. However, most *Actinomyces* is a transient colonizer of the lower genital tract with an increase in prevalence with prolonged IUD use. If it is found on a routine pap test in an asymptomatic woman, consideration may be given to a course of antibiotics if the IUD is to be retained. In Europe, surveillance alone is also accepted as safe practice. However, removal or replacement of the IUD does eradicate cytological evidence of *Actinomyces*.

Pathology

Endometritis, characterized by a plasma cell infiltration, is found in all cases of salpingitis. The tubal inflammation starts in the mucosal layer and extends to the subepithelial tissue with eventual epithelial ulceration. The pathologic spectrum of PID is quite diverse. In mild cases there may only be a mild edema and erythema of the tube. A purulent

exudate may be identified from the fimbriated end of the tube. In severe cases there may be intense congestion and fibrin deposits. The omentum can adhere to the pelvic structures, thus limiting the peritonitis to the pelvic cavity. However, generalized intraperitoneal spread of infection can occur and lead to perihepatitis (Fitz–Hugh–Curtis syndrome). Perihepatitis can also occur via a hematogenous or lymphatic pathway. Tubal damage after resolved PID can manifest itself in several ways:

- epithelial mucosal damage (deciliation);

- intraluminal adhesion formation and occlusion (proximal and/or distal);

- formation of hydrosalpinges;

- peritubal adhesions.

Genital tuberculosis

Genitourinary tuberculosis causes PID by hematogenous spread after a primary lung infection. Although uncommon, it should be considered in women from areas of the world where tuberculosis is endemic, as well as in HIV-positive patients. The primary site of genital tuberculosis is the fallopian tube. Most cases will also have endometrial and occasionally cervical spread. Most tubal infections with tuberculosis will present with chronic pelvic pain or infertility. Menstrual abnormalities can also occur. If suspected, a tuberculin test should be performed. A negative test excludes tuberculosis. If positive, an endometrial biopsy

should be performed in the week prior to menses. Histology may show granulomas and cultures are usually positive. Many cases in North America are diagnosed by serendipity in the course of an infertility evaluation by hysterosalpingography, endometrial biopsy or diagnostic laparoscopy. The latter may show extensive pelvic adhesions and peritoneal nodularity. Treatment is with standard antituberculosis medications.

Diagnosis

The physical manifestations of infection with *N. gonorrhoeae* and *C. trachomatis* in males and females are listed in Table 18.2. The primary clinical syndromes are not organism specific. The clinical criteria for diagnosing PID have not been standardized or validated in a large prospective study. The signs and symptoms are variable, may be very subtle and none are pathognomonic (Table 18.3) [17]. A comprehensive analysis of signs, symptoms and laboratory data was unable to develop an algorithm to yield a reliable clinical diagnosis of PID [18]. Of the several proposed clinical guidelines for diagnosing PID, the Centers for Disease Control and Prevention (CDC) recommendations are currently the most widely used (Box 18.1) [19]. Policies for screening for chlamydia and gonorrhea are listed in Box 18.2.

Sweet et al. [20] compiled data from their study and two earlier reports that compared laparoscopic findings in patients with clinically diagnosed PID. Of 1066 patients, 62% had laparoscopic confirmation of

Table 18.2 Gender manifestations of infection with *N. gonorrhoeae* and
C. trachomatis

	Male	Female
Most common site(s) of infection	Urethra	Cervix and urethra
Other sites	Pharynx; anus and rectum[a]	Pharynx; anus and rectum[b] Bartholin's gland
Most common symptoms	Dysuria and urethral discharge	Dysuria and vaginal discharge, menstrual disorder (e.g. menorrhagia, and intermenstrual bleeding)
Common complications	Epididymitis	Salpingitis, perihepatitis Bartholinitis, tubo-ovarian abscess
Uncommon complications	Prostatitis[c], urethral stricture[c] Disseminated gonococcus[c] Reactive arthritis and Reiter's syndrome[d]	Bartholin gland abscess Disseminated gonococcus[c]

[a]Usually in homosexual men; symptomatic if infected.
[b]Usually asymptomatic if infected.
[c]*N. gonorrhoeae* only.
[d]*C. trachomatis* only.

PID, 22% had normal findings, and 5% or less each had ovarian cysts, ectopic pregnancy, appendicitis or endometriosis. Thus, approximately one third of the patients with presumed PID would have been subjected to unnecessary antibiotic therapy. Conversely, laparoscopy for other clinical diagnoses may disclose unsuspected PID as many patients have subclinical PID with vague or very mild symptoms. These patients may not receive necessary antibiotic treatment, leaving them vulnerable to complications and long-term sequelae. 'Silent' PID can only be detected by targeted screening (Box 18.2).

Laparoscopy is the gold standard for diagnosing PID and provides for microbiologic culturing of the tubal exudate. It may be very helpful when the diagnosis is in doubt, but the cost effectiveness of its routine use in the diagnosis of PID is debated. The presence of endometritis on endometrial biopsy or a complex adnexal mass on pelvic sonography provides further support for a diagnosis of PID. Clearly, better techniques are required to improve our diagnostic accuracy and to screen asymptomatic patients at risk. Until then, it seems prudent to maintain a low threshold for initiating treatment. It should also be kept in mind that patients with PID are at risk of other STDs. In addition to cervical cultures for *N. gonorrhoeae* and *C. trachomatis*, such patients should be screened for syphilis, hepatitis and HIV, and a pap smear performed for human papilloma virus (HPV) and dysplastic changes.

Chlamydia and gonorrhea in men

The usual presentation of acute attacks in men is urethral discharge and/or dysuria. These are the features of non-specific urethritis (NSU) which in 50% of cases is chlamydial. Other causes of NSU include *Ureaplasma urealyticum* and *Trichomonas vaginalis*. Gonorrhea is more likely to present as a purulent discharge.

Treatment

Figure 18.1 Summarizes the management of PID.

Approximately 75% of PID patients are managed in an outpatient setting. Although many experts advocate inpatient management with parenteral antibiotics for all patients with PID, prospective data comparing outcomes of inpatient versus outpatient treatment are lacking. The CDC guidelines for hospital admission are as follows.

• The diagnosis is uncertain, and surgical emergencies such as appendicitis and ectopic pregnancy cannot be excluded.

Table 18.3 Clinical findings in 623 patients with laparoscopically confirmed PID

Sign/symptom	Number of patients (%)
Lower abdominal pain	585 (94)
History of vaginal discharge	340 (55)
History of fever or chills	257 (41)
Irregular bleeding	221 (36)
Urinary symptoms	116 (19)
Gastrointestinal symptoms	64 (10)
Adnexal tenderness	573 (92)
Abnormal vaginal discharge	394 (63)

Reproduced from Jacobson L, Westrom L. Objectivized diagnosis of acute PID. Diagnostic and prognostic value of routine laparoscopy. *Am J Obstet Gynecol* 1969;105:1088–98.

Box 18.1   Criteria for the clinical diagnosis of PID

Minimum criteria (all three should be present with no competing diagnosis):
• Lower abdominal tenderness
• Adnexal tenderness
• Cervical motion tenderness

Additional criteria
• Routine
  • Oral temperature >38.3°C
  • Abnormal cervical or vaginal discharge
  • Elevated erythrocyte sedimentation rate and/or C-reactive protein
• Elaborate
  • Endometritis on endometrial biopsy
  • Tubo-ovarian abscess on sonography or other radiological tests
  • Laparoscopic abnormalities consistent with PID

Modified from CDC MMWR 1993;42:1–102

• Pelvic abscess is suspected.

• The patient is pregnant.

• The patient is an adolescent.

• The patient has HIV infection.

• Severe illness or nausea and vomiting preclude outpatient management.

• The patient is unable to follow or tolerate an outpatient regimen.

• The patient has failed to respond clinically to outpatient therapy.

• Clinical follow-up within 72 h of starting antibiotic treatment cannot be arranged.

(Reproduced from Centers for Disease Control. *MMWR* 1993; 42: 75–81 [19].)

Early diagnosis and prompt treatment of PID provide the optimal chance to preserve reproductive capacity. Delaying treatment by 3 or more days after the onset of symptoms results in nearly a threefold increase in subsequent infertility [21].

Since PID is a polymicrobial infection and cultures from the upper genital tract are not easily accessible, antibiotic treatment must be of sufficiently broad spectrum to include coverage for *N. gonorrhoeae*, *C. trachomatis*, Gram-negative facultative rods, anerobes, mycoplasmas and streptococci. Several antibiotic regimens have been shown to achieve clinical resolution of PID and reversal of positive cervical cultures, but eradication of

infection from the endometrium and fallopian tubes, and reduction of late sequelae has not been adequately assessed. The current CDC recommendations for inpatient and outpatient treatment (Box 18.3) [19] remain the standard against which other regimens are compared. If a patient develops PID with an IUD in place, it should be removed after antibiotic therapy is initiated and alternative contraception provided.

Outpatients should be monitored within 72 h after initiating treatment. In the absence of clinical improvement, hospitalization is indicated to reassess the diagnosis and to begin parenteral antibiotics. Hospitalization also allows for bedrest, hydration and analgesia. Hospitalized patients who fail to improve after 48–72 h on antibiotics require further evaluation with pelvic ultrasonography and/or laparoscopy to confirm the diagnosis. Laparoscopy also allows for the drainage of purulent material, blunt lysis of the early fibrinous adhesions and copious irrigation of the peritoneal cavity. Proponents of routine laparoscopic management of PID claim more rapid clinical improvement, reduced pelvic adhesions and better preservation of fertility, although comparative studies with medical treatment have not been reported. Laparoscopy should be avoided in the presence of generalized peritonitis and/or an ileus.

TOAs develop in up to 34% of hospitalized PID patients. Medical treatment is effective in over 75% of patients. Further intervention is required for patients who do not respond adequately. If the abscess

Box 18.2   Policies for screening for chlamydia and gonorrhea

1. Target for screening
• Women with a recent change of partner/or had two or more partners in the past 12 months
• Women presenting for a termination of pregnancy
• Women <25 years of age
• Those requesting IUDs in a high prevalence area
• Young women with intermenstrual bleeding
• Contacts of cases

2. Improve technique for sample collection

3. Use ligase chain reaction/polymerase chain reaction urine testing as appropriate

4. Contact tracing essential to reduce prevalence

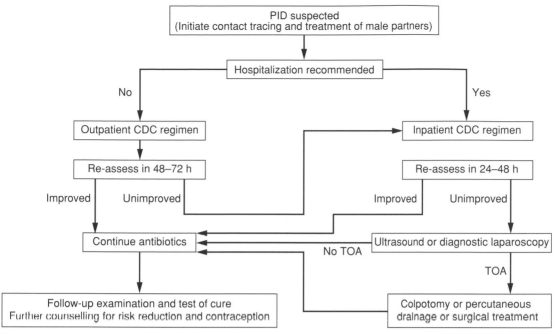

Fig. 18.1 Algorithm for the management of PID.
TOA = Tubovarian abscess.

Box 18.3   Treatment of PID

Inpatient treatment

- *Regimen A*
  Cefoxitin 2 g iv every 6 h or cefotetan 2 g iv every 12 h
  plus
  Doxycycline 100 mg iv or orally every 12 h
- *Regimen B*
  Clindamycin 900 mg iv every 8 h
  plus
  Gentamicin 2 mg/kg iv or im loading dose followed by 1.5 mg/kg
  every 8 h

Note: Both regimens should be continued for at least 48 h after the
patient demonstrates substantial clinical improvement, followed with
doxycycline 100 mg orally twice daily to complete a total of 14 days of
therapy. In regimen B, clindamycin 450 mg orally 4 times a day may be
substituted for doxycycline. Recently, the combination of
ampicillin/sulbactam was shown to be equally efficacious and better
tolerated than either of the above regimens [22].

Outpatient treatment

- *Regimen A*
  Cefoxitin 2 g im plus probenecid 1 g orally, or ceftriaxone 250 mg im
  or other parenteral third-generation cephalosporin (e.g. ceftizoxime
  or cefotaxime)
  plus
  Doxycycline 100 mg orally twice daily for 14 days
- *Regimen B*
  Ofloxacin 400 mg orally 2 times a day for 14 days
  plus
  Either clindamycin 450 mg orally 4 times a day, or metronidazole 500
  mg orally twice daily for 14 days

Modified from CDC MMWR 1993;42:75–81.

---

is fluctuant and dissecting the
rectovaginal septum, it may be
drained via a colpotomy incision.
Treatment options for other
TOAs include percutaneous
drainage under computed
tomography or ultrasound
guidance [23], and laparoscopic
drainage. Drainage of pelvic
abscess by interventional
radiology is acceptable, even if the
cause is an appendiceal abscess.
Therefore, knowledge of the
specific etiology of the pelvic
abscess is not essential before
drainage, as long as the patient
responds clinically. Adnexectomy
(unilateral for one-sided TOAs)
may be performed via laparoscopy
or laparotomy. Total abdominal
hysterectomy with bilateral
salpingo–oophorectomy (TAH–
BSO) is reserved for patients with
severe disease who are no longer
desirous of future childbearing.
Approximately 3–15% of TOAs
rupture, creating a life-threatening
surgical emergency for which

TAH-BSO has long been the standard treatment. In recent years, more conservative fertility-preserving surgery has been shown to be effective [24].

Following effective inpatient or outpatient treatment, some authorities advise sexual abstinence for at least 6 weeks. A test of cure should be performed 1 week after treatment if a culture test is used, or after 3 weeks if the more sensitive polymerase (PCR) or ligase chain reaction (LCR) assays are employed. All male partners should be tested for *N. gonorrhoeae* and *C. trachomatis*. Over half will test positive and approximately 50% will be asymptomatic [19]. They should all be treated empirically with ceftriaxone 125 mg intramuscularly then doxycycline 100 mg orally twice daily for 7 days, regardless of symptomatology or culture status.

Principles of counseling

Prevention is the fundamental basis of counseling. Patient education is the most important tool to achieve this goal. Knowledge of high-risk sexual behavior and adoption of a preventative health behavior can be achieved through public awareness programs as well as individual counseling.

The components of public awareness programs are as follows:

- the prevalence of STD;
- the potential for serious consequences;
- high-risk sexual behavior;
- seeking medical evaluation promptly;

- emphasizing the importance of barrier methods (condoms).

The patient who has been treated for PID should be counseled as to the risk of recurrence, possible sequelae to the infection, as well as the following issues:

- identification and treatment of sexual partners;
- discuss medication, dosage, length of treatment and side effects;
- avoidance of sex while infectious or if symptoms recur;
- avoidance of sex with partner until he is treated;
- assure follow-up;
- adoption of low-risk sexual behavior, including use of condoms;
- discuss recurrence;
- discuss long-term sequelae: infertility, ectopic pregnancy and chronic pelvic pain.

There is a high rate of recurrence of PID. Specific rates are difficult to obtain, especially with the trend towards outpatient treatment. However, it is estimated that one third of patients will have a second episode of PID. The second and subsequent episodes are less likely to recover gonorrhea or chlamydia from the sites of infection. Prevention of recurrence assumes proper identification and treatment of sexual partners. Patient responsibility assumes that she will play a role in contact tracing with the healthcare professional. Since the desired result is the

treatment of all infected partners, the particular situation will dictate the degree of involvement of the patient and doctor. This should be explicitly detailed and specific time limits discussed. Test of cure cultures for patients with PID are recommended.

The risk of recurrence can be diminished by adopting low-risk sexual behaviors that will decrease the probability of reinfection with an STD. Although abstinence and fidelity of both partners are clearly ideal behaviors to avoid STD, they are unlikely to be an effective strategy. Therefore, the adoption of low-risk sexual behavior, such as the use of condoms, should be implemented. The value of routine screening for cervical *Chlamydia* infection in a high-risk group of patients has been demonstrated [25]. The number of cases of PID can be reduced significantly by implementing this strategy. Strategies to combat the global threat of sexually transmitted infections are as follows [26]:

- syndromic treatment for those with symptoms and signs of infection;
- screening for those without symptoms;
- STD risk assessment to guide contraceptive counseling;
- dual protection in family planning programs.

Sequelae of PID

Infertility

STDs are not a common cause of infertility in men, in contrast to women. The dramatic increase in infertility is attributed to a significant degree, to the increase in prevalence of STDs. PID will cause tissue damage with pronounced deciliation of the tubal epithelium. This is often accompanied by tubo–ovarian adhesions and distal tubal obstruction. Unfortunately, previous asymptomatic PID is a common cause of this tubal-factor infertility [27]. In one series, only 25% of patients with tubal-factor infertility at the time of diagnostic laparoscopy for infertility had a history of PID. There was a high prevalence of chlamydial antibodies despite the lack of previous symptoms of PID [28].

Westrom et al. [29] have documented the close association between salpingitis and infertility. They showed that the infertility rate increased with the number of episodes of acute PID. It was predicted that tubal-factor infertility occurred in 10% of patients after one episode of PID, 20% after a second episode and 40% after a third episode. The following factors modified these figures:

- the number and severity of PID episodes;
- the age of the patient;
- the choice of contraceptive method;
- delay of treatment.

Increasing age and severity of disease are associated with a higher probability of infertility. The use of oral contraceptives may be associated with a lower incidence and milder form of PID and consequently, lower rates of tubal-factor infertility

[30]. The fact that delay in treatment is associated with a higher incidence of tubal-factor infertility emphasizes the need for a high index of suspicion, especially in the patients with risk factors. The type of organism that is isolated with PID does not appear to influence the incidence of infertility.

Ectopic pregnancy

The increase in incidence of ectopic pregnancy has mirrored the increase in incidence of acute PID and STD. As discussed above, acute PID is associated with damage to the tube, including loss of cilia. Ciliary movement contributes to the orderly movement of the zygote towards the uterus. It is presumed that, when there is no overt disease, there is still ciliary damage that predisposes to ectopic pregnancy. Westrom et al. [29] have shown that the risk was related to the number of episodes of PID with 6% after the first episode, 12% after two episodes and 22% after three or more episodes.

Chronic pelvic pain

Pelvic adhesions and distorted pelvic anatomy are common causes of chronic pelvic pain. High rates of surgical intervention, such as multiple laparoscopies for adhesiolysis, are reported in these patients. The prevalence of chronic pelvic pain is reported to be approximately 20% after a history of treated PID [31]. This rate is modified by the number and severity of PID episodes.

Perinatal complications

include preterm rupture of membranes and neonatal conjunctivitis.

Future developments

These fall mainly in the sphere of prevention and screening:

- Aggressive dissemination of information through public awareness programs. Access to the Internet may assist this process.
- This information should focus on safe sex practices, as well as results of surveillance programs.
- Improved screening programs to detect asymptomatic cervical carriers of STD.
- Development of better detection methods of asymptomatic patients with PID. PCR/LCR techniques are 100% sensitive and can be carried out on urine samples.

Tips for safe practice

- Maintain knowledge base of STD trends.
- Update knowledge of recent treatments of PID.
- Assess patient risk factors/case finding.
- Maintain a high index of suspicion; diagnose and treat quickly.
- Apply aggressive follow-up and treatment of sexual partners.
- Arrange for appropriate counseling/education.
- Prevent re-exposure.

Resource list

- Patient education pamphlets on PID, and another on gonorrhea and chlamydia, can be obtained at this address: American College of Obstetricians and Gynecologists, 409 12th Street SW, Washington, DC, 20024–2188, USA.

- Recommendations on current PID treatment can be obtained from:
  - Morbidity and Mortality Weekly Report, Massachusetts Medical Society, PO Box 9120, Waitham, MA 02254–9120, USA.
  - The UK Women's Health, 52–54 Featherstone Street, London ECIY 8RT, UK. (Tel. 0207–251–6580

- Information leaflets provided to the public

Appendix 1

Toxic shock syndrome (TSS)

TSS is an acute multisystem disorder caused by a toxin-producing strain of *Staphylococcus aureus*. The most commonly isolated toxin is called TSST-1. A peak in incidence occurred in 1980–1 with the introduction of a new hyperabsorbable tampon on the market. The onset of disease was mainly during menses. Removal of that particular brand of tampon has decreased the incidence of disease and increased the relative frequency of the non-menstrual type of TSS. These include postpartum patients, post-cesarean section, post-abdominal surgery and post-abortal cases [32]. It is presumed that, in these patients, the infection is acquired in hospital. The clinical profile of menstrual-associated TSS is:

- elevated temperature (>38.9°C);
- systolic blood pressure less than 90 mmHg;
- erythematous rash with a desquamative reaction 1–2 weeks later;
- multiorgan involvement (gastrointestinal, muscular, mucous membranes, kidney and liver failure, blood and central nervous system).

Diagnosis of TSS requires a high index of suspicion and exclusion of Rocky Mountain spotted fever, leptospirosis and measles. Management consists of aggressive fluid management, removal of the tampon and vaginal culture for *Staphylococcus*. Antibiotics should be initiated with a beta-lactamase-resistant penicillin. Recurrence is unusual after antibiotic treatment and cessation of tampon use.

Appendix 2

Perioperative antibiotic prophylaxis

The generally accepted concept of perioperative antibiotics to prevent wound infections is dependent on the presence of adequate tissue levels at the time of incision (skin or vagina). Most infections after gynecological procedures arise from bacteria, which are generally present in the vagina. Therefore, antibiotics, such as a first-generation cephalosporin (cefazolin 1 g iv) are acceptable [33]. Patients allergic to penicillin can be given vancomycin. One dose 30 min preoperatively followed by additional doses intraoperatively for procedures longer than 4 hours is usually adequate. Prolonged use of the antibiotic is the major problem with 'prophylactic' antibiotics because of the potential to select for resistant micro-organisms.

In high-risk patients for PID (see above) who are undergoing a first-trimester therapeutic abortion, doxycycline should be given (100 mg 1 h before and 200 mg 30 min after the procedure) [33]. Penicillin G one million units can also be used. Second-trimester abortion patients should receive cefazolin 1 g iv.

References

1. Jones OG, Saida AA, St John RK. Frequency and distribution of salpingitis and pelvic inflammatory disease in short stay hospitals in the USA. *Am J Obstet Gynecol* 1980;138:905–9.

2. Rolfs RT, Galaid EI, Zaidi AA: PID: trends in hospitalizations and office visits, 1979 through 1988. *Am J Obstet Gynecol* 1992;166:983–90.

3. Washington AE, Katz P. Cost of and payment source for PID: trends and projections, 1983 through 2000. *JAMA* 1991; 266:2565–9.

4. Washington AE, Aral SO, Wolner-Hanssen P, Grimes DA, Holmes KK. Assessing risk for pelvic inflammatory disease and its sequelae. *JAMA* 1991; 266:2581–6.

5. Rowe PJ. You win some and you lose some: contraception and infection. *Aust NZ J Obstet Gynaecol* 1994;34:299–305.

6. Sinei SKA, Schulz KF, Lamptey PR, et al. Preventing IUCD-related pelvic infection: the efficacy of prophylactic doxycycline at insertion. *Br J Obstet Gynaecol* 1990;97:412–19.

7. Soper DE, Brockwell NJ, Dalton HP, Johnson D. Observations concerning the microbial etiology of acute salpingitis. *Am J Obstet Gynecol* 1004; 170:1008–17.

8. Patton DL, Halbert SA, Kuo CC, Wang SP, Holmes KK. Host response to primary *C. trachomatis* infection of the fallopian tube in pig-tailed monkeys. *Fertil Steril* 1983;40:829–40.

9. Patton DL, Kuo CC, Wang SP, Halbert SA. Distal obstruction induced by repeated *C. trachomatis* salpingeal infection in pig-tailed macaques. *J Infect Dis* 1987;155:1292–9.

10. Witkin SS, Jeremias J, Toth M, Ledger WJ. Cell mediated immune response to the recombinant 57 KD heat shock protein of *C. trachomatis* in women with salpingitis. *J Infect Dis* 1993;167:1379–83.

11. Hook EW, Reichart CA, Upchurch DM, et al. Comparative behavioral epidemiology of gonococcal and chlamydial infections among patients attending a Baltimore Maryland, STD clinic. *Am J Epidemiol* 1992;136:662–72.

12. Nettleman MD, Jones RB, Roberts SD, et al. Cost effectiveness of culturing for *C. trachomatis*. A study in a clinic for STD. *Ann Intern Med* 1986; 105:189–96.

13. Sackel SG, Alpert S, Fiunara NJ, et al. Orogenital contact and the isolation of *N. gonorrhea*, *Mycoplasma hominis* and *Ureaplasma urealyticum* from the pharynx. *Sex Transm Dis* 1979;6:64–68.

14. Westrom L. Incidence, prevalence and trends of acute PID and its consequences in industrialized countries. *Am J Obstet Gynecol* 1980; 138:880–92.

15. Kessel E. PID with intrauterine device use: a reassessment. *Fertil Steril* 1989;51:1–11.

16. Lee NC, Rubin GL, Borucki R. The intrauterine device and PID revisited. New results from the Women's Health study. *Obstet Gynecol* 1988;72:1–6.

17. Jacobson L, Westrom L. Objectivized diagnosis of acute PID. Diagnostic and prognostic value of routine laparoscopy. *Am J Obstet Gynecol* 1969; 105:1088–98.

18. Kahn JG, Walker CG, Washington AE, et al. Diagnosing pelvic inflammatory disease. A comprehensive analysis and considerations for developing a model. *JAMA* 1991;266:2594–604.

19. Centres for Disease Control. 1993 Sexually Transmitted Diseases treatment guidelines. *MMWR* 1993;42:75–81.

20. Sweet RL, Mills J, Hadley KW, et al. Use of laparoscopy to determine the microbiologic etiology of acute salpingitis. *Am J Obstet Gynecol* 1979;134:68–74.

21. Hillis SD, Joesoef R, Marchbanks PA, Wasserheit JN, Willard C, Westrom L. Delayed care of PID as a risk factor for impaired fertility. *Am J Obstet Gynecol* 1993;168:1503–9.

22. McGregor JA, Crombleholme WR, Newton E, Sweet RL, Tuomala R, Gibbs RS. Randomized comparison of ampicillin-sulbactam to cefoxitin and doxycycline or clindamycin and gentamicin in the treatment of PID or endometritis. *Obstet Gynecol* 1994;83:998–1004.

23. Casola G, vanSonnenberg E, D'Agostino HB, et al. Percutaneous drainage of tubo-ovarian abscesses. *Radiology* 1992;182:399–402.

24. Rivlin ME, Hunt JA. Ruptured tubo-ovarian abscess: is hysterectomy necessary? *Obstet Gynecol* 1977;50(S):518–22.

25. Scholes D, Stergachis A, Heidrich F, Andulla H, Holmes KK, Stamm WE. Prevention of PID by screening for cervical chlamydia infection. *N Engl J Med* 1996;334:1362–6.

26. Cates W. How much do condoms protect against sexually transmitted diseases? *IPPF Med Bull* 1997;31:2–3.

27. Rosenfeld LD, Seidman SM, Bronson RA, Scholl GM. Unsuspected chronic pelvic inflammatory disease in the infertile female. *Fertil Steril* 1983;39:44–8.

28. Sellors JW, Mahony GB, Chernesky MA, Roth DJ. Tubal factor infertility. An association with prior chlamydial infection and asymptomatic salpingitis. *Fertil Steril* 1988;49:451–7.

29. Westrom LV, Joesoef R, Reynolds G. PID with infertility. A cohort of 1,844 women with laparoscopically verified disease and 657 control women with normal laparoscopy results. *Sex Transm Dis* 1992;19:185–92.

30. Svensson L, Mardh PA, Westrom L. Infertility after acute

salpingitis with special reference
to *C. trachomatis. Fertil Steril*
1983;40:322–9.

31. Safrin S, Schachter J, Dahrouge
D, Sweet R. Long-term sequelae
of acute pelvic inflammatory

disease. *Am J Obstet Gynecol*
1992;166:1300–5.

32. Karin KC, Schulzer M, Chow
AW. Clinical spectrum of
nonmenstrual toxic shock
syndrome (TSS): comparison

with menstrual TSS by
multivariate discriminant analyses.
Clin Infect Dis 1993;16:100.

33. Antimicrobial prophylaxis in
surgery. *Med Lett Group Ther*
1992;34:5.

HIV and AIDS

Valerie S Kitchen FRCP

Introduction

The acquired immunodeficiency syndrome (AIDS) is caused by infection with the human immunodeficiency virus (HIV). Most HIV disease is caused by HIV 1; HIV 2 is essentially confined to West Africa. Three routes of viral transmission are now recognized: (1) sexual transmission through either anal or vaginal intercourse; (2) parenteral transmission as a result of transfusion of infected blood products; and (3) perinatal transmission from mother to child. When AIDS was first described in the early 1980s, it was initially thought to occur exclusively in male homosexuals but the disease was then quite quickly diagnosed in other risk groups, namely haemophiliacs and intravenous drug users, and their female sexual partners.

In the 1990s, approximately 70% of infections worldwide are acquired heterosexually and, correspondingly, increasing numbers of women are becoming infected. It is estimated that 40% of adult infections occur in women at the present time, with women comprising approximately 10–20% of the infected population in North America and Europe, and about 50% of adults infected in sub-Saharan Africa. The US

Centers for Disease Control and Prevention (CDC) ranks AIDS as the third leading cause of death among American women aged 25–44 years. In the UK, new cases of HIV infection continue to rise, although at a rate lower than the projections of the mid-1980s.

The majority of infected women are young adults and many are parents. In view of this and the fact that most infected individuals are asymptomatic and unaware of their HIV status, they are at risk of transmitting the infection to their sexual partners and to their children. Early diagnosis provides an opportunity to interrupt horizontal and vertical transmission, and also allows appropriate therapy to be instigated in order to delay disease progression. Box 19.1 provides information about the HIV test.

Pathogenesis of HIV infection

HIV is a retrovirus which predominantly infects CD4-positive T lymphocytes and macrophages. Like all other retroviruses, HIV transcribes its genetic material, which exists in the form of RNA, to DNA by the action of the viral enzyme, reverse transcriptase. In this way, the genetic material of the virus is incorporated into the infected cells as proviral DNA and this becomes a component of the host cell genome. Here it remains latent prior to cell activation, when DNA transcription to viral RNA leads to the production of viral progeny and consequently the infection of further CD4+ lymphocytes and macrophages, leading to their eventual destruction and depletion.

Box 19.1   The HIV test

- Pretest counselling can be done by a knowledgeable primary care physician, gynaecologist or staff within Sexual Health Services.
- The test picks up an HIV antibody response usually within 3 months after exposure. It would not exclude infection from more recent exposure.
- A practitioner should keep a record of the test. If the patient objects, he or she is best tested in a specialist facility e.g. a Genito-Urinary Medicine Clinic.
- Discuss the potential benefits to the patient of HIV testing. If negative – reassurance and discussion about risk reduction. If positive – prevention of sexual transmission, prevention of mother/child transmission and access to affected therapy.
- A person newly diagnosed with HIV infection needs appropriate support personally and in terms of breaking the news to others who may be infected also.

Following initial infection, HIV spreads to the regional lymph nodes and thence to circulating immune cells and the thymus. The acute viraemia that follows initial infection provokes a host immune response that leads to containment of viral load and the production of anti-HIV antibodies. Initially it was thought that viral replication was low during the clinically latent period following seroconversion, but recent studies of viral dynamics suggest that viral production is active and extensive from the onset of infection, with the production of 10^9 viral progeny per day, and the loss and subsequent replacement of similar numbers of CD4+ lymphocytes. Over time, however, there is a gradual attrition of CD4+ cell numbers. Acceleration of CD4+ cell loss reflects an increase in viral load and heralds the onset of symptomatic disease and AIDS (Figure 19.1).

Clinical features of HIV infection

Seroconversion to HIV-antibody positivity usually occurs between 3 and 12 weeks after infection, and in a proportion of individuals (approximately 50%) is accompanied by a glandular fever-like illness, characterized by a truncal maculopapular rash, fever and generalized lymphadenopathy. Other features may include a sore throat, aseptic meningitis and mucosal ulceration in the mouth, pharynx or genital region. The CD4+ cell count during seroconversion may be sufficiently low for opportunistic infections such as oral candidiasis and *Pneumocystis carinii* pneumonia to occur prior to immune containment with subsequent rebound in CD4+ cell numbers, sometimes to transiently supranormal levels.

This self-limiting illness is followed by an asymptomatic period of variable duration (2–15 years), with approximately 50% of patients progressing to AIDS within 10 years of infection. During this clinically latent period, a large proportion of those infected will have persistent generalized lymphadenopathy (PGL) but in some there will be no evidence of HIV infection on examination. The first evidence of immunosuppression may be the development of shingles, recurrent and/or severe episodes of genital herpes, recalcitrant genital wart virus infection or recurrent oral and/or vaginal candidiasis. Some individuals present with unexplained fevers, weight loss and/or diarrhoea – clinical features which represent a condition known as AIDS-related complex (ARC), a forerunner to the development of AIDS. The diagnosis of AIDS is defined by the occurrence of one of a designated list of opportunistic infections and malignancies first drawn up by CDC Atlanta in 1987 and later revised in 1992 [1]. Box 19.2 lists AIDS-defining conditions. This revised AIDS definition also includes the laboratory finding of a CD4+ lymphocyte count less than 200 per µl, an inclusion criterion that is now widely used in the USA, but one that has been slow to gain acceptance in Europe.

Management principles

At present there is no cure for HIV infection and currently prospects for an effective vaccine in the medium term are bleak. However, it is now clear that disease progression can be delayed, and both survival and quality of life improved significantly by combination antiretroviral therapy and prophylaxis against common life-threatening opportunistic infections, notably *Pneumocystis carinii* pneumonia (PCP) (see 'Maternal disease' and 'Mother to child transmission'). Median survival following diagnosis of AIDS is about 20 months in those receiving treatment [2]. The principle of drug therapy of HIV

Fig. 19.1 Natural history of HIV infection.

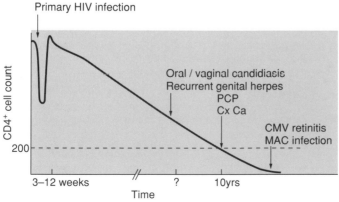

PCP = *Pneumocystis carinii* pneumonia; CaCx = carcinoma of the cervix; CMV = cytomegalovirus; MAC = *Mycobacterium avium* complex.

Box 19.2 AIDS-defining conditions
- Kaposi's sarcoma
- Non-Hodgkins lymphoma
- *Pneumocystis carinii* pneumonia
- Systemic candidiasis
- Tuberculosis
- Cryptococcal meningitis
- HIV-related dementia
- CMV retinitis
- Primary cerebral lymphoma
- Carcinoma of the cervix

infection is to reduce viral load. Three categories of drugs are available, nucleoside analogues, protease inhibitors and non-nucleoside reverse transcriptase inhibitors.

Every opportunity should be taken to give advice on prevention of HIV transmission, including the avoidance of high-risk activities such as unprotected vaginal or anal intercourse (see 'Contraception' and 'Planned pregnancies in discordant couples'), and in the case of intravenous drug users, the sharing of needles and syringes. In addition, where appropriate, women should be given relevant information with regard to maternal health and the prevention of mother to child transmission (see below).

It is important to remember that HIV infection is a sexually transmitted disease, and patients should therefore be screened for the presence of other, more common infections of this type, such as gonorrhoea, chlamydil infection, syphilis and hepatitis B. In addition, cervical cytology screening should be undertaken annually in HIV infection, in view of the increased risk of cervical intraepithelial neoplasia (CIN) developing as a result of HIV-related immunosuppression [3] (see 'Cervical intraepithelial neoplasia').

Patients often require additional support and counselling which should be linked to their medical care. In particular, they may welcome advice and practical help in informing sexual partners of their diagnosis, and provision should be made for partners to attend for counselling and testing if required.

Gynaecological issues

Vulvovaginal infections

Vulvovaginal infections are a common and troublesome feature of HIV infection. Recurrent, severe vaginal candidiasis often occurs as the first manifestation of HIV disease in women and should alert the clinician to the possibility of HIV infection. Treatment in the first instance should be with intermittent topical antifungal pessaries. Intermittent oral azole therapy is indicated when topical therapy has proven unsuccessful. The use of long-term systemic antifungal prophylaxis should now be avoided as this has led to the development of fungal resistance, which presents an increasing clinical problem in later stage disease and one that is made worse by improved survival.

Herpes simplex (HSV) and human papilloma viruses (HPV) may evade immune control and cause persistent lesions; as HIV infection progresses these may prove resistant to standard management. Where recurrent episodes of genital herpes are frequent and/or prolonged, it may be appropriate to consider long-term prophylaxis with aciclovir at a dose of 400 mg twice daily. Aciclovir-resistant HSV mutants have been occasionally described in patients with AIDS and may respond to treatment with intravenous foscarnet sodium.

Vulval genital warts should be treated aggressively, preferably with electrocautery to prevent the development of large confluent areas of disease which then require surgical excision or, excision by high-frequency ultrasound.

Pelvic inflammatory disease (PID)

It has been suggested that PID is more common in women with HIV infection than in the population at large. To some degree this may reflect the fact that both infections are sexually transmitted. However, HIV infection may affect the course of PID. In one study, HIV-positive women were more likely to develop tubo-ovarian abscesses and require surgical drainage than their seronegative counterparts [4]. The management of PID in the context of HIV disease should include administration of intravenous antibiotics with activity against *C. trachomatis*, *N. gonorrhoeae* and anaerobic bacteria. Care should be taken to treat the sexual partner appropriately in order to avoid reinfection, and advice regarding condom use should be reinforced.

Cervical intraepithelial neoplasia

Current estimates suggest that HIV seropositive women have a tenfold increased risk of developing CIN in comparison to that seen in the general population [5]. This increased risk is seen in women with HIV infection who are immunosuppressed, supporting the hypothesis that the immunodeficiency rather than HIV itself is the predisposing factor for the development of cervical neoplasia in these individuals [3]. In recognition of this association, cervical cancer was added to the revised list of AIDS-defining conditions drawn up by CDC Atlanta in 1992 [1]. In patients with early HIV disease, cervical cytology screening should be undertaken annually, but with the development of significant immunosuppression, screening should take place at 6-monthly intervals and should incorporate colposcopy in view of the increased risk of multifocal disease [6].

Treatment of CIN in HIV-infected individuals is by loop diathermy excision of the transformation zone, a procedure which is best performed in the controlled environment of the operating room to reduce infection risk to healthcare personnel. Overt cervical neoplasia should be treated aggressively and HIV disease *per se* should not be considered a contraindication to surgery [7]. A higher than average recurrence rate of CIN is seen in HIV infection and 6-monthly review following treatment is therefore recommended [8].

Menstrual function

Anecdotal reports have suggested that HIV-seropositive women are at increased risk of menorrhagia, oligomenorrhoea and amenorrhoea. However, intravenous drug use, methadone maintenance therapy, oral ketoconazole and weight loss are all independently associated with oligomenorrhoea and amenorrhoea. The only controlled study to take account of these confounding variables showed no difference in menstrual function between women who were infected with HIV and those who were not, regardless of the degree of immunosuppression [9]

A further study of endocrine function showed no difference in hypothalamo-pituitary function between HIV-seropositive and HIV-seronegative women. However, a trend was seen between HIV-related immunosuppression and raised follicle-stimulating hormone (FSH) and reduced oestradiol (E2) levels (features of a premature menopause) [8].

Contraception

Firstly, it is important not to assume that HIV infection will necessarily lead to a decision to avoid pregnancy (see 'Planned pregnancy in discordant couples'). However, those keen to pursue pregnancy should be fully informed with regard to the relevant risks (see 'Maternal disease' and 'Mother to child transmission'). Where contraception is required, the need to reduce the risk of sexual transmission of HIV infection should be stressed and the contraceptive method selected accordingly. The risk of sexual transmission of HIV infection from male to female is approximately twice that of female to male in Europe [10], whereas in sub-Saharan Africa the ratio is approximately equal [11].

Barrier methods

Patients should be advised that the male condom used together with a water-based lubricant throughout intercourse provides excellent protection against the sexual transmission of HIV. Great care should be taken in the case of anal intercourse as condom breakage occurs more frequently than during vaginal intercourse – the use of thicker latex condoms should be advised.

Male (and female) condoms, when used *consistently* and *correctly*, offer reliable protection against both pregnancy and sexually transmitted infections (STIs); the latter include gonorrhoea, non-gonococcal urethritis and, more importantly, HIV as recently reviewed by Cates [12]. Cates was impressed by work on HIV-discordant couples even with typical imperfect use of condoms. He concludes that, while sexual abstinence is risk-free, the use of condoms reduces by 70% the total risk between unprotected sex and abstinence. The 30%

failure reflects the cumulative condom failure over time.

The recently introduced female condom provides a female-controlled method of contraception which has similar contraceptive efficacy to the male condom, based on a limited number of studies. It is likely with correct use to have similar efficacy against HIV transmission, although at present there are no data published to support this view. The use of other female-controlled barrier methods, namely the cap or diaphragm, should not be advised as an appropriate method to reduce the risk of HIV transmission, as it is not yet known whether infection can occur across intact vaginal epithelium.

The intrauterine contraceptive device (IUD)

The IUD is contraindicated in HIV infection owing to its association with an increased risk of PID immediately post-insertion. PID, increased duration or volume of menstrual bleeding, and the risk of micro-abrasions to the penis may facilitate HIV transmission.

Hormonal methods

Cervical ectropion associated with the use of the combined oral contraceptive may render women more vulnerable to infection [13], and predisposes to bleeding on intercourse, which may facilitate female to male transmission. Progestogen-only preparations may theoretically lead to increased susceptibility to HIV acquisition as a result of vaginal mucosal thinning and frequent bleeding, although amenorrhoea is an advantage in users of depot medroxy progesterone acetate (DMPA). If hormonal methods are used in the context of HIV infection, the additional use of condoms for every episode of intercourse should be stressed. Where the oral contraceptive pill is prescribed in HIV disease, it is important to recognize the risk of potential drug interactions with the instigation of HIV-related therapy.

Spermicides

There is *in vitro* evidence that some spermicidal agents are capable of inactivating HIV. Nonoxynol-9 (N9) is the most extensively investigated agent of this type. At present, results of clinical trials investigating the efficacy of this compound in HIV prevention are contradictory; some studies suggest a reduction in transmission risk [14,15], whilst others have suggested that N9, being a detergent, when used frequently at high dose, may lead to vaginal epithelial disruption which may facilitate HIV transmission [16]. The use of N9 as a means of preventing HIV transmission cannot, therefore, be recommended at the present time (see 'Vaginal microbicides'). However, there is some evidence for a protective effect against *N.gonorrhoea* and *C.trachomatis*, and thus may reduce HIV risk indirectly.

Infertility

Women with HIV infection suffering from infertility present complex dilemmas in terms of their optimal management [17]. Patients often find it reassuring to know the reason for their infertility, although once a diagnosis is made, most gynaecologists feel unable to participate in active management because of the risk of vertical transmission, and the ethical and potential legal issues surrounding their involvement in the birth of an infected child.

Obstetric issues

Planned pregnancy in discordant couples

The desire for pregnancy in couples where one partner is HIV infected presents particular problems, as the couple's wishes need to be considered in the light of reducing the risk of HIV transmission to the uninfected partner and to the unborn child.

Positive woman–negative man

Artificial insemination by the husband (AIH) should be considered as a means of preventing exposure of the uninfected male to potentially infectious cervicovaginal secretions. However, if the couple insist on pursuing unprotected vaginal intercourse as a means of achieving pregnancy, they should be strongly advised to limit such exposure to the most fertile time of the menstrual cycle.

Positive man–negative woman

Under these circumstances, unprotected intercourse will put the female at risk of infection. Furthermore, if the female partner seroconverts at around the time of conception, the fetus may be at increased risk of acquiring HIV as a result of the high viral load that accompanies primary infection. Artificial insemination with donor sperm (AID) should be considered as a safe alternative in this setting. If this is not acceptable, then, once again, the couple should be encouraged to have unprotected intercourse only during the time of ovulation.

The possibility of 'sperm washing' as a means of removing HIV-infected lymphocytes from seminal fluid and thereby reducing the risk of male to female transmission where pregnancy is the goal, is currently under investigation [18]. It is as yet too early to determine the efficacy of this method. However over 200 women have now received a total of over 600 artificial inseminations and no seroconversions to date (E. Semprini, personal communication). It could be argued, therefore, that this method appears to be at least as safe as unprotected sex, where the risk is estimated at 1 in 500 sexual encounters. If pregnancy is achieved, the woman should be offered HIV testing at 12 weeks' gestation in order for her to consider the possible interventions available if she is found to be infected (see 'Mother to child transmission'). In women who test negative with a continuing pregnancy, repeat serological testing should be offered in the third trimester in order to inform decisions with regard to mode of delivery and breastfeeding (see 'Mother to child transmission').

Antenatal HIV testing

It is well-recognized that in the absence of routine antenatal HIV testing, a large proportion of HIV-seropositive women will remain undiagnosed [19]. However, until recently there has been a great deal of reluctance on the part of many midwives and obstetricians to instigate a policy of routine testing, with the need for complex and time-consuming pretest counselling being stressed as a prerequisite for such testing to be conducted. There is now, however, increasing recognition that a great deal can be gained from such a policy in the light of the fact that it may be possible to reduce the risk of vertical transmission to less than 2% (see 'Mother to child transmission') [20]. Appropriate information must be given by suitably trained personnel prior to testing, and the necessary support should be readily available for those found to be infected [21]. With the provision of these features it may be appropriate to offer an 'opt-out' in place of the previous 'opt-in' policy, which resulted in unacceptably high rates of vertical transmission, and of maternal morbidity and mortality [22]. Some women who discover they are infected with HIV early in pregnancy will decide after appropriate counselling to terminate the pregnancy. However, current evidence suggests that the majority decide against the option of therapeutic abortion under these circumstances (D. Gibb, personal communication).

Practitioners who argue against routine HIV testing antenatally do so largely on the grounds that those found to be infected may be subject to discrimination and believe that, on balance, there is little to be gained for the individual by adopting such a policy. However, this latter view was more appropriate to the early days of the epidemic when little or nothing (other than termination) could be offered and when fear on the part of the healthcare worker may have led to prejudicial treatment of those found to be infected.

Confidentiality is extremely important but should not lead to a circumstance whereby those immediately involved in the care of the HIV-infected woman remain ignorant of her serostatus, as this is not in the interest of her optimum care.

It should be stressed that routine antenatal HIV testing in no way precludes the need for a universal infection control policy, which is required for the protection of staff and patients alike from the risk of transmission of all blood-borne pathogens, including HIV.

It has been suggested that routine antenatal testing becomes appropriate where seroprevalence rates of HIV in the population exceed 1 in 1000 [23]. However, as HIV antibody tests are now highly sensitive and specific, and many urban areas of industrialized countries have seroprevalence rates in excess of those quoted, it seems likely that HIV testing will in due course become absorbed into the battery of antenatal tests currently offered.

Maternal disease

The antenatal care of the HIV-infected pregnant woman is best provided jointly by her physician and obstetrician, who should liaise closely on management issues throughout her pregnancy. The frequency with which she should be seen by her physician during this period will depend to some degree on the stage of her disease. Where there is evidence of clinically significant immunosuppression, 4–6 weekly medical review is likely, and therapeutic intervention may be required to reduce the risk of disease progression and opportunistic infection. It is generally considered appropriate to instigate antiretroviral therapy to reduce the risk of maternal disease progression when the CD4+ lymphocyte count is in the region of 200 per µl or less. However, earlier antiretroviral therapy is now commonly offered as this has been associated with a marked reduction in vertical HIV transmission (see 'Mother to child transmission'). At present the data on the use of antiretroviral drugs in pregnancy are limited. Where clinical experience exists it is mostly of zidovudine. This agent is now licensed for use in pregnancy, and to date it has not been associated with abnormalities in the newborn other than occasional reports of transient anaemia [24]. Prophylaxis against the common, life-threatening opportunistic infection, *Pneumocystis carinii* pneumonia should be started when the CD4+ lymphocyte count is in the region of 200 per µl, as the risk to both mother and fetus from the fever and hypoxia associated with this condition considerably outweighs the risk to the fetus from the prophylactic regimen.

There are no data available from appropriately controlled studies to suggest that the course of HIV disease is accelerated by pregnancy. Common recurrent genital infections seen in pregnancy, such as vaginal candidiasis and genital herpes, are likely to be more troublesome and severe in the presence of HIV disease.

Mother to child transmission

The World Health Organization (WHO) currently estimate that, of the 21 million individuals worldwide thought to be infected with HIV, approximately 2 million are children who have acquired the infection from their mothers. The risk of vertical transmission is usually quoted as being approximately 15% in Europe, 25% in the USA and 30% in Africa [25]. Three modes of vertical transmission are recognized: (1) *in utero* as a result of HIV transmission across the placenta; (2) intrapartum following contact of the fetus with infected cervicovaginal secretions and maternal blood; and (3) postpartum as a result of breastfeeding.

Risks and interventions for vertical transmission

In utero
HIV infection has been detected in fetuses aborted as early as a week's gestation, providing good evidence that, although apparently unusual, transplacental infection does occur [26]. In contrast to this finding, placental infection is a not infrequent occurrence and it has been argued that the placenta often functions as a barrier to fetal infection unless disturbed [25]. Serum viral load studies have not shown any specific level which is associated with vertical transmission. However, there is good evidence for increased transmission of HIV where the mother has advanced HIV disease [27]. No fetal syndrome has been shown to be associated with HIV infection.

Intrapartum
It is now widely accepted that the greatest risk of vertical transmission occurs during labour and delivery (50–70%) [28]. This view is supported by the finding that HIV can be detected in the cervicovaginal secretions of up to 50% of infected women [29] and data showing that duration of membrane rupture greater than 4 h is associated with transmission [30]. Added to this is the evidence from a meta-analysis of data from a number of studies showing a reduction in transmission risk for those infants delivered by elective caesarean section (ELCS) [31]. This risk may be further reduced by the use of a 'bloodless' operative technique [32]. Prompt washing of the baby and suction to remove infected serosanguinous secretions is advised. A study of birth canal cleansing with chlorhexidine solution at the onset of labour suggested a reduction of HIV transmission where membrane rupture had occurred more than 4 h before delivery (see vaginal microbicides).

Postpartum
It has been shown that an additional risk of vertical transmission of approximately 14% (95% CI 7–21) is conferred by breastfeeding [33]. The risk is considered to be greatest with high circulating maternal viral load. The current advice of the WHO is that, where formula

feeding can be undertaken safely and is sustainable, this should replace breastfeeding in the context of HIV infection [34].

Antiretroviral therapy

It is now clear that zidovudine therapy given during pregnancy after the first trimester, and to the infant for 6 weeks postdelivery, can reduce vertical transmission by two-thirds (from 25% to 8%) [24]. Where women have had prolonged exposure to zidovudine prior to pregnancy, viral resistance may reduce efficacy in terms of vertical transmission risk. It may be then be advisable to consider the addition of another antiretroviral agent – lamivudine (3TC) has been suggested as the most appropriate choice.

Future prospects

Vaccination

Prophylactic vaccination remains a key objective in the fight against further global spread of AIDS. A number of candidate vaccines are currently under evaluation; however, results so far are not promising. It is not yet clear which vaccine construct is likely to provide the best protection against subsequent infection, and the results of clinical trials in volunteers have raised the vexed question as to what level of humoral or cellular immunity is associated with protection. The prospect of an effective HIV vaccine is now widely viewed as a long-term objective; few would consider this feasible within the next 10 years.

Vaginal microbicides

The most exciting prospect in the field of HIV prevention is currently the potential for the development of intravaginal agents with the capacity to inactivate the virus, thus providing a female-controlled method of preventing sexual transmission. At present, prevention of sexual transmission is very largely dependent on the successful negotiation of condom use by the male partner, and women often have too little power within their sexual relationships to achieve this. The female condom has to some degree addressed the issue of the need for a female-controlled method of protection; however, it is expensive in comparison to its male counterpart and it is not possible for this method to be used covertly where the male partner objects to the principle of protection, as is often the case.

Ideally, vaginal microbicides should be cheap, stable compounds which are easy to use. They should be colourless, odourless and tasteless to prevent detection during covert use, and should have a broad range of activity against other STIs in addition to HIV. Such broad microbicidal activity could greatly reduce the burden of disease caused by gynaecological infection, the pathological consequences of which are particularly prevalent in the developing world. In addition, these agents should not exhibit any potentially detrimental effects on the vaginal epithelium or normal vaginal ecology, as disruption of these may enhance sexual transmission of HIV [35].

In addition, vaginal microbicides should be free from side effects in either the female or the male partner, so as not to affect their acceptability and thereby their efficacy adversely. Finally, there is a need for microbicides to be developed that will permit conception, as the contraceptive effect of the spermicidal agents investigated to date is also likely to serve as a disincentive to their consistent use in some populations.

A range of products are currently under investigation in clinical trials. These include the widely used spermicidal agent N9 (see 'Spermicides'), which exerts its potent antiviral effect through a non-specific disruption of the bilipid membrane. In addition, many novel agents are in preclinical development or early clinical trials. Some of these compounds produce viral disruption (e.g. myeloperoxidases and the amphoteric surfactant C31G) whereas others interfere with viral binding or entry into susceptible cells (e.g. the sulfated polysaccharide dextrin-2-sulphate). Alternative novel agents currently under evaluation potentially enhance the natural protection offered by a healthy vaginal environment and these include acid-buffering agents and hydrogen peroxide producing lactobacilli. However, it would seem unlikely at this stage that any novel microbicidal agent would reach the market in under 10 years.

Vaginal microbicides are also likely to play an important role in the prevention of vertical transmission in the future. It is now clear that prolonged exposure of the fetus to infected cervicovaginal secretions is likely to be the principal route of mother to child transmission. Therefore agents with the capacity to reduce viral load markedly at this site are likely to reduce the risk of the fetus becoming infected. This method has the considerable advantage of being both cheap and simple, in contrast to the use of combination antiretroviral therapy or elective caesarean section. In addition, it does not require antenatal testing to be performed prior to use. However, there are currently only limited data regarding the potential efficacy of such an intervention using chlorhexidine as the virucidal agent [36]. In this study, a reduction in HIV transmission was seen where membrane rupture exceeded 4 h duration. In addition, there was a reduction in infant morbidity and mortality due to sepsis amongst the offspring of the mothers given intravaginal chlorhexidine, and reduced maternal morbidity.

Risk of HIV transmission in the healthcare setting

Reducing the risk to the healthcare worker

It has been shown that the average risk of seroconverting for HIV following a percutaneous injury contaminated with infected material is in the region of 0.2–0.4% [37]. The likelihood of transmission in individual circumstances is largely determined by a number of important variables. These include the level of viral load in the index patient, the nature of the body fluid involved and the volume of the inoculum. The injury most frequently associated with subsequent seroconversion is deep percutaneous inoculation with a wide-bore hollow needle, or needle and syringe, involving injection of a quantity of infected blood. In contrast, the risk following contamination of intact skin with infected fluids appears to be extremely small, and seroconversion has only clearly been documented following prolonged exposure to large volumes of infected blood, typically with an identifiable portal of entry [38]. An intermediate risk is posed by percutaneous injury with a suture needle. In this circumstance, a significant amount of infected blood is removed from the needle surface as it passes through the latex glove prior to skin puncture.

Universal precautions are essential in the prevention of transmission of all blood-borne pathogens, including HIV. Such precautions should involve the routine use of gloves, with the addition of masks and spectacles and disposable plastic aprons, where appropriate, to prevent splash injury. Other precautions include the use of blunt-tipped suture needles, which dramatically reduce the risk of skin puncture and which are considered suitable for suturing most tissues, and the use of a kidney dish for the transfer of sharp instruments including needles. In addition, a newly designed needleholder has been developed to protect the point of the suture needle whilst tying knots, and during transfer of the needle between the surgeon and the scrub nurse (Femcare™ Ltd).

Post-exposure prophylaxis

The use of zidovudine given as post-exposure prophylaxis has been associated with a decrease of approximately 79% in the risk of seroconversion following percutaneous exposure to HIV-infected blood [39]. In HIV-infected patients, the combination of two or more antiretroviral agents has a greater impact on circulating viral load than the use of monotherapy. It is therefore reasonable to suppose that the use of combination therapy as post-exposure prophylaxis may have a greater impact on seroconversion than zidovudine given alone. The additional benefit of combination therapy in this context is the potential for improved efficacy against transmission of zidovudine-resistant viral strains from infected patients who have been previously heavily treated with zidovudine monotherapy. For these reasons, it is our current practice to offer combination therapy with two nucleoside reverse transcriptase inhibitors and a protease inhibitor over a period of 4 weeks following a significant occupational exposure.

Reducing the risk to the patient

There remains only one case report in the literature of a healthcare worker who has transmitted HIV infection to patients in his care. This is the well-cited case of the Florida dental surgeon; the circumstances of transmission remained unclear after the look-back procedure and it was concluded that this represented a distinctly idiosyncratic case. As no other cases of transmission of HIV from healthcare worker to patient have been identified, it can be assumed that such a route of transmission is exceptionally rare in clinical practise. The consistent use of universal precautions (as listed above) would further reduce this already minimal risk.

Resources

For the general public (UK)

- The National AIDS Helpline: 0800 567123 (24 hours, free)

- The Terence Higgins Trust, 52–54 Gray's Inn Road, London WCIX 8JU. Housing, benefits and legal advice. Helpline: 0207–242 1010 (daily 10am–12 midnight)

- Body Positive, 51b Philbeach Gardens, London SW5 9EB. Support and advice for people affected by HIV. Office telephone 0207–835 1045; helpline: 0207–373 9124

- Red Admiral Project, 51a Philbeach Gardens, London SW5 9EB. Free specialist counselling. (Tel: 0207–835 1495)

- London Lighthouse, 111–117 Lancaster Road, London W11 1QT. Residential and support centre offering a wide range of services. (Tel: 0207–792 1200)

- BHAN (Black HIV/AIDS Network), St Stephen's House, 41 Uxbridge Road, London W12 8LH. Welfare rights advice and multilingual counselling. (Tel: 0208–749 2828)

- Mainliners, 205 Stockwell Road, London SW9 9SL. Support and advice for drug users affected by HIV. Office telephone: 0207–737 7472. Helpline: 0207–737 3141

- Scottish AIDS Monitor, 26 Anderson Place, Edinburgh EH6 5NP. Support groups and services in Scotland. (Tel: 0131–555 4850)

References

1. Centers for Disease Control (CDC). Revised classification system for HIV infection and expanded surveillance case definition for AIDS among adolescents and adults. *MMWR* 1992;41:1–18.

2. Mocroft A, Youle M, Morcinek J, et al. Survival after diagnosis of AIDS: a prospective observational study of 2625 patients. Royal Free/Chelsea and Westminster Hospitals Collaborative Group. *Br Med J* 1997;314:409–3.

3. Smith JR, Kitchen VS, Botcherby M, et al. Is HIV infection associated with an increase in the prevalence of cervical neoplasia? *Br J Obstet Gynaecol* 1993;100:149.

4. Hoegsberg B, Abulafia O, Sedlis A, et al. Sexually transmitted diseases and human immunodeficiency virus infection among women with pelvic inflammatory disease. *Am J Obstet Gynecol* 1990;163:1135–9.

5. Mandelblatt JS, Fahs M, Garibaldi K, et al. Association between HIV infection and cervical neoplasia: implications for clinical care of women at risk of both conditions. *AIDS* 1992;6:173–8.

6. Byrne M, Taylor-Robinson D, Munday PE, et al. The common occurrence of human papilloma virus and intraepithelial neoplasia in women infected by HIV. *AIDS* 1989;3:379.

7. Minkoff HL, DeHovitz JA. Care of women infected with the human immunodeficiency virus. *JAMA* 1991;266:2253–8.

8. Smith JR, Shah P, Stafford M. HIV in obstetrics and gynaecology. *J Bellevue Obstet Gynecol Soc* 1996;XII:22–30.

9. Shah P, Smith JR, Wells C, et al. Menstrual symptoms in women infected by the human immunodeficiency virus. *Obstet Gynecol* 1994;83:397.

10. European Study Group of Heterosexual Transmission of HIV. Comparison of female to male and male to female transmission of HIV in 563 stable couples. *Br Med J* 1992;304:809–13.

11. Anderson RM, May RM, Boily MC et al. The spread of HIV-I in Africa – sexual contact patterns and the predicted demographic impact of AIDS. *Nature* 1991;352:581–9.

12. Cates W. How much do condoms protects against sexually transmitted diseases? *IPPF Med Bull* 1997;31:2–3.

13. Moss GB, Clemetson D, D'Costa L, et al. Association of cervical ectopy with heterosexual transmission of human immunodeficiency virus: results of a study in Nairobi, Kenya. *J Infect Dis* 1991;164:588–91.

14. Feldblum PJ, Hira S, Goodwin S, et al. Efficacy of spermicide use and condom use by HIV

discordant couples in Zambia. 8th International Conference on AIDS/III STD World Congress. Amsterdam, July 1992: Abstract WeC 1085.

15. Zekeng L, Feldblum PJ, Oliver RM, et al. Barrier contraceptive use and HIV infection among high risk women in Cameroon. *AIDS* 1993;7:725–31.

16. Kreiss J, Ngugi E, Holmes K, et al. Efficacy of nonoxynol-9 contraceptive sponge use in preventing heterosexual acquisition of HIV in Nairobi prostitutes. *JAMA* 1992;268:477–82.

17. Smith JR, Foster GE, Kitchen VS, et al. Infertility management in HIV seropositive couples; a dilemma. *Br Med J* 1991; 302:1447–50.

18. Semprini AE, Levi-Setti P, Bozzo X, et al. Insemination of HIV negative women with processed semen of HIV positive partners. *Lancet* 1992;340:1317–9.

19. MacDonald MG, Ginzburg HM, Bolan JC. HIV infection in pregnancy; epidemiology and clinical management. *J AIDS* 1991;4:100–8.

20. Bryson Y. Perinatal transmission – associated factors and therapeutic approaches. XI International Conference on AIDS. Vancouver, 1996. Plenary session Tu 07.

21. Riva M, Lipman M. HIV pretest discussion. *Br Med J* 1996;313:130.

22. Smith JR, Barton SE, Boag F, et al. To opt in or opt out – that is the question. *Br J Obstet Gynaecol* (in press).

23. Minkoff RL, Landesman SH. The case for routinely offering prenatal testing for human immunodeficiency virus. *Am J Obstet Gynecol* 1988;159:793–6.

24. Connor E, Sperling R, Gelber R, et al. Reduction in maternal–infant transmission of human immunodeficiency virus type I with zidovudine treatment. *N Engl J Med* 1994;331:1174–80.

25. Stafford MK, Shah P, Smith JR. HIV: who to screen, how to manage. In: Yearbook of the RCOG 1995:191–205.

26. Lewis SH, Reynolds-Kohler C, Fox HE, et al. HIV-1 in trophoblastic and villous Hofbauer cells, and haematological precursors in eight week fetuses. *Lancet* 1990;335:565–8.

27. Tibalidi C, Tovo PA, Ziarati N, et al. Asymptomatic women at high risk of vertical transmission to their fetuses. *Br J Obstet Gynaecol* 1993;100:334–7.

28. Peckham CS, Newell ML and European Collaborative Study. Perinatal findings in children born to HIV infected mothers. *Br J Obstet Gynaecol* 1994; 101:135–41.

29. Wofsy CB, Cohen JB, HaVer LB, et al. Isolation of AIDS-associated retrovirus from genital secretions of women with antibodies to the virus. *Lancet* 1986;1:527–9.

30. Sheldon H, Landesman ND, Leslie A, et al. Obstetrical factors and the transmission of human immunodeficiency virus type I from mother to child. *N Engl J Med* 1996;334:1617–23.

31. Dunn DT, Newell XL, Mayaux MJ, et al. Mode of delivery and vertical transmission of HIV-1; a review of prospective studies.

Perinatal AIDS Collaborative Transmission Studies. *J AIDS* 1994;10:1064–6.

32. Towers CV, Devekis A, Asrat T, et al. Role of 'bloodless C section' to decrease maternal–child HIV transmission: a pilot study. Proceedings of the 9th International AIDS Conference, Berlin, 1993, Abstract PO C16–2978.

33. Dunn DT, Newell ML, Ades AE, et al. Risk of human immunodeficiency virus type I through breast feeding. *Lancet* 1992;340:585–8.

34. Consensus statement from the WHO/UNICEF constitution on HIV transmission and breast feeding. *Weekly Epidemiol Rec* 1992;67:177–84.

35. Stone AB, Hitchcock PJ. Vaginal microbicides for preventing the sexual transmission of HIV. *AIDS* 1994;8(Suppl 1):5285–93.

36. Biggar RJ, Miotti PG, Taha E, et al. Perinatal intervention trial in Africa: effect of a birth canal cleansing intervention to prevent HIV transmission. *Lancet* 1996;347:1647–50.

37. Tokars JI, Bell DM, Culver D, et al. Percutaneous injuries during surgical procedures. *JAMA* 1992;267:2899–904.

38. Centers for Disease Control. 1992 surveillance for occupationally acquired HIV infection: United States. *MMWR* 1981–1992;41:823–5.

39. Update: Provisional public health service recommendations for chemoprophylaxis after occupational exposure to HIV. *MMWR* 1996;45;22:468–72.

Sexual therapy

Fran Reader FRCOG MFFP BASRT Accred

Introduction

Sexual expression and intimacy are a fundamental part of the human experience. We have a drive to procreate but we also use sexual expression recreationally and to confirm bonding in a non-exploitative environment of trust and affection. However, sexual expression has a darker side and can be used or withheld to demonstrate domination or humiliation. Art and literature of all cultures throughout history display the ecstasy, fear, successes, failures, light and darkness of human sexuality. This century has seen the opening up of the previously private arena of sexual behaviour. It has been analysed and medicalized and confronts us through the media every day. Knowledge has broadened, expectations have been raised and limits extended. This has led to attempts to bring back control and provide boundaries by defining 'normality' from a variety of cultural and religious perspectives.

So what is sexual normality, and what constitutes a sexual problem? The shift in the last 20 years has been away from imposed definitions and to an individualized definition. Sex therapy has developed to help individuals who identify themselves as having a sexual problem. This may be a discrepancy with their ability to respond sexually, and thus presents as a sexual dysfunction, or a problem of their sexual identity or orientation.

Background

Freud's theories on libido catalysed thinking in the emerging world of psychoanalysis and opened the door to psychodynamic concepts of how childhood experiences can affect the adult subconscious and underlie adult sexual difficulties.

Human sexual behaviour became a legitimate topic for research after the pioneering work of Kinsey in the USA [1]. The door of understanding of human sexuality opened wider with the publication in 1970 of Masters and Johnson's book *Human Sexual Inadequacy* [2]. Masters and Johnson went on to develop behavioural programmes for the management of specific sexual dysfunctions. In 1974, Dr Helen Singer Kaplan published *The New Sex Therapy* [3], which integrated a variety of therapeutic models including analysis, behavioural therapy, family and marital therapy, group therapy and psychosomatic medicine. Throughout the 1970s and 1980s, sex therapy has evolved further away from Masters and Johnson's initial simplistic behavioural approach.

In the UK, the field of sex therapy has developed in three ways. During the 1950s, doctors working with the Family Planning Association began seminars under the leadership of Dr Michael Balint who was a trained analyst. Further seminars were led by Dr Tom Maine [4] who went on to develop a training scheme for doctors (based on 2 years basic and 2–3 years advanced seminars). From this, the Institute of Psychosexual Medicine (IPM) was formed in 1974. The emphasis of training through the IPM is to work with the doctor–patient relationship to help uncover emotional blocks that may be unconsciously contributing to the individual's sexual problem. The genital examination is used as a window to understanding anxieties, fears and fantasies about sexuality.

Parallel to the work of the IPM, a multidisciplinary organization was developed in 1976 as the Association of Sexual and Relationship Therapists. In

1991 this became the British Association for Sexual and Relationship Therapists (BASRT). BASRT has seven approved training courses. BASRT members come from a variety of backgrounds including psychology, psychotherapy, counselling, social work, medicine and nursing. The organization has an accreditation process and accredited members register with the United Kingdom Council for Psychotherapy (UKCP). The third group are psychiatrists, psychologists or psychotherapists who work with sexual problems as their special interest.

In the USA, UK and Europe, there is an active debate about the uniqueness of sex therapy and the respective importance of counselling and psychotherapeutic skills versus medical knowledge. Another debate has been between those who prefer to work with individuals, and those who work primarily with relationships and therefore with couples. The trend in the 1990s is to see better understanding and respect for these different approaches, and acceptance that, regardless of the primary focus of the work, a basic understanding of the physical, psychological, social and ethical dimensions is essential (Figure 20.1).

Sex therapy today

Most of the work in sex therapy is with individuals or couples who present with sexual dysfunction. Catalan et al. [5] reported erectile dysfunction as the most commonly presenting problem in men, followed by premature

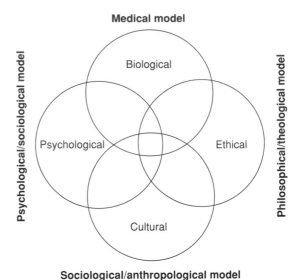

Fig. 20.1 Dimensions relevant to a holistic approach to sex therapy.

ejaculation, low sexual desire and retrograde or inability to ejaculate. In women, the most frequent presentation was low sexual desire, followed by vaginismus, dyspareunia and orgasmic dysfunctions. Female arousal disorder was not identified as a separate category. The work of Jehu [6] drew attention to the special needs of individuals with a past history of sexual abuse who may present with any dysfunction but particularly sexual aversion. Sexual identity and orientation problems may also present.

Table 20.1 lists the non-organic sexual dysfunctions as classified by the International Classification of Disorders (ICD-10) [7] and identifies recommended texts, listed in the reference section, that provide information about current sex-therapy approaches.

Effectiveness of sexual therapy

Masters and Johnson reported their failure rate as 18.9% [2]. However, such low failure rates

Table 20.1 ICD-10 classification of sexual dysfunctions and recommended references

Sexual dysfunction	Recommended reference
Lack or loss of sexual desire	Kaplan [8]
Sexual aversion and lack of sexual enjoyment	Kaplan [9]
Failure of genital response	Male – Gregoire and Pryor [10]
	Padma-Nathan and Elstrom [11]
	Goldstein and Lue [12]
	Female – Hiller [13]
Orgasmic dysfunction	Male – Zilbergeld [12]
	Female – McCarthy [15]
Premature ejaculation	Zilbergeld [14]
Vaginismus	Goldsmith [16]
Dyspareunia	Graziottin [17]
Excessive sexual drive	Carnes [18]

have never been replicated. This has called into question the validity of their results. Bancroft reported that outcome research in the field of sex therapy is notoriously difficult [19]. Many couples and individuals present with more than one dysfunction and with mixed organic and psychogenic factors. The variables involved are complex and confuse outcome results. Further confusion has arisen because of failure to define dysfunctions by internationally agreed classifications. Finally, a successful outcome defined by the patient may not be a resolution of the dysfunction. Sometimes the individual or couple find ways of adapting to the dysfunction and therefore satisfaction with the outcome maybe more relevant than 'success'. Table 20.2 summarizes research findings related to the effectiveness of sex therapy.

Aetiology of sexual problems

Sexual problems can be caused by a number of factors.

Physiological factors

Examples of physiological factors are childbirth or the menopause in women and the ageing process in men.

Organic or iatrogenic factors

These can cause sexual problems through:

- directly affecting the sexual response, e.g. diabetes;
- alteration of genital anatomy affecting sexual response post-surgery, e.g. vulvectomy;

- mobility for sexual activity affected, e.g. spinal cord injury;
- pain limiting sexual activity, e.g. rheumatoid arthritis;
- general ill health leading to fatigue, e.g. renal failure;
- those side effects secondary to medication.

It is important to remember that, although organic or iatrogenic factors can affect sexual function, there may be a psychological component.

Psychosocial factors

Lack of or incorrect information about sex
Even in the 1990s it is unsafe to assume that individuals are knowledgeable about sexual anatomy, physiology and behaviour. They may have received inadequate information owing to a restrictive upbringing, or incorrect information from peers and dirty jokes, etc. Alternatively they may have a false impression of sexual behaviour from media sensationalism.

Sexual myths and taboos
Our value systems, beliefs and attitudes develop within our family, and through social, cultural and religious experiences. Myths and taboos about sexual behaviour evolve within different cultural frameworks, and perpetuate guilt and shame about sexual activity.
Examples of sexual myths are:

- performance is everything;
- the man is responsible for the woman's orgasm;

Table 20.2 Research findings related to the effectiveness of sex therapy

Parameter studied	Research/review Reference	Comment
Sex therapy clients compared to waiting list clients	Heiman and LoPiccolo [20], Bancroft, Dickson et al [19]	Sex therapy beneficial
Response of dysfunction to sex therapy	Bancroft and Coles [21]	Good response – vaginismus and impotence
	Hawton and Catalan [22]	Poor response – low sexual desire, especially in men
Frequency of therapy	Clement and Schmidt [23], Heiman and LoPiccolo [20]	Weekly therapy optimal during the initial phase
Co-therapists/individual therapists	Crowe et al. [24]	No difference; therefore, for cost effectiveness individual therapist preferred except in training situations
Specific therapy	Whitehead and Mathews [25]	Lack of enjoyment in female partner Couple approach more effective, but individual approach reasonable
Prognostic indicators	Hawton (review) [26]	Good general relationship Motivation of partners Physical attraction Early compliance

- the woman is responsible for the man's erection;

- good sex is spontaneous sex;

- only loose women initiate sexual activity;

- sex equals intercourse;

- mind reading – when you are in love you don't need to tell your partner what you want because they already know.

Communication problems

The mind-reading myth frequently underlies sexual problems. Talking about sex can be embarrassing and one partner may fear hurting the other's feelings. Alternatively, there may be general communication problems. Fear, anger, resentment or guilt can build up because of communication problems, and these can be carried into the bedroom and be acted out as sexual avoidance.

Predisposing, precipitating and perpetuating factors

Past experiences, life events and behaviour patterns for dealing with problems can all contribute to the onset and maintenance of sexual problems (Table 20.3).

Differing and unrealistic expectations

Problems can arise when partners have a different need for sexual expression. For example, one partner may want to have sex every night and the other partner once a month. Alternatively, problems can arise due to unrealistic expectations. This can lead to performance pressure and fear of failure.

Examples of unrealistic expectations are:

- expecting no change in sexual interest when ill, tired or bereaved;

- expecting always to achieve orgasm during intercourse;

- expecting mutual orgasm on every occasion;

- expecting to return to the same interest in sex after childbirth;

- expecting performance to remain unchanged by age.

Assessment

Taking a sexual history

Whenever there is a sexual problem, there is likely to be embarrassment when talking about the problem with a health professional. It is therefore important that health professionals are trained to be self-aware so they can develop an open non-judgemental style that encourages talking about such delicate matters as sexual orientation, masturbation, fantasies, affairs and fetishes.

The practice of taking a sexual history varies between different models of therapeutic practice. Some therapists begin by taking a full assessment consisting of history, examination and investigations, while other therapists have a less structured approach, working with the here and now and evolving the history as it is presented.

Therapists who adopt the structured assessment approach are likely to cover the following aspects while taking a sexual history.

Childhood experiences

- family background and relationships;

- educational, cultural and religious background;

- attitudes to sexuality, intimacy and expression of emotion;

- traumatic sexual or other life experiences.

Adolescent experiences

- sex education;

- experience of puberty – menses, wet dreams, etc.;

- sexual opportunities, masturbation, non-coital and coital experiences;

- traumatic sexual and other life experiences.

Adult experiences

- past relationships;

- past medical and surgical history;

Table 20.3   Common precipitating and predisposing factors for sexual problems

Precipitating factors	Predisposing factors
Parenthood	Physical, emotional or sexual abuse in childhood
Illness	Restrictive upbringing
Random failure	Lack of information
Life stresses	Poor self-esteem
Performance pressure	Poor body image
Traumatic sexual experience	Communication problems
Loss of trust in relationship	Uncertain sexual identity
	Psychiatric illness

- past gynaecological and obstetric history;
- traumatic life events.

Current experiences

- history of the presenting problem;
- details of the current sexual dysfunction;
- present sexual practices and preferences including masturbation;
- present relationship(s);
- sexual orientation;
- use of fantasy, erotic material or sex aids;
- drug history, both social and therapeutic;
- contraception/infertility.

Couple assessment

It is common practice to take most of the history conjointly, which gives the opportunity to assess the relationship and communication. This is followed by individual sessions which provide an opportunity to assess each partner's motivation, and for the individual to open up on issues that may have been difficult to disclose with the partner present.

Use of language

It is important to be confident about the use of language and sexually explicit words. It can be helpful to check out the understanding of words that are used to ensure words will be understood by the client and help him or her to feel comfortable in explaining the details of their sexual problem.

The verbal and body language

of the client can be a window into their belief systems, their fears and their shame. The information gained from observing how clients answer specific questions can be used diagnostically and therapeutically.

Examination

Examination of patients with a sexual problem is limited to therapists with a medical background. Non-medically trained therapists usually work by referral to an appropriate medical professional when the history suggests it is necessary to exclude organic factors.

Medical professionals examining patients with sexual problems need to be able to put the patient at ease and progress with the examination at a pace the client can cope with. This is particularly important in patients who give a past history of sexual abuse. The client needs to feel that they remain in control of the situation.

Sex therapists trained through the Institute of Psychosexual Medicine are particularly skilled at working with the insights into the sexual problems that are exposed by the client's response to the genital examination [27].

Investigations

Investigations should be performed selectively depending on the possible underlying causes for a sexual problem, e.g. checking for diabetes, thyroid disorders, etc.

Box 20.1 lists assays of sex hormones that are useful for excluding endocrine disorders.

Box 20.2 lists specific investigations for erectile problems.

Sexual therapy options

Psychological approaches

These include education, advice and guidance, brief counselling/therapy or long-term psychotherapy.

Models of therapeutic intervention
Psychodynamic psychotherapies

These look into the meaning of symptoms in terms of the individual's past and present experiences. Childhood experiences are seen as particularly relevant in establishing unconscious strategies for survival that may be appropriate to surviving a

---

Box 20.1   Sex Hormone Assays

Prolactin
- Loss of libido (male and female)
- Erectile dysfunction

FSH
- Possibility of menopause (female)
- Male infertility

LH
- Male erectile problem if testosterone low

Testosterone
- Low desire, erectile problems

FSH = follicle-stimulating hormone; LH = luteinizing hormone.

Box 20.2 Specific investigations for erectile dysfunction

Diagnostic injection:	Papaverine/prostaglandin E₁
Arteriogenic impotence:	Doppler ultrasound
	Arteriography
Venous impotence:	Cavernosometry
	Cavernosonography
Neurogenic impotence:	Test of nerve conductivity
Endocrine impotence:	Serum testosterone

dysfunctional childhood, but which can disrupt and interfere with successful adult living. The relationship between the client and the therapist is used to gain insights into the client's belief systems (personal scripts) and associated feelings. This approach is useful for intrapersonal issues, especially when they underlie sexual desire difficulties.

Cognitive/behavioural psychotherapies

These use the here and now of the individual's thinking, feeling and behaviour to develop a problem-solving approach to bring about change through structured exercises. The exercises are targeted at changing beliefs and behaviour, and consequently modifying associated feelings to release the individual from fear, anger, grief, guilt or shame.

Systemic psychotherapies

These are particularly applicable to family and group therapy, but have also found a role in the management of couple therapy and hence in sexual work with couples. The sexual problem is viewed as part of a system with positive and negative feedback loops that can be identified and altered.

Humanistic or existential psychotherapies

These work with the here and now. The humanistic approach covers a wide range of philosophies and styles of practice,

including art therapy, drama therapy, music therapy, Gestalt therapy, body work therapy, etc. Common to all is the belief that the client contains within himself or herself the necessary seeds for growth and development into a fulfilled person. This approach is useful when there is a past history of sexual abuse.

Sex therapy has developed an integrative approach with the emphasis of the theoretical model underlying the therapy determined by the problems presented by the client(s) during the assessment. The approach that is most likely to bring about change is chosen.

Medical approaches

Tables 20.4–20.7 outline the treatment options that are available for sexual dysfunctions. With the development of new drug treatments for impotence [10,11] and especially the oral preparation sildenafil (Viagra) [12], more men are coming forward for help. Sildenafil is the first of a new class of oral drugs for the treatment of erectile dysfunction and it is anticipated that more 'designer drugs' will follow that will have benefits for both men and women and will target different phases of the sexual response cycle.

Simple strategies for common problems

The sexual response staircase (Figure 20.2)

Information about the human sexual response can be given as an analogy to going up stairs.

Table 20.4 Medical options for low sexual desire and sexual aversion

Sexual dysfunction	Treatment	Comment
Low sexual desire	Testosterone injections/oral	Male hypogonadism
	Testosterone implant/oral	Female post-oophorectomy/ post-menopause
	Bromocriptine	Hyperprolactinaemia
Sexual aversion and phobias	Serotonin reuptake inhibitors	To reduce physiological effects of adrenaline release during desensitization
	β blockers	

Table 20.5 Medical treatment options for erectile disorders

Treatment option	Comment
Sildenafil (Viagra)	Type 5 cGMP phosphodiesterase inhibitor useful for all forms of impotence
Transurethral alprostadil (Muse) and Intracavernosal injections of alprostadil (Caverject)	Used therapeutically for psychogenic, mild arteriogenic and neurological impotence
Penile rings and vacuum pumps	Useful for all forms of impotence
Testosterone	Hypogonadism
Penile implants	Last resort if other options fail
Cardiovascular surgery	For arterial or venous problems

Table 20.6 Medical treatment options for orgasmic disorders

Problem	Treatment	Comment
Premature ejaculation	Oral – chlorimipramine /serotonin reuptake inhibitors	Therapeutic use of their side effect of delaying ejaculation
Inhibited orgasm	Use of vibrators	Effective in male and female

Table 20.7 Medical treatment for female dyspareunia and vaginismus

Treatment	Comment
Topical oestrogen/HRT	Atrophic changes
Topical steroids	Dermatological conditions, e.g. vestibulitis, lichen sclerosis
Synthetic lubricants	KY Jelly, Replens
Local anaesthetic gel	Use cotton bud to apply to trigger points
Amitryptiline (nocte)	Vulvodynia
Vaginal trainers	Gradual desensitization

- *Ground level* is non-sexual.

- *Step 1:* is desire without any physical change.

- *Step 2:* arousal begins. The woman begins to lubricate and for the man the penis begins to become firm but not firm enough for penetration.

- *Step 3:* arousal progresses and for the woman there is more

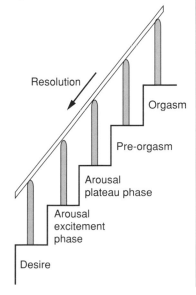

Fig. 20.2 The sexual response staircase.

lubrication and vaginal ballooning. For the man there is a firm erection that could penetrate.

- *Step 4:* orgasm is recognized as being imminent.

- *Step 5:* orgasm itself.

Sliding down the banisters is a process of returning back to the ground – you can climb on to the banister from any step on the staircase. As you slide you take with you all the thoughts and feelings surrounding that particular sexual encounter. It is normal for both men and women to spend time going up and down the steps and not go directly to step 5 in one dash up the stairs.

Men and women often progress up the stairs at different rates. Physiologically a man on step 3 can penetrate a woman who can still be on step 1 or even on the ground level. The reverse is impossible. A common problem occurs when the man is ahead of his partner and reaches step 5, to slide down the banisters leaving her to feel frustrated still on step 1 or 2.

The important concept for both partners to understand is that each is responsible for their own progression up the stairs. The woman is responsible for her orgasm and the man for his. Communication is therefore essential. There is no need to aim for synchronicity. What is important is that each individual feels comfortable with their own progress and if they do not wish to reach orgasm on that occasion this is also all right. For sex to be seen as a positive experience, the thoughts and feelings that are around when we are returning down the banisters need to be those of fulfilment and contentment, and not anger, resentment or a sense of failure.

The sexual arousal circuit
(Figure 20.3)

Imagine sexual energy flowing freely around a circuit and that with each turn more energy is added until there is sufficient energy to build up to release a surge of energy or orgasm. Then imagine the effects of having blocks in the circuit preventing this progression:

- Block 1 depends on the quality and type of initial sensory input. What is heard, seen, smelt, touched or tasted. Body odour, bad breath, too much or too little light, what is worn or not worn can all affect the initial progression from desire to arousal. The use of fantasy can also play an important role at this point.

- Block 2 depends on feelings. The typical feelings that are likely to sabotage the energy in the circuit are fear, anger, sadness and shame.

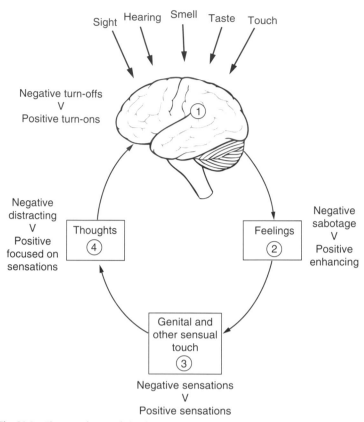

Sight Hearing Smell Taste Touch

Negative turn-offs
V
Positive turn-ons

①

Negative
distracting
V
Positive
focused on
sensations

Thoughts
④

Feelings
②

Negative
sabotage
V
Positive
enhancing

Genital and
other sensual
touch
③

Negative sensations
V
Positive sensations

Fig. 20.3 The sexual arousal circuit.

- Block 3 depends on the quality and quantity of tactile sensations coming from the genitals and other erogenous zones. The tactile input may be too little, too much, too soft, too ticklish or even painful.

- Block 4 depends on distracting thoughts. Typical intrusive thoughts are worries about work, family or finances. Another distraction can be performance anxiety: 'am I scxy?' or 'am I pleasing my partner?'. Sometimes people will describe a sense of being outside themselves, watching the performance: this is called spectatoring.

Understanding the concept of this circuit can help diagnostically to highlight blocks and to plan an appropriate course for future management.

Self-discovery and self-pleasuring

Understanding how the body works during the sexual response cycle is frequently a revelation for men and women. With this new knowledge, they can relate to themselves and embark on learning about their own body and sexual needs through a process of self-discovery and self-pleasuring. Progress can be made by encouraging self-discovery and self-pleasuring as something they can experiment with privately through structured 'homework' tasks which will give insights into their sexual needs. These insights can be communicated to their partner.

Sensate focus

This is an extension of the self-discovery programme into couple work. It is a strategy for overcoming sexual problems by addressing all the possible blocks to arousal outlined in the sexual arousal circuit. 'Homework' assignments are set for the couple and can be tailored to meet specific needs.

Step 1 (Non-genital sensate focus)

Sexual intercourse is banned, thus removing performance pressure. The couple set 2–3 1-hour sessions during the week to be together. Failure to find this time may highlight other issues such as privacy or a busy schedule.

Setting the scene is important. Ensuring privacy, choosing the room, lighting, clothing, etc. are an important part of setting the scene. The couple take turns to touch and be touched in all areas of the body excluding the breasts and genitals. Ideal timing would be for each partner to have 20 minutes as giver and 20 minutes as receiver. The final 20 minutes is for talking about the experience.

Focusing on the sensation of touch and being touched helps overcome distracting thoughts. Each individual focuses on getting pleasure from the experience for themselves but not at the expense of the partner. In this way, each person takes responsibility for their own enjoyment but also cares about the other person's enjoyment. It is often the negative feedback that is most difficult. It is therefore important to remember that negative feedback is about an action and not a rejection of the person. If talking is difficult, then feedback can be given by the receiver moving the hands of the giver to achieve the desired effect.

Step 2

Once the couple are comfortable with step 1, then they can move on to introduce genital touching. Arousal is still not the goal and it is important for the couple to discuss what they will do should the exercise lead to arousal in one or other of the partners. It is important to continue the ban on sexual penetration so that the couple experience the pleasure of arousal for its own sake and trust is maintained.

Step 3

Steps 1 and 2 may be sufficient in their own right. From these steps the couple may gain insights into each other's likes and dislikes. The final step is to remove the ban on intercourse and bring back the concept of pleasure leading to arousal. When there has been a problem with penetration, a further sequence of gradual steps may be required before full penetrative sex can be achieved.

The future

As sexual dysfunction joins the mainstream components of sexual health, we hope to see consolidation of many current initiatives.

- Society to develop a stratified approach to teaching about human sexuality and relationships from nursery school through to higher professional training.

- Improved sex education in schools addressing both the knowledge and social skills required for the individual to learn how to use their adult sexuality pleasurably and responsibly without causing or suffering physical or mental harm.

- Improved basic training in human sexuality and relationships for all health professionals, teachers, social workers and other relevant professionals.

- Improved basic training in human sexuality and relationships for all counsellors, psychotherapists, psychologists and psychiatrists.

- Improved in-depth understanding of human sexuality for health professionals in specific specializations, such as obstetrics and gynaecology, sexual health, urology and general practice.

- Continued training of specialist sex therapists and specialists in sexual medicine.

- Improved audit and research.

Tips for safe practice

- Abide by codes of ethics and codes of practice of the profession or the organization.

- Be aware of one's own limits and know about referral options.

- Be aware of the law regarding confidentiality and regarding sexual offences.

- Always consider all possible dimensions of the aetiology and avoid focusing on the medical to the exclusion of the psychosocial or vice versa.

- Awareness of self in relation to others (in the context of working with patients/clients with sexual and relationship problems).

- In-depth work with sexual problems to be undertaken by appropriate specialists trained in sexual medicine or sexual therapy.

- Trained sex therapists/ counsellors to maintain supervision and ongoing professional development.

Resource list

Books for professionals

- Hawton K. Sex therapy – a practical guide. Oxford: Oxford Medical Publications.
- Woody D. Treating sexual distress – integrative synthesis therapy. London: Sage Publications.

- Rosen Leiblum SR. Principles and practice of sex therapy, 2nd edn. Guilford Press.

- Bancroft J. Human sexuality and its problems. Edinburgh: Churchill Livingstone.

- Crowe M, Ridley J. Therapy with couples. Oxford: Blackwell.

- Wellings K, Field, Johnson A, Wadsworth. Sexual behaviour in Britain – the national survey of sexual attitudes and lifestyles. London: Penguin.

- Lincoln R. Psychosexual medicine. London: Chapman and Hall.

- Rosen Leiblum SR. Sexual desire disorders. Gilford Press.
- Riley AJ, Peet M, Wilson C. Sexual pharmacology. Oxford: Oxford Medical Publications.
- Rako S. The hormone of desire. Harmony Books.

Self-help books

Couples

- Litvinoff S. The Relate guide to sex in loving relationships. London: Vermillion, 1998.
- Brown, Faulder. Treat yourself to sex. London: Penguin, 1989.

Women

- Dickson A. The mirror within. Optimum Press, 1985.
- McCarthy and McCarthy, Female sexual awareness. Virgin Books, 1991.
- Heiman JR and Lo Piccolo J. Becoming Orgasmic: A sexual and personal growth program for women. Piatkus, 1988.

Men

- Zilbergeld B. Men and sex. London: HarperCollins, 1995.
- Yaffe and Fenwick. Sexual happiness for men. London: Dorling Kindersley.

Sexual abuse

- Bass E, Davis L. Courage to heal. London: Harper and Row, 1991.

Ageing

- Greengross S, Greengross W. Living, loving and ageing: sexual and personal relationships in later life. Age Concern, 1989.

Childbirth

- Rix J. Is there sex after childbirth? Thorsons, 1995.

Sex education

- Harris RH. Let's talk about sex. Walker Books, 1995.

Videos

- Stanway A. Lovers guide videos (Series of 3). Pickwick Videos, The Hyde Industrial Estate, The Hyde, London NW9 6JU (Tel: 0208 200 7000).
- Sex: a lifelong pleasure (Series of 5). NTV Entertainments Ltd, Russell Chambers, The Piazza, Covent Garden, London WC2E 8AA, UK.

Bookshops/booksellers (UK)

- Healthwise, Family Planning Association Bookshop (Tel. 0207 837 5432).
- Abbey Books (Conference and mail order booksellers) (Tel. 01332 290021).

Medical suppliers (UK)

- Owen Mumford (Amielle vaginal trainers, penile rings and vacuum devices), Brook Hill, Woodstock, Oxford, OX20 1TU (Tel. 0199 381 2021).
- Genesis Medical Ltd (Erection assistance systems), Freepost WD 1242, London NW3 4YR (Tel. 0207 284 2824).

Medical suppliers (USA)

- The Townsend Institute, PO Box 8855, Chapel Hill, NC 27515 (Tel. 800–888–1900).
- Good Vibrations, 938 Howard Street, San Francisco, CA 94103 (Tel. 800–289–8423).

Organizations (UK)

- British Association for Sexual and Relationship Therapists, PO Box 13686 London SW20 9ZH.
- Institute of Psychosexual Medicine, 11 Chandos Street, London W1M 9DE (Tel. 0207 580 0631).
- Relate, Herbert Gray College, Little Church Street, Rugby CV21 3AP (Tel. 0207 857 3241)
- SPOD (Association to aid sexual and personal relationships of people with a disability), 286 Camden Road, London N7 0BJ (Tel. 0207 607 8851/2)

Organizations (USA)

- American Association for Marriage and Family Therapy, 1100 17th St NW, Tenth Floor, Washington, DC 20036 (Tel. 202–452–0109)
- AASECT (American Association of Sex Educators, Counselors and Therapists), 435 N. Michigin Avenue, Suite 1717, Chicago, IL 60611 (Tel. 312–644–0828).

References

1. Kinsey AC, Pomeroy WB, Martin CE. Sex behaviour in the human male. London: WB Saunders, 1948

2. Masters WH, Johnson VE. Human sexual inadequacy. London: Churchill, 1970.

3. Kaplan HS. The new sex therapy: active treatment of sexual dysfunction. New York: Brunner/Mazel, 1984.

4. Maine TF. Training for the acquisitions of knowledge or the development of skill. In: Draper KC (ed.) The practice of psychosexual medicine. London: John Library, 1982.

5. Catalan J, Hawton K, Day A. Couples referred to a sexual dysfunction clinic: psychological and physical morbidity. *Br J Psychiatr* 1990;156:61–7.

6. Jehu D. Beyond sexual abuse. Therapy with women who were childhood victims. Chichester: Wiley, 1989.

7. World Health Organisation (WHO) International Classification of Disorders-10 Geneva: WHO, 1994.

8. Kaplan HS. Disorders of sexual desire. New York: Brunner/Mazel, 1995.

9. Kaplan HS. Sexual aversion, sexual phobias and panic disorders. New York: Brunner/Mazel, 1987.

10. Gregoire A, Prior J. Impotence: an integrated approach to clinical practice. London: Churchill Livingstone, 1993.

11. Padma-Nathan H, Hellstrom W, Kaiser FE, et al. Treatment of men with erectile dysfunction with transurethral alprostadil. *N Engl J Med* 1997;336:1–7.

12. Goldstein I, Lue T, Padma-Nathan H, et al. Oral Sildenafil in the treatment of erectile dysfunction. *N Engl J Med* 1998;338:1 397–404.

13. Hiller J. Female sexual arousal and its impairment: the psychodynamics of non-organic coital pain. *Sex Marital Ther* 1987;11:55–76.

14. Zilbergeld B. Men and sex. London: HarperCollins, 1995.

15. McCarthy B and McCarthy E. Female sexual awareness. London: Virgin Books 1993.

16. Goldsmith M. Painful sex: a guide to causes, treatment and prevention. London: Thorsons 1995.

17. Graziottin A. Organic and psychological factors in vulval pain: implications for management. *Sex Marital Ther* 1998;13(3):329–338.

18. Carnes P. Don't call it love. Recovery from sexual addiction. London: Piatkus, 1992.

19. Bancroft J, Dickerson M, Fairburn CG, et al. Sex therapy outcome research: a reappraisal of methodology. *Psychol Med* 1985;16:851–63.

20. Heiman J, LoPiccolo J. Clinical outcomes of sex therapy. *Arch Gen Psychiatr* 1983;40:443–9.

21. Bancroft J, Coles M. Three years experience in a sexual problems clinic. *Br Med J* 1976;1:1575–7.

22. Hawton K, Catalan J. Prognostic factors in sex therapy. *Behav Res Ther* 1986;24:377–85.

23. Clement U, Schmidt G. The outcome of couple therapy for sexual dysfunctions using three different formats. *J Sex Marital Ther* 1983;9:67–78.

24. Crowe MJ, Gillan P, Golombuk S. Form and content in the conjoint treatment of sexual dysfunction: a controlled study. *Behav Res Ther* 1981;19:47–54.

25. Whitehead A, Mathews A. Factors related to successful outcome in the treatment of sexually unresponsive women. *Psychol Med* 1986;16:373–8.

26. Hawton K. Treatment of sexual dysfunction by sex therapy and other approaches. *Br J Psychiatr* 1995;167:307–14.

27. Tunadine P. Insight into troubled sexuality. Chapman and Hall, London, 1992.

Section 5:
Office gynecology

Pediatric and adolescent gynecology

Joseph Sanfilippo MD FACOG
George Creatsas MD FACS

Introduction

The adolescent population has continued to grow and flourish. According to the US Bureau of Census, the number of women between 15 and 19 years of age will increase from 8.5 million in 1990 to 9.2 million in 2010 [1]. A significant proportion of this population is the female adolescent. Pediatric and adolescent gynecology (PAG) continues to evolve as an area of subspecialized services in obstetrics and gynecology. Expertise in gynecological disease is an appropriate prerequisite for gynecological care. However, a different approach is required owing to the sensitive psychology of the child, and the need for preservation of the anatomy and normal function of the reproductive system. PAG encompasses obstetrics, namely adolescent pregnancy and abortions. It is also concerned with adolescent sexual education, sexually transmitted diseases and contraception during adolescence.

Adolescence is a transitional period which coincides with several biological, social and psychological changes [2]. The most important are the endocrinological alterations during maturation of the hypothalamic–pituitary–ovarian axis, ultimately resulting in the culmination of pubertal development, namely menarche.

History and physical examination

Pediatric

The logical place to begin is with a discussion of pediatric gynecology in the newborn infant, in which case the history has been obtained from the parent(s), followed by a general physical examination. The examination begins with a general inspection of the body. As our primary focus in this segment is assessment of the neonate, it is appropriate that attention be centered on evaluation of the external genitalia and abdominal examination. The latter begins with inspection, followed by gentle palpation for evidence of abdominal mass or other acute injury. The external genitalia are assessed for signs of any lacerations, edema, palpable mass or other abnormality. The labia are gently grasped and separated for easier inspection of the introital–hymenal area. Upon completion of vaginal inspection, the anal opening is evaluated.

On recto-abdominal bimanual examination, a midline structure indicative of the uterus is palpable; however, the adnexa should *not* be palpable. Inadequate examination of the neonate can result in an individual being faced with a lifelong problem such as congenital adrenal hyperplasia or other life threatening circumstance.

For the preadolescent patient, one objective during the examination should be to win the child's confidence. A 'show and tell' approach is often effective. The history is obtained primarily from the parent(s) who, for this age group, ideally are integrally involved in the child's physical examination. The two most significant ingredients in performing a genital examination in children include: (1) the patient must have a sense of control and experience no discomfort – ideally, the goals are accomplished via an adequate explanation prior to the examination in order to eliminate any 'surprises' for the child during the examination process; and (2) the patient, no matter what age, should be actively involved in the examination.

The prepubertal child's genital

examination includes use of several concepts: (1) 'just looking', when visualization alone frequently can provide the appropriate diagnosis in the majority of children; and (2) placement of the patient in the frog-legged position is especially helpful for the inspection phase of the examination. A knee–chest position with the Valsalva maneuver will permit further assessment of the introital lower third of the vagina. Magnification, especially with use of a colposcope or a hand-held magnifying lens, is useful; visualization of the vestibule allows further assessment of the lower vagina. An otoscope and/or vaginoscope or other light source is particularly helpful. Gentle traction on the labia, upward and outward, will further expose the introital hymenal area and permit appropriate assessment. The clinician should be aware of the various 'normal' hymenal configurations. A number of 'breaks and bumps' can provide minute variations with respect to the 'normal hymen'; an imperforate, microperforate or septated hymen should be identified. For all age groups, when evaluation is warranted, it is requisite that an adequate gynecological examination be carried out.

Adolescent

Obtaining a history in the adolescent age group may occur initially in the presence of the parent(s). However, the clinician must provide the adolescent adequate time to convey her own concerns regarding sexuality, her specific medical problems, etc.

The clinician also must win the confidence of the adolescent, just as with the pediatric patient, and ideally approach the situation in a relaxed manner that provides the best opportunity for obtaining information.

During the examination, the adolescent must be informed, ideally just prior to the performance of the examination, regarding specific aspects of the examination process. It is best that the healthcare team avoid a 'hand-holding' approach and explain that it is better that the parent(s) not be present during the examination. Continued communication thoughout the process tends to alleviate anxiety in the patient. The adolescent is placed in the dorsal lithotomy position for the examination, with an effort made on the physician's part to maintain eye contact during the pelvic examination. It is imperative that appropriate-sized specula be available, including the small Pedersen (8 cm depth). The 4–5 cm pediatric

speculum is inadequate for appropriate visualization of the cervix (Figure 21.1).

Inspection of the vulva is followed by palpation of Bartholin's and urethroskenes glands. The clitoris normally is 2–4 mm wide; hymenal configuration should be evaluated. Trauma to the urethra or fourchette area should be carefully ascertained and documented. Upon completion of the speculum portion of the examination, a single digital bimanual (in the virginal female) is sufficient for proper assessment of the pelvic organs. A recto-vaginal examination is performed to complete the bimanual assessment.

Menstrual disorders

Menstrual disorders are the most common gynecological abnormality during adolescence, mainly due to the incomplete maturation of the hypothalamic–

Fig. 21.1 Pederson speculum.

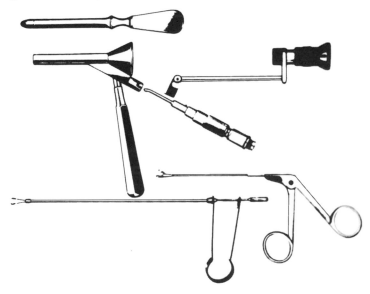

pituitary–ovarian (HPO) axis. Environmental factors such as stress and malnutrition and a number of chromosomal disorders interfere with the normal function of the menstrual cycle.

Amenorrhea

Amenorrhea is characterized as primary (PA) if the patient has never reached menarche, or secondary (SA) if menstrual periods have ceased for at least 6 months. Primary amenorrhea may be related to anatomical and/or endocrinological problems or to specific genetic disorders.

Primary amenorrhea of anatomical origin includes cases with normal development of secondary characteristics (SC) and absence of the vagina and/or the uterus (Rokitansky–Kuster–Hauser syndrome). In obstruction of the vaginal outflow tract due to a septum or absence of the cervix, PA is clinically associated with recurring pain and occasionally with foul-smelling vaginal discharge. A didelphic uterus with obstruction of one segment of the vagina is a clinically more confusing circumstance because the patient menstruates normally from one side and may present with signs of obstruction on the other [3]. This condition is often misdiagnosed as a pelvic ovarian mass [4]. A common complication of this deformity is the development of (pelvic) endometriosis [5]. The medical history, gynecological examination, pelvic ultrasound and occasionally magnetic resonance imaging are important in assessing PA that appears to be

of anatomic origin, as mullerian anomalies are associated with urinary system anomalies in 20% of patients (Box 21.1) [6].

The management of PA due to obstruction is considered an emergency; it includes incision of the obstruction within the vaginal canal, canulation of the cervical route and reconstruction of the genital tract so as to preserve reproductive potential and prevent juvenile endometriosis.

If anatomical reasons are excluded and the secondary sex characteristics are absent, or poorly developed or heterosexual, endocrinological investigation is indicated. Delayed puberty may be of central (hypothalamic or pituitary) or ovarian origin (gonadal dysgenesis, GD) (Box 21.2) or may be due to extragenital reasons such as thyroid dysfunction. The possibility of a constitutionally delayed puberty should also be taken into account if no significant pathology is identified. Finally, the presence of PA associated with heterosexual characteristics may be related to an androgen-secreting ovarian tumor, congenital adrenal hyperplasia or to an androgen insensitivity syndrome (Box 21.2). Box 21.3 summarizes the differential diagnoses of primary and secondary amenorrhea.

Treatment of PA should be individualized. Classification of cases according to Box 21.3

would facilitate the choice of treatment. Estrogen therapy is indicated in hypoestrogenic conditions. Treatment should be initiated early to avoid osteoporosis. Estrogen treatment will also increase vaginal epithelialization. Estrogens may be administered orally or transdermally. Cyclical progestins should be added to prevent endometrial hyperplasia and ensure regular menstruation. Ultrasonography is useful to assess endometrial lining thickness. If it is greater than 10 mm, there should be concern for endometrial hyperplasia and the rare but possible carcinoma. Thus, sampling would be indicated [7].

Treatment of the young GD patient with growth hormone alone or in combination with low doses of ethinyl estradiol has also been advocated [8,9]. The results regarding the final height are promising.

Secondary amenorrhea is much more common than primary amenorrhea. In this age group, anorexia nervosa/weight loss amenorrhea are common presentations. In managing such patients with psychological problems, coordination of care with the adolescent psychiatry team is desirable. Another common cause of SA is athletic amenorrhea, which is very much related to stress conditions and is dependent on the degree of exercise [10]. In all cases, reassurance of the patient and the

---

Box 21.1 Basic evaluation of primary amenorrheic adolescents

- Medical history
- Physical examination
- Complete blood count
- Follicle stimulating hormone (FSH)
- Prolactin
- Imaging studies (as indicated)

Box 21.2 Causes of primary amenorrhea during adolescence

Normal development of secondary characteristics
- Vaginal agenesis
- Vaginal and uterine aplasia
- Deformities with obstruction

Poor development or absence of secondary characteristics
- Constitutional delayed puberty
- Delayed puberty of central origin
- Delayed puberty of ovarian origin
- Extragenital reasons of delayed puberty

Presence of heterosexual characteristics
- Androgen insensitivity (testicular feminizing) syndrome
- Congenital adrenal hyperplasia
- Ovarian tumor

family as well as a frank explanation of the problem are advised to improve compliance with treatment.

Treatment of primary amenorrhea is dependent on the underlying etiology. Treatment with regard to anatomic causes of primary amenorrhea should be initiated if there is absence of menarche by 12.5 years of age (mean age of menarche). Failure to reach menarche at a bone age of 13 establishes appropriate priority to proceed with evaluation/treatment.

Treatment of vaginal agenesis as in the Mayer-von Rokitansky-Kuster-Hauser syndrome requires the use of Frank dilators, ideally with use of a bicycle seat at regular time intervals to generate pressure at the vaginal dimple. Perserverance in this approach may well lead to a functional vagina. In cases where the patient is unable to carry out such an approach or when there is development of an inadequate vagina, surgical treatment is in order.

With functional causes of

primary amenorrhea such as hyperandrogenism of ovarian origin, as in the case of polycystic ovarian syndrome, treatment is predicated upon menses being induced on a routine basis, i.e. ideally at least every 3 months with a progestin or, as an alternative, prescription of an estrogen-dominant oral contraceptive. For the patient who has complete absence of secondary sex characteristics, menstrual induction can be accomplished with the use of ethinyl estradiol 5–10 mg daily dosages or conjugated equine estrogens 0.3 mg daily. In addition, transdermal 17β-estradiol (0.025 mg) can be prescribed. After 12–18 months of unopposed estrogen therapy or after the occurrence of vaginal bleeding, a progestin should be added cyclically in the form of medroxyprogesterone acetate 5 mg or cyproterone acetate at similar dosages to prevent the unopposed estrogen effect, i.e. endometrial hyperplasia [11].

Dysfunctional uterine bleeding

Dysfunctional uterine bleeding (DUB) and oligomenorrhea due to chronic anovulation are the most common types of menstrual disturbances, accounting for more than 40% of menstrual irregularities during the first 2 postpubertal years [12]. A common pattern is of periods of amenorrhea and DUB alternating. The normal menstrual cycle ideally would be of a mean interval of 26–28 days with a mean duration of 3–7 days and a menstrual flow between 30–80 ml per cycle. DUB may

Box 21.3 Differential diagnosis of primary and secondary amenorrhea based on clinical presentation

Heterosexual clinical signs
- Congenital adrenal hyperplasia
- Ovarian or adrenal tumor
- Chronic anovulation syndrome
- Polycystic ovarian disease
- Cushing's disease or syndrome
- Pituitary tumor

Abnormal stature
- Gonadal dysgenesis
- Pituitary lesions
- Extragenital disease (thyroid, malnutrition)

Galactorrhea
- Post-pill amenorrhea
- Hyperprolactinemia (due to pharmacologic or pathologic causes)
- Hypothyroidism

Other symptoms and conditions
- Periodic pelvic pain (cryptomenorrhea)
- Nutritional (anorexia nervosa, obesity)
- Anemia
- Iatrogenic
- Adolescent pregnancy

present as metrorrhagia, menorrhagia, menometrorrhagia or polymenorrhea. The disease may appear as an urgent gynecological problem, in which case the healthcare provider should be aware of the diagnosis and management of the disease entity.

Creatsas et al. reported that DUB accounted for 46.5% of all pubertal vaginal bleeding [13], occurred at a median age of 12 years and presented a 'seasonal distrubution' with over 55% occurring during the winter months. Nearly 50% of adolescent DUB was associated with anovulation. Intermenstrual bleeding caused by inadequate hormonal replacement or non-compliance with hormonal therapy accounted for 8.4% of consultations.

DUB is mainly due to incomplete maturation of the HPO axis and is particularly related to the lack of positive feedback. This leads to anovulatory cycles often associated with hyperplastic endometrium owing to an unopposed estrogen effect. The degree of endometrial shedding is related to the preceding endometrial proliferation. Prostaglandins (PGs) are also implicated in the pathophysiology of this dysfunction. Alterations of the $PGF_{2\alpha}$ (vasoconstrictor) and PGE_2 (vasodilator) ratio have been reported in both ovulatory and anovulatory DUB. The proposed mechanism is that increased levels of arachidonic acid saturate the $PGF_{2\alpha}$ pathway, thus increasing PGE_2 formation and altering the ratio of vasoconstriction to vasodilation [14]. Box 21.4 lists the

---

Box 21.4 Basic evaluation of adolescents with dysfunctional uterine bleeding

- Medical history
- Physical examination
- Gynecological examination
- Blood cell count, coagulation profile
- Thyroid function tests
- Beta-human chorionic gonadotropin
- Prolactin
- Pelvic ultrasound
- Other diagnostic procedures – including vaginoscopy, hysteroscopy (used very occasionally)

---

components of the clinical evaluation of DUB.

The clinical classification of the disease depends on the hemoglobin levels and cycle patterns. DUB is classified as mild, moderate or severe if hemoglobin levels are more than 12 g/dl, 10–12 g/dl or less than 10 g/dl, respectively; moderate DUB is associated with prolonged profuse and irregular menstrual periods, while severe cases present with heavy and prolonged vaginal bleeding.

Coagulopathies account for 19% of abnormal bleeding in teenagers, being the second most common cause after anovulatory DUB [15]. Coagulation disorders include idiopathic thrombocytopenic purpura, von Willebrand's disease and leukemia. Several of these blood dyscrasias are discovered during the first menstruation. Other systemic diseases such as hepatic/renal failure, malignancies, thyroid and adrenal disorders, and iatrogenic causes such as inappropriate contraceptive devices as well as adolescent pregnancy should be ruled out. The medical history may point to one or other of these conditions.

Organic disease may involve trauma, infections or neoplasia of the reproductive system. Trauma

from sexual intercourse may be the cause of bleeding since the vagina is still immature. Uterine pathology is an uncommon cause for teenage menorrhagia/abnormal bleeding. Conditions such as endometritis, polyps, submucosal leiomyomata, uterine malignancies and mullerian anomalies may present as abnormal uterine bleeding.

Treatment of DUB depends on the severity of the problem and includes several modalities such as the administration of hemostatic estrogen/progestin preparations, cyclic progestins alone or combined oral contraceptives (Box 21.5). The goal of treatment is to increase endometrial thickness, induce stromal stability, and to 'engineer' a controlled withdrawal bleed. Prostaglandin synthetase inhibitors may be used as primary therapy or as an adjunct to hormones. Dilatation and curettage is a last resort, performed in a very limited number of cases. The use of GnRH analogs, danazol and clomiphene citrate is not recommended. Finally, iron supplements are prescribed to correct anemia. Explanation and reassurance given to both the adolescent and the parent are essential bases for management. The long-term prognosis in most cases is excellent, for although

Box 21.5 Management of dysfunctional uterine bleeding

Hemoglobin > 12 g/100 ml
- Reassurance
- Menstrual calendar
- Iron supplements
- Periodic re-evaluation

Hemoglobin 10–12 g/100 ml
- Reassurance and explanation
- Menstrual calendar
- Iron supplements
- Cyclic progestin therapy or oral contraceptives
- Re-evaluation in 6 months

Hemoglobin < 10 g/100 ml
1. No active bleeding
   - Explanation
   - Transfusion/iron supplements
   - Oral contraceptives
   - Re-evaluation in 6–12 months
2. Acute hemorrhage
   - Transfusion
   - Fluid replacement therapy
   - Hormonal hemostasis (intravenous or oral conjugated estrogen)
   - Intensive progestin therapy
   - Curettage when hormonal hemostasis fails
   - Oral contraceptives for 6–12 months

Reproduced with permission from Muram D, Sanfilippo JS, Hertweck P. Vaginal bleeding in childhood and menstrual disorders in adolescence. In: Sanfillipo J, Muram D, Lee P, Dewhurst J (eds) Pediatric and adolescent gynecology. Philadelphia: WB Saunders, 1994: 230.

50% of cases may still have persistent problems 4 years later, no more than 5% of patients present with further bleeding episodes later in their reproductive life [16].

Breast disorders

Breast examination

Breast examination in adolescent patients should be performed as an integral part of the general physical examination. Tanner staging should be addressed from the perspectives of both visual inspection and palpation of the breasts. Adolescents should receive instruction regarding breast awareness in an effort to increase chances for early identification of specific abnormalities. Normally, thelarche occurs between 8 and 14 years of age with a mean age of 11 years. Thelarche is usually the first sign of pubertal development and in general is followed within 6 months by pubarche and within 2–4 years by menarche.

Breast development and growth have their genesis during the embryonic phase with the presence of a mammary ridge. The embryonic ridge extends from the axilla to the groin and develops at 5–6 weeks' gestation. This entity later involutes in all but the thoracic area. Remnants of the anlage can be identified in the form of polythelia and/or polymastia. In addition to congenital factors, a number of other abnormalities including endocrinopathies and chromosomal defects can affect breast development. Several congenital breast abnormalities have been reported (Box 21.6).

Mammary gland development in the newborn can be identified as a reflection of maternal estrogen production; elevation of the glands in both male and female neonates is often noted. Histologically, there is evidence that the alveoli in the neonate have secretory activity. This stimulation can result in the appearance of 'witch's milk' in 80–90% of newborns [17]. The phenomenon is a manifestation of

Box 21.6 Classification of primary congenital breast anomalies

Congenital anomalies of the nipple and areola
1. Disorders of absence/excess
   - Amastia
   - Polythelia
   - Athelia
2. Disorders of size/shape
   - Inversion
   - Herniation
   - Hypertrophy
   - Hypoplasia

Congenital anomalies of the breast
1. Disorders of absence/excess
   - Amastia (e.g. Poland syndrome)
   - Polymastia
2. Disorders of shape/size
   - Hypertrophy
   - Hypoplasia
   - Combined hypertrophy/hypoplasia
   - Asymmetry
   - Abnormal shape (tuberous, conical, goat-udder breast)
3. Congenital breast hemangioma

hormone withdrawal, coupled with stimulation by prolactin, which results in neonatal secretion of milk for up to 3–4 weeks postpartum.

During early childhood, only a minor amount of ductal branching occurs; the breast is otherwise quiescent. In the typical sequence of pubertal development, thelarche (onset of visible breast growth) is the earliest sign. The mean age of onset of thelarche in the USA is 9.8 years [18]. The endocrinological phenomena associated with breast development are a reflection of increasing estrogen production from the ovary. Estrogens stimulate the mammary ducts to elongate and reduplicate their epithelial lining and induce proliferation of the terminal ducts resulting in formation of breast lobules. Volume and elasticity of the periductal tissues seem to respond to estrogen. This hormonal stimulation also results in mammary vascularization and fat deposition.

Pubertal breast development occurs in a horizontal 'disk-like' fashion, as well as in a vertical direction, with dichotomy of sprouting of primary and secondary milk ducts. Mammary ducts grow and differentiate into lobular-areolar structures. Development revolves around five distinct stages:

- Stage I: Pre-adolescent elevation of papilla (nipple).
- Stage II: Mammary growth with further development of subareolar area, resulting in formation of the breast bud.
- Stage III: Further growth and development of the papilla.

- Stage IV: Accelerated development of subareolar area with elevation of the nipple and areolae with the breast taking on a 'globular' shape.
- Stage V: Mature breast which reflects estrogen and progesterone effect (Tanner classification).

Dependence upon a normal hypothalamic–pituitary–ovarian interaction is critical and frequently 18 months after onset of menarche the breasts will undergo cyclical changes in response to the ovarian hormones. Final breast maturity and formation are usually attained toward the end of the second decade, a time course that should be taken into consideration prior to any surgical intervention in adolescents.

Congenital breast anomalies

Amastia

The congenital absence of one of both breasts, or one or both nipples, is the rarest of the congenital anomalies. The condition is usually unilateral and often associated with other anomalies, such as abnormal development of the chest musculature, shoulder girdle and arm (Poland syndrome). Treatment is surgical.

Polythelia and polymastia

Abnormal regression of the mammary ridge may lead to retention of accessory breast tissue (polymastia) or acessory nipples (polythelia). The phenomenon of polythelia is the most common congenital breast anomaly, occurring in 1–5% of all females [19,20]. It appears to be more common in Oriental and Black patients. Polythelia and polymastia can occur simultaneously.

Polymastia is less common than polythelia. The accessory breast tissue is usually identified in the axilla and may or may not have an associated nipple. It may enlarge premenstrually as well as during pregnancy. It is more commonly a cosmetic problem than a source of other bothersome symptoms. Excision of accessory breast tissue can be performed, if indicated, especially during pregnancy when the accessory tissue is well outlined.

The presence of polymastia and/or polythelia provides suggestions for other congenital anomalies [21,22].

Renal anomalies, including agenesis, renal cell carcinoma, supernumerary kidneys, cardiac anomalies (septal defects, conduction defects), limb and vertebral anomalies have all been associated with increased incidence of polymastia and/or polythelia.

Hypertrophy

Excessive breast growth may be unilateral or bilateral (virginal hypertrophy, unilateral hypertrophy with contralateral hypoplasia or amastia). The exact etiology of breast hypertrophy remains a point of controversy. The most frequent type of true hypertrophy occurs during adolescence and is not associated with obvious pubertal or endocrinological abnormalities. Excessive breast growth poses both psychological and physical difficulties in the developing adolescent. Enlarged breasts are often a source of discomfort, mastalgia and other associated problems. When there is no regression of adolescent breast hypertrophy, reduction mammoplasty is required.

Breast hypoplasia

Decreased quantity of breast tissue is a subjective perception by the affected individual. Whereas amastia may be an obvious end to the spectrum of breast size, any completed breast development may be defined as 'too small' by the beholder. The incidence of true breast hypoplasia cannot be accurately discerned.

Breast asymmetry

All females experience some degree of breast asymmetry. When it is quite noticeable, intervention is indicated. In general, significant asymmetry is noted in 4% of patients [23].

Abnormal breast shape has been reported. The nipple and areola complex may enlarge and comprise much of the substance of the breast (nipple breast) [24]. The areola complex may herniate and produce a sessile protrusion from the breast mound. Other abnormalities in shape include the conical breast (sharply tapering) [25]. In addition, tuberous breasts resembling a tuberous root or a cylinder as well as the goat udder-like breast have been reported [26,27]. Surgical correction of these abnormal breast shapes is the most feasible approach.

Contraception during adolescence

Adolescent contraception usage differs from that of adults. Many adolescents do not seek medical advice for contraception until they have been sexually active or following an accidental pregnancy. Another challenge is that, when adolescents start a contraceptive method (CM), their compliance is often poor. The determinants of compliance are attitudes to sexuality, the previous history of contraception, socioeconomic and environmental factors, and access to sex education and to contraception. The attitudes of parents and healthcare providers influence whether a teenager uses them as a resource for advice [28–30].

Concerns about breach of confidentiality are an important barrier. Guidelines have been drawn up in the UK to guide the provision of contraceptive care to adolescents under 16 years (Box 21.7). Compliance is expected to be higher when the suggested CM is also indicated for medical reasons, i.e. when oral contraceptives (OCs) are used to regulate the menstrual cycle. The use of peer counselors may be an effective strategy. Other factors affecting contraceptive use are adverse publicity about contraceptives, misconceptions about side effects (weight gain) or risks (cancer), the shift to barriers because of concerns about sexually transmitted diseases (STDs) and human immunodeficiency virus (HIV), and national or local abortion legislation and facilities [29–31].

Hormonal and non–hormonal methods may be used for contraception during adolescence. Oral contraceptives seem to be favored among adolescents. In a European multicenter study conducted by the International Federation of Infantile and Juvenile Gynecology (FIGIJ), it was found that in 6 out of 11 European countries participating in the study, OCs were the most common contraceptive method utilized. However, poor compliance remains a problem. Among the barrier methods used, the condom was the most common [31].

A significant number of adolescents during the first 2–3 postpubertal years present with menstrual irregularities. Oral contraceptives can have a dual

---

Box 21.7 Factors to remember when choosing a contraceptive method for the adolescent

- Acceptability: is it a method the patient will continue to use consistently?
- Effectiveness of method and frequency of intercourse: does the method lend itself to the 'unplanned' coital episode often seen in this age group?
- Number of partners/concerns about sexually transmitted disease: is the patient adequately protected?
- Cost/access to medical care: can the patient afford the method on a long-term basis?
- Motivation/self-discipline of patient and male partner: will reluctance to interrupt foreplay result in non-use of the method?
- Safety/risk: will short-term convenience result in long-term drawbacks?
- Personal and family religious and ethical philosophy: will it influence usage?

Reproduced with permission from Slupik R. Contraception. In: Sanfilippo J, Muram D, Lee P, Dewhurst J (eds) Pediatric and adolescent gynecology. Philadelphia: WB Saunders, 1994: 290.

role in regulation of the menstrual cycle and providing contraception [32,33]. The benefits associated with OCs when used during adolescence can be summarized as follows:

- a decreased risk of functional ovarian cysts;

- menstrual cycle regulation/ prevention of anemia;

- control of dysmenorrhea;

- a lower incidence of pelvic inflammatory disease;

- a long-term reduction in ovarian and endometrial carcinoma;

- a lower incidence of ectopic pregnancy;

- a lower incidence of benign breast disease.

Hormonal contraception is best initiated after menses are established. There is no evidence that low-dose combined pills affect epiphyseal growth. Most epiphyseal growth occurs premenarche and only about an extra inch in height is added after menarche.

Other hormonal CMs include depot medroxyprogesterone acetate (Depo-Provera®, DMPA) and the Norplant subdermal implant system. DMPA is given in a standard dose of 150 mg intramuscularly every 12 weeks and yields a rate of 0.5–1 pregnancies per 100 woman-years. DMPA suppresses the preovulatory surge of luteinizing hormone and follicle-stimulating hormone and therefore inhibits ovulation. The Norplant subdermal implant system contains six slow-releasing silastic capsules (rods) which release

levonorgestrel over 6–7 years, although it is licensed for use for 5 years. The World Health Organization (WHO) reported a cumulative pregnancy rate over 5 years of 2.6. Both methods are not user dependent and therefore have low user-failure rates [34].

A combination of 35 μg of ethinylestradiol and 2 mg cyproterone acetate (CPA) is one contraceptive and can be used in young women with significant acne. CPA blocks androgen receptors and reduces androgen production while ethinyl estradiol raises sex hormone-binding globulin thereby 'mopping up' free circulating androgens. Other non androgenic low-dose pills are also appropriate for teenagers with acne.

Among the non-hormonal contraceptive methods, the condom is very popular. In many countries it is offered free by family planning and other sexual health services. All healthcare providers should be able to instruct in the correct use of the condom. Adolescents are advised to use approved lubricated latex condoms, preferably those with a spermicidal lubricant [35]. HIV has changed the sexual behavior of many teenagers. The fear of STDs has made the condom a popular method among adolescents. In addition, the condom is available without medical intervention, has a low cost and presents virtually no side effects [36].

Female barrier methods are less commonly used by adolescents. Diaz et al. reported the use of the sponge by 1.9% of 208 adolescents who completed a 54-item questionnaire [37]. Other researchers have drawn similar

conclusions [38]. Intrauterine devices (IUDs) are not recommended during the adolescent years, although in Europe they are used for emergency contraception. In a study of 120 adolescents who received the Copper 7 IUD, satisfaction with the method was reported by 72% of the users, and the pregnancy rate was 2 per 100 woman-years [39].

Finally, it should be mentioned that many adolescents often use less effective methods, such as periodic abstinence and coitus interruptus.

Chronic pelvic pain

Chronic pelvic pain (CPP), defined as 6 months or longer of lower abdominal discomfort, is a phenomenon observed in adolescents [40].

When an adolescent presents with a specific complaint of CPP, she should be evaluated among other things for any history of sexual abuse. A high incidence of childhood sexual abuse has been reported in adults and also has been noted in adolescents with CPP; behavioral patterns differ significantly, with respect to life control, punishing responses to pain, and higher levels of somatization and 'global distress' between abused and non-abused adolescents with CPP [40].

Diagnosis

When a clinician determines that CPP is the most obvious primary complaint of the adolescent, a multisystem approach is most efficacious. Determination must be made as to whether the pain results from: (1) gynecologic; (2) gastrointestinal; (3) genitourinary; (4) musculoskeletal; or (5) psychological causes [41–44] (Boxes 21.8–21.10) The history will undoubtedly help establish the most obvious diagnosis along with the physical examination that follows. Identification of any 'trigger points' eliciting the pain, the presence of any flank or costovertebral angle tenderness, or a well-delineated pelvic–rectovaginal examination are of paramount importance. In addition, assessment of the extremities, with tests such as leg-raising etc., is recommended.

Completion of assessment, with identification of a primary source of the pain, should be followed by appropriate evaluation, the basic tests being:

- complete blood count;

- urinalysis;

- sedimentation rate.

The history and physical examination findings will direct the clinician towards further investigations, such as ultrasound (for assessment of any mass), computed tomography, magnetic resonance imaging, radiological imaging (such as barium enema, intravenous pyelogram etc.), neurologic opinion/trigger point injection and, as indicated, operative intervention [45] primarily in the form of diagnostic laparoscopy.

A multidisciplinary approach to CPP holds the most therapeutic promise. The importance of the adolescent's insight into her own disease process and pain management must be emphasized.

Treatment

Treatment modalities include non-steroidal drugs (Table 21.1). A distinct effort to avoid narcotics is strongly advised. In addition, the use of antidepressants such as fluoxetine 20 mg/day appears to be effective in the treatment of chronic pelvic pain [46]. Anxiolytics such as alprazolam (Xanax) and triazolo-benzodiazepine (with added antidepressant effects) also appear to be effective. Non-medical treatments including the use of biofeedback, transcutaneous electrical nerve stimulation (TENS) units, relaxation training and psychological counseling with an effort made to change the lifestyle of the adolescent should also be considered.

Sexual abuse

One out of every four females is the victim of sexual abuse [47].

Box 21.8   Gastrointestinal causes of pelvic pain

Irritable bowel syndrome
1. *Symptoms*
   - crampy, colicky lower abdominal pain
   - pain – hours or days
   - exacerbations – diet related, high-fat diets, stress, anxiety depression, menses
2. *Treatment*
   - reassurance – education, stress reduction
   - bulk-forming agents
   - anxiolytics
   - low-dose tricylate antidepressants
   - avoid anticholinergic agents

Inflammatory bowel disease
- Crohn's disease
- Diagnosis – upper gastrointestinal, small bowel follow-through
- Colonoscopy

Ulcerative colitis
1. *Symptoms*
   - Acute pain, diarrhea, hematochezia
2. *Diagnosis*
   - Sigmoidoscopy
   - Rectal biopsy

Diverticular disease
- Diverticulosis
- Diverticulitis

Infectious enterocolitis

Intestinal neoplasms

Carcinoma
- Colon or rectum
- History – adenomatous polyps
- Family history – first-degree relatives

Appendicitis

Hernia

Ischemic bowel disease

Intestinal endometriosis

Reproduced with permission from Summitt RL Jr. Urogynecologic causes of chronic pelvic pain. *Obstet Gynecol Clin North Am* 1993;20:688.

Box 21.9 Urologic causes of pelvic pain

Acute causes
- Acute cystitis
- Acute urethritis
- Urethral diverticulum
- Urolithiasis
- Radiation cystitis

Chronic causes
- Interstitial cystitis
- Urethral syndrome
- Urethral diverticulum
- Urolithiasis
- Radiation cystitis
- Urethral caruncle
- Neoplasm
- Detrusor–sphincter dyssynergia

Reproduced with permission from Summitt RL Jr. Urologic causes of chronic pelvic pain. *Obstet Gynecol Clin North Am* 1993;20:688.

Unfortunately, child sexual abuse is recognized as a problem that affects children independent of age, sex, socioeconomic status or geographic location. There is evidence that younger children (4–9 years of age) are at a higher risk because of their naive, trusting approach to adults, and thus their vulnerability with respect to sexual activities [47]. It has been estimated that 1% to 38% of all females younger than 18 years have been victims of child sexual abuse [48]. In the United States, the National Center on Child Abuse and Neglect compiles data regarding the number of child victims which is currently estimated at 200 000 per year [49]. Among adolescents, date rape is an area of increased concern. There seems to be a fine line between what constitutes 'consent' versus forced rape.

Date rape

The National Institute of Mental Health reports that one in every four women has been a victim of rape or attempted rape [50]. Sadly date rape usually goes unreported [51]. Reluctance to report such events is common. For this reason, strong emphasis must be placed on the need for teenagers to report rape as well as attempted rape to responsible authorities. In a survey of middle and high school students, 12% of males and 18% of females reported 'unwanted sexual activity', with a majority of these episodes occurring between 13 and 16 years of age [52]. Of interest, 25–47% of date rapes occur on the first date, with a statistically increased risk of rape if the male has initiated the date, driven the car and paid for the entertainment [53,54]. An association has been identified between the incidence of alcohol/substance abuse and date rape [54]. Correlation between impairment of judgement in sexual relationships and use of alcohol remains a concern.

When date rape is reported, prophylaxis for sexually transmitted infections is appropriate [55]. In addition, pregnancy prevention in the form of emergency contraception should be offered to the patient. The current recommended treatment within 72 h of the rape is 50 µg ethinyl estradiol and 0.5 mg norgestrel, two tablets immediately followed by two tablets 12 h later. Antiemetics may also be prescribed. A number of other regimens, including mifepristone (RU486), have been evaluated.

Date rape in association with flunitrazepam, a hypnotic, has been reported in recent years. While this medication has never been marketed in the USA, as well as in a number of other countries, it is nevertheless 'smuggled' into many countries and used to facilitate date rape [56]. As a prelude to an assault, flunetrazepam, a benzodiazepine, is rapidly dissolved in any solution, and it is colorless, odorless and tasteless. Its primary

Box 21.10 Diagnosis of musculoskeletal-associated pelvic pain

Musculoskeletal pain
- Identify trigger points
- Referred pain
- Poor posture

Diagnostic assessment
- Physical therapy evaluation
- History
- Postural examination
- Active and passive range of motion
- Palpation examination
- Muscle strength testing
- Neurologic screening
- Gait

Reproduced with permission from Baker PK. Musculoskeletal origins of chronic pelvic pain. *Obstet Gynecol Clin North Am* 1993;20:719–42.

Table 21.1 Specific-dose medical therapy for chronic pelvic pain

Drug	Initial dose (mg)	Subsequent dose (mg)	Frequency
Acetic/salycylic acids			
Indomethacin	25	25	t.i.d.
Tolmetin	400	400	t.i.d.
Sulindac	200	200	b.i.d.
Diflurisal	1000	500	q.d. 12 h
Diclofenac	75–100	75	b.i.d.
Etodolac	400	400	q.d. 4–6 h
Ketrolac	10	10	q.d. 4–6 h
Propionic acids			
Ibuprofen	400	400	q.d. 4 h
Naproxen	500	250	q.d. 6–8 h
Naproxen sodium	550	275	q.d. 6–8 h
Fenoprofen calcium	200	200	q.d. 4–6 h
Ketoprofen	75	75	t.i.d.
Fenamates			
Mefenamic acid	500	100	t.i.d.
Meclofenamate	100	50–100	q.d. 6 h
Pyrazolones			
Oxyphenbutazone	100	100	t.i.d.
Phenylbutazone	100	100	t.i.d.
Oxicams			
Piroxicam	20	20	q.d.

Reproduced with permission from Smith R. Cyclic pelvic pain and dysmenorrhea. *Obstet Gynecol Clin North Am* 1993;20:761.
t.i.d. = three times daily; b.i.d. = twice daily; q.d. = every day.

manifestations include drowsiness, impaired motor skills and anterograde amnesia. Clinicians should be aware that patients with a complaint of sexual assault who appear intoxicated or have anterograde amnesia may have been exposed to flunitrazepam [57].

A number of programs addressing prevention of acquaintance (date) rape through education have been implemented. Focus is placed on identification of the 'general likeability and aggressiveness' components of the perpetrator's personality. Such programs focus on techniques such as debunking rape mythology, generating participant interaction, providing sexuality education and a feminist orientation, all of which serve to avoid confrontational approaches. Avoidance of alcohol and substance use is also emphasized [58,59].

Incest is one subcategory of sexual abuse and is defined as inappropriate sexual behavior within the context of a pre-existing family relationship. This can include relatives, step-parents–stepchild or a number of other sexual companions of a parent, such as a common-law spouse. It may be that initially the sexual acts are limited to exposure, light touch, etc. These can rapidly progress to overt sexual activity, the most common of which is oral penetration. The next most common is sodomy; vaginal penetration in the very young child is the least common. However, rubbing of the perpetrator's penis against the child's genitalia, an act known as 'dry intercourse', has been reported with increasing frequency [60]. When a history is obtained from a child sexual abuse victim, a number of guidelines are recommended. These are included in Box 21.11. The physical examination requires an overall inspection for any trauma; specific injuries must be identified and appropriately addressed. Magnifying devices (magnifying glass, otoscope or colposcope) enhance anogenital assessment. Documentation with photographs via the colposcope remains a controversial area. Abnormal findings must be appropriately classified (Table 21.2).

Absence of any physical

Box 21.11 Obtaining a history from child victims of sexual abuse

General measures
• Provide a comfortable environment
• Language and technique should be developmentally appropriate
• Allow sufficient time to avoid any coercive quality to the interview
• Establish a rapport with the child

Questioning
• The initial questions should be non-directive to elicit spontaneous responses
• Leading questions should be avoided. If such questions are used, responses should be carefully evaluated
• Non-verbal tools (e.g. anatomically detailed dolls or drawings) may be used to assist the child in communication
• Anatomically detailed dolls should be used primarily for the identification of body parts and clarification of previous statements
• Psychological testing is not required for the purpose of proving sexual assault
• At some point, the child should be questioned directly about the abusive relationship

Reprinted with permission from Muram D. Sexual abuse. In: Sanfilippo J, Muram D, Lee P, Dewhurst J (eds) Pediatric and adolescent gynecology. Philadelphia: WB Saunders, 1994: 365.

Table 21.2 Medical evaluation of abused children: classification of abnormal findings

Category	Abnormalities
1. Normal examination	No abnormalities detected Variations of normal
2. Non-specific abnormalities	Friability of the posterior fourchette Labial adhesions, hymenal tags, hymenal bumps and clefts Non-specific infections Bruising of the external genitalia
3. Specific findings	Hymenal–vaginal tear Hymenal–perineal tear Sexually transmitted disease Bite marks on the genitalia
4. Definitive abnormalities	Presence of sperm Pregnancy in an adolescent

Reprinted with permission from Muram D. Sexual abuse. In: Sanfilippo J, Muram D, Lee P,

findings should not be interpreted as lies on the child's part or incorrect answers. One study attests to the fact that often there is complete absence of any physical findings, but clear evidence of child sexual abuse [61]. Perineal findings frequently take the form of erythema and venous congestion as well as dilatation of the anal area. Table 21.3 conveys the frequency of perianal findings with child sexual abuse.

Collection of evidence

It is of paramount importance that the appropriate mechanism be established to secure information that is possible to evaluate. Ideally, this is accomplished within 72 h of an assault. Each item should be appropriately identified with the patient's name, type of specimen, site from which the specimen was collected, date and time collected and the examiner's initials. A forensic evaluation is suggested as shown in Box 21.12.

Treatment has the objective of removing the child from the victimization situation, repairing of injuries, treatment for sexually transmitted diseases (as appropriate) and psychological support for the victim and family.

Expressive art therapy has proven to be a method of communication. The tools utilized include human figure drawings, in which the child victim is asked to express the abuse via a drawing. Emotional indicators can be used as has been previously established [62]. The indicator has proven to be a clinically valid entity. Kinetic family drawings are also a tool which allows communication of how the individual perceives herself with respect to other family members. This specific information can often be helpful for assessment of psychological pathology and allows further family-centered orientation to treatment strategies. Art therapy continues to be a tool utilized for a myriad of psychobiological issues with regard to child sexual abuse.

Vulvo-vaginitis in children and teenagers

Vaginitis in teenagers differs from that found in the prepubertal child in both etiology and clinical manifestation. The latter presents as

Table 21.3 Frequency of perianal findings

Findings in sexual abuse	Number of subjects observed[a]	Subjects with positive findings	Percentage with positive findings (%)
Erythema	168	68	41
Pigmentation	251	74	30
Venous congestion			
Beginning	113	8	7
Midpoint	113	59	52
End	113	83	73
Anal dilatation	267	130	49
Intermittent anal dilatation	130	81	62
Configuration during			
dilatation	94	84	89
Oval	94	8	9
Round	94	2	2
Irregular			
Smooth area	81	21	26
Dimple/depression	81	15	18
Skin tags	164	18	11
Scars	240	4[b]	2

[a]The number of observed subjects varied because of missing data as a result of changes over time in the number of variable assessed. Includes only those subjects whose anus dilated.
[b]May include 'smooth area' on anal verge. No photographs were available to recheck findings.
Reprinted with permission from Muram D. Sexual abuse. In: Sanfilippo J, Muram D, Lee P, Dewhurst J (eds) Pediatric and adolescent gynecology. Philadelphia: WB Saunders, 1994: 373.

Box 21.12   The forensic evaluation specimens to be collected

General
- Outer and underclothing if worn during or immediately after the assault
- Fingernail scrapings
- Dried and moist secretions and foreign material observed on the patient's body. Use Wood lamp to detect semen

Oral cavity
- Swabs for semen (two) if within 6 h of the assault
- Culture for gonorrhea and other sexually transmitted diseases
- Saliva (for reference)

Genital area
- Dried and moist secretions and foreign material
- Comb pubic hair; collect all loose hair and foreign material
- Vaginal swabs (three)
- Dry mount slides (two)
- Culture for gonorrhea and other sexually transmitted diseases

Anus
- Dried and moist secretions and foreign material
- Rectal swabs (two)
- Dry mount slides (two)
- Culture for gonorrhea and other sexually transmitted diseases

Blood
- Blood type
- RPR
- Pregnancy test (blood or urine)
- Alcohol/toxicology evauation (blood or urine)

Urine
- Urinalysis

Blood or urine
- Pregnancy test
- Alcohol/toxicology evaluation

Other
- Saliva: use clean gauze or filter paper
- Head hair: cut and remove sample
- Pubic hair: cut and remove sample

Reprinted with permission from Muram D. Sexual abuse. In: Sanfilippo J, Muram D, Lee P, Dewhurst J (eds) Pediatric and adolescent gynecology. Philadelphia: WB Saunders, 1994: 376.

vulvo-vaginitis, represents 85% of the gynecologic problems during childhood and involves both vagina and vulva [63]. Teenagers may present with vaginitis following coitarche, with or without unprotected sex and its risk of unwanted pregnancy [64–66].

Pathogenesis

Glycogen concentration in the vaginal epithelium varies according to age and maintains the low vaginal pH. Glycogen levels are low prepuberty and postmenopause [67,68].

The 'normal' vaginal flora contains organisms such as *Staphylococcus epidermidis*, diphtheroids, lactobacilli and anerobes, such as the *Bacteroides*. *Candida* species are the most frequent cause of infection of the genital tract during adolescence. Recurrent candidiasis should raise suspicion of diabetes or immunocompromise [69,70]. Bacterial vaginosis is also seen in sexually active adolescents. Vaginal trichomoniasis is relatively rare in young girls. *Chlamydia trachomatis* and *Mycoplasma* are also causes of vulvo-vaginitis post puberty. The highest risk is in sexually active teenagers presenting for termination of pregnancy.

Diagnosis

The patient's history is the primary step for making the diagnosis. This should be handled delicately. Questions should deal with sexual activity and recent partners, menstrual hygiene, systemic illness and concurrent medications. Identification of the offending pathogen is a prerequisite before antibiotic treatment.

Vaginal examination is undertaken to collect specimens for microbiology and to exclude a foreign body, a common cause of vaginitis in children. In virginal teenagers, the vaginoscope may be an alternative to the ordinary speculum (Figure 21.1).

Management

Management incorporates education, reassurance of parents and treatment of infections identified. Compliance may be a problem and preference should be given to shorter treatment courses, whether systemic or topical.

References

1. Trussel J, Vaughan B. Contraceptive use projections: 1990 to 2010. *Am J Obstet Gynecol* 1992;167:1160–4.

2. Creatsas G. Adolescent gynecology and obstetrics. *Eur J Obstet Gynecol* 1955;58:107–9.

3. Creatsas G, Sideromenos P, Kaskarelis D. Uterus double associé a un imperforation d'un col ou un hemivagin borgne. *Gynecologie* 1984;34:43–7.

4. Creatsas G, Cardamakis E, Hassan E, Deligeoroglou E, Salakos N, Aravantinos D. Congenital uterine anomalies with obstructed cervix, hemivagina, or both during adolescence: report of 22 cases. *J Gynecol Surg* 1994;10:159–67.

5. Sanfilippo JS, Wakinn NG, Schikler KN, Yussman MA. Endometriosis in association with uterine anomaly. *Am J Obstet Gynecol* 1986;154:39–43.

6. Creatsas G, Malhotra N, Malhotra J, Malhotra P, Malhotra RM. Vaginal agenesis associated with renal ectopia. *Adolesc Pediatr Gynecol* 1990;3:103–5.

7. Creatsas G. Hormone replacement therapy in gonadal dysgenetic cases. 5th World Cong Gynecol Endocrinol, Barcelona, 1996.

8. Werther AG, Dietsch S. Multicenter trial of synthetic growth hormone and low dose of estrogen in Turner syndrome: analysis of final weight. In: Albertsson-Wikland K, Ranke M (eds) Turner syndrome in a life-span perspective. New York: Elsevier, 1995:105–12.

9. Nilsson KO, Albertsson-Wikland K, Alm J, et al. Growth hormone treatment in girls with Turner syndrome: final height results according to three different Turner syndrome growth standards. In: Albertsson-Wikland K, Ranke M (eds) Turner syndrome in a life-span perspective. Elsevier, 1995:89–94.

10. Creatsas G, Salakos N, Averkiou M, Miras K, Aravantinos D. Endocrinological profile of oligomenorrheic strenuously exercising adolescents. *Int J Gynecol Obstet* 1992;38:215–18.

11. Creatsas G. Menstrual disorders during adolescence. Personal communication.

12. Kantero R, Widholm D. Correlation of menstrual traits between adolescent girls and their mother. *Acta Obstet Gynecol Scand* (Suppl) 1971;14:1.

13. Deligeoroglou E. Dysfunctional uterine bleeding. Proc 3rd Int Cong 'Update on Adolescent Gynecology–Endocrinology', Athens, 1995. *Ann NY Acad Sci*

14. Creatsas G, Deligeoroglou E, Zachari E, Louradis D, Papadimitriou T, Miras K, Aravantinos D. Prostaglandins PGF2a, PGE2, 6-keto-PGF1a and TXB2 serum levels in dysmenorrheic adolescents before, during and after treatment with oral contraceptives. *Eur J Obstet Gynecol Reprod Biol* 1990;36:283–98.

15. Claessens EA, Cowell CA. Acute adolescent metrorrhagia. *Am J Obstet Gynecol* 1981;139:277–81.

16. Southam AL, Richart RM. The prognosis for adolescents and menstrual abnormalities. *Am J Obstet Gynecol* 1966;24:637–40.

17. Vorherr H. The breast: morphology, physiology and lactation. San Diego: Academic Press, 1974.

18. Speroff L, Glass R, Kase N (eds). Clinical gynecologic endocrinology and infertility, 5th edn. Baltimore: Williams & Wilkins, 1994:336.

19. Haagensen CD. Diseases of the breast, 2nd edn. Philadelphia: WB Saunders, 1971.

20. Mimouni F, Merlob P, Reisner SH. Occurrence of supernumerary nipples in newborns. *Am J Dis Child* 1983;137:952–3.

21. Mehes K. Association of supernumerary nipples with other anomalies. *J Pediatr* 1979;95:274–5.

22. Carella A. Supernumerary breasts associated with multiple vertebral malformations. Case report. *Acta Neurol* 1971;26:136–8.

23. Pitangui I. Surgical treatment of breast hypertrophy. *Br J Plast Surg* 1967;20:78.

24. Longcare J. Correction of the hypoplastic breast with special reference to reconstruction of nipple-type breast with local dermo-fat pedicle flaps. *Plast Reconstr Surg* 1976;3:339.

25. Glaesmer E, Amersback A. Die pathologie der Hangerbrust and ihr moder operative behandlung. *MMW* 1927;74:1171.

26. Reese T, Aston S. The tuberous breast: description and surgical correction. *Clin Plast Surg* 1976;3:339.

27. Deaver JB, McFarlane J. The breast. Its anomalies, its diseases, and their treatment. Philadelphia: Blackston, 1917.

28. Creatsas G. Sequelae of premature sexual life. *J Roy Soc Med* 1995;8:369–71.

29. Creatsas G. Sexuality: sexual activity and contraception during adolescence. *Curr Opin Obstet Gynecol* 1993;5:774–83.

30. Brown RT, Cromer BA, Fischer R. Adolescent sexuality and issues in contraception. *Pediatr Adolesc Gynecol* 1992;19:177–91.

31. Creatsas G, Vekemans M, Horejsi J, et al. Adolescent sexuality in Europe. Multicentric study. *Adolesc Pediatr Gynecol* 1995;8:59–63.

32. Creatsas G, Adamopoulos P, Eleftheriou N, et al. Clinical and metabolic effects of the monophasic gestodene/ethinyl estradiol pill for contraception during adolescence. *Adolesc Pediatr Gynecol* 1991;4:76–9.

33. Creatsas G. Progestogens in reproductive endocrinology. *Eur J Obstet Gynecol Reprod Biol* 1991;41:28.

34. Miller M. Depot levonorgestrel (Norplant) use in teenagers. *West J Med* 1993;158:183.

35. Weisberg E, North P, Buxton M. Sexual activity and condom use in high school students. *Med J Aust* 1992;156:612–3.

36. Elfenbein DS, Weber T, Grob G. Condom usage by a population of delinquent southern male adolescents. *J Adolesc Health Care* 1991;12:35–7.

37. Diaz A, Jaffe LR, Leadbeater BJ, Levin L. Frequency of use, knowledge and attitudes toward the contraceptive sponge among inner city black and hispanic adolescent females. *J Adolesc Health Care* 1990;11:125–7.

38. Psychoyos A, Creatsas G, Hassan E, Georgoulias V, Gravanis A. Spermicidal and antiviral properties of cholic acid. Contraceptive efficacy of a new vaginal sponge (Protectaid), containing sodium cholate. *Hum Reprod* 1993;866–9.

39. Kulig JW. Adolescent contraception: nonhormonal methods. *Pediatr Clin North Am* 1989;36:717–30.

40. ACOG Technical Bulletin no. 129. Chronic Pelvic Pain. June, 1989.

41. Baker PK. Musculoskeletal origins of chronic pelvic pain. Diagnosis and treatment. *Obstet Gynecol Clin North Am* 1993; 20:719–42.

42. Steege JF. Assessment and treatment of chronic pelvic pain. TeLinde's Operative Gynecol Updates 1993;1:1–10.

43. Fordyce WE. Behavioral methods of control of chronic pain and illness. St Louis: CV Mosby, 1976.

44. Milburn A, Reiter RC, Rhomberg AT. Multidisciplinary approach to chronic pelvic pain. *Obstet Gynecol Clin North Am* 1993;20:643–61.

45. Candiani GB Fedele L, Vercellini P, Bianchi S, DiNola G. Presacral neurectomy for the treatment of pelvic pain associated with endometriosis: a controlled study. *Am J Obstet Gynecol* 1992;167:100–3.

46. Eisendrath SJ, Kodama KT. Fluoxetine management of chronic abdominal pain. *Psychosomatics* 1992;33:227.

47. Diesendorf R. The incidence and prevalence of intrafamilial and extrafamilial sexual abuse of female children. *Child Abuse Negl* 1983;7:133.

48. Gelinas D. The persisting negative effects of incest. *Psychiatry* 1983;46:312.

49. National Center on Child Abuse and Neglect (NCCN). Child sexual abuse: incest, assault, and exploitation. Special Report, Washington, DC: HEW, Children's Bureau, August 1978.

50. US Department of Justice, FBI. Crime in the United States: uniform crime reports 1990. Washington, DC, US Government Printing Office, 1991:23–6.

51. Finkelson L, Oswalt R. College date rape: incidence and reporting. *Psychol Rep* 1995;75:526.

52. Committee on Adolescence. Sexual assault and the adolescent. *Pediatrics* 1994;94:761–5.

53. Hibbard RA. Sexual abuse. In: McAnarney ER, Kreipe RE, Orr DP, Comerci GD (eds) Textbook of adolescent medicine. Philadelphia: WB Saunders, 1992:1123–7.

54. Simon T. Violence and sexual assault on college campuses. In: Principles and practices of student health, Vol 3: College health. Oakland: Third Party Publishing Co, 1992: Chapter 20.

55. CDC Guidelines, 1993.

56. Woods JH, Winger G. Abuse liability of flunitrazepam. *J Clin Psycopharmachol* 1997;17(3 Suppl. 2):1S–57S.

57. Anglin D, Spears KL, Hutson HR. Flunitrazepam and its involvement in date or acquaintance rape. *Acad Emerg Med* 1997;4:323–6.

58. Lonsway KA. Preventing acquaintance rape through education: what do we know? *Pychol Women Quart* 1996;20:229–65.

59. Alicke MD, Yurak TJ. Perpetrator personality and judgements of acquaintance rape. *J Appl Soc Psychol* 1995;25:1900–21.

60. Muram D. Child sexual abuse. In: Sanfilippo JS, Muram D, Lee P, et al. (eds) Pediatric and adolescent gynecology. Phildadelphia WB Saunders, 1994.

61. Muram D. Child sexual abuse: relationship between sexual acts and genital findings. *Child Abuse Negl* 1989;13:211–6.

62. Coppitz E. Psychological evaluation of children's human figure drawings. New York: Grune and Stratton, 1986.

63. Koumantakes EE, Hassan EA, Deligeoroglou EK, Creatsas GK. Vulvovaginitis during childhood and adolescence. *J Pediatr Adolesc Gynecol* 1997;10:39–43.

64. Creatsas G. Sequelae of premature sexual life. *J Roy Soc Med* 1995;88:369–71.

65. Creatsas G. Sexuality: sexual activity and contraception during adolescence. *Curr Opin Obstet Gynecol* 1993;5:774–83.

66. Creatsas G, Vekemans M, Horejsi J, Uzel R, et al. Adolescent sexuality in Europe: a multicentric study. *Adolesc Pediatr Gynecol* 1995;8:59–63.

67. Creatsas G. Neonatal pediatric and adolescent gynecology. Creatsas G (ed.). Entopia Publications, 1987:76.

68. Albritton WL, Brunton JL, Meier M, et al. Haemophilus influenzae: comparison of respiratory tract isolates with genitourinary trat isolates. *J Clin Microbiol* 1982,16:826–7.

69. Paradise JE, Campos JM, Frishmuth G. Vulvovaginitis in premenarchal girls. Clinical features and disgnostic evaluation. *Pediatrics* 1982;70:193–8.

70. McFarlane DE, Shanna DP. Haemophilus influenzae and genital tract infections in children. *Acta Pediatr Scand* 1987;76:363–4.

Preconception care, pregnancy diagnosis and management of early pregnancy complications

Gillian E Robinson MD MRCOG MFFP

Introduction

The benefits of antenatal care to both a mother and her baby are widely acknowledged. In contrast the role of preconception care, a logical extension of antenatal care, is yet to be realized partly because at least half of all pregnancies are unplanned.

Pregnancy is a normal, natural event, the outcome of which may be influenced by many diverse factors including behavioural, psycho-social, genetic and medical conditions. The challenge of preconceptual care is to ensure that appropriate advice is readily available to modify these influences without causing unnecessary anxiety (Box 22.1).

The role of a designated preconception clinic, particularly within a hospital setting, is limited. Many consultations will occur on an opportunistic basis in a general practice setting or in a Family Planning Clinic, e.g. for cervical screening, postnatal check, after negative pregnancy test, etc. A structured discussion can be centred around the general headings of lifestyle, previous reproductive history and medical conditions. All women should have their rubella status determined and be encouraged to accept immunization if non-immune. Those women at risk of haemoglobinopathies or disorders such as Tay–Sachs disease should be offered screening as required. Couples who have had a baby with an abnormality, a complicated obstetric history or a chronic medical condition should be offered referral to a specialist to discuss the management of future pregnancies. Even within this selected group, few routine investigations prove abnormal and subsequent pregnancy outcome has only been found to be improved in those with chronic medical disease [1]. However, the opportunity to discuss maternal and fetal risks in a future pregnancy, together with the support and counselling given should not be underestimated. A

Box 22.1 The 'Cs' of preconception care

Contraception – how to stop/when to start 'after'/any obstacles

Child care

Career – leave, benefits, working hours

Cigarette, alcohol and other lifestyle issues

Chronic disease – control before pregnancy

Calories – weight/nutrition

Chlamydia and other STIs, also immunization against rubella

Condoms –? to be used/safer sex

Classes – aerobics, relaxation, parent craft

Capsules, tablets and other drugs – teratogenicity, interactions

Chromosomes/CVS/screening and diagnosis of inherited defects (e.g. cystic fibrosis, Tay–Sachs)

Choice – of maternity care

Culture and religion

Conflict – family/partner/domestic violence

Chaps – role of the partner

Chat – about anxieties, support groups, literature, etc.

Cervical cytology

Check blood pressure

Consideration of socioeconomic status/education/housing, etc.

Chemicals/radiation/workplace hazards/other environmental hazards

Clotting disorders – venous thromboembolism risk much higher in pregnancy and puerperium

22

Preconception
care,
pregnancy
diagnosis and
management
of early
pregnancy
complications

preconceptual health appraisal should have questions on nutrition, social and lifestyle, personal, medical and family, reproductive, and drug and allergies histories. Many of the historical elements can be obtained with a questionnaire completed by the couple themselves.

Lifestyle

The lifestyle of a couple may affect a pregnant woman and her baby. These influences are potentially changeable and are the ones for which pre-pregnancy counselling may be most effective.

Smoking

Smoking in pregnancy is common. In the UK at least one-third of pregnant women smoke. Those that continue to do so throughout their pregnancy are younger, have a poorer education and socioeconomic background, and smoke more heavily.

Smoking affects all aspects of reproductive health. Ovulation is less frequent, the menopause occurs several years earlier and, in men, the number of abnormal spermatozoa is increased and their fertilization capacity is reduced. Smoking in pregnancy increases the risk of spontaneous abortion by 25% and there may be an association with congenital abnormality in the fetus. The risk of premature labour and delivery is increased twofold and birthweight at term is reduced. Also the incidence of placenta praevia and abruption is raised.

Smoking may also cause a delay in fetal maturation which can impair the child's subsequent development. Babies born to mothers who smoke have an increased risk of sudden infant death and respiratory disease in the first years of life. Smokers' children have an impaired reading ability and perform less well in educational testing up to the age of 11 years [2].

Women should be encouraged to stop, or if they are unable to do so, to reduce the number of cigarettes smoked in pregnancy. Those who are able to stop prior to 16 weeks' gestation have heavier babies than those unable to do so. Sadly, many women claim never to have been counselled about smoking during their pregnancy.

Alcohol

Alcohol remains widely accepted within present society; 90% of women consume alcohol when not pregnant and 50% do so during pregnancy. However, it is teratogenic and has serious effects upon fetal growth and development. Excessive alcohol consumption in pregnancy may result in fetal structural and developmental malformations as well as increasing the risks of pregnancy complications. It remains one of the most common causes of mental retardation.

Women who drink heavily in pregnancy have an increased risk of spontaneous abortion (2–3 times higher than non-drinkers), an increased risk of intrauterine growth retardation and a probable increase in preterm birth.

The fetus may demonstrate a variety of morphological and developmental defects (Box 22.2).

Pre-pregnancy advice is difficult. The fact that only one-third of babies of mothers who drink heavily demonstrate

---

Box 22.2 The spectrum of fetal alcohol effects

Altered facial features[a]
- Elongated mid-face
- Short palpebral fissures
- Ptosis
- Thin upper lip
- Short nose – underdeveloped philtrum
- Low set/rotated ears

Cardiac defects
- Ventricular or atrial septal defect are the most common

Skeletal defects

Renal/urogenital defects
- Hydronephrosis
- Renal hypoplasia
- Labial hypoplasticity
- Undescended testis

Central nervous system defects[a]
- Microcephaly
- Neurodevelopmental delay
- Sleep dysfunction
- Hearing loss
- Intellectual impairment

Fetal growth retardation[a]

[a]Components of fetal alcohol syndrome

adverse effects makes giving exact advice difficult as the cause is believed to be multifactorial. One study has shown no demonstrable effect on pregnancy of alcohol levels below 100 g/week [3]. Mothers should be counselled to drink less than 15 units of alcohol per week whilst pregnant [1 unit of alcohol = 8 g]. Consumption of 15 or more units has been associated with low birth weight. Taking 20 or more units of alcohol per week is associated with intellectual impairment; the effect of binge drinking is unknown.

Exercise

Moderate exercise is not only safe in pregnancy but may improve the psychological well-being of the mother. When maternal exercise is prolonged or the maximum exercise capacity is reached, the fetal heart rate can alter, but generally it remains within the normal range [4]. Women who exercise excessively often have a reduced caloric intake, which could result in babies with asymmetrical growth retardation [5]. This would suggest that such exercise causes a reduction in uterine blood flow and should be discouraged in those women already at risk, such as those with diabetes and pre-eclampsia. Exercise hyperthermia should be avoided.

Sports to be avoided include scuba diving (where the fetus is at risk of hypoxia, hypercapnoea and possible congenital malformations), water skiing (with the risk of high pressure vaginal douching which may cause infection and preterm labour), and sports where bodily contact or trauma to the abdomen carry a risk of placental detachment.

Work

Quantifying the effect of working in pregnancy is difficult, and dependent on the type of employment and whether travel is involved. Many mothers without employment work at home – the work involved in looking after children and maintaining a household should not be underestimated.

Studies have demonstrated that the risk of premature delivery is increased if the mother works more than 40 h a week. This risk is increased if the woman is subjected to occupational fatigue, such as working an industrial machine, physical exertion or mental stress (such as noise, cold temperatures and a wet atmosphere). The risk is further increased in those with a previous preterm delivery [6].

Certain industrial hazards pose a particular risk. Exposure to anaesthetic gases in operating room staff leads to a higher rate of miscarriage and low birth weight [7].

In recent years, concern about adverse effects of working with computer video display units in pregnancy has not been borne out by scientific evidence [8].

Nutrition/diet

The relationship between nutrition, health and reproductive performance is well recognized. Low body fat results in delayed menarche and disordered ovulation, which reduces fecundity and fertility.

The famines in the USSR and Holland in World War II demonstrated that food shortage was followed by an increase in perinatal mortality and congenital malformation. The Dutch famine led to a reduction in the birth rate of 50% owing to an increase in miscarriage and stillbirth. The highest incidence of congenital malformation was found in those conceived during or in the 4 months following the famine. Those conceived during the famine also had a higher incidence of low birth weight. This suggests that the fetus is at greater risk if the mother is deprived of food at the time of conception rather than during the pregnancy [9]. A female fetus born after a famine has an increased risk of premature delivery in her pregnancies.

Pre-pregnancy weight has an important effect on pregnancy outcome. Women with amenorrhoea due to low body mass have a 25% risk of delivering an infant which is of low birth weight should they conceive; this risk increases to 54% if ovulation is induced [10]. Women who are underweight should be encouraged to achieve normal weight prior to conception. The practice of ovulation induction in women who are anovulatory due to low body mass is questionable. It is suggested that maternal dieting, particularly in the third trimester, reduces maternal weight gain and the birth weight of the infant. On the other hand, maternal obesity should be tackled prior to conception because of the associated risk of hypertension, diabetes and fetal macrosomia.

Vitamin supplementation is of limited value except in those

cases where the woman has had a previous pregnancy where the baby had a neural tube defect (NTD). Folic acid supplementation reduces the recurrence of NTD by 72% [11] (Box 22.3). Doses of vitamin A higher than 15 000 iu are suspected to be associated with neural crest defects.

All women trying to conceive or who are pregnant should avoid unpasturized soft cheese products, pate (unless tinned) and chilled foods sold without reheating (quiche, coleslaw), which may harbour *Listeria*.

Sexually transmitted infections (Table 22.1)

Women infected with the human immunodeficiency virus (HIV) have a higher risk of an adverse pregnancy outcome such as stillbirth or prematurity compared to women without the virus. In the UK the risk of transmission of the virus to the child during pregnancy is 15–20%. If the mother breastfeeds, this risk is increased by a further 10–20%. Vertical

Table 22.1 Genital tract and other infections in pregnancy[a]

Infection	Treatment	Comments
Candidiasis	Vaginal clotrimazole or econazole or miconazole	Common in pregnancy
Bacterial vaginosis	Vaginal clindamycin or oral metronidazole after the first trimester	Risk of preterm labour
β-Haemolytic streptococci	Broad-spectrum penicillin	Treat if high-risk situation, e.g. premature rupture of membranes
Trichomonas vaginalis	Oral metronidazole	Marker for other STIs Little neonatal risk
Chlamydia	Erythromycin	Tetracycline is contraindicated
Primary herpes	Aciclovir	50% risk of fetal infection
Recurrent herpes	Aciclovir	Not a risk unless vaginal delivery imminent
Gonorrhoea and syphilis	Penicillin	
Cytomegalovirus	No specific antiviral, so prevention is the only available strategy	Affects 1% of infants Maternal CMV presents non-specific symptoms

CMV = cytomegalovirus.
[a]For HIV, see text and Chapter 19.
Note: The aim of preconception care is to diagnose and treat infection *before* conception; the treatment suggestions in this table are for *pregnant* women.

transmission may be reduced by the administration of antiretroviral therapy during pregnancy and by bottle feeding. The place of routine caesarean section in reducing transmission is unclear [12].

It is debatable whether all pregnant women should be screened for HIV status; however, the knowledge of serostatus may benefit the unborn child. It is suggested that such screening be considered in those presenting for prenatal diagnosis, since knowledge at this stage will allow such issues as to whether to proceed with a pregnancy to be discussed.

Rubella

The majority of women of child-bearing age are immune to rubella because of either immunization or previous infection. However, since the effects of rubella infection in pregnancy are devastating, with 80% of fetuses becoming infected if the mother contracts the illness in the first trimester [13], serological testing of all women on an opportunistic basis is recommended.

Box 22.3 Periconceptual folic acid supplementation

- Reduces recurrence rates of NTD by 72%
- Reduces NTD occurrence and possibly other major non-genetic abnormalities
- All women should take an extra 0.4 mg folic acid daily before conception to the end of the first trimester (neural tube closes day 26–27 of embryonic life)
- Women should be advised to take folic acid supplement from the time they stop contraception to the end of the 12th week of pregnancy
- Women with NTD or whose previous child had NTD should take 5 mg folic acid daily until the 12th week of pregnancy (4 mg is the recommended dose in the USA)
- Women should be made aware of folate-rich foods and fortified breads and cereals and avoid overcooking them
- Epileptics should take folic acid throughout the pregnancy and at the higher dose (5 mg daily) if taking anticonvulsants

(The average dietary intake of folates in USA and UK is 0.2 mg/day.)

Toxoplasmosis

Toxoplasmosis infection is usually asymptomatic, leading to 'silent' congenital infection which causes ocular and auditory abnormalities. Countries with a high prevalence of toxoplasmosis, such as France, offer antenatal screening of the mother and fetal blood sampling if required. In the UK chemoprophylaxis with spiromycin is offered to seroconverters. General advice is to avoid raw and undercooked meat, and to avoid contamination with soil and cat litter.

Recreational drugs

Cocaine use in pregnancy is associated with prematurity, reduced fetal growth, placental abruption, microcephaly and possible congenital abnormalities of the urinary tract. The neonate may also display neuro-behavioural deficits [14]. Eliciting a substance misuse history may be difficult. The use of all recreational drugs including amphetamines and marijuana should be discouraged.

Pre-existing medical disorders

Women with a chronic medical disease may consult their primary care physician prior to a pregnancy for information regarding the effects of the disorder upon the fetus. It must also be recognized that the pregnancy may potentially have deleterious effects upon the mother. Whilst this doctor may give general advice, help should be sought from an obstetrician/physician with a special interest in the dual effects of pregnancy and medical disease. The drugs a woman is taking prior to pregnancy should be reviewed to ensure that none are teratogenic.

There are a few medical disorders where a pregnancy would be contraindicated. These include Eisenmenger's syndrome, primary pulmonary hypertension, moderate and severe renal disease, and severe diabetes with vascular complications.

Epilepsy

Epileptics have a slightly higher rate of miscarriage, and a doubling of the perinatal mortality rate and congenital malformation rate. For epileptics the preconception period is vital to establish optimal drug regimens, commence folic acid and agree plans for prenatal screening and diagnosis. The relationship between epilepsy, anticonvulsants and congenital fetal abnormality is controversial. Sodium valproate and carbamazepine are associated with NTDs, while phenytoin is associated with cleft lip. As a precaution, women should be advised to take folic acid 5 mg daily for 3 months prior to conception. In addition, anticonvulsants should be continued, since the risk of seizures is probably greater than any due to the anticonvulsant.

Overall, 10% of women experience an increase in seizure frequency in pregnancy.

Hypertension

Women with previous pre-eclampsia or chronic hypertension have a higher risk of developing pre-eclampsia in a subsequent pregnancy. Those whose hypertension is controlled with ACE inhibitors or beta blockers should have their therapy reviewed. The former affect fetal kidneys, the latter fetal growth.

Renal disease

Those with mild chronic renal disease have few problems in pregnancy. In those with moderate and severe impairment, pregnancy, should it occur, may cause severe maternal complications. It is advisable to consider dialysis/transplantation to stabilize the condition prior to conception.

Diabetes

Whilst the need for preconception advice and assessment of blood pressure and vasculopathy is obvious, the value of specific preconceptual diabetic clinics has been questioned [15]. All diabetics should be controlled with insulin prior to pregnancy. Insulin allows tighter diabetic control, thereby improving fetal and maternal outcomes, and reduces the possibility of transplacental drug passage. Maternal retinopathy should be treated, by laser coagulation, prior to pregnancy. Good control prior to conception reduces the risk of congenital malformation and early pregnancy loss [16].

Haemoglobinopathies

Sickle cell disease and thalassaemia are autosomal recessive conditions. Prenatal diagnosis by chorionic villus sampling is possible. For this to be offered 'in time', the carrier status of both parents must be ascertained.

Recurrent spontaneous abortion

Sporadic miscarriage is common, affecting 25% of pregnancies. In contrast, recurrent miscarriage, which is defined as three or more consecutive pregnancy losses, is much less common, affecting 1% of women. The risk of a further spontaneous abortion increases after each pregnancy lost, from over 20% after one miscarriage to over 40% after three consecutive losses [17].

The aetiology of recurrent spontaneous abortion is diverse, including chromosomal, uterine, immunological, endocrinological and environmental causes (Table 22.2).

Prenatal diagnosis/antenatal screening

Unfortunately, fetal malformation is not uncommon. The aim of antenatal screening is to identify pregnancies at high

Table 22.2 Causes and management of recurrent spontaneous abortion

Condition	% of abortions due to condition	Investigation	Management
Genetic	5%	Peripheral blood karyotyping	Genetic counselling and prenatal diagnosis
Thrombophilic defects	15% [17]	Antiphospholipid antibody, lupus anticoagulant, anticardiolipin antibodies	Low-dose aspirin Low-dose aspirin+ heparin [18]
Polycystic ovarian syndrome	3%	Mid-follicular LH + FSH measurement Pelvic ultrasound	? GnRH analogues
Anatomical	10% (2nd trimester)	Ultrasound Hysterosalpingogram + hysteroscopy	? Hysteroscopic surgery ? Coincidental
Cervical incompetence	30% (2nd trimester)	Ultrasound, HSG	Cerclage
Infection	15%	Cause of sporadic miscarriage except ? bacterial vaginosis	Awareness ? Screening and eradication
Idiopathic	?	By exclusion	Counselling and support

LH = luterinizing hormone; FSH = follicle-stimulating hormone; GnRH = gonadotrophin-releasing hormone; HSG = hysterosalpingography.

risk of congenital abnormalities so that a woman can be offered appropriate tests and, if confirmed, a termination of pregnancy. It has been claimed that 85% of first trimester spontaneous pregnancy loss is associated with a structural abnormality. Furthermore, malformations account for up to 25% of pregnancy loss, perinatal mortality and childhood death up to the age of 10 years. Approximately one in 40 babies has a major malformation which is detected at birth. Many of these anomalies are potentially detectable prior to birth. A few, such as neural tube defect and Down's syndrome, are sufficiently common that screening tests are available for their detection. The anxiety caused by the availability of screening tests and the ethical issues raised should not be overlooked. All couples should be fully aware of the advantages, limitations and implications of

the results prior to undertaking the tests.

Down's syndrome

Down's syndrome (DS) is common, with a worldwide frequency of approximately 1.3 per 1000 births. It is the commonest single cause of severe mental retardation in schoolchildren. It arises from trisomy of chromosome 21, which usually results from non-disjunction of this chromosome in the ovum. Rarely, it may be the result of inheritance from a balanced translocation in an apparently normal parent.

The risk of a mother carrying a child with Down's increases with maternal age (Table 22.3)

The majority of babies with Down's syndrome do not survive to term. More than 50% are miscarried in the first trimester and a further 23% die between 15

Table 22.3 Risk of Down's syndrome by maternal age

Maternal age at delivery	Risk of any chromosomal defect	Risk of Down's syndrome at term
25		1 in 1376
30		1 in 960
35	1 in 110	1 in 424
36	1 in 90	1 in 341
38	1 in 70	1 in 212
40	1 in 45	1 in 126
45	1 in 15	1 in 50

weeks' gestation and term. Thus, at any given maternal age, the incidence of DS is higher in the first and second trimester of pregnancy than it is at term, a fact that needs to be considered when interpreting results of screening tests, which may either quote the rate at the gestation when the test was performed or the rate at term.

Screening for Down's syndrome may involve one of two methods: biochemical markers in maternal blood or an ultrasound scan.

Biochemical markers

In 1984 an association between trisomies 18 and 21 and low maternal alpha fetoprotein was reported. Subsequent studies suggested other fetal and placental products might be altered in DS and therefore provide the basis for a screening test.

The triple test (also called Bart's or Leeds test) utilizes alpha fetoprotein (AFP, a globulin synthesized in the fetal liver), oestriol (a steroid product of the feto-placental unit) and human chorionic gonadotrophin (HCG, a placental-derived glycoprotein). The levels of these in maternal serum at around 16 weeks' gestation (may require a 'dating' scan), together with maternal age, form the basis of the screening

test. When applied to the antenatal population, a typical programme will detect 60% or more of DS cases with a false-positive rate of 5% [19]. Vaginal bleeding or multiple pregnancy affect the test result.

Some units use a double test employing AFP and HCG alone, others use the free beta component of HCG. Research continues and inhibin A has recently been added to the triple test, with claims that the detection rate of DS is increased.

Biochemical markers are also being developed for the first trimester. The four most promising are free βHCG, unconjugated oestriol, AFP and plasma protein A. It is said that, if all four markers are assumed to be independent measures of risk, first-trimester screening could detect 70% DS with a 5% false-positive rate [20].

Ultrasound

A new method of screening for DS using ultrasound scanning between 10 and 13 weeks' gestation has been described. The method measures nuchal translucency which has been associated with chromosomal defects (particularly trisomies 21, 18 and 13, as well as triploidy) and structural cardiac defects.

Screening has been introduced in many centres utilizing this

technique. It is claimed that the sensitivity for trisomy 21 is 80% with a false-positive rate of 5%. These initial results are encouraging but require confirmation outside of specialist centres in a low-risk population.

The future will probably see a combination of biochemical testing together with ultrasound scanning in the late first trimester.

Neural tube defects

In the UK the prevalence of a neural tube defect at birth is 2–3/10 000, but without antenatal diagnosis and termination of pregnancy is nearer 3–4/1000 births. The incidence shows a geographic variation with a higher incidence in the North and Western regions than the South of the British Isles. A parent with one affected child has a 4% risk of a future pregnancy being similarly affected.

The three types of neural tube defect are considered individually in the following paragraphs.

Anencephaly

Anencephaly is a lethal abnormality and is thought to result from failure of the rostral portion of the neural tube to close. The cerebral hemispheres and often the midbrain are absent, but remnants of the forebrain and medulla may be present.

Open spina bifida

Spina bifida (SB) is a defect in the spine resulting from a failure of both halves of the vertebral arch to fuse with each other. The lesion is usually in the lumbosacral or cervical region, but may involve any or all of the spine. The meninges and/or neural tissue may protrude through the defect.

The 5-year survival rate is 36%; of these, 82% are severely handicapped and 10% are moderately handicapped.

Closed spina bifida

The defect in the neural canal is covered by skin. The 5-year survival rate is 60% with a third being severely handicapped and a third moderately handicapped.

If there is an *open* SB lesion, AFP leaks into the amniotic fluid and across the amniotic membrane into the maternal circulation. At 16–18 weeks, the levels in maternal serum are four times greater in affected than unaffected pregnancies, which forms the basis of the screening test. Women who screen positive are offered amniocentesis.

In recent years, high-resolution ultrasound has largely superseded screening maternal serum for AFP.

Ultrasound screening for fetal anomaly

Up to 90% of congenital anomalies occur in couples with no known risk factor. Ultrasound scanning can detect the majority of these malformations and is increasingly offered to women between 18 and 20 weeks of pregnancy. The scan aims to estimate gestational age, locate placental site and pick up anatomical abnormalities. For advantages and drawbacks of second trimester scanning, see Table 22.4.

Diagnostic tests

Amniocentesis

Amniocentesis is the most common invasive procedure used in prenatal diagnosis. It was first described in the last century for the management of polyhydramnios. In the 1960s it became possible to culture and karyotype desquamated fetal cells in amniotic fluid and amniocentesis became popular as a method of genetic prenatal diagnosis.

The technique is performed aseptically, a 22-gauge needle being introduced into the amniotic fluid under ultrasound guidance. Up to 20 ml of amniotic fluid is withdrawn. The cells take about 12 days to harvest and the result is available within 2–3 weeks. The procedure is usually performed at 16 weeks'

gestation. Early amniocentesis, where the technique is performed between 10 and 14 weeks, has an unacceptably high miscarriage risk and, in one study, the risk was higher than chorionic villous sampling [23].

Maternal complications are very rare but include maternal infection and rhesus iso-immunization. To prevent the latter, all rhesus-negative mothers should be given anti-D prophylactically at the time of the procedure. Fetal effects include intrauterine death (which is rare), direct fetal trauma and an excess spontaneous abortion risk of 1%. Late fetal complications include increased rate of respiratory distress at term and a possible increase in preterm labour. In cases of elevated maternal AFP, a detailed anomaly scan is the preferred investigation as the risk of miscarriage with amniocentesis is high.

Chorionic villus sampling

Chorionic villus sampling (CVS) has a major advantage over amniocentesis as a diagnostic test in that it is performed in the first trimester of pregnancy and thus the result is available to the parents sooner.

CVS is performed either transabdominally (local anaesthetic required) or transcervically (discomfort similar to having a smear): the former technique is becoming more popular. In both techniques the procedure is accomplished under ultrasound control and a sample from the chorion frondosum (which later develops into the placental site) is aspirated using a fine cannula. A direct chromosome preparation result is available within 24 h, but has the

Table 22.4 Advantages and drawbacks of the second trimester scan (anomaly scan)

Advantages	Drawbacks
Detects major abnormalities	Parental anxiety
Improves the diagnosis and dating of multiple pregnancy and dating of singleton pregnancy	Questionable value in low-risk population
Reassures parents/confirms viability	Sensitivity in District General Hospital 74.4% [21] Only 35% of major malformations detected in USA [22]
A baseline for further assessments	Precise diagnoses not always possible

drawback of a risk of contamination by maternal cells and low reliability. In 1% of cases mosaicism is diagnosed, but the abnormal karyotype is actually confined to the placenta and does not affect the fetus. This later problem is reduced by half if the results of long term (10 days) culture are used.

Complications of CVS include transient cramping, vaginal bleeding (in 30% of transcervical samplings), infection and rhesus sensitization. Whether CVS carries an inherently higher risk of fetal loss compared with amniocentesis is subject to debate. The MRC trial [24] found a higher risk of spontaneous miscarriage (3%), and late fetal loss (0.5%) and termination for abnormality rate (0.5%), resulting in an overall increased loss rate of 4% compared with amniocentesis. This was not found in American studies. More recently, there has been concern that CVS increased the rate of fetal malformation, particularly limb defects. Most of these abnormalities resulted from the procedure being performed at less than 9 weeks' gestation. Most centres now defer CVS until 10–11 weeks.

Pregnancy diagnosis and the management of early pregnancy complications

Pregnancy diagnosis

The diagnosis of early pregnancy is not always straightforward. Clinical history, symptoms and signs are not diagnostic. Biochemical tests and ultrasound scan are helpful but do not always distinguish between a viable intrauterine, an ectopic and a non-viable pregnancy.

History

Nearly all women who are pregnant do not bleed and thus a missed period is the first sign of a pregnancy.

Symptoms

The symptoms of pregnancy are non-specific and include nausea, vomiting, breast enlargement and pain. Whilst they often occur after the first missed period, some women notice them before and realize they are pregnant before a pregnancy test is positive.

Signs

The signs of early pregnancy include breast enlargement and prominent veins. On pelvic examination, the uterus is softer and has a globular shape.

Tests

A pregnancy test measures the β-subunit of human chorionic gonadotrophin which is produced by the placenta. It may be measured on blood or urine. Modern tests may detect very low levels, which lowers specificity and may result in 'positive' tests from non-pregnant and postmenopausal women. This rarely interferes in clinical practice since most of the currently commercially available tests have a lower level of detection of 25–50 iu.

Modern tests are either dipstick methods or immunofluorometric assays, which may give both qualitative and quantitative results. It is often assumed that testing maternal serum is more sensitive than urine but levels of HCG in blood are similar to those in urine. A single estimate of HCG should only be considered diagnostic of pregnancy if it is greater than 25 iu. A lower level would be expected to double within 3 days.

Ultrasound

An abdominal or transvaginal ultrasound scan will diagnose an intrauterine pregnancy. The latter will confirm a pregnancy up to 7 days earlier than the abdominal route. Transvaginally, a yolk sac will be detected at 33 days, embryonic echoes at 28 days and a viable heart beat at 43 days from the last menstrual period.

Ultrasound is not as good in the diagnosis of a spontaneous abortion or an ectopic pregnancy.

Bleeding in early pregnancy (Figure 22.1)

The differential diagnoses of bleeding in early pregnancy include spontaneous miscarriage, (threatened, incomplete or complete), missed abortion and ectopic pregnancy. The latter is still potentially life-threatening and, in addition, carries significant morbidity. Women who have had a previous ectopic and wish to conceive have a 15% risk of a further ectopic and only 35% will achieve a viable intrauterine pregnancy [25].

The classic presentation of a ruptured ectopic as a profoundly shocked woman owing to massive haemorrhage is fortunately rarely seen. However, such acute presentations require urgent resuscitation and surgical intervention. Diagnostic procedures/tests should aim not to delay management. More commonly the clinical picture is that of a young woman

22

**Preconception
care,
pregnancy
diagnosis and
management
of early
pregnancy
complications**

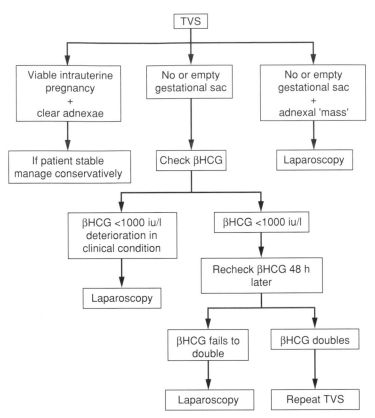

Fig. 22.1 Bleeding in early pregnancy – management flow chart. TVS = transvaginal sonography.

embryo within a gestation sac situated in the adnexa is only seen in less than 20% of women with an ectopic after 7 weeks' amenorrhoea. Furthermore, in at least 25% of women with an ectopic pregnancy, the scan is reported as normal.

Hyperemesis gravidarum

Nausea and vomiting are very common in pregnancy. Hyperemesis gravidarum may be defined as vomiting, of sufficient severity, prior to the 20th week of pregnancy, to require hospital admission.

The symptoms are most common in the first few weeks of pregnancy but in 20% vomiting may persist into the second and third trimester. The aetiology remains unclear but postulated causes include: altered gastric emptying, a central role for oestrogen and a raised βHCG.

The differential diagnoses include:

Thyrotoxicosis	Intestinal obstruction
Pyelonephritis	Appendicitis
Hepatitis	Pancreatitis
Cholecystitis	Addison's disease
Raised intracranial pressure	

Management in mild cases involves supportive therapy and a bland diet. Women who are dehydrated require hospital admission, intravenous fluids and electrolyte replacement. If vomiting persists an antiemetic (cyclizine or promethazine) should be used. Refractory vomiting may respond to oral glucocorticoid administration. In severe cases there may be gastrointestinal bleeding due to Mallory Weiss tears. Very

presenting with vaginal bleeding together with little if any abdominal pain, with a positive pregnancy test. A pelvic ultrasound and βHCG estimation establish the diagnosis and may reduce the indiscriminate use of laparoscopy. The diagnostic capability of either a single βHCG estimation or an ultrasound scan may be limited in the one-third of cases where the date of the last menstrual period is unclear and therefore the gestational age uncertain.

The rate of rise of serum βHCG is lower in cases of spontaneous abortion and ectopic pregnancy than in those with a viable intrauterine pregnancy. In a viable intrauterine pregnancy, the serum βHCG should double in 48–72 h. Conversely, the half-life of βHCG falls rapidly in complete abortion. βHCG levels may vary slightly on repeated measurement, the so-called 'plateau effect', which is highly suggestive of ectopic pregnancy. A βHCG level of 100 iu/ml should be accompanied by a demonstrable intrauterine gestation sac on transvaginal scan. Unfortunately, there is no pattern of βHCG production that will diagnose an ectopic with certainty.

Transvaginal ultrasound is a useful diagnostic tool and will demonstrate an intrauterine pregnancy and a missed abortion. However, it does not distinguish between spontaneous abortion and ectopic pregnancy. A live occasionally parenteral nutrition may be required. Thiamine should be given to prevent the development of neurological disturbances such as Wernicke's encephalopathy.

There are usually no side effects for the fetus. If the vomiting is severe enough to cause protracted and significant maternal weight loss, the baby may be small for dates.

Urinary tract infection

Asymptomatic bacteriuria

In asymptomatic bacteriuria the woman has no symptoms or signs of urinary tract infection (UTI) but culture of the urine reveals significant bacterial growth. Up to 5% of women are susceptible to bacteriuria. Up to 40% of those with asymptomatic bacteriuria develop an acute asymptomatic urinary tract infection; if treated, this will prevent 70% of all acute UTIs in pregnancy. Other postulated benefits of treatment, such as prevention of prematurity, preeclampsia and fetal loss, remain speculative.

The optimal time for testing is at 16 weeks' gestation. The most common micro-organism is *E. coli* but *Klebsiella*, *Proteus*, staphylococci and *Pseudomonas* are also found.

Those women who develop an acute UTI or in whom there is difficulty eradicating the organism should be referred for further investigations in the postpartum period.

Symptomatic UTI

Symptomatic UTI may involve the lower part of the urinary tract, when it is termed cystitis, or the upper part, when it is termed acute pyelonephritis. The latter may cause preterm labour and is associated with intrauterine growth retardation and fetal death.

Cystitis should be treated with appropriate antibiotics to relieve symptoms and prevent the development of pyelonephritis.

The differential diagnosis of acute pyelonephritis includes causes of fever (respiratory tract infection, viraemia) and abdominal pain. The diagnosis is made by culture of a midstream urine specimen. Treatment should be aggressive and often initially in hospital. Intravenous fluid replacement should be given if the woman is vomiting. Regular assessment of renal function is important because, in pregnancy, pyelonephritis may cause transient reduction in the glomerular filtration rate. Antibiotic treatment should be continued for at least 2 weeks and a repeat urine sample checked 1 week post-treatment and then at every antenatal visit.

Counselling tips

- Provide written information before any test.

- A screening test provides an *estimate* of risk only.

- A negative test does not nullify risk, low risk is not zero risk.

- Give a numerical absolute risk (i.e. 1 in 100), a risk of ≥1.250 is 'high'.

- Be non-directive; advice may need to be repeated.

- Discuss the tests' intended benefits, limitations, adverse effects and options for action if it proves positive.

- Use diagrams.

Resources

UK

- Regional Genetics Centres and Fetal Medicine Units provide verbal information, literature and leaflets.

- SAFTA (Support around Termination for Abnormality), 73 Charlotte Street, London W1P 1LB (Helpline: + 44 (0) 207–631 0285).

- Down's Syndrome Association, 155 Mitcham Road, London SW17 9PG (Helpline +44 (0) 208–682 4001).

- Miscarriage Association, Clayton Hospital, Northgate, Wakefield WF1 3JS.

USA

- Local teratogen registers, hotlines.

- Environmental Teratology Information Center, PO Box 12233, National Institute of Environmental Health Sciences, Mail Drop 18–01, Research Triangle Park, North Carolina 27709.

References

1. Cox M, Whittle MJ, Byrne A, et al. Pre pregnancy counselling; experience from 1075 cases. *Br J Obstet Gynaecol* 1992;99:873–8.

22

Preconception
care,
pregnancy
diagnosis and
management
of early
pregnancy
complications

2. Butler NR, Goldstein H. Smoking in pregnancy and subsequent child development. *Br Med J* 1973;iv:573–5.

3. Sulaiman NB, Forey VC Du, Taylor DJ, et al. Alcohol consumption in Dundee primigravidas and its effects on outcome of pregnancy *Br Med J* 1988;296:1500–3.

4. McMurray RG, Mottola MF, Wolfe LA, et al. Recent advances in understanding maternal and fetal responses to exercise. *Med Sci Sports Exec* 1993;25:1305–21.

5. Hatch MC, Shu XO, McLean DE, et al. Maternal exercise during pregnancy, physical fitness and fetal growth. *Am J Epidemiol* 1993;137:1105–14.

6. Mamelle N, Laumon B, Lazar P. Prematurity and occupational activity during pregnancy. *Am J Epidemiol* 1984;119:309–22.

7. Vessey HP, Nunn JF. Occupational hazards of anaesthesia. *Br Med J* 1980;281:696–8.

8. Royal College of Obstetricians and Gynaecologists. Working with visual display units in pregnancy. London: RCOG, 1996.

9. Wynn M, Wynn A. The case for preconception care of men and women. Oxford: AB Academic Publishers, 1991.

10. Van der Spuy ZH, Steer PJ, McKuster M, et al. Outcome of pregnancy in underweight women after spontaneous and induced abortion. *Br Med J* 1988;296:962–5.

11. MRC Vitamin Study Research Group. Prevention of neural tube defects: results of the Medical Research Council vitamin study. *Lancet* 1991;338:131–7.

12. Johnstone FD. HIV and pregnancy. *Br J Obstet Gynaecol* 1996;103:1184–90.

13. Miller E, Craddock-Watson JE, Pollock TM. Consequences of confirmed maternal rubella at successive stages of pregnancy. *Lancet* 1982;ii:781–4.

14. Volpe JJ. Effect of cocaine use on the fetus. *N Engl J Med* 1992; 327:399–407.

15. Gregory R, Tattersall RB. Are diabetic pre-pregnancy clinics worthwhile? *Lancet* 1992;340: 656–8.

16. Miller E, Hare JW. Elevated maternal haemoglobin A1$_c$ in early pregnancy and major congenital anomalies in infants of diabetic mothers. *N Engl J Med* 1981;304:1331–4.

17. Clifford KA, Regan L. Recurrent pregnancy loss. In: Studd J (ed.) Progress in obstetrics and gynaecology, Vol. 11. Edinburgh: Churchill Livingstone, 1994.

18. Rai R, Cohen H, Dave M, et al. Randomised controlled trial of aspirin and aspirin plus heparin in pregnant women with recurrent miscarriage associated with phospholipid antibodies (or anti phospholipid antibodies). *Br Med J* 1997;314:253–6.

19. Wald NJ, Cuckle HS, Densem JW, et al. Maternal serum screening for Down's syndrome in early pregnancy. *Br Med J* 1988;297:883–7.

20. Wald NJ, Kennard A, Smith D. First trimester biochemical screening for Down's syndrome. *Ann Med* 1994;26:23–9.

21. Luck CA. Value of routine scanning at 19 weeks: a four year study of 8849 deliveries. *Br Med J* 1992;302:1474–8.

22. Crane JP, Le Fevre ML, Winborn RC, et al. A randomised trial of prenatal ultrasonographic screening: impact on the detection, management and outcome of anomalous fetuses. *Am J Obstet Gynecol* 1994;171:392–9.

23. Nicolaides K, Brizot MDL, Patel F, et al. Comparison of chorionic villus sampling and amniocentesis for fetal karyotyping at 10–13 weeks gestation. *Lancet* 1994;344: 435–9.

24. MRC European Trial of Chorion Villus Sampling. *Lancet* 1991;337:1491–6.

25. Lavy G, Diamond HP, De Cherney AH. Ectopic pregnancy: its relationship to tubal reconstructive surgery. *Fertil Steril* 1987;543–56.

Infertility management options

Talha Shawaf MBChB FRCS(Ed) FRCOG

Background

A total of 15% of couples fail to conceive after 1 year of unprotected intercourse. A joint World Bank and World Health Organization (WHO) analysis made apparent that reproductive ill health accounts for over 30% of reported disease among women and for 12% among men. The United Nations International Conference on Population and Development (September 1994) declared that 'Reproductive health therefore implied that people are able to have a satisfying and safe sex life, and that they have the capability to reproduce and the freedom to decide if and when and how often to do so'. With the third millennium looming, reproductive health providers are faced with a formidable task and challenge. The WHO [1] estimated that there are 60–80 million infertile couples worldwide. The impact this has on the mental and social well being of society, as well as the probable physical ill health it will produce, is obvious. However, the significance of the incidence, the cost and the perception that infertility is not an illness have led national and international health agencies to assign infertility management a low priority.

With this in mind, primary health care providers need to join forces with specialists to provide cost–effective, low-risk and above all compassionate care plans for their infertile population.

Definitions

Infertility is not a diagnosis. It is a state of failure of the male and/or female reproductive systems. Subfertility is the term defining the failure of a couple to achieve a pregnancy within 2 years of unprotected regular coital exposure. Sterile men or women are those in whom there is no possibility of natural pregnancy. Together these groups comprise the infertile population. Fecundability is the probability of achieving a pregnancy or conceiving within one menstrual cycle. Fecundity is the ability to achieve a live birth from one cycle's exposure to the risk of pregnancy.

Primary subfertility describes a couple who never achieved a pregnancy, while secondary subfertility relates to a couple who have had one or more prior pregnancies. The definition of primary or secondary infertility could similarly be applied to the man or woman in that relationship.

Prevalence and epidemiology

Male or female infertility cannot be considered separately. The estimated prevalence will differ in a monogamous society from that in a society where the male has many partners. In addition, the distinction between voluntary and involuntary infertility poses a limitation on the estimation of prevalence.

The prevalence (percentage) of primary infertility by region was estimated to be 10.1 in Africa, 6.5 in the Caribbean, 4.8 in Asia and Oceania, 3.1 in Latin America, 3 in the Middle East, 5.4 in Europe and 6 in North America [2]. There are wide intercountry variations. Secondary infertility estimates are much more difficult to quantify because of the influence of family planning methods or lactation. Coital frequency is an important determinant of fertility.

Minor degrees of fertility impairment are common in either partner. When these are present in one partner they may not result in infertility. Hence the distinction between subfertility and sterility. In a WHO study [3] of 5713 infertile couples, 14.1% had no demonstrable cause (male partners with normal semen quality and sexual function, female partners with regular menses and ovulation, normal endocrine profile and tubal patency). Only 5.9% of males were deemed to be sterile (aspermia or azoospermia), and only 15.9% of females were sterile (bilateral tubal occlusion, amenorrhoea with elevated follicle-stimulating hormone, FSH) and in 19% both partners had minor factors. In this study it was estimated that 78.6% of couples had minor or no demonstrable factor in one or both partners.

Diagnosis and planned management

It is imperative to develop a common plan for early diagnosis and management (Box 23.1). In general, it is easy to diagnose sterility but may be hard to diagnose subfertility. This is due to a lack of an agreed value for a diagnostic test (Box 23.2).

Diagnostic protocols

Owing to the increased pressure upon healthcare funding for infertility management, a common diagnosis and relevant investigations plan is required. Protocols need to satisfy the local needs reflecting the prevalence of various aetiological factors. A needs-driven model based on UK purchasing health authorities has been outlined [4]. A joint primary care, reproductive medicine and endocrinology plan may be much more cost effective in establishing diagnoses and outlining planned management.

The standard tests that have

Box 23.1   Schematic plan for infertility diagnosis in primary care (by special interest care provider)

(a) Woman

History and advice
- Menstrual history/dysmenorrhoea
- Amenorrhoea/oligomenorrhoea
- Coital history/dyspareunia
- Systemic chronic disease/intercurrent illness
- Sexual history – STIs, PID
- Previous surgery
- Previous pregnancies, complications and ectopics
- Previous contraception
- Drugs – folic acid awareness/smoking

Examination
- Body mass index
- Galactorrhoea
- Hirsutism
- Pelvic examination

Tests
- Screening (rubella, haemoglobinopathies)
- LH/FSH/E_2 (days 2–4 unless amenorrhoeic)
- Progesterone (7 days before expected menses)
- Arrange hysterosalpingo contrast sonography or hysterosalpingogram[a]
- Thyroid stimulating hormone/prolactin in amenorrhoea/oligomenorrhoea (cycles >42 days)
- *Chlamydia* screen/hepatitis/? HIV screen

(b) Man

History and advice
- History of parenthood
- History of acute or chronic diseases/surgery
- History of orchitis, maldescended testes
- Sexual history – STIs, erectile dysfunction
- Lifestyle – smoking, alcohol, anabolic steroids

Examination
- Testicular size/volume/consistency
- Testicular/scrotal swelling (varicocoele/epididymal pathology)
- Phimosis/balanitis

Tests
- Semen analysis (repeat if abnormal)[a]
- *Chlamydia* screen/hepatitis/? HIV screen

Specialist care protocol

- Repeat any of the primary care tests
- Tubal/pelvic disease – laparoscopy, hysteroscopy + corrective surgery
- Female-basal endocrinology: early follicular-phase profile (serum FSH, LH, E_2)
- Thyroid function tests, prolactin
- Transvaginal pelvic ultrasound

In selected cases:

- Monitoring ovulation cycles by serial scans and hormone measurement
- Female endocrinology: FSH, LH, prolactin, thyroid function tests, testosterone and sex hormone-binding globulin
- Male endocrinology: FSH, LH, testosterone
- Surgical scrotal exploration and surgical correction, if deemed possible, combined with facilities for surgical retrieval of sperm and cryopreservation for assisted reproduction treatment

STIs = sexually transmitted infections; PID = pelvic inflammatory disease; LH = luteinizing hormone; FSH = follicle-stimulating hormone; E_2 = oestradiol; TSH = thyroid-stimulating hormone; HIV = human immunodeficiency syndrome.
[a]Carried out in reproductive medicine centre.

been evaluated and shown to be effective in the investigation of infertility include: laboratory assessment of ovulation, evaluation of tubal patency and semen analysis. Other additional investigations contribute relatively little to the effective diagnosis and hence to cost-effective management. The three cardinal tests are listed below.

Assessment of ovulation

There is no ideal method of evaluating normal ovulation in the infertile couple. Measurement of serum progesterone in the mid-luteal phase may be the most cost-effective method. Repeated values exceeding 16 nmol/l, or a single value exceeding 32 nmol/l, are indicative of ovulation. Serial ultrasound assessment of follicular maturation in the menstrual cycle combined with the use of over the counter luteinizing hormone (LH) surge predictor urine tests followed by serum progesterone (8 days later) may be more effective in confirming a woman's normal ovulatory process, but it is costly.

Tubal patency tests

Hysterosalpingography is ideal as a cost-effective primary test in cases in which the clinical evaluation does not indicate tubal disease. Ultrasonography utilizing echogenic contrast media instilled in the uterus and followed along the fallopian tubes (hysterosalpingo contrast sonography) has been used to evaluate not just patency of the fallopian tubes, but also more accurately the uterine cavity, reducing the need for hysteroscopy and laparoscopy. Through the use of ultrasonography the ovaries can be evaluated; in addition, their function can be assessed by detecting the number of primordial follicles present and the ovarian volume. This type of investigation, apart from reducing the risk of radiation, is also cost effective.

Laparoscopy remains the gold standard for diagnosis of pathology of female pelvic organs. However, to utilize this tool efficiently, it is best used, not just as a diagnostic procedure, but as a therapeutic one in the same setting.

Semen analysis

This is evaluated by applying WHO recommendations (Table 23.1).

Determination of treatment and prognosis

Once the fertility assessment is complete, various therapeutic options are discussed with the couple. Couples need full information and counselling to enable them to weigh the benefits and risks of each option. The final choice/decision is theirs to make. The degree of urgency and concern may influence the choice. A valid choice may be to defer or reject treatment. Factors to consider include/duration of infertility, whether the cause indicates sterility or subfertility, and if the infertility is primary or secondary.

Finally, the specific option is determined by its cost effectiveness and the availability of a healthcare system to provide the treatment. The worry for some is that recent advances in fertility treatment present an open-ended financial commitment without a guarantee of success. Managed care plans are one way of providing effective treatment [7]. This needs to be audited regularly to establish whether or not targets are met.

Causes of infertility – female

Table 23.2 details the main causes of infertility and their management.

Disorders of ovulation

Table 23.3 details the causes and diagnosis of anovulation.

Table 23.1 Normal values of semen variables standard tests [6]

Variable/test	
Volume	2.0–5 ml
pH	7.2–8.0
Sperm concentration	$> 20 \times 10^6$ spermatozoa/ml
Total sperm count	$> 40 \times 10^6$ per ejaculate
Motility	$> 50\%$ with forward progression (categories 'a' or 'b') *or* 25% with rapid progression (category 'a') within 60 min of ejaculation
Morphology	$> 30\%$ normal forms
Vitality	75% live, i.e. excluding dye[a]
White blood cells	$<1 \times 10^6$/ml
Mixed agglutination reaction test	<10% spermatozoa with adherent particles
Fructose	Present
Nomenclature for normal and pathological findings in semen analysis [6]:	
Normozoospermia:	normal ejaculate (as above)
Oligozoospermia:	sperm concentration $<20 \times 10^6$/ml
Asthenozoospermia:	<50% spermatozoa with forward progression (categories 'a' and 'b') or < 25% spermatozoa with category 'a' movement
Teratozoospermia:	<30% spermatozoa with normal morphology
Oligoasthenoteratozoospermia:	all three variables (concentration, progression and morphology) are abnormal
Azoospermia:	no spermatozoa in the ejaculate (even after spinning)
Aspermia:	no ejaculate

[a]Using staining procedure the live sperm do not stain, i.e. they exclude dye.

Hyperprolactinaemia

Hyperprolactinaemia causes oestrogen-deficient amenorrhoea, galactorrhoea in up to 80% of cases and loss of libido (often neglected); it can be physiological (lactation, hypothyroidism, stress) or drug induced (e.g. phenothiazines). The normal circulating level of prolactin in an amenorrhoeic, hypo-oestrogenic woman is 400–500 mIU/ml, while in normal oestrogenic (menstruating) women it is 600–800 mIU/ml. Levels beyond 800 mIU/ml are pathological. When elevated levels are noted, the test must be repeated together with an assessment of thyroid function. A careful history must be taken to rule out drug-related hyperprolactinaemia. Its association with polycystic ovarian syndrome (PCOS) is well recognized. Computerized tomography (CT) or magnetic resonance imaging (MRI) should

Table 23.2 Main causes of infertility – therapeutic options

Disorder of ovulation	Tubal/Peritoneal	Male
Correct body weight – obesity or underweight	Operative laparoscopy – good prognosis in 50% of selected cases	Azoospermia: • IUI with donor (IUID) • Surgical reconstruction (+ cryopreservation of sperm retrieved). If no pregnancy after 1 year – IVF/ICSI
Improve lifestyle (e.g. stop smoking, drugs, alcohol)	If no pregnancy after 6–12 months – IV F× 3 cycles	
Antioestrogens (clomiphene citrate) × 6 cycles with pelvic ultrasound monitoring	Poor prognosis or not suitable for surgery – IVF × 3 cycles	• If poor prognosis for surgical reconstruction, ICSI with surgically retrieved sperm, or IUID
Gonadotrophin therapy and/or ovarian diathermy in selected cases which do not respond to antioestrogens		Severe abnormality of sperm parameters – ICSI × 3 IUID 6–10 ×
Bromocriptine × 6 cycles		Moderate to mild abnormality of sperm parameters – IVF ± ICSI
Gonadotrophin-releasing hormone × 6 cycles If not pregnant with any of the above (30% of cases): • IUI × 3 cycles • IVF/GIFT if not pregnant after IUI or as an alternative × 3 cycles		

IUI = intrauterine insemination; ICSI = intracytoplasmic sperm injection; IVF = *in vitro* fertilization; GIFT = gamete intrafallopian transfer.

Table 23.3 Causes and diagnosis of anovulation [8]

	FSH	LH	Prolactin	E_2	Testosterone

Gonadotrophin deficiency
  Pituitary tumour
  Pituitary necrosis or
  thrombosis
	Reduced	Reduced	Unchanged	Reduced	Unchanged

Disorders of gonadotrophic action					
Polycystic ovary syndrome	Unchanged	Unchanged /increased	Unchanged /increased	Unchanged	Increased
Multifollicular ovary	Unchanged	Unchanged	Unchanged	Unchanged	Unchanged

Intrinsic ovarian failure
  Genetic
  Autoimmune disease
  Others (e.g. cytotoxic
  chemotherapy)
	Increased	Increased	Unchanged	Reduced	Unchanged

Secondary ovarian dysfunction
  Disorders of gonadotrophin
  regulation					

(a) Specific					
• Hyperprolactinaemia	Unchanged	Unchanged	Increased	Reduced	Unchanged
• Kallman's syndrome	Reduced	Reduced	Unchanged	Reduced	Unchanged
(b) Functional					
• Weight loss	Reduced	Reduced	Unchanged	Reduced	Unchanged
• Intensive exercise	Reduced	Reduced	Unchanged	Reduced	Unchanged
• Idiopathic	Reduced	Reduced	Unchanged	Reduced	Unchanged
• Drugs[a]	Reduced	Reduced	Unchanged	Reduced	Unchanged

[a]Endocrine changes depends on drugs used.

be carried out if persistent elevated levels are noted, to exclude microprolactinoma (<10 mm) or macroprolactinoma (> 10 mm).

Bromocriptine is the most widely used dopamine agonist in treating hyperprolactinaemia. Escalating dosage to 2.5 mg twice daily is prescribed until the prolactin levels are normal. A higher dosage may be required and bromocriptine can be given vaginally to reduce gastrointestinal side effects. Other drugs have been used in resistant cases, such as the long-acting cabergoline. Women with hyperprolactinaemia ideally should receive specialized care especially during pregnancy. Some cases may require surgery if tumour extension has been identified and neurological symptoms appear.

If ovulation does not occur, an antioestrogen such as clomiphene citrate can be added and, if this combination fails, then gonadotrophins may be administered with the bromocriptine. If after 6–8 months of ovulatory cycles pregnancy does not occur, the couple need to be re-evaluated.

Hypogonadotrophic hypogonadism (WHO group 1)

The presentation is amenorrhoea, the serum oestradiol is < 110 pmol/l, with low FSH and LH, and no withdrawal bleed in response to progestogen challenge. The primary aim is correction of causative factors such as low body mass, malnutrition, drugs, excessive exercise and stress. If there is a specific primary pituitary failure, for instance post-surgery, the treatment is with gonadotrophins under ultrasound monitoring. Pituitary failure secondary to hypothalamic disorders is best treated with subcutaneous pulsatile gonadotrophin-releasing hormone (GnRH) in a dose of 10 µg every 90 min via a pump, under specialist care. If this fails to induce ovulation, which is uncommon, then gonadotrophin stimulation may be used, but the risk of ovarian hyperstimulation is real and careful monitoring is essential. Table 23.4 details the effectiveness of ovarian stimulation regimens.

Hypergonadotrophic hypogonadism

A combination of low oestrogen, elevated plasma FSH (> 20 IU/ml), no response to progestogen challenge and amenorrhoea indicates premature ovarian failure (premature menopause) in women under 40 years of age. If the woman is less than 24 years old, karyotyping should be performed.

Spontaneous regnancy is rare, but not impossible, after this diagnosis. No practical treatment is available. Ovum donation, through assisted conception, is the only option. Hormone

Table 23.4 Effectiveness of ovarian stimulation in WHO group 1 anovulatory women

Treatment	Probability of pregnancy per treatment cycle	Cumulative pregnancy rate after six cycles
Gonadotrophins	25%	72%
Gonadotrophin-releasing hormone	27%	96%

replacement therapy must be offered to prevent premature ageing, osteoporosis and cardiovascular disease in these women.

Normogo-gonadotrophic anovulation (WHO group 2)

The majority of these patients have polycystic ovaries (PCO). Polycystic ovaries are diagnosed in 20% of the population; the aetiology and pathophysiology remain unknown, hence management is imprecise. Women with PCO syndrome have oligomenorrhoea, hirsutism, obesity and high free androgen levels. Weight gain may trigger PCOS symptoms. A variant of PCO is multifollicular ovaries (MFO) with normal androgens [9]. Both PCO and MFO have a less favourable response to all forms of ovulation induction and higher risk of ovarian hyperstimulation to gonadotrophins. PCOS women also have insulin resistance [10], which increases the chance of developing diabetes and cardiovascular disease later in life, although the latter may be mitigated by their relative hyperoestrogenicity. High levels of LH and free androgens are responsible for poor ovarian function, infertility and high miscarriage rates. Table 23.5 lists the infertility treatment options in women with PCOS.

Weight reduction improves the symptoms and the endo-crinological pathology, but can be problematic. The body mass index (BMI) needs to be reduced to <25 in overweight women to enhance the effect of other modalities of treatment. Antioestrogens, such as clomiphine citrate or tamoxifen, are the first-choice modalities of therapy. The dose of clomiphene is 50 mg/day for 5 days, starting any day between cycle days 2–5, but usually from the second to the sixth day of the cycle. The dose can be increased by 50 mg daily up to 200 mg/day if ultrasound and plasma progesterone monitoring show no ovulation. If ovulation occurs, the dose can be maintained for a maximum of 6–8 cycles. Follicular cysts may develop with clomiphene treatment and, if this is noticed on ultrasound, treatment must be discontinued until the cysts regress. The alternative is to use tamoxifen 20–40 mg/day for 5 days beginning on cycle day 3 or 4. A total of 80% of women ovulate on clomiphene, 75% conceive with a spontaneous abortion rate of 30–40%.

The risk of hyperstimulation with antioestrogens is negligible in comparison with gonadotrophins. There is a risk of a small increase (5%) in twinning and no increase in ectopic pregnancy or miscarriage. However, women with PCOS have an increased risk of spontaneous abortion if they conceive. Other side effects include vasomotor symptoms (hot flushes), visual disturbance, urticaria and loss of hair in a small group of patients.

Patients who fail to ovulate on

Table 23.5 Treating Infertility in polycystic ovarian syndrome (WHO group 2)

Treatment options	Remarks
Weight adjustment	BMI 20–25
Clomiphene citrate	Primary treatment Six cycles Cumulative successful pregnancy 50%
Clomiphene citrate + hCG	Non-ovulation on ultrasound Risk of multiple pregnancy
hMG/FSH	If Clomiphene resistant Chronic low-dose, 18% pregnancy/cycle
GnRHa + hMG/FSH	?those who miscarry with above treatment No controlled or large studies available Risk of multiple pregnancy and OHSS
Ovarian diathermy or laser drilling	Clomiphene resistant ? 50% pregnancy rate over 1 year ? risk of adhesion formation No controlled trial
IVF/GIFT	Failure to ovulate with above treatment Six cycles of ovulation but no pregnancy

BMI = body mass index; hCG = human chorionic gonadotrophin; hMG = human menopausal gonadotrophin ; FSH = follicle-stimulating hormone; GnRHa = gonadotrophin-releasing hormone analogue; OHSS = ovarian hyperstimulation syndrome; IVF = *in vitro* fertilization; GIFT = gamete intrafallopian transfer.

antioestrogens may be offered low-dose gonadotrophins or laparoscopic ovarian diathermy. They also need to be investigated for adrenal dysfunction. All these are the domain of specialist care.

Low-dose gonadotrophins require intensive monitoring, have a higher risk of multiple birth, high pregnancy rates and high cost. Ovarian diathermy, however, has a 50% spontaneous pregnancy rate over 1 year with no increase in multiple pregnancy or miscarriage. This technique has not been evaluated in a prospective comparative study [11] and there is a risk of postoperative adhesions in about 20% of cases.

Conditions associated with ovulation induction

Ovarian hyperstimulation syndrome (OHSS)

This condition was initially described in the 1960s. It is a rare but dangerous consequence of gonadotrophin therapy. It is most commonly seen in women with PCO or MFO, following gonadotrophin stimulation. Its incidence has risen sharply since *in vitro* fertilization (IVF) and other assisted reproductive technologies (ART) became widely practised, and also with the introduction of GnRH agonist (GnRHa) stimulation protocols, which led to the use of high doses of gonadotrophins. In its severe form it can be potentially fatal; the severe form requiring hospitalization and intensive care is seen in 0.5–1% of cases of controlled ovarian stimulation. The pathophysiology of OHSS is not clear. Human chorionic gonadotrophin (HCG), both exogenous in

ovulation induction regimens and endogenous from pregnancy, acts as a triggering mechanism. A vascular permeability factor has been isolated in high concentrations in women with OHSS. Increased vascular permeability leads to fluid shift from the intravascular to the extravascular compartments and hence haemoconcentration. The fluid shift leads to ascites, hydrothorax and dependent oedema. The haemo-concentration may affect the renal flow, and also induce thrombosis and intravascular coagulation, with potentially fatal consequences. The syndrome comprises, in addition, gross ovarian enlargement. The other features of OHSS are abdominal pain, nausea and vomiting, abdominal distension and breathlessness.

The risk factors for OHSS are as follows:

- GnRHa/gonadotrophin ovulation stimulation;
- PCO/MFO;
- youth;
- high-dose gonadotrophin;
- HCG for luteal support;
- multiple gestation.

Identifiable features:

- large numbers of follicles (>20);
- serum oestradiol > 13 000 pmol/l.

Ovarian cancer

The use of ovarian stimulation drugs has been speculated to increase the incidence of ovarian cancer later in life by 2.8-fold

[12]. Another case-control study estimated a relative risk of developing ovarian cancer with the use of clomiphene to be 2.3. When it was used for more than 12 cycles, the relative risk increased to 7 [13]. These speculations led to the advice that clomiphene use should be limited to 6–8 cycles. Large multicentre studies are needed to elucidate an association/causal effect between fertility drugs and ovarian cancer.

Tuboperitoneal infertility

Prevention of sexually transmitted infections (STIs), especially *Neisseria gonorrhoeae* and *Chlamydia trachomatis*, can have a profound influence on the incidence of tuboperitoneal infertility. Tubal pathology follows laparoscopically verified pelvic infection in 12% of patients compared to 0.8% of controls. An ectopic pregnancy rate of 1 in 11 is seen in women with STIs compared with 1 in 73 of controls [14] and 14% of patients were infertile compared with 2% of controls.

Diagnosis

Hysterosalpingography (HSG) and hysterosalpingo contrast sonography (HyCoSy), also termed sonohysterography, are the preliminary tests to examine the uterine cavity, tubal patency and rouge (mucosal folds). Both have good specificity (0.83) and sensitivity (0.65) to detect tubal patency, but are not as accurate regarding peritoneal (peritubal or periovarian) adhesions. These tests are performed in the follicular phase of the cycle usually unless strict contraceptive measures are taken during the cycle. If oil-based contrast fluid is used in HSG, this may have a therapeutic value.

Laparoscopy and hysteroscopy

This is the gold standard to evaluate the reproductive system, but it is costly, and requires general anaesthesia and hospital facilities. It can be reserved as a secondary procedure with the ability to use the facility for therapeutic advantage as well as a diagnostic tool, making it more cost effective.

The limitation of laparoscopy is its inability to visualize the tubal lumen and mucosa. Falloposcopy (salpingoscopy) is still a research tool.

Treatment

It is evident that careful selection of patients for either of the two main treatment options of tubal infertility, surgery or IVF, will ensure better results and cost effectiveness. The degree of severity of tubal disease, the luminal diameter, mucosal damage and age of the patient help determine the preferable option.

Laparoscopic surgery has produced similar results to open microsurgery in cases of adhesiolysis, neosalpingostomy and fimbroplasty, but reversal of sterilization and proximal (cornual) reanastomosis are more complex and not yet evaluated in a randomized study. The overall intrauterine pregnancy rate after tuboplasty is 26%, spontaneous abortion 5% and ectopic pregnancy 8% [15].

The cost effectiveness of IVF treatment per initiated cycle was estimated to be similar to that of tubal surgery, despite the IVF success rate being calculated at 10% (in some groups the IVF success rate was superior to this [15]). The utilization of both modalities of treatment after proper selection should reduce unnecessary tubal surgery and ensure more effective IVF treatment.

Endometriosis may be associated with infertility. Treatment can be medical through ovulation suppression or surgical laparoscopic ablation. There are protagonists for each treatment. In general, moderate and severe endometriosis requires a surgical approach. Assisted reproduction treatment may be recommended; also, if no other symptoms are present, a combination of medical and surgical approach is sometimes utilized.

Causes of infertility – male

The evaluation of the male is based on taking a comprehensive history, which may suggest a cause (Box 23.3), on physical examination, semen analysis and ancillary tests such as scrotal ultrasound. The semen analysis provides the basis for the diagnosis and treatment. However, the predictive value of subnormal semen parameters is limited when compared with severe abnormalities such as azoospermia. A cost-effective, highly predictive test of fertilizing capacity of spermatozoa is not available.

STDs are the largest single preventative cause. There has been a concern about a decline in sperm count and quality in the last half-century but there is no consistent proof of this decline. Various factors such as water contamination with oestrogenic byproducts, environmental pollution, dietary changes and others are considered to be contributing factors.

Damaged spermatogenesis can be diagnosed when azoospermia is present with small firm testes and raised serum FSH. When azoospermia is found with normal size testes and a normal level of FSH, an obstructive cause (including congenital absence of vas) or hypothalamic hypo-pituitarism should be suspected.

The role of varicocoele in male infertility is still controversial. Varicocoele was the most common abnormality found in a WHO study (present in 12% of men with abnormal semen parameters). Box 23.4 lists the causes of male subfertility. Vasectomy appears to be increasingly reported as a cause because of change in lifestyles and increase in divorce.

Laboratory identification of male genital infection as a cause of male infertility is difficult. Immature germ cells are confused

---

Box 23.3   Recognized risks for male subfertility

- Undescended testes
- Testicular torsion
- Chronic disease
- Previous surgery or radiotherapy
- Mumps orchitis
- Drugs – alcohol, nicotine, marijuana

Box 23.4	Causes of male subfertility
Idiopathic	31.7%
Endocrine	9%
Infective	9%
Maldescended testicle	8.5%
Ejaculatory/erectile dysfunction	6%
General disease	5%
Sperm antibodies	4%
Obstruction	1.5%
Testicular tumours	2.3%
Varicocoele	16.6%
Other causes	6%

with white cells unless a special stain (e.g. peroxide stain) is used and semen samples are always contaminated, making bacterial culture growths inconclusive.

Prevention

The most important means of prevention concerns the prevention of STIs. Varicocoele ligation is not recommended for the prevention of infertility. Cryopreservation of sperm prior to cancer treatment is very appropriate, even in adolescents.

Treatment and prognosis

Empirical use of antioestrogens or gonadotrophins in oligospermia or asthenozoospermia has no proven benefit in controlled studies. Similarly, intrauterine insemination in male factor infertility has resulted in low pregnancy rates. Ligation of varicocoele may improve pregnancy rate in oligozoo-spermic men. Mild abnormalities of sperm may respond to conventional IVF.

Intracytoplasmic sperm injection (ICSI) is now considered of proven value in moderate and severe male infertility [16]. This technology is an extension of IVF, where a single sperm (selected as the most motile and most normal in morphology) is injected into an oocyte retrieved following ovarian stimulation. Following fertilization and cell multiplication, it is placed *in utero*. Sperm used can be selected from the ejaculate or surgically retrieved. The sperm can be retrieved from the epididymis in cases of obstructive azoospermia or from the testicular tissue in obstructive and non-obstructive azoospermia. Concern has been raised regarding the genetic safety of ICSI procedures, but this has not been substantiated. Further, genetic counselling and assessment is required in cases of severe oligospermia (total count < 3–5 million sperm/ml) or in cases of surgical retrieval of sperm in bilateral congenital absence of the vas deferens and in non-obstructive azoospermia. Increased prevalence of aneuploidy has been found in cases of non-obstructive azoospermia and severe oligozoospermia. A gene (azoospermia factor) mutation has been identified in some cases of severe oligozoospermia.

The use of donor sperm has declined in recent years since the advances of ICSI, but a substantial minority of men with severe oligozoospermia or azoospermia may request or can only have their fertility resolved with donor sperm usage. Counselling in these cases is mandatory and the welfare of the unborn child should be high on the agenda.

Unexplained infertility

When the standard tests (ovulation assessment, tubal patency and semen analysis) are normal and the couple have been trying for more than 2 years, the condition is labelled unexplained infertility. Luteal phase deficiency, abnormal postcoital test, immunological causes, sperm mucus contact tests and zona-free hamster egg penetration test have not been proven to aid in fertility prognosis assessment.

The prognosis in untreated cases of unexplained infertility is determined by the woman's age. Women > 30 years are considered to have a lower chance of pregnancy. The other factor affecting the rate of spontaneous conception is duration of infertility, with infertility of over 3 years having a worse prognosis. Secondary infertility has twice higher pregnancy rates than primary infertility. Couples may have below average fecundity, although they have normal fecundity parameters. Others may have low fecundity because of latent or undetectable defects, e.g. the inability of spermatozoa to fertilize the partner's eggs. Follow-up of couples with unexplained infertility over 1 year reported a spontaneous conception rate between 15% and 60%, and this rose to 40–80% at 3 years.

Treatment

Since no clear cause can be identified, treatment strategies become more empirical. Well-designed studies showing clinical effectiveness are scarce. It is hence practical, if age and duration of infertility permit, to allow a period of observation while improving lifestyle. Clomiphene citrate used empirically is of little benefit. A maximum of six cycles is recommended. Ultrasonography to monitor follicular and endometrial development and timed sexual intercourse should be considered. The use of gonadotrophins can increase the pregnancy rate, but also results in higher multiple pregnancy rates and ovarian hyperstimulation.

If pregnancy does not follow ovarian stimulation alone, then it can be combined with intrauterine insemination with prepared spermatozoa which is a much more effective treatment. After six cycles of IUI, treatment with IVF or gamete intrafallopian transfer (GIFT) should be considered.

Assisted reproduction technology

Boxes 23.5 and 23.6 show the indications for ART and ART treatment modalities, respectively.

The standard ART consists of controlled ovarian stimulation (COS) to induce multiple follicles, oocyte harvesting (or retrieval), preparation of a suspension of motile sperm, approximation of male and female gametes, either gamete transfer (in GIFT) or *in vitro* incubation (IVF) and later transfer of fertilized zygotes (ZIFT) or embryo transfer (ET). The most widely used ovarian stimulation regimen in ART is a combination of GnRH analogue and gonadotrophins, either human menopausal urinary or the newly introduced recombinant type. Monitoring of COS is mostly by vaginal ultrasonography and measurement of serum oestradiol. Oocytes are retrieved with vaginal ultrasound control, or in some cases laparoscopically, as in GIFT. In the UK, a maximum of three embryos (or oocytes) are transferred. It is also reasonably argued to limit the number of embryos transferred to two embryos in young women below 35 years of age to reduce multiple pregnancy risk and its sequelae.

Intracytoplasmic sperm injection has transformed the treatment of male infertility [16]. A viable normal sperm is injected into a mature oocyte under microscopic control using fine glass needles (Figure 23.1). Resulting embryos are then transferred to the uterus. The results of ICSI in terms of pregnancies have equalled and even superseded those of conventional IVF, largely due to the younger age and normal fertility of the women. Until recently, azoospermia was treated by donor insemination. Many cases now can be treated with surgical retrieval of epididymal or testicular sperm followed by ICSI.

Couples opting for ICSI should be informed about the relatively limited data on this procedure and its potentially

---

Box 23.5 Indications for assisted reproduction technology

Absolute indications
- Tubal disease not corrected by surgery
- Moderate to severe male infertility

Relative indications
- Unexplained infertility
- Endometriosis not responsive to surgical and/or medical therapy
- Repeated failure of ovulation induction treatment
- Last resort in protracted subfertility

Other indications
- Ovum donation to women with premature ovarian failure
- Surrogacy in women with no uterus

Box 23.6   ART treatment modalities

Established treatment modalities
- *In vitro* fertilization and *in utero* embryo transfer (IVF–ET)
- Intracytoplasmic sperm injection (ICSI)
- Gamete intrafallopian transfer (GIFT) (can be combined with IVF of supernumerary oocyte and ET)
- Cryopreserved embryo transfer

Other treatment modalities
- Zygote intrafallopian transfer (ZIFT)
- Assisted hatching (AH)

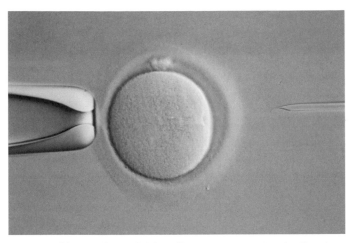

Fig. 23.1 A viable normal sperm is injected into a mature oocyte using fine glass needles

unknown aspects. Parental karyotyping may be recommended in severe oligozoospermia and in non-obstructive azoospermia. Results of about 500 prenatal karyotypes and the prospective follow-up of 750 children resulting from ICSI have not indicated an increase in abnormal fetal karyotypes or in major congenital malformation [17]. However, an increase in prevalence of chromosomal aneuploidy and mutation of the azoospermic gene on the Y chromosome have been reported in men with severe oligozoospermia and obstructive azoospermia. It is, therefore, prudent to follow-up pregnancies resulting from ICSI and the children born, and to collate national and multinational data to ensure long-term safety.

Risks induced by ART

These include risks related to gonadotrophin stimulation as OHSS and cancer risk (see earlier text). There is a minimal risk of pelvic infection or exacerbating an already present chronic pelvic infection. There are specific risks related to pregnancy outcome. These include multiple pregnancies, also influenced by the woman's age and the number of embryos (or oocytes) transferred. Multiple pregnancy, and specifically high order ones (triplets and over), increases the risk of pregnancy wastage, prematurity and consequently perinatal death. The implementation of selective fetal reduction in high-order multiple pregnancies adds further to the dilemma faced by couples: while reduction cuts the overall pregnancy wastage, it does carry its own risk of spontaneous abortion.

There are other manageable risks in pregnancies resulting from ART, such as an increased risk of fetal growth retardation and a higher caesarean section rate. Since women undergoing ART are older, and especially if they are around 40 years of age and over, their pregnancies may be complicated further with a higher incidence of chromosomal abnormalities, perinatal mortality and even maternal mortality. Ovum donation reduces the problems related to old oocytes, but not to pregnancy complications.

Outcome

ART has changed the lives of many infertile women and men, and transformed the management of infertility, but the expectations are still not fully met. Further advances should improve outcome and meet patients' expectations. The UK Human Fertilisation and Embryology Authority (HFEA) is mandated to publish yearly results of all UK centres. Despite some deficiencies, these publications are seized on by purchasers and patients to select centres with acceptable results. In the USA, similar national results are published by the American Society of Reproductive Medicine and its affiliated Society for Assisted Reproductive Technology (SART). Furthermore, the US Congress demands that each clinic provide results to be scrutinized by the public.

Outcome measures seem to be improving slowly. In the UK, the delivery rate per cycle of IVF initiated was 14.5% in 1995–96, as reported by the HFEA last survey [18]. In the USA, SART reported a delivery rate of 22.5% per oocyte retrieved for IVF in 1995. The same year, results per initiated cycle were 19.35% in IVF/ET and 23.9% for GIFT [19]. Standardization of reporting ART outcomes nationally and internationally is needed to compare results and audit treatment.

One of the important impediments to achieving higher pregnancy rates is age. This seems to affect all modalities of assisted conception. It has been suggested that women perform best at childbearing when they are young, just as they do in athletics and marathon running. When a woman approaches 40, IVF success rates plummet down and similarly the GIFT rates. This is the reason why many managed care plans seem to discriminate in accepting women who are approaching 40 years of age for treatment of their infertility. Another important factor is cigarette smoking, which may compound the age effect and negatively influence ovarian reserve. If ART can be provided without delay to women who need appropriate infertility treatment, this can boost the success rate of IVF and, in the long run, reduce the cost of the fertility service. Waiting until a woman is over 35 years will negatively influence the pregnancy potential for the couple.

Counselling

Counselling is an integral part of any fertility treatment and specifically in those attempting ART. The typical reaction to infertility in the majority of patients is distress of varying degrees, which could manifest as a life crisis experience. The failure to attain one of life's goals, parenting, can lead to deep bereavement. This results in isolation, lack of control and a stressed relationship.

Counselling can be offered at varying stages. Supplying information on procedures, treatment options and choices is the initial stage, provided by the clinician. Understanding these issues, and accepting particularly a choice, is often difficult for the patient. Counselling by other staff and by special fertility counsellors can assist the decision-making process. The choice is further influenced by family, cultural and religious values. A therapy plan is then developed to take into account the patient's present and future aims.

The stress of infertility can bring forward many other issues. Professional, independent counselling is needed to explore issues and help couples come to terms with distressing feelings. Supportive and confidential counselling helps couples face the continuing uncertainty of their childlessness. Counselling is also important when the couple have a pregnancy loss, with its consequent despair. Subfertile couples who fail and discontinue therapy must be supported in their decision and encouraged to feel that they have 'done their best' and given permission to 'let go'.

Couples who are planning to undergo gamete (oocyte or sperm) donation or embryo donation, and especially those who are going to use a host (surrogacy), are best served by detailed counselling by a specialist in the field. Issues of future conflict must be explored as well as present difficulties that may arise during treatment. The law, especially in cases of oocyte donation and surrogacy, has been laid in statute in the UK, but it is still controversial. Specialist clinics are licensed for these emotionally difficult treatment modalities and they need to have in place exhaustive and expensive counselling before accepting such couples for treatment.

References

1. World Health Organisation. Achieving reproductive health for all. Geneva: WHO/FHE, 1995.

2. Farley TMM, Belsey FH. The prevalence and aetiology of infertility. In: Biological components of fertility, Vol. 2. Proceedings of the African Population Conference, Dakar, Senegal, November 1988. Liege: International Union for the Scientific Study of Population, 1988:15–30.

3. Farley TMM. The WHO standardised investigation of the infertile couple. In Ratnam SS, Reah E-S, Ananda Kumar C (eds) Infertility male and female. Proceedings of the 12th World Congress on Fertility and Sterility, Singapore, October 1987. Carnforth, UK: Parthenon, 1987:123–35.

4. Hull MGR. Managed care of infertility. *Curr Opin Obstet Gynaecol* 1996;8:305–13.

5. Crosignani PG, Rubin B. The Eshre Capri Workshop. Guidelines to the prevalence, diagnosis, treatment and management of infertility. *Hum Reprod* 1996;11:1775–807.

6. World Health Organisation. WHO laboratory manual for the examination of human semen and sperm–cervical mucus interaction, 3rd edn. Cambridge: Cambridge University Press, 1992:44–5.

7. Bates GW, Bates SR. Infertility services in a managed care environment. *Curr Opin Obstet Gynaecol* 1996;8:300–4.

8. Franks S. Diagnosis and treatment of anovulation. In: Hillier SG (ed.) Ovarian endocrinology. Oxford: Blackwell Scientific, 1991:227–38.

9. Filicori M, Flamigni C, Cognigni G, Dellai P, et al. Increased insulin secretion in

patients with multifollicular and polycystic ovaries and its impact on ovulation induction. *Fertil Steril* 1994;62:279–85.

10. Dunaif A, Segal KR, Futterweit W, et al. Profound peripheral insulin resistance, independent of obesity, in polycystic ovary syndrome. *Diabetes* 1989;38:1165–74.

11. Donesky BW, Adashi EY. Surgically induced ovulation in the polycystic ovary syndrome: wedge resection revisited in the age of laparoscopy. *Fertil Steril* 1995;63:439–63.

12. Whittemore AS, Harris R, Intyre J, Halprin J and the Collaborative Ovarian Cancer Group. Characteristics relating to ovarian cancer risk: collaborative analysis of 12 US case-control studies. *Am J Epidemiol* 1992;136:1175–1183.

13. Rossing MA, Daling JR, Weiss NS, et al. Ovarian tumors in a cohort of infertile women. *N Engl J Med* 1994;331:771–6.

14. Westrom L. Sexually transmitted disease and infertility. *Sex Transm Dis* 1994;21:532–7.

15. Marana R, Quagliarello J. Distal tubal occlusion: microsurgery versus in vitro fertilisation – a review. *Int J Fertil* 1988; 33:107–15.

16. Van Steirteghem A, Nagy ZP, Joris H, et al. High fertilisation and implantation rates after intracytoplasmic injection. *Hum Reprod* 1993;8:1060–6.

17. Van Steirteghem A, Tournaye H, Van der Elst J, et al. Intracytoplasmic sperm injection three years after the birth of the first ICSI child. *Hum Reprod* 1995; 10:2517–28.

18. Human Fertilisation and Embryology Authority. Sixth annual report. London: HFEA, 1997.

19. Assisted reproductive technology in the United States and Canada: 1995 results generated from the American Society for Reproductive Medicine/Society for Assisted Reproductive Technology Registry, Birmingham, Alabama. *Fertil Steril* 1998;69:389–98.

Additional Resource

In October 1998 the RCOG (UK) published two guidelines: (1) The initial investigation and management of the infertile couple, and (2) the management of infertility in secondary care.

Further information from: Clinical Guidelines, RCOG, 27 Sussex Place, Regent's Park, London NW1 4RG. E-mail: clinicalguidelines@rcog.org.uk

Breast disease

William H Hindle MD

Motivated by fear of breast cancer, many women will seek medical advice and evaluation for their perceived breast symptoms and concerns. Primary healthcare providers for women can appropriately evaluate such symptoms and concerns, diagnose and treat benign breast conditions, and judiciously refer suspicious (for cancer) lesions to the appropriate medical consultant. Optimally, the initial breast evaluation is performed in a convenient and comfortable outpatient setting.

The incidence of invasive breast cancer, as measured by reliable statistics worldwide, has been increasing for the past several decades. Although environmental factors are suspect, the etiology of this progressive increase remains undetermined. Simply by virtue of being female and advancing in age, all women are at notable risk for breast cancer; while the disease-free (or controlled) survival has increased with adjuvant therapy and irradiation, the mortality rate (overall survival) has essentially remained the same for the past half-century. Nevertheless, effective local control is now achievable with breast-conserving therapy for the majority of stage I and II breast cancers.

The predominant presenting breast complaint is a perceived palpable breast mass or breast pain. A systematic diagnostic approach to these symptoms will allow reassurance to those women without breast pathology, specific treatment of benign breast conditions, and pertinent referral of suspicious and undiagnosed lesions. The primary diagnostic goal of the initial evaluation is to identify a palpable dominant breast mass or masses (if present) and to order mammography as indicated. Subsequently, the primary therapeutic goal is reassurance of those women with no evidence of malignancy, and treatment of benign symptoms or lesions. Owing to the frequency and indolent biologic behavior of breast cancer, women who present with breast problems should receive long-term follow-up and be re-evaluated promptly for any new breast findings.

Breast diagnostic techniques

The diagnostic triad for the investigation of breast symptoms consists of the clinical breast examination (which includes a 'breast' history), mammography and fine-needle aspiration of a dominant mass. Diagnostic techniques can be summarized as follows:

1. clinical examination, including breast-oriented history;
2. mammography;
3. fine-needle aspiration:
   - cyst
   - solid mass;
2. ultrasound
3. tissue core-needle biopsy:
   - ultrasound-guided
   - stereotactic mammography-guided;
4. Open surgical biopsy:
   - palpable mass
   - mammographic needle localization of non-palpable lesion.

'Breast' history

The assessment interview should be conducted without interruption in a private, comfortable surrounding. The critical points to be covered in a woman's breast-oriented history are:

1. age;
2. the date of last menstrual period;
3. the chief complaint;

4. any family history of breast cancer, particularly of first-degree relatives (mother and sisters) with their age at diagnosis;

5. personal history of breast cancer;

6. history of breast surgery including aspirations;

7. date of her last mammogram, if applicable, and the results;

8. current and past hormone therapy.

Oral contraceptive therapy, estrogen replacement therapy and estrogen/progestin therapy can be related to breast symptoms (such as mastalgia), and can alter the mammographic density in some women. However, the evidence that hormonal therapy relates to a clinically meaningful change in the risk of breast cancer is debatable.

Clinical breast examination

The clinical breast examination should be conducted under lighting equivalent to sunlight without shadows. Throughout the examination, one side of the breast should be compared to the other and specific areas to the remainder of the same breast (e.g. with respect to nodularity). Inspection of the breast begins with the patient in the upright position, sitting or standing. Inspection proceeds with the patient: (1) at ease; (2) with her hands behind her head; (3) with her hands pressing on her hips; and (4) leaning forward. Asymmetry of the nipple or breast, skin changes (e.g. dimpling), skin appearance (e.g. erythema) and localized lesions

are noted. While the patient is upright, the examiner should palpate the axillary and supraclavicular areas with the pads of the fingers, held flat. Palpation of the breast is performed with the patient lying flat with the arm on the side being examined bent palm up (pronated), at right angles to the shoulder. The entire anterior chest should be palpated on each side utilizing the vertical strip method. Palpation is performed with the pads of the second, third and fourth fingers of the examiner's dominant hand moving in concentric 1.5 cm circles with varying degrees of pressure (light, medium and firm) until the underlying ribs are felt. Abnormal findings should be recorded on a preprinted breast diagram in the patient's medical record, or described and located using a clock-face identification and noting distance from the areolar–skin margin (e.g. 3 cm at 3 o'clock).

Mammography

Mammography may be indicated in women aged over 30 who present with breast symptoms for evaluation. In women younger than 30, a diagnostic mammogram should also be ordered if there is clinical suspicion of breast malignancy, but probably special arrangements should be made with the mammographer. Besides giving a mammographic impression of the primary lesion, diagnostic mammography is clinically useful to evaluate the remainder of the breast and the contralateral breast. On the other hand, screening mammography

(for women without breast symptoms or findings) should follow established regional/national guidelines.

Fine-needle aspiration

The presence of a palpable dominant mass is the indication for fine-needle aspiration. There are no contraindications. Ecchymosis or hematoma formation are possible complications of the procedure. Pneumothorax has been reported but should be readily avoided by the technique of compressing the mass over an underlying rib. Fine-needle aspiration can be effectively performed with or without an attached syringe, and negative pressure in the syringe during the actual aspiration. There are various pistol-type syringe holders that assist the aspirator in maintaining negative pressure during the actual aspiration. A three-finger control syringe can be used for the same purpose. A 22-gauge needle with a clear (translucent) plastic hub is commonly used. The equipment for a fine-needle aspiration used by the author is listed below:

- alcohol skin wipe;

- 22-gauge 1-inch needle with a clear plastic hub;

- 4 × 4 inch sterile gauze pad;

- Bandaid/Elastoplast;

- 10 ml syringe;

- Inrad (pistol-type syringe holder).

The most difficult aspect of fine-needle aspiration of a

palpable mass less than 4 cm in diameter is the complete immobilization of the mass during the aspiration. The fingers of the aspirator's non-dominant hand are used to stretch and compress the skin above the mass and position it over a rib. Trapped in such a position, the mass will not move. The initial entry of the needle into the mass should be a slow exploration of the tactile resistance, which assures that the needle tip is centered within the mass. If the mass is a cyst, fluid will flow up the needle and out of the hub. In such case, a syringe is attached and all the fluid withdrawn from the cyst. Thus, the initial free flow of fluid is diagnostic of a cyst and the complete withdrawal of all the cyst fluid becomes therapeutic.

Normal breast is mostly adipose tissue which offers little or no tactile resistance to the needle after the skin puncture. With fibrocystic changes (nodularity), intermittent fibrous bands may be perceived using the needle-alone technique. A fibroadenoma is typically dense and resists the needle thrusting, both in and out. The consistency has been likened to that of a pencil eraser. Carcinomas are usually vascular and gritty with a consistency similar to a raw potato.

With the needle-alone (without syringe) aspiration technique, the aspirator should make 30 sharp thrusts while the needle tip is within the mass. When a syringe and negative pressure are used, 20 such thrusts are usually adequate. With both techniques, the needle hub should be continuously observed for gross blood. The presence of some foamy blood often permits

adequate cellular smears but gross blood will clot, making cellular recovery and interpretation difficult if not impossible. However, carcinomas are typically vascular and the aspirator must make a judgment as to how many strokes to take and how much blood can be allowed to accumulate in the needle hub.

The steps in the performance of fine-needle aspiration of a palpable dominant breast mass (solid) are listed below.

1. Immobilize the mass over a rib while compressing the tissue above the mass and hold the skin taut. (This is done with the second and third fingers of the non-aspirating hand.)
2. Cleanse the skin over the mass with an alcohol (or equivalent) skin wipe.
3. Insert the needle through the skin with a sharp thrust and then slowly press the needle tip into the center of the mass, taking note of the tissue resistance to the needle and watching for fluid in the needle hub.
4. With the needle-alone technique, move the needle tip up and down 30 times keeping the tip within the mass. All the thrusts are made in the same direction in sharp jackhammer-like motions, which allows exfoliated cellular material into the barrel of the needle.
5. With the needle and syringe aspiration technique, negative pressure in the syringe is created only after the needle tip is within the mass. Twenty thrusts similar to those described in step 4 are made. Then, the negative pressure in

the syringe is released.
6. Remove the needle from the breast and quickly prepare the cytologic slides. The smears should be prepared and fixed immediately, unless the slides are to be air dried.
7. Air within a syringe is used to eject the drop of tissue 'juice' within the barrel of the needle forcefully on to the slide (the needle tip touching the center of the slide).
8. Another slide is gently placed over the first and then quickly drawn apart lengthwise as in the preparation of a hematology smear).

Ultrasound

Real-time ultrasound, with a 7.5 MHz linear array nearfield transducer, is useful in the clinical outpatient setting to delineate vague palpable possible masses, to determine if a palpable dominant mass is cystic or solid, and to assist in the aspiration of cyst fluid when the aspiration (drainage of the cyst fluid) seems incomplete.

Tissue core-needle biopsy (Trucut biopsy)

Tissue core-needle biopsy is a popular method of histologic sampling of non-palpable breast lesions. Guidance can be by ultrasound or stereotactic mammography. The use of spring-loaded core-needle guns and #14 gauge needles, and the collection of five or more tissue samples is common. Local anesthesia, a skin stab wound and insertion of the needle parallel to the chest wall are standard procedures. The technique is particularly effective for a 'mass' lesion.

Open surgical biopsy

Open surgical biopsy is the final diagnostic procedure when an adequate fine-needle or tissue core-needle diagnosis has not been obtained. If there is a question of malignancy, an excision biopsy following National Surgical Adjuvant Breast Project (NSABP) lumpectomy technique should be performed [3]. Alternatively, a cytologically diagnosed fibroadenoma can be appropriately enucleated with complete removal of the neoplasm through a cosmetically acceptable incision (e.g. circumareolar).

Benign versus malignant breast disease

Breast cancer is much more common in older (peri-menopausal and postmenopausal) women. The risk in a 35-year-old is 1 in 500 rising to 1 in 100 in those aged 45 years.

Benign breast disease is mostly hormonal driven and is therefore more common in perimenopausal women. In communicating this to women, one can simply say that benign breast disease is an aberration of physiology, while breast cancer is a true 'pathology'.

Mastalgia

Most women experience bothersome intermittent cyclic breast pain sometimes during their menstruating years and many, propelled by an underlying fear of breast cancer, will seek medical evaluation. The essential questions in the history are: (1) is the pain cyclic or non-cyclic (constant or intermittent) – this is best verified with a breast pain chart; and (2) is the pain diffuse or localized? Physiologic mastalgia is cyclic (premenstrual), diffuse and, most often, bilateral. Pain from intrinsic breast pathology, such as duct ectasia, is usually non-cyclic and localized, although a cyst or fibroadenoma can be painful during the premenstrual phase. Mastalgia as the sole symptom of breast cancer is rare, being seen in only 7% of presentations.

The breasts are innervated by branches of the anterior and lateral intercostal nerves arising from T2 to T6, but mostly from T3 to T4 [4]. Although pain can be referred to other areas, the innervation of the breast *per se* does not produce shoulder, arm, neck, back or radiating pain. However, owing to her fear of breast cancer, the patient may perceive any discomfort in the anterior chest area to be of breast origin. Careful questioning and examination should identify anterior chest pain which is of non-breast etiology. Some of the etiologies of anterior chest pain (usually non-cyclical) that have been perceived by patients to be mastalgia are:

- achalasia;
- cervical radiculitis/spondylosis;
- cholecystitis;
- cholelithiasis;
- coronary artery disease;
- costochondritis (Tietze's syndrome);
- hiatal hernia;
- myalgia (along lateral border of pectoralis major);
- neuralgia;
- osteomalacia;
- phantom pain;
- pleurisy;
- psychological pain;
- rib fracture;
- trauma;
- tuberculosis;
- iatrogenic, e.g. hormone replacement therapy.

A detailed history, supplemented by a pain chart, and a complete and careful bilateral clinical breast examination should assist in the diagnosis of true mastalgia and give a clear clinical impression of the etiology. However, tenderness (or lack thereof) upon examination may or may not correlate with the patient's complaint, and the clinical or pathologic diagnosis. Except with obviously advanced disease, breast cancer rarely presents with a complaint of pain without an associated suspicious mass. However, as with all breast complaints, it is medically imperative and essential for the patient's reassurance to rule out any evidence of breast cancer. This can be accomplished by the judicious application of the diagnostic triad of clinical breast examination (including pertinent history), mammography and fine-needle aspiration of a dominant breast mass.

The treatment of mastalgia should proceed in a stepwise fashion (Box 24.1) beginning with explanation and reassurance.

Box 24.1 Therapies for mastalgia

- Reassurance
- Mechanical measures (e.g. change of clothing, shoulder purse, wearing a firm supporting bra)
- Premenstrual salt restriction
- Intermittent non-steroidal (NSAID) analgesia for true diffuse breast pain
- Evening primrose oil (EPO) 3 g q.d.s. or gammolenic acid in EPO (120 mg b.d.)[a]
- Low-dose oral contraceptive therapy
- Danazol (100–200 mg/day)[b]
- Progesterone (e.g. continuous oral or intramuscular)
- Bromocriptine (5 mg o.d.)[c]
- Tamoxifen
- Gonadotropin-releasing hormone analogs
- Injection of local anesthetic/steroids (2 ml lidocaine + 40 mg methylprednisolone in 1 ml) – suitable for trigger spots

[a]Response within 3–4 months. Suitable for moderate pain. As side effects are few, this should be first-line treatment.
[b]Therapeutic response highest (over 75% for cyclic mastalgia).
[c]Dosage to be increased gradually.

More than 75% of women presenting with breast pain will be satisfied and appropriately treated by reassurance and explanation after a complete breast evaluation has excluded cancer [5]. However, as with all women seeking medical attention for breast complaints, the patient should be instructed to monitor her symptoms, perform monthly breast self-examination and return promptly if her symptoms progress or if she perceives a dominant mass.

Iatrogenic mastalgia associated with initiating hormone replacement therapy, especially in premenopausal women, tends to settle with continued use.

Mastitis

Breast infections are most commonly related to pregnancy and/or lactation and usually caused by *Staphylococcus aureus*. Dicloxacillin/cloxacillin or equivalent antibiotics achieve effective and prompt clinical response. Antibiotic therapy should be initiated as soon as there is clinical suspicion of mastitis. The patient should be re-evaluated about every 3 days to ascertain if the infection is responding to treatment and that there is no evidence of abscess formation. If an abscess does form, it should be drained immediately. This can usually be accomplished by needle (e.g. 18-gauge) aspiration although the procedure may have to be repeated [6]. If the infection does not respond to the initial antibiotics, therapy should be changed to a broader spectrum (e.g. amoxycillin/clavulanate and metronidazole) which covers anerobic bacteria [7]. This combination of antibiotics (or dicloxicillin and metronidazole) is usually effective for chronic mastitis [7]. However, recurrent subareolar fistulae most often require surgical excision as definitive treatment.

If diffuse erythema persists in spite of appropriate antibiotic therapy, a skin biopsy (e.g. punch biopsy) should be performed to evaluate the dermal lymphatics and rule out histologic inflammatory carcinoma.

Nipple discharge

Nipple discharge is not a common presenting complaint. Most women during the menstruating years can occasionally elicit some nipple discharge, usually from multiple duct openings on the nipple [8]. Except for puerperal nipple discharge, which is usually milky, the color of the elicited discharge is often clear, cloudy or serosanguinous.

Pathologic nipple discharge is spontaneous and usually unilateral. Except for periductal mastitis, pathologic discharge is from a single lobe opening on the nipple. Intraductal papillomas are the etiology of more than 60% of spontaneous unilateral single duct nipple discharge [9]. The rare intraductal papillary carcinoma produces grossly bloody or serosanguinous nipple discharge. In such malignant cases, there may be a palpable mass.

The diagnosis of pathologic nipple discharge can be established by galactography (ductography) with precise localization of the lesion within the involved duct [10–12]. If this mammographic technique is not available, a lacrimal probe placed down the involved duct can identify the affected lobe anatomically. In all cases of pathologic nipple discharge, the involved duct should be completely excised and histologically evaluated to ascertain definitely whether the lesion is a benign process or a rare intraductal papillary carcinoma. Focused ultrasound can identify the characteristic dilated ducts below the areola.

Periductal mastitis (mammary ductal ectasia, plasma cell mastitis) causes dark greenish or occasionally black discharge from multiple lobe openings on the nipple. Sometimes the discharge is bilateral. Although the distended ducts filled with amorphous debris are surrounded by an inflammatory reaction, etiologic bacteria have not been identified and antibiotic therapy has proven to be ineffective. If the patient's symptoms warrant it, surgical excision of all the involved ducts will eliminate the symptoms.

All women with pathologic nipple discharge should receive long-term follow-up after treatment, with annual clinical breast examinations and annual mammography for women 40 years of age and older. However, once completely excised, intraductal lesions rarely recur.

Palpable dominant breast mass

The pre-eminent objective of clinical breast examination is the identification of a dominant breast mass. Once identified, a persistent dominant breast mass must be investigated definitively and expeditiously (within 3 months). In most breast centers, about 20–25% of dominant breast masses prove to be malignant. The ratio of benign to malignant masses is directly related to age with cancer becoming the most common diagnosis in postmenopausal women.

Fibrocystic change

The most common diagnoses of dominant breast masses in premenopausal women are

distinct nodular formations (fibrocystic changes) and fibroadenomas. Fibroadenomas are most common in the teenage and early reproductive years of a woman's life. Cysts occur most commonly in the later reproductive years. The diagnosis of breast cancer most frequently occurs in the perimenopausal and immediate postmenopausal years. The incidence and rate of breast cancer rises continuously as a woman ages.

Fibrocystic change, in some shape or form, is almost universally present within the female breast [13,14]. Unfortunately, in some women, these changes present as a palpable dominant breast mass. Concordance of the diagnostic triad (clinical breast examination, mammography, and fine-needle aspiration cytology) will provide the diagnosis in most cases [15,16]. Open surgical biopsy provides a definitive histologic diagnosis and reassurance when necessary to allay any remaining doubts on the part of either the patient or physician.

Fibroadenoma

Serial mammograms have provided insight into the biologic behavior of fibroadenomas. Lesions may remain small and non-palpable or they may be multiple and indeed bilateral in some cases. Palpable fibroadenomas have a characteristic cellular pattern by fine-needle aspiration. When all the cytologic criteria are met, including an abundant cell sample, the cytologic diagnosis of fibroadenoma is definitive and reliable. Fibroadenomas tend to be

estrogen related, and to diminish in size and become non-palpable in the perimenopausal years. Some atrophic fibroadenomas calcify with a characteristic popcorn pattern seen on mammography. Although fibroadenomas have a characteristic appearance on mammography and ultrasound, neither technique is clinically diagnostic.

Fibroadenomas are not premalignant [17,18]. However, since there are abundant ductal epithelial cells within a fibroadenoma, it is not surprising that the occurrence of carcinoma within fibroadenomas has been reported. In 1985 a comprehensive review of the English language medical literature revealed 120 published cases of carcinoma within a fibroadenoma [19]. Of the 104 cases that could be histologically analysed, 73 (70%) were lobular carcinoma *in situ*, 11 (10%) were ductal carcinoma *in situ* and 19 (18%) were invasive carcinoma. Nine of the 27 malignancies that were not confined to the fibroadenoma were invasive carcinoma. Thus, some surgeons view the excision of a cytologically (by fine-needle aspiration) diagnosed fibroadenoma as a patient's elective choice [20–22]. Annual clinical examination and appropriate breast imaging, when indicated, are adequate follow-up. However, if the patient perceives a significant change in the palpable mass, prompt medical re-evaluation is indicated.

Breast cyst

It is likely that all women have microscopic microcysts (non-palpable) within their breasts. Some will develop microcysts, which can be seen on mammography or ultrasound. Some microcysts will enlarge and become palpable macrocysts that can be readily diagnosed by fine-needle aspiration (Haagensen et al. reported that 7% of women presenting to Western World hospitals have a palpable breast cyst [23]). Some palpable cysts become symptomatic and require therapeutic fine-needle aspiration.

Although mammography is useful in detecting a benign-appearing, well-marginated mass of low density, ultrasound is required to differentiate a cyst from a solid mass. If the mass is palpable, however, fine-needle aspiration is the diagnostic procedure of choice because the cyst can thereby be thera-peutically drained as well as diagnosed.

Cytologic evaluation of cyst fluid is not cost effective [24]. The only cyst aspirate that should be sent for cytologic evaluation is a grossly (old) bloody fluid which may be associated with intracystic carcinoma. The occurrence of intracystic carcinoma is reported to be about 1:1000 cysts [25,26]. Most clinicians and many breast clinics will never see an intracystic carcinoma. Such a malignancy becomes clinically apparent as a palpable mass after complete cyst fluid aspiration or when the cyst refills (usually with grossly bloody fluid) within a 3-month period. Pneumocystography and ultrasound are reported to demonstrate intracystic lesions, which require surgical excision for definitive histologic diagnosis [10,27].

Once a cyst has been diagnosed and completely drained of non-bloody fluid with no residual palpable mass and it has not reformed (refilled) within 3 months, the patient can be followed as if she had not had the cyst.

A summary of benign breast disease is given in Table 24.1.

Breast cancer

A global view of breast cancer

Breast cancer is the most prevalent female cancer in developed countries and the second most common in developing countries. The highest incidence of breast cancer is in women in the USA. Every year over 500 000 new cases of breast cancer are reported worldwide. The age-standardized mortality from breast cancer is about 40%. Geographical differences in incidence apply mainly to postmenopausal disease. Risk factors are listed in Table 24.2.

Non-palpable lesions

Identification and evaluation of non-palpable breast lesions is the purview of the breast imager (mammographer). The screening or diagnostic mammography report should indicate the imaging impression (diagnosis) and give specific recommendations for further evaluation or follow-up. Ultrasound is utilized as a focused examination of a suspect mammographic lesion or as guidance for tissue core-needle biopsy. Ultrasound is particularly effective in differentiating a cyst from a solid mass and can be useful in the evaluation of mammographically dense breasts.

Mammographically placed needle/wire localization and open surgical excision (usually with a specimen radiograph to ascertain if the radiographic lesion is in the tissue excised) with subsequent histologic diagnosis has been the standard approach to indeterminate and suspicious non-palpable breast lesions. However, tissue core-

Table 24.1 Benign breast disease

Condition	Average age at presentation	Presentation
Microfibroadenoma	20s	Subclinical
Macrofibroadenoma	20s	A lump
Fibrocystic change	Reproductive years (average age 30)	Diffuse nodularity/a lump with or without atypia
Cyclic mastalgia	Reproductive years (mid-30s)	Cyclical pain from midcycle to menses Described as 'heavy', tender to touch, increased by physical activity and usually lateral aspect
Non-cyclic mastalgia	Late reproductive years (mid-40s)	Persistent or episodic pain usually localized, described as 'burning'
Breast cysts	Late reproductive years (mid-40s)	Micro- or macrocysts

Table 24.2 Breast cancer risk factors

Factor	Relative risk
Age	10
Geographical (developed versus developing countries)	5
Early menarche (before 11 years)	3
Late menopause (after 54 years)	2
Delayed first term pregnancy (>35 years)	3
Family history of first-degree relative	2
Atypical hyperplasia	4
High saturated fat diet	1.5
BMI > 35 in premenopause	0.7
BMI > 35 in postmenopause	2
Oral contraceptives	1.24
HRT > 10 years	1.3
High alcohol intake	1.3

BMI = body mass index;
HRT = hormone replacement therapy.

needle biopsy has become popular in many breast centers. The appropriate treatment and follow-up depends on the specific histologic diagnosis and status of the surgical margins.

Palpable lesions

Palpable breast cancer is readily, efficiently and effectively diagnosed in the outpatient setting by the application of the diagnostic triad (clinical breast examination, fine-needle aspiration and mammography) for a persistent palpable dominant breast mass. Further specific testing for breast cancer includes a chest film and liver function tests (e.g. alkaline phosphatase). The initial clinical staging is followed by precise surgical/pathological staging, the outcome of which defines the therapy.

A multidisciplinary treatment planning conference is optimum for individualized therapeutic recommendations. It is common for breast cancer patients to seek (request) second opinions. The patient and her family can be overwhelmed by the options of therapies with unknown risks and indeterminable prognoses.

Counseling, the provision of clear unbiased information, and emotional support are important components of the patient's treatment, in which her primary care physician can and should actively participate.

The preferred treatment of stage I and II breast cancer is breast conserving therapy: lumpectomy with clear surgical margins, anterior chest irradiation to control local recurrence and axillary lymph node dissection for prognostic information [28]. Modified radical mastectomy is the traditional therapy. Each newly diagnosed breast cancer patient should make her own informed choice of therapy after being given full current information about the options of treatment, and carefully considering her own risk tolerance and quality of life issues. The primary care physician can be a resource and counselor for the woman and her family during the decision-making process.

Radiation therapy utilizing multiple radiation ports is usually given in daily treatments over a 6-week period. Erythema, skin changes (sometimes resembling a second-degree burn) and fatigue are common side effects of

irradiation. With current dedicated equipment, the side effects are often mild and in most cases subside spontaneously with time.

Adjuvant therapy is given when the axillary lymph nodes are involved with the cancer. Premenopausal women usually have cancer that is estrogen-receptor negative and are given multidrug chemotherapy in serial courses over a 6-month interval. Postmenopausal women usually have estrogen-receptor-positive cancers and are treated with oral tamoxifen daily for 5 years. Again, the adjuvant therapy is tailored to the specific details and circumstances of each patient.

After her treatment is completed, a woman with breast cancer should be followed with annual clinical breast examinations, annual mammography and periodic chest X-rays and liver function tests. Psychological morbidity is common in women with breast cancer. Up to 30% of sufferers present with anxiety/depression. Post-mastectomy a quarter of women develop negative body image and sexual dysfunction. The primary health care team should target those at risk and enlist the help of specialist nurses, self-help groups and other dedicated personnel.

Counseling and health education

Most women have concerns and questions about their breasts and breast cancer, and their primary care physicians can be the optimum medical source of current accurate information, the presentation of which should be in an empathetic non-judgmental fashion without haste or personal bias. A compassionate nurse often can initiate the discussion of a patient's breast concerns and uncertainties. When the media represent medical data as crises requiring urgent, dramatic action, primary healthcare providers for women should furnish an overview in readily understood language of all the known data, emphasizing the impact (or lack thereof) of the data upon the healthcare of the individual patient.

Genetic testing for breast cancer raises ethical, economic and propriety issues. A detailed pedigree, i.e. for breast, ovarian and colon cancer with verification of the diagnoses, should precede the medical recommendation about genetic testing (e.g. *BRCA1*, responsible for 4% of all breast cancers; Table 24.3). Furthermore, the physician should be clear as to exactly what she wants to know and what the patient thinks the results will achieve. Currently, there is no clear consensus as to the indication for breast cancer genetic testing, much less any specific appropriate recommendation when the result is determined.

The criteria for referral to a cancer family clinic are:

- one first-degree relative with breast cancer at age <40 years;

- two first-degree relatives with breast cancer at age < 60 years;

- three first-degree relatives with breast cancer at any age.

Screening for breast cancer

There is no evidence that clinical examination, breast ultrasonography and teaching breast self-examination are effective in screening for breast cancer. Breast self-examination or breast awareness can be adjuncts to screening to pick up interval cases of those who do not attend (Box 24.2).

Screening mammography is the generally accepted procedure for the early diagnosis of breast cancer. Film screen mammography with dedicated equipment and specialized film processing, backed by trained radiologists, has been shown to be the most effective procedure for population screening. Double reading of films, i.e. by two independent mammographers, can increase the cancer detection rate and reduce the number of imaging work-ups [29]. Screening mammography is the norm for women aged 50–75 years. The indications for screening mammography of women aged 40–49 and older than 75 remains controversial, and should be individualized after discussion of the data currently available with the patient (and/or her family as appropriate).

Clinical breast examination should accompany mammography in the screening for breast cancer as 10% of palpable breast cancers will not be evident in the mammogram [30,31]. Annual clinical breast examinations are an important part of the many medical health maintenance programs for women, but their value in reducing mortality from breast cancer remains unproven.

Breast self-examination is a useful technique to familiarize a woman with her breasts, to detect changes in her breast and to facilitate her seeking medical attention for breast symptoms. Most breast lumps are discovered by their owners. Breast self-examination is best done postmenstruation in premenopausal women and monthly in postmenopausal women. It consists of systematic inspection and palpation of both

Table 24.3 Family History and *BRCA1* gene carriage

Number of family members with breast cancer	Age at diagnosis	Risk of *BRCA1* carrier state (%)
2	≤25	100
3	<60	35
3	<50	40
2	<60	20
2	<50	37
2	<40	46

breasts. 'Breast awareness' focuses on maximizing the opportunities in a woman's daily routine (changing, having a bath or shower) to encourage her to be breast aware. Box 24.3 gives the criteria for and attributes of mammographic screening for breast cancer.

Box 24.3 Criteria for and attributes of mammographic screening for breast cancer

- Allows early detection of breast tumors. At the initial screen, up to 20% of cases will be *in situ* and another 20–25% will be <1 cm in diameter.
- UK screening between the ages of 50 and 70 years results in a drop of up to 10% in mortality compared with an unscreened population.
- The UK breast screening program (Forrest) aims to screen women aged 50–65 years every 3 years. In the USA, screening is recommended to age 75 years. In the UK, women over 65 may be screened on request.
- Mediolateral oblique views are the standard in the USA; single oblique view mammography is still in use in some other programs, including that in the UK.
- Frequency of screening has to ensure a positive cost–benefit ratio: the 3-year screening interval adopted by the UK screening program satisfies this requirement, but interval cancers are known to occur after 2 years. In the USA, annual mammograms are advocated. A happy medium may be an 18-month to 2-year interval.
- Mammography misses 5% of cancers in women >50 years and 20% in women <50 years.
- The benefit of mammographic screening of women aged 40–49 is still debatable especially in North America. It is recommended by the AMA and American Cancer Society, opposed by the American College of Physicians and not yet endorsed by the National Institutes of Health. The benefit from mammographic screening of 40–49-year-olds is slower (seen after 8 years of screening) and smaller (picking up more *in situ* cancers), while having more false-positive and false-negative lesions, and a consequent smaller reduction in mortality.

Resource list

For clinicians

- Dixon JM. The ABC of breast diseases. London: BMJ Publications, 1995.
- NHS Breast Screening Programme/Cancer Research Campaign. Guidelines for referral of patients with Breast Problems. Sheffield, NHS Breast Screening Programme, 1995.
- Lee L, Stickland V, Wilson ARM, Roebuck EJ. Fundamentals of mammography. London: WB Saunders, 1995.

Resources for patients

Breast cancer self-help groups

- Breast Cancer Care (UK Freephone 0500 245 345)

- Cancer Link (UK) (Tel. 0207-833 2451/0131-228 5557)
- Cancer Relief Macmillan Fund, Anchor House, 15–19 Britten Street, London SW3 3TZ, UK
- American Cancer Society (ACS), Reach to Recovery Program, American Cancer Society (USA) (Tel. 1-800-ACS-2345).
- USA Cancer Information Service (CIS) of the National Cancer Institute (Tel. 1-800-4-CANCER)
- US National Alliance of Breast Cancer Organizations (NABCO) (Tel. 1-212-719-0154)
- CANCER-NET of the National Cancer Institute: e-mail: cancernet@icicc.nci.nih.gov with the word HELP (for English) or SPANISH (for Spanish)

Reading for patients

A woman's guide to breast cancer diagnosis and treatment by Breast Cancer Treatment Options, Medical Board of California, 1426 Howe Avenue, STE 54, Sacramento, CA 95825, USA (Fax: 1-916-263-2479.)

References

1. Hindle WH. The diagnostic evaluation. In: Marchant DJ (ed.) Breast disease I: benign disease. *Obstet Gynecol Clin North Am* 1994;21:499–517.

2. Zajdela A, Zillhardt P, Voillemot N. Cytological diagnosis by fine needle sampling without aspiration. *Cancer* 1987; 59:1201–5.

3. Margolese R, Poisson R, Shibata H, Pilch Y, Lerner H, Fisher B. The technique of segmental mastectomy (lumpectomy) and axillary dissection: a syllabus from the National Surgical Adjuvant Breast Project

workshops. *Surgery* 1987;102:823–34.

4. Sarhadi NS, Dunn JS, Lee FD, Soutar DS. An anatomical study of the nerve supply of the breast, including the nipple and areola. *Br J Plast Surg* 1996;49:156–64.

5. Pye JK, Mansel RE, Hughes LE. Clinical experience of drug treatments for mastalgia. *Lancet* 1985;ii:373–7.

6. Dixon JM. Repeated aspiration of breast abscesses in lactating women. *Br Med J* 1988; 297:1517–8.

7. Edmiston CE Jr, Walker AP, Krepel CJ, Gohr C. The nonpuerperal breast infection: aerobic and anaerobic microbial recovery from acute and chronic disease. *J Infect Dis* 1990; 162:695–9.

8. Devitt JE. Management of nipple discharge by clinical findings. *Am J Surg* 1985;149:789–92.

9. Gulay H, Bora S, Kilicturgay S, Hamaloglu E, Goksel HA. Management of nipple discharge. *J Am Coll Surg* 1994;178:471–4.

10. Fajardo LL, Jackson VP, Hunter TB. Interventional procedures in disease of the breast: needle biopsy, pneumocystography and galactography. *AJR* 1992; 158:1231–8.

11. Tabar L, Dean PB, Pentek Z. Galactography: the diagnostic procedure of choice for nipple discharge. *Radiology* 1983; 149:31–8.

12. Diner WC: Galactography: mammary duct contrast examination. *AJR* 1981; 137:853–6.

13. Love SM, Gelman SR, Silem W: Fibrocystic 'disease' of the breast – a nondisease. *N Engl J Med* 1983;307:1010–14.

14. Frantz VK, Pickren JW, Melcher FW, Auchincloss H Jr. Incidence of chronic cystic disease in so-called 'normal breasts': a study based on 225 postmortem examinations. *Cancer* 1951; 4:762–83.

15. Hindle WH. Breast masses. In-office evaluation with diagnostic triad. *Postgrad Med* 1990;88:85–7.

16. Hermansen C, Poulsen HS, Jensen J, et al. Diagnostic reliability of combined physical examination, mammography, and fine-needle puncture ('triple test') in breast tumors: a prospective study. *Cancer* 1987;60:1866–71.

17. Dupont WD, Page DL. Risk factors for breast cancer in women with proliferative disease. *N Engl J Med* 1985;312:146–51.

18. College of American Pathologists. Is 'fibrocystic disease' of the breast precancerous? *Arch Pathol Lab Med* 1986;110:171–3.

19. Yoshida Y, Takaoka M, Fukumoto M. Carcinoma arising in fibroadenoma: case report and review of the world literature. *J Surg Oncol* 1985;29:132–40.

20. Hindle WH, Alonzo LJ. Conservative management of breast fibroadenomas. *Am J Obstet Gynecol* 1991;164: 1647–50.

21. Dent DM, Cant PJ. Fibroadenoma. *World J Surg* 1989;13:706–10.

22. Wilkinson S, Anderson TJ, Rifkind E, Chetty U, Forrest AP. Fibroadenoma of the breast: a follow-up of conservative management. *Br J Surg* 1989;76:390–1.

23. Haagensen CD, Bodian C, Haagensen DE. Breast carcinoma risk and detection. Philadelphia: WB Saunders, 1981.

24. Rosemond FP, Burnett WE, Caswell HT. Aspiration of breast cysts as a diagnostic and therapeutic measure. *Arch Surg* 1955;71:223–9.

25. Rosemond GP, Maier WP, Brobyn TJ. Needle aspiration of breast cysts. *Surg Gynecol Obstet* 1969;128:351–4.

26. Abramson DJ. A clinical evaluation of aspiration of cysts of the breast. *Surg Gynecol Obstet* 1974;139:531–7.

27. Tabar L, Pentek Z Dean PB. The diagnostic and therapeutic value of breast cyst puncture and pneumocystography. *Radiology* 1981;14:659–63.

28. NIH Consensus Conference. Treatment of early-stage breast cancer. *JAMA* 1991;265:391–5.

29. Brown J, Bryan S, Warren R. Mammography screening: an incremental cost effectiveness analysis of double versus single reading of mammograms. *Br Med J* 1996;312:809–12.

30. Edeiken S. Mammography in the symptomatic woman. *Cancer* 1989;63:1412–14.

31. Baker LH. Breast cancer detection demonstration project: five-year summary report. *Cancer* 1982;32:194–225.

Therapeutic termination of pregnancy

Anna Glasier BSc MD FRCOG

Introduction

Abortion is common. It has been estimated that 50 million abortions occur worldwide annually – 40% are illegal and around 20 million unsafe. Abortion accounts for between 60 and 120 000 maternal deaths each year (20% of total maternal deaths); almost all are in developing countries and almost all are preventable.

Abortion rates are usually expressed as the number of abortions per 1000 women of reproductive age (15–44 years). Worldwide the average abortion rate is thought to be 32–46/1000 and 10–30/1000 in developed countries. There are wide variations in abortion rates with the lowest being found in the Netherlands (5/1000) and the highest in parts of the former USSR (186/1000). In 1990, in the USA and UK, the rates were 24/1000 and 15.8/1000, respectively.

Abortion rates are related to contraceptive prevalence. Countries with low contraceptive prevalence tend to have higher rates than those where contraceptive use is widespread. In a recent review of the subject, Kulcyzyki and colleagues [1] point out that 'no society has achieved low fertility without recourse to abortion'. Abortion is an intrinsic element of fertility regulation and, as contraceptive prevalence rises in developing countries, so eventually abortion rates fall. However, even in countries where contraceptive prevalence is high and couples have access to methods with low failure rates, abortion is still common. In the UK, where contraception is free of charge and without consultation fees, it has been estimated that 47% of all pregnancies are unintended and 43% of these are terminated [2], amounting to one in five conceptions ending in an abortion. In England and Wales, a woman's average lifetime risk of abortion was calculated by the UK Birth Control Trust to be 43% based on 1995 figures.

After the 1967 Abortion Act in England and Wales, there was a rapid rise in the abortion rate which reached a plateau in the late 1980s. Since then there has been a gradual rise in the rate each year until 1993 when a small downward trend began. In 1994, 166 876 abortions were performed in England and Wales, a 1.1% fall compared with 1993. However, since 1972 the proportion of abortions to conceptions has remained constant at 8% for married women and 37% for single women [3]. In 1996, England and Wales witnessed an 8.3% rise in abortions compared with 1995 (Figure 25.1). The rise was attributed to the 'pill scare' of October 1995, which led to an estimated 5% of women discontinuing their oral contraceptive pills.

Demographics of abortion

The risk of abortion is related to age, parity, ethnicity and socioeconomic status. Cultural values, laws and policies obviously also play a role. In Western countries the peak age for abortion is 20 and the tendency for young women to be most at risk of abortion is universal. Women over the age of 35 are also more likely to have a pregnancy terminated, perhaps because of the catastrophic domestic and medical consequences of unplanned pregnancy for many women and the decline in the prevalence of effective contraception among this age group.

Marital status also has an effect on abortion risk. In Europe, most women undergoing abortion are

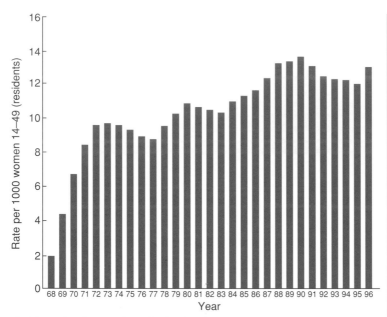

Fig. 25.1 Abortion rates in England and Wales 1968–1996.

unmarried. In England and Wales in the early 1990s, eight pregnancies were terminated for every 100 births among married women compared with 52 per 100 births among unmarried women. In contrast, in Asia, most women are married, while in Africa and Latin America, slightly more married than unmarried women are at risk. The effect of parity is closely related to marital status.

Although data on socioeconomic status are scarce, in general it is true to say that women who are better educated and those who live in urban areas are most likely to undergo abortion. In a recent Scottish survey, Smith and co-workers [4] demonstrated that unplanned pregnancies are commoner among teenagers who live in socially deprived areas than among teenagers from more affluent areas, who, when they do conceive, are more likely to have their pregnancy terminated than their economically deprived

peers. In the USA, non-Whites are nearly three times more likely to have a therapeutic abortion, while in the Netherlands, immigrants are significantly more at risk than Dutch women.

With the legalization of abortion and improvements in service delivery, the average gestation at which abortion is performed has fallen. Figures may be misleading, however, since in some countries, abortion may be illegal after 12 weeks, while elsewhere, although legal, it may be much more difficult to obtain after the first trimester.

Legal issues

From the mid-19th to the mid-20th centuries most developed countries had restrictive or very restrictive abortion laws. Concern about the harmful effects of illegal abortion led to liberalization of the laws. Abortion became legal for 'social reasons' in the USSR in 1920 and

in Iceland, Sweden and Denmark in the 1930s, with almost all developed countries, together with China and India, following in the 1960s and 1970s. In the USA, access to abortion, at least during the first trimester, became a constitutional right in 1973. More recently, a swing towards less liberal attitudes and laws has occurred in the USA, and in some central and eastern European countries, particularly Poland and Hungary. Most developing countries have restrictive abortion laws. In Bangladesh, while abortion is illegal, menstrual extraction is available in government clinics up to 8–9 weeks' gestation as long as the pregnancy has not been confirmed.

It has been estimated that 63% of women in the world have access to abortion on request, 12% on broad medical grounds only, while 25% of women must continue the pregnancy unless their life is endangered. Most countries in which abortion is legal require assessment and agreement by at least one doctor, although this may change in the future at least for abortions in the first trimester. In South Africa, recent abortion legislation does not require agreement by a doctor for pregnancies of less than 8 weeks' gestation.

Legalized abortion does not guarantee access to safe abortion. In some countries, such as India, services may be inadequate or too expensive to meet the demand. In the USA, 84% of counties have no specialist medical provider of abortion services. In contrast, in Brazil, where abortion is illegal, it is available in clandestine but safe clinics to women who can afford to pay. In the UK, the law defines specific indications for abortion which reflect the reasons why a woman finds herself with an unwanted pregnancy. The 1967 Abortion Act and its amendment in the Human Fertilisation and Embryology Act of 1990, states that abortion can be performed if two registered medical practitioners acting in good faith, agree that the pregnancy should be terminated on one or more of the grounds shown in Box 25.1.

The 1990 amendment reduced the upper limit from 28 to 24 weeks' gestation for clauses C and D, reflecting the lowering of the limits of fetal viability resulting from advances in neonatal care. It also included selective reduction in multiple pregnancy cases and authorized the Secretary of State for Health to licence premises for the sole purpose of providing medical termination of pregnancy.

The 1967 Abortion Act does not apply to Northern Ireland, where abortion is only legal under exceptional circumstances, e.g. to save the life of the mother. The law recognizes that some doctors have ethical objections to abortion. Doctors who do have objections should refer women to another colleague who does not hold similar views.

Adolescents

One-fifth of the world's population is aged between 10 and 19 years, and in some developing countries the majority of the population is under 20 [5]. Everywhere age at first intercourse is falling, while age at marriage is increasing. As a result, teenage pregnancy is becoming common and is widely regarded in many countries as a significant sociomedical problem. In the USA, one million women under 20 become pregnant each year and 82% of these pregnancies are unintended. In Kenya, the percentage of pregnancies among 15–19-year-olds which are mistimed or unwanted is 47% among married women and 74% among those not married.

Young people are less likely to use contraception because they do not expect to have sex, do not know about contraception, lack access to it or lack the ability or power to make decisions. In developing countries, adolescents are more likely to suffer pregnancy-related complications and to die in childbirth than women in their 20s. Abortion-related complications and deaths are also thought to be more common among adolescents than older women. In many countries unwanted pregnancy in an adolescent presents problems with the issue of consent, since the law may require parental consent for the procedure. However, in the UK, if the termination is lawful, consented to by a competent patient and if considered in the teenager's best interests, then a doctor may proceed with the operation if forbidden or unable to obtain parental consent. The issue of competency of minors to give consent is defined in the UK in the Children's Act.

Counselling for abortion

The decision to have a pregnancy terminated is never an easy one. All women should have access to abortion counselling, which should provide opportunities for discussion, information, explanation and advice in a manner which is both non-judgemental and non-directive. The way in which counselling is provided will vary; in some developed countries it is mandatory. Whatever the format of counselling, every woman should be given the opportunity to explore her feelings and anxieties, and to make an informed choice. She may be sad about her decision but she should have no long-term regrets. Box 25.2 outlines the management

---

Box 25.1 Clauses under which abortion is legal in the UK

A. The continuance of the pregnancy would involve risk to the life of the pregnant woman greater than if the pregnancy were terminated.

B. The termination is necessary to prevent grave permanent injury to the physical or mental health of the pregnant woman.

C. The pregnancy has *not* exceeded its 24th week and the continuance of the pregnancy would involve risk, greater than if the pregnancy were terminated, of injury to the physical or mental health of the pregnant woman.

D. The pregnancy has *not* exceeded its 24th week and that the continuance of the pregnancy would involve risk, greater than if the pregnancy were terminated, of injury to the physical or mental health of the existing child(ren) of the family of the pregnant woman.

E. There is substantial risk that if the child were born it would suffer from such physical or mental abnormalities as to be seriously handicapped.

Box 25.2 Management and care of the unplanned pregnancy

1. 'Counselling' – risks and alternatives; inform her that she can change her mind.
2. Assessment of gestation:
   - History
   - Clinical examination
   - Pregnancy test, if indicated
   - Ultrasound, especially if discrepancy between dates and size, suspected adnexal mass or questionable viability
3. Explain:
   - Procedure – medical, surgical, admission and discharge
   - Anaesthetic – GA, LA
   - After effects
   - Complications
   - Contraception
   - Follow-up
4. Document:
   - Reason for termination of pregnancy
   - Gestational age and date of pregnancy test
   - Informed choice with alternatives
   - Discussion of complications and possible sequelae
   - Contraceptive care
   - Tests carried out/offered
5. Tests:
   - Mandatory – haemoglobin, blood group and rhesus status, sickle screen (if indicated) and rubella screen (if indicated, and if follow-up immunization, if required, is feasible)
   - *Chlamydia* and other STD screening, especially in women under 25 years and those who have had a recent change of partner
   - Opportunistic – cervical cytology
   - ?HIV
6. Supply contraception

GA = general anaesthesia; LA = local anaesthesia; STD = sexually transmitted disease; HIV = human immunodeficiency virus.

and care of the unplanned pregnancy at the abortion facility.

Counsellors should encourage the woman to think of both the practical and emotional consequences of all the possible options: abortion, continuing with the pregnancy and adoption. Unless a woman is quite certain of her decision, she will be more likely to regret it later. A few women will need more time and perhaps more counselling to help them make up their minds. Some women will change their minds. The incidence of long-term regret/emotional sequelae is low.

Even in countries where abortion is legal and accessible, many women fear they may be refused an abortion and, perhaps, for some, it is not possible to make the final decision until they are quite certain that they really do have a choice. For others, the reality of abortion may not become apparent until they are faced with the practicalities of undergoing the procedure. In some countries, such as France, statute demands a waiting period between the time the abortion has been agreed and the time it is carried out, to allow women the opportunity to reflect on their decision free from the worry that the request may be refused.

The majority of women (around 80%) have made their decision before they see a doctor. Seeing the doctor is usually a necessary part of obtaining an abortion and women attend expecting confirmation of their pregnancy, information and referral to an abortion provider.

The skill of the counsellor lies in the ability to detect those women who need lengthy discussions and more support, and those who may be at risk of severe regret.

The different techniques, together with their advantages and disadvantages, should be discussed to enable a choice to be made where available and appropriate. The risks of abortion together with the effect of abortion on future fertility should be covered. Women also need to receive information about what happens after the abortion, the expected duration of bleeding, when to have intercourse and even such details as when to have a bath. The decision to have a termination has often arisen because a relationship has ended and the woman may not see an immediate need for future contraception. While discussion about future contraception prior to or even immediately after the abortion may not be ideal, in some cases it may be the only chance the professional has. Contraception is an important issue in post-abortion care and follow-up.

Medical assessment

Medical history
Particular attention should be paid to conditions such as asthma, which may influence the choice of method of abortion, and to factors which may increase the risks of the procedure such as previous thromboembolic disease.

Gestation
Gestation should be determined by menstrual history and pelvic examination. A pelvic ultrasound

scan is unnecessary unless there is doubt about the gestation or ectopic pregnancy is suspected.

Genital tract infection (*particularly* Chlamydia)

Whether screening is performed or everyone is treated with prophylactic antibiotics depends on the background incidence of infection in the local population and on the relative costs. If screen is positive, antibiotic therapy should be started *before* the abortion is performed. In high-risk populations, both screening (and wherever possible, contact tracing) and antibiotic prophylaxis may be justified. Antibiotic prophylaxis should comprise anti-chlamydial and antianaerobic infection agents. There is evidence that antibiotic prophylaxis for high-risk cases reduces the incidence of infection [6].

Hepatitis B and HIV

Women considered to be at high risk of hepatitis B or HIV should be offered screening with appropriate counselling. Women who refuse screening should be treated as high risk during the abortion procedure.

Cervical screening

Cervical screening is not essential and may not be practical, but should be offered in accordance with national screening policies.

Haemoglobin and blood group

Haemoglobin concentration and blood group should be determined. Women who are rhesus negative should be injected with anti-D immunoglobulin (1250 IU) before or within 48 h of the abortion to prevent the development of rhesus isoimmunization.

Box 25.3   Methods for inducing abortion

Early first trimester (≤ 9 weeks)

Surgical
- Menstrual regulation
- Vacuum aspiration

Medical
- Antiprogesterones + prostaglandins
- Methotrexate + prostaglandins
- Prostaglandins alone (not currently recommended)

Late first trimester (9–14 weeks)

Surgical
- Vacuum aspiration

Second trimester (beyond 14 weeks)

Surgical
- Dilatation and evacuation
- Hysterotomy

Medical
- Intrauterine irritants
- Prostaglandins

Methods of terminating pregnancy

There is a variety of methods available for termination of pregnancy (Box 25.3). The method chosen depends largely on gestation and availability of methods (Figure 25.2). The woman's parity, medical history and her wishes are other issues to consider.

Early first trimester (up to 9 weeks)

Surgical methods

Menstrual regulation

In some countries women who have missed a menstrual period

Fig. 25.2   Methods of termination of pregnancy by gestational age. PG = prostaglandin.

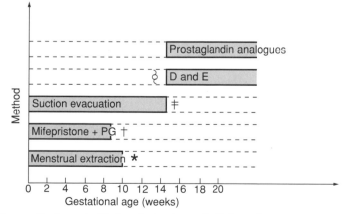

*No anaesthesia required to 6 weeks, local anaesthetic thereafter.
†Mifepristone is also licensed in UK for medical termination of pregnancies 12–20 weeks' gestation.
‡Can be done under local or general anaesthetic. Cervical priming using prostaglandins, mifepristone or hydrophilic dilators is recommended for nulliparous women over 10 weeks' gestation.
§Cervical priming essential.

have access to menstrual regulation, when suction evacuation of the uterine cavity is performed usually without confirmation of pregnancy. This method is common in China, where abortion is legal, and in Bangladesh up to 6–9 weeks of amenorrhoea. Usually undertaken very soon after the missed menstrual period, it is done with a hand-held syringe attached to a manual or electrical aspiration pump.

Vacuum aspiration

Vacuum aspiration has been the method of choice for early surgical termination of pregnancy in most developed countries for over 20 years. Dilatation and curettage is not recommended as it requires a greater degree of cervical dilatation, and is associated with a significantly higher incidence of uterine injury and of retained products of conception. Vacuum aspiration can be performed under either local paracervical block (LA) or general anaesthesia (GA). Some evidence suggests that local anaesthesia may be safer: in the USA, the mortality rate is 2–4 times greater when general rather than local anaesthesia is used for first-trimester abortion. In the UK, where most abortions are performed under general anaesthesia, there has not been an abortion-related maternal death in many years. In developing countries, economic considerations and the availability of skilled personnel may influence the choice of anaesthetic.

Preoperative treatment with a cervical priming agent reduces the risk of haemorrhage and genital tract trauma.

Prostaglandins, bougies and the antiprogesterone RU486 (mifepristone) are all effective, but prostaglandins probably have a faster onset of action. Pretreatment of the cervix increases the cost of the procedure and may be difficult to organize when abortion is performed as a day case. As cervical trauma is commoner in women under the age of 17 years and uterine perforation is associated with increasing parity and increasing gestation, efforts to arrange cervical ripening should be concentrated on very young women, highly parous women and those presenting at later gestation.

A curette of 6–10 mm internal diameter is passed through the cervix and the contents of the uterus aspirated using negative pressure. It is advisable to use the smallest diameter curette which is adequate for the gestation – 8 mm at 8 weeks, 10 mm at 10 weeks. The curette may be made of metal or plastic, curved or straight, and either flexible or rigid.

Vacuum aspiration at this stage of pregnancy is safe, with an incomplete abortion rate of less than 2%. Failure is more likely to occur before 7 weeks' gestation when the fetus may be missed by the curette. Thus it may be better to defer operation until after 7 weeks or to use medical methods. The mortality from vacuum aspiration in the first trimester is less than about 1 per 100 000, considerably less than the maternal mortality from continuing pregnancy.

Medical methods

A variety of compounds have been used to induce abortion medically rather than surgically (Figure 25.2).

Prostaglandins

Prostaglandins stimulate uterine contractions, and can be administered orally, vaginally, extra-amniotically, intra-amniotically or by intramuscular injection. In the early first trimester, prostaglandins alone will induce complete abortion in up to 95% of cases, but the duration of treatment and the incidence of side effects militate against their routine use.

Antiprogesterones

Antiprogesterones are synthetic steroids which block the action of progesterone by binding to its receptor. Mifepristone (RU486, Mifegyne) is the only such compound yet marketed and is used in France, China, UK and Sweden. In 1996 it was recommended to the US Food and Drugs Administration as a safe and effective means of inducing abortion, although it is as yet not available for use in the USA. Mifepristone also binds to the glucocorticoid receptor and blocks the action of cortisol.

When mifepristone is used alone, for pregnancies with up to 63 days of amenorrhoea, complete abortion only occurs in around 60% of cases. The antiprogesterone itself stimulates some uterine contractility but also greatly enhances the sensitivity of the myometrium to prostaglandins. The rate of complete abortion rises to over 95% if a prostaglandin analogue is given 36 or 48 h after the administration of mifepristone. In the UK, the recommended regimen is mifepristone given as a single oral dose of 600 mg (3 × 200 mg tablets) followed 48 h later by a 1 mg vaginal pessary of the prostaglandin Cervagem (gemeprost) (Figure 25.3). Mifepristone 200 mg has been shown to be equally effective and since this makes the regimen considerably cheaper, the lower dose is now widely used. In the UK, mifepristone is also licensed for use with gemeprost for termination of second-trimester pregnancies and for management of death *in utero* in the third trimester. Its use in the pretreatment of the cervix prior to surgical termination has already been discussed.

Misoprostol, an oral prostaglandin E₁ analogue, marketed for the treatment of peptic ulcer, has been shown to be effective in combination with mifepristone, although efficacy may decline after 7 weeks' gestation. Unlike gemeprost, it does not require refrigeration and 'thawing' for an hour prior to administration. Misoprostol can be administered vaginally or orally, and may be more effective vaginally, but randomized controlled studies are few. In the

> **Box 25.4   Contraindications to first-trimester medical abortion using antiprogesterone + prostaglandins**
>
> Absolute contraindications
> - > 9 weeks' gestation
> - Suspected ectopic pregnancy
> - Active asthma
> - Liver and/or renal disease
> - Suspected adrenal insufficiency
> - Heavy smoking (>15 cigarettes per day) *and* > 35 years
> - Unavailability for follow-up within 2 weeks
> - Anaemia (Hb < 10 g/dl)
> - Haemolytic disease or taking anticoagulants
>
> Relative contraindications
> - > 8 weeks' gestation
> - Hypertension (diastolic pressure > 100 mmHg)
> - Heavy smoking (> 15 cigarettes per day)
> - > 35 years
> - Women taking systemic steroids

UK, misoprostol is not licensed for termination of pregnancy. The cost of misoprostol is 50 times less than gemeprost. Misoprostol has also been used with mifepristone in the termination of second-trimester pregnancies.

Not all women are suitable for medical abortion. The contraindications are shown in Box 25.4.

There are very few side effects following the administration of mifepristone. The fetus is usually aborted following the administration of prostaglandins, and this is accompanied by bleeding and pain. The bleeding is usually like a heavy period, although rarely (<1%) there may be very heavy bleeding requiring resuscitation. The amount of bleeding is related to gestation, since the size of the placental site increases as pregnancy advances. Nulliparous women and those with a history of dysmenorrhoea are more likely to experience severe pain and 10–20% of women may need opiate analgesia; the rest will cope with paracetamol alone. Prostaglandin synthetase inhibitors, such as aspirin or mefenamic acid, should be avoided. Bleeding can continue for up to 20 days after the abortion, although in most women bleeding stops after 10 days. The total amount of blood lost is similar to that occurring at the time of vacuum aspiration.

A follow-up visit about 2 weeks after administration of the prostaglandin is essential because 30% of women do not pass an identifiable fetus and/or placental tissue. Ongoing pregnancy occurs in only 1% of cases; however, evacuation of the uterus will be

Fig. 25.3 Protocol for medical termination of early pregnancy (≤ 63 days' amenorrhoea)

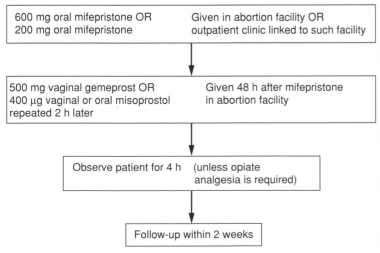

| 600 mg oral mifepristone OR 200 mg oral mifepristone | Given in abortion facility OR outpatient clinic linked to such facility |

| 500 mg vaginal gemeprost OR 400 µg vaginal or oral misoprostol repeated 2 h later | Given 48 h after mifepristone in abortion facility |

Observe patient for 4 h (unless opiate analgesia is required)

Follow-up within 2 weeks

necessary in up to 5% because of incomplete abortion. These figures are no different from those associated with surgical abortion.

The risk of fetal malformation following RU486 alone or in combination with prostaglandins is unknown. Women should be advised that medical abortion is a two-stage procedure, and that it is not possible to have a change of heart after taking RU486 and before prostaglandin administration. In the event of a failed medical abortion, the woman must be strongly advised to have vacuum aspiration, although babies born to the few women who have chosen to continue with the pregnancy, after medical abortion has failed, have been normal. Misoprostol is teratogenic; however, any congenital defect may partly be the consequence of the failed abortion.

In France and the UK, around 20–25% prefer medical abortion. Women often choose the medical method because it usually avoids an anaesthetic and because they feel more in control of the situation. Some women, however, find the two stages a disadvantage. The incidence of serious complications is probably similar to that associated with surgical abortion but, because 95% of women need neither anaesthesia nor instrumentation of the uterus, large randomized trials may eventually show medical abortion to be safer.

Methotrexate

The cytotoxic drug methotrexate has recently been used in the medical management of ectopic pregnancy. In the USA, methotrexate has been proposed as an effective adjuvant to prostaglandins used for first-trimester abortion. Unlike RU486, methotrexate is known to be teratogenic, thus risking fetal malformation and inevitable litigation in the event of ongoing pregnancy.

Late first trimester (9–14 weeks)

At this stage of pregnancy, the method of choice is vacuum aspiration, which can be done under local or general anaesthesia. Although abortion can be induced by antigestagens and prostaglandins, the incidence of incomplete abortion is high. The cervix should be pretreated at gestations of greater than 10 weeks in nulliparous women. Although vacuum aspiration is an extremely safe operation, the incidence of complications rises as gestation advances.

Beyond 14 weeks

Surgical methods

Dilatation and evacuation (D&E)

In some countries, including the USA, D&E is commonly used for terminating pregnancies up to 20 weeks' gestation. It should only be performed by experienced surgeons. Under local or general anaesthetic, the cervix is dilated to 14 mm or more to allow removal of relatively large fetal parts. Pretreatment cervical priming is essential and an oxytocin infusion during D&E is advisable to reduce blood loss. Fetal parts should be kept so that the completeness of the procedure can be checked before evacuating the cavity with a 12 mm suction curette. D&E is thought to be safer than intra-amniotic instillations up to 16 weeks' gestation, although the procedure has not been compared with vaginal prostaglandins.

Hysterotomy

The removal of the uterine contents via laparotomy and a vertical or transverse uterine incision is associated with relatively high mortality and is rarely necessary, particularly as the presence of a uterine scar may compromise future pregnancies.

Medical methods

Intrauterine irritants

Hypertonic saline and urea can be administered intra-amniotically to induce late abortion. The procedure is prolonged but can be shortened by pretreatment cervical priming and the use of intravenous oxytocin to enhance uterine contractions. The incidence of infection, haemorrhage and retained products of conception is higher than with prostaglandins but the fetus is rarely delivered alive. Rarely, disseminated coagulopathy may occur and the inadvertent systemic administration of hypertonic saline may lead to cardiovascular collapse. Another agent, ethacridine lactate (Rivanol) is an acridine dye which can be inserted into the extra-amniotic space. It is cheap, safe and weakly antiseptic and, for these reasons, is popular in some developing countries. There is some evidence of acute toxicity in animals and, for this reason, WHO has denied permission for clinical trials.

Prostaglandins

Prostaglandins alone have been widely used in the termination of second-trimester pregnancy. Intra-amniotic administration requires skilled personnel. Rarely, acute systemic absorption may cause hypotensive crisis, myocardial infarction, cerebral haemorrhage, bronchospasm and death. The induction–abortion interval is prolonged with a concomitant increase in the risk of infection. The experience is painful. The vaginal administration of pessaries containing a prostaglandin E_1 analogue or misoprostol is safer and less unpleasant. In the UK, this approach is now routinely preceded by pretreatment with the antiprogesterone RU486 (mifepristone), which significantly shortens the interval between administration of the prostaglandin and abortion of the fetus to 6–8 hours. Mifepristone 600 mg is given 36 h before vaginal insertion of a 1 mg gemeprost pessary repeated at intervals of 3 and 6 h until expulsion of the fetus occurs. Infusion of prostaglandin E_2 into the extra-amniotic space can be used if pessaries are not available. Overall, 30% of women retain all or part of the placenta, and require surgical evacuation of the uterus.

Despite some disadvantages, medical abortion with prostaglandins alone, or preferably in combination with mifepristone, is very effective and associated with a very low incidence of complications. Because it requires less surgical skill, the potential for serious complications is probably less than for D&E and hence, it will continue to be used in many parts of the world.

Abortion beyond 18 weeks' gestation is rare and is usually reserved for pregnancies complicated by severe fetal malformation. Particularly distressing for both the mother and the staff, these late abortions are often effectively managed with vaginal prostaglandins in combination with RU486, with intra-amniotic urea or fetal intracardiac injection of potassium to minimize the chances of expulsion of a live fetus (see Chapter 33 for information about anaesthesia for termination of pregnancy). Box 25.5 gives details of cervical preparation.

Sequelae of abortion

In developed countries where abortion is legal, associated mortality and morbidity have fallen over the last two decades. In Europe and the USA, the risk of death is less than 2 per 100 000 procedures; in Sweden, abortion is ten times safer than childbirth. The risks rise with gestation. Serious complication rates for first-trimester abortions are less than 1% (Box 25.6), with fewer than 1 in 1000 women needing hospitalization; beyond 10 weeks' gestation the health risks of abortion rise with each week. The risk of late second-trimester abortion is up to four times higher than that for first-trimester abortion. Complications are usually divided into immediate (during or within 3 h of the procedure), delayed (3 h to 28 days) and late (>28 days) (Box 25.7).

Box 25.5 Preparation of the cervix

I. Hydrophilic dilators
Reduce the force needed for dilatation

(a) Laminaria tents:
- Stems of seaweed
- Radial force on the cervix
- Swell to 3–4 × their size
- Cheap
- Never 100% sterile
- Slow action (6–48 h)

(b) Synthetic dilators:
- Rapid dilatation
(i) Lamicel
  - Polyvinyl sponge containing 450 mg of $MgSO_4$; 3 and 5 mm sizes
  - Force not radial, therefore not useful for late abortions
  - Maximum action after 2 h
(ii) Dilapan
  - Hypan dilator – radial force
  - Quick action
  - 4–8 mm in 30 min
  - 12 mm in 1 h

II. Prostaglandins
e.g. Gemeprost 1 mg pessary 1–3 h preoperatively produces dilatation of 7–9 mm; or misoprostol orally

III. Foley catheter
Inserted intracervically and balloon inflated with 20–30 ml of water; left overnight

IV. Mifepristone

Box 25.6   Complication rates (first-trimester abortion)

Infection	2–5%
Cervical laceration	<1–3.5%
Incomplete abortion	<1–19%
Uterine perforation	<1–1.3%
Haemorrhage	<1–2.5%

Immediate complications

Trauma

Cervical laceration occurs usually when the tenaculum pulls off the cervix during dilatation. The risk is reduced by preoperative cervical priming and by placing the tenaculum vertically with one tooth in the os and the other high on the anterior lip, taking a 'big bite' of tissue. If laceration occurs, it may require suturing but, more commonly, simple postoperative observation is all that is needed.

Uterine perforation probably occurs more commonly than is apparent: perhaps as many as one in six perforations goes undiagnosed. When recognized, perforation is usually without complications and the patient should simply be observed. If intra-abdominal trauma is suspected – more likely during

Box 25.7   Sequelae of induced abortion

Immediate
• Trauma
• Haemorrhage
• Amniotic fluid embolism
• Anaesthetic complications

Delayed
• Incomplete abortion
• Unrecognized ectopic pregnancy
• Infection
• Venous thromboembolism

Late
• Reproductive sequelae
• Psychological sequelae

second- than first-trimester termination – laparoscopy and/or laparotomy should be performed and the damage repaired by a competent surgeon.

Haemorrhage

The true incidence of haemorrhage depends on the definition used. Management includes blood transfusion, paracervical injection of vasopressin solution, hysteroscopy and internal compression of the uterine cavity with the balloon of a Foley catheter or with a pack soaked in vasopressin solution. Coagulopathy rarely complicates abortion.

Amniotic fluid embolism

This is a rare but potentially fatal complication of second-trimester abortion. The risk may be reduced by draining the amniotic fluid at the beginning of the procedure.

Anaesthetic complications

In the USA, complications of general anaesthesia are the leading cause of abortion-related death. In a recent review of the subject, Grimes [7] concluded that abortion under local anaesthesia is preferable in terms of both safety and cost. Abortion in the UK is still predominantly managed with general anaesthesia. Offered the choice, some women would certainly find the idea of being awake during the procedure quite unacceptable. However, up to 30% of women in the first trimester choose local anaesthesia when offered.

Venous thromboembolism

Pregnancy increases the risk of thromboembolism; so does

general anaesthesia. Most women undergoing termination of pregnancy are young and physically fit, and surgical abortion is rarely a prolonged procedure. Nonetheless, the risk of venous thrombosis should never be overlooked and a previous history of thromboembolism might determine the choice of anaesthetic and, if practical and available, the method of inducing abortion.

Delayed complications

Incomplete abortion

The commonest complication following abortion is the persistence of placental and/or fetal tissue. Up to 5% of women undergoing first-trimester medical abortion will require surgical re-evacuation of the uterus within the first month.

The incidence of incomplete abortion after vacuum aspiration rises with gestation. Bleeding 2 weeks after a medical or surgical abortion is not in itself an indication to evacuate the uterus. Ultrasound scans often show residual trophoblastic tissue even in women who have stopped bleeding. Although an ultrasound scan of the uterus and the measurement of human chorionic gonadotrophin (HCG) in plasma may be helpful in diagnosing an ongoing pregnancy, the decision to evacuate the uterus should be made on clinical grounds, i.e. continued heavy or persistent bleeding from a bulky uterus in which the cervix is still dilated. The majority of women with an incomplete or missed abortion will pass the residual tissue with time if they will wait. The belief that all women with an incomplete abortion have a high risk of intrauterine infection until the uterus is evacuated probably stemmed from the time when illegal abortion was common.

Unrecognized ectopic pregnancy

Examination of aspirated tissue for chorionic villi and fetal parts should reduce the risk of unrecognized ectopic pregnancy which may be fatal. Microscopic (pathological) examination of the specimen is only indicated if a molar pregnancy is suspected.

Infection

Post-abortion infection is probably also under-reported but should be suspected in a woman with prolonged heavy vaginal bleeding as well as those with classical symptoms of pain and pyrexia. Established pelvic inflammatory disease with pyrexia, abdominal pain and offensive vaginal discharge occurs in around 1% of women whatever method of abortion is used. The risk can be reduced by pre-abortion screening and/or prophylactic antibiotics as discussed earlier.

Late complications

Reproductive sequelae

Almost all studies [8,9], agree that neither vacuum aspiration nor second-trimester prostaglandin abortion is associated with a significant increase in secondary subfertility. There is a 30% risk of tubal infertility following severe post–abortion infection. The latter is uncommon occurring in <0.5% of cases. There are as yet insufficient data on first-trimester medical abortion, but there is no reason to suspect that the risk will be different. Uncomplicated induced abortion does not increase the risk of ectopic pregnancy, nor of spontaneous abortion unless sharp curettage is used. Abortion has no effect on the outcome of subsequent pregnancies continued to childbirth, such as low birth weight or premature delivery. The data on the increased risk of placenta praevia following induced abortion are inconclusive. Ashermann's syndrome is a rare complication of abortion where intrauterine adhesions follow vigorous curettage of the uterine wall. Management is hysteroscopic division of the adhesions, placement of a Foley catheter or an intrauterine device *in utero* and treatment with a short course of oestrogen/progestogen.

Psychological sequelae

Many women feel emotional for a few days following the abortion. Many studies have, however, demonstrated a significant improvement in psychological well-being by 3 months after, compared with before the abortion [10]. There is no evidence of an increase in the incidence of serious psychiatric problems following abortion: indeed a recent review of the subject [11] concluded that 'there is, as yet, no credible evidence for the existence of post–abortion syndrome'. In contrast, the incidence of depression, suicide and child abuse is higher in women who have continued with the pregnancy because abortion was refused [12]. In the same study, the children born to women refused abortions had higher incidences of psychopathology and educational and social problems than their matched contemporaries, and these differences persisted into adulthood.

Breast cancer

Induced abortion does not seem to increase the risk of breast cancer [13].

Follow-up

All women should have their questions answered and receive contraceptive advice (Table 25.1) and, if appropriate, supplies before leaving the abortion facility. All

Table 25.1 Post-TOP contraception

Method	When to start?
Combined pill	Day of operation or following day
Progestogen-only pill	Day of operation or following day
Condom	Advisable whenever intercourse occurs for STI prevention
IUD	At operation (if ≤ 12 weeks) or at next menses
Diaphragm	Check size ≥ 2 weeks post-TOP
Depo-Provera	Within 5 days of TOP
Norplant	At operation
Sterilization	Discussed as for interval procedures

STI = sexually transmitted infection; IUD = intrauterine device; TOP = termination of pregnancy should be given a follow-up appointment within 3 weeks, either with the clinic which carried out the abortion or with a suitable alternative doctor. At follow-up, a pelvic examination should aim to confirm complete abortion and the absence of infection. Discussion should include contraceptive advice and post-abortion counselling if required.

The future

In the foreseeable future, the important changes in the management of unwanted pregnancy are likely to be political rather than clinical. Clinical scientists will continue to tinker with regimens for medical abortion in an attempt, for example, to find the 'perfect' prostaglandin, which is free from side effects or to develop slow-release prostaglandins to be given at the same time as mifepristone.

A number of pharmaceutical companies have antiprogesterone drugs which may be superior to mifepristone. Most, however, seem reluctant to develop them as abortifacients because of the politics of abortion.

Women's health advocates and some non-governmental organizations are pressing for widespread availability of medical abortion, particularly in developing countries where surgical techniques may be dangerous, and where abortion-related morbidity and mortality are high. In this context, there is also a move to facilitate the use of medical methods by individual women in their own homes. Many doctors have concerns about the safety of do-it-yourself medical abortion but, seen as a wider public health imperative, persuasive arguments can be made at least for reducing the need for medical supervision for some stages of medical

abortion procedures. There is, however, a risk that moves to allow abortion at home will increase popular support of the anti-abortion lobby and, in developed countries, where safe abortion is available and accessible, it may be sensible not to 'rock the boat'.

Finally, it is likely that abortion legislation will continue to change throughout the world. In developing countries, where abortion is currently illegal, the inevitable processes of liberalisation – as in South Africa – may result in legalisation. In Europe, where birth rates have fallen in some countries to below replacement level, it is equally possible that governmental concerns about demographic changes may result in abortion becoming less easily available. Whatever happens, we can rest assured that in no country will abortion ever be out of the headlines.

Resource list

Further reading for healthcare professionals

- Baird DT, Grimes DA, Van Look PFA (eds). Modern methods of inducing abortion. Oxford: Blackwell Science, 1995.

- Bygdeman M (ed.). Medical induction of abortion. Bailliere's Clinical Obstetrics and Gynaecology, Vol. 4. London: Bailliere Tindall.

- Huggins GR, Cullins VE. Fertility after contraception or abortion. *Fertil Steril* 1990:54:559–73.

- Templeton A. Mini-symposium: therapeutic

abortion. *Curr Obstet Gynaecol* 1993;3:1–27.

References

1. Kulkczycki A, Potts M, Rosenfield A. Abortion and fertility regulation. *Lancet* 1996;347:1663–8.

2. Allaby MAK. Risks of unintended pregnancy in England and Wales in 1989. *Br J Fam Plann* 1995;21:93–4.

3. Paintin D. Abortion in the first trimester. *Br Med J* 1992; 305:967–8.

4. Smith T. The influence of socio-economic factors on attaining targets for reducing teenage pregnancies. *Br Med J* 1993;306:1232–5.

5. Population Reports. Meeting the needs of young adults. Population Reports 1995, Vol.

XXIII, no. 3, Series J, no. 41. Baltimore: Population Information Program, The Johns Hopkins School of Public Health.

6. Penney QC, Thomson M, Norman J, et al. A randomised comparison of strategies for reducing infective complications of induced abortion. *Br J Obstet Gynaecol* 105; 599–604.

7. Grimes DA. Sequelae of abortion. In: Baird DT, Grimes DA, Van Look PFA (eds) Modern methods of inducing abortion. Oxford: Blackwell Science, 1995;95–111.

8. Frank P, McNamee R, Hannaford PC, Kay CR, Hirsh S. The effect of induced abortion on subsequent fertility. *Br J Obstet Gynaecol* 1993; 100:575–80.

9. World Health Organisation Task Force on Sequelae of Abortion. Secondary infertility following induced abortion. *Stud Fam Plann* 1984;15:291–5.

10. Adler NE, David HP, Kajor BN, Roth SH, Russo NF, Wyatt GE. Psychological responses after abortion. *Science* 1990;268:41–4.

11. David HP. Comment: post-abortion trauma. Abortion review no. 59 1–2. London Birth Control Trust, 1996.

12. Matejcek Z, Dytrych Z, Schuller V. Follow up study of children born to women denied abortion. In: Porter R, O'Connor M (eds) Abortion: medical progress and social implications. Ciba Foundation Symposium 115. London: Pitman, 1985:136–46.

13. Westoff C. Abortion and breast cancer: good data at last. *IPPF Med Bull* 1997;31:1–2.

Premenstrual syndrome

Janet Barter MBChB MRCOG MFFP

Background

Although the effect of the menstrual cycle and menstruation on a woman's feelings and behaviour has been discussed since the time of Hippocrates, premenstrual tension as an entity was first described by Frank in 1931 [1]. The name was changed to premenstrual syndrome (PMS) in the 1970s because of the recognition that there were more symptoms than simply tension. In 1987, late luteal phase dsyphoric disorder was accepted into the third edition of the American Psychiatric Association diagnostic and statistical manual (DSM111-R). There is, however, still a debate as to whether this is a true 'disease', a variant of normal or a psychological problem, perhaps stemming from the demands placed on women by Western culture. Many causes have been suggested, including endocrine abnormalities, such as oestrogen excess, oestrogen deficiency and progesterone deficiency, nutritional inadequacies, psychological disorder and neurotransmitter abnormalities. To date, no one aetiological theory has been accepted, but recent research is beginning to add to our understanding of the syndrome, and thereby helping us to treat it more effectively.

It does seem that 95% of women of reproductive age can recognize some physical and/or emotional differences premenstrually, and that the pattern does not occur in 'low hormone level' conditions such as before puberty, or after the menopause, be it surgical or natural. PMS does not occur in pregnancy, a 'high hormone level' condition. In relatively few women (most sources estimate 30–40%), these differences are extreme enough to be called symptoms, and to cause distress and handicap. In 2.5% of women, the syndrome may be a causative factor in depression, violence, child abuse, and other antisocial and criminal behaviours. It is likely that this exacerbation is due to a combination of factors, biochemical and psychological, and the most successful management will be a strategy that recognizes this multifactorial aetiology. No clear association has been demonstrated between PMS and age or other demographic variables. However, PMS sufferers have a higher prevalence of past affective disorders than the general population; whether a genetic factor is involved is unclear, although adolescent daughters of PMS mothers are more likely to experience PMS.

Definition

The fact that the incidence of PMS is quoted in different sources as being between 10% and 90% of the female population illustrates that there is no one accepted definition. However, the following is a useful working definition:

> The repeated occurrence of symptoms in the luteal phase of the menstrual cycle, which are sufficiently severe to interfere with a woman's ability to function within her social framework.

A National Institute for Mental Health conference in 1983 [2] recommended that diagnostic criteria should be made more precise and based on a prospective documentation of symptoms for at least two menstrual cycles, and a 30% increase in symptom intensity when menstrual cycle days 5 to 10 are compared with the 6 days prior to menses.

It is important to note that, although the classical group of symptoms (Table 26.1) occurs in most cases of PMS, these symptoms are not definitive and the diagnosis must rest on the cyclical pattern and persistence of symptoms over at least three

Table 26.1 'Classical' symptoms of PMS

Physical	Emotional	Other
Breast tenderness	Depression	Forgetfulness
Abdominal bloating	Anxiety	Poor concentration
Clumsiness	Irritability/aggression	Food cravings
Headache	Lack of control	Increased alcohol
Physical anxiety symptoms	Paranoia	intake
Lethargy	Low self-esteem	Insomnia
Constipation		
Weight increase		

cycles. The guidelines for diagnosis laid down by Dalton remain useful [3]:

1. symptoms are cyclical, occurring only in the second half of the cycle;
2. symptoms increase in severity as the cycle progresses;
3. symptoms are relieved with the onset of menstrual flow, with complete relief within 2–3 days;
4. there must be at least 7 days, usually 9 or 10, completely clear of symptoms, after menstruation;
5. symptoms must be present for at least three cycles;
6. symptoms interfere with work, usual social activities or relationships with others.

This would now be accepted as primary PMS. Most specialists would now also recognize 'secondary' PMS as consisting of an underlying symptom, usually depression or anxiety, but sometimes a physical problem, which is exacerbated in the luteal phase to the extent that the symptoms become a problem at that time. Women with secondary PMS are often difficult to manage, and usually treatment of the underlying condition is most successful in the long term. However, luteal exacerbations of, for example, rheumatic pain,

asthma or epilepsy, may respond well to hormonal manipulation of the menstrual cycle.

Symptoms of PMS

Any symptom which occurs according to the guidelines above may be part of the syndrome. The commonest are included in Table 26.1.

Aetiology

PMS is a psychoneuroendocrine disorder. The cyclical hormonal changes of the 'normal' cycle act

as a trigger for neurotransmitter changes in the central nervous system (CNS).

Normal effects of the menstrual cycle

The key to understanding PMS is to understand the changes that occur during the 'normal' menstrual cycle, and how these are mediated. One can then look at how and why these mechanisms can generate symptoms. The hormonal changes of the menstrual cycle are explained in Chapter 4 and the mechanisms of their effects are given in Table 26.2.

Exacerbating factors

There is no evidence to suggest that there is any abnormality of hormone levels in women suffering from PMS compared to those who do not suffer. It appears that the symptoms are due to an

Table 26.2 Mechanism of luteal-phase symptoms

Luteal change	Mechanism
Mastalgia	Effect of oestrogen and progesterone: increased activity of glandular and ductal elements of breast Mediated by prostaglandin E$_1$
Abdominal bloating, constipation	Progesterone-induced relaxation of the smooth muscle of the gut wall May cause bloating and reduced transit time
Nausea	May be an effect of progesterone on gut transit time or a prostaglandin effect
Swelling ankles/fingers	Oestrogen effect on kidney: increase in renin, angiotensin II and aldosterone Results in mild fluid retention
Headaches	Possibly reducing oestradiol level or progesterone and/or prostaglandin effect
Lethargy, less 'buoyant'	Progesterone effect: direct sedative effect on central nervous system Possibly via GABA receptors
Depression, irritability, clumsiness	Correlation with serotonin levels being lower in luteal phase

GABA = gamma aminobutyric acid.

exaggerated response to the changing levels of oestrogen and progesterone within their normal range. Thus, the normal tendency to be less buoyant in the luteal phase becomes exhaustion and lethargy, abdominal bloating and mastalgia become disabling, and headaches become troublesome.

End-organ response to sex steroids is mediated via essential fatty acids and their metabolites the prostaglandins. Sex steroid levels also affect the central neurotransmitter activity. Thus, changes in the levels of these hormones affect almost every system of the body via different mechanisms. This makes it much less surprising that the presentation of PMS varies so widely from one woman to another.

Although the aetiology of the problem is by no means clear, several mechanisms are being explored and deserve recognition. These are considered in detail below.

Oestrogen and progesterone

Although there is no evidence of consistent abnormalities in the levels of these hormones in PMS, there is no doubt that both have profound effects on cerebral function. In at least some cases of PMS, there may be a relative oestrogen deficiency in the late luteal phase which could cause depression by reducing serotonin receptors in some areas of the brain [4]. This fact may be helpful in the management of some women with the condition. It has also been suggested that progesterone withdrawal may be the cause as the symptoms increase as the progesterone level drops in the luteal phase [5]. These two theories form the rationale for treatment with either luteal phase oestrogen or progesterone. High enough doses of oestrogen will, of course, also inhibit ovulation and reduce the cyclical variation of both hormones. Paradoxically, the use of cyclical progestogen in hormone replacement therapy (HRT) in menopausal women causes PMS-like symptoms in up to 40% of women.

Serotonin

Both human and animal work has demonstrated the effect of oestrogen and progesterone on serotonin metabolism, with the suggestion that oestrogen increases serotonin activity, whilst progesterone reduces it. Low CNS serotonin levels have been implicated in the aetiology of major depressive illness, and in addition to depression are recognized to cause anxiety, social withdrawal and clumsiness. In major depression, there is a debate as to whether the decreased serotonergic activity is a response to chronic raised cortisol levels due to long-term social stress, or a primary deficiency perhaps because of low levels of the substrate, L-tryptophan, or defects in the process which transports L tryptophan through the blood–brain barrier.

Brain serotonin levels cannot be measured directly but measurement of whole blood serotonin level and platelet uptake of serotonin are accepted as markers. Studies [6–8] have demonstrated lower levels of both during the luteal phase in women with PMS compared with those without PMS. Studies of L-tryptophan and its carrier protein suggest that the cause of the reduction is different in PMS from that in depression, and that reduced serotonin activity in PMS is not due to substrate deficiency [9].

The strongest evidence for serotonin deficiency being a major factor in the causation of PMS is the efficacy of the serotonin agonist fenfluramine and the serotonin reuptake inhibitor fluoxetine in improving the condition. In particular, fluoxetine has been shown to be more effective than placebo in several randomized placebo-controlled trials [10–12].

Endorphins

Beta endorphins are produced when pro-opiomelanocortin is cleaved to produce adrenocorticotrophic hormone (ACTH) during the hypothalamic–pituitary–adrenal axis response to stress. Various psychological states have been linked with abnormal endorphin levels, and inhibition of endorphin with naloxone has been shown to produce PMS-like symptoms [13]. The level of beta endorphins in the peripheral blood is higher during the luteal phase of the menstrual cycle than the follicular phase [14], and women with PMS have been shown to have lower levels of endorphin in the luteal phase than controls [15]. Exercise increases endorphin release and may have a useful part to play in the management of PMS.

Prostaglandins

Many hormones act peripherally via secondary messenger systems. One of these is the synthesis of prostaglandin E_1 (PGE_1) from the essential fatty acid dihomogammalinolenic acid, which derives from dietary linoleic acid. There is a suggestion that deficiency of PGE_1 could affect the peripheral activity of prolactin, opioids, dopamine, serotonin and luteinizing hormone, resulting in an exaggerated end-organ response. In the breast, oestradiol esterifies to essential fatty acids and, the more saturated the fats in the resulting complex, the more potent the effect of the hormone. One study [16] has suggested that there is no difference in dietary fat between women with and without PMS, and speculates whether there may be a problem with the metabolic step from linolenic acid to gammalinolenic acid (GLA). The findings of this study were not corroborated by a study by O'Brien and Massil [17] but these authors agree that addition of essential fatty acids to the diet may be helpful in the treatment of some women with PMS. Many workers recommend that women with PMS increase the amount of GLA in their diet, either by dietary means or by taking supplements. Studies are conflicting on the issue of whether or not this is helpful, but randomized controlled trials do show that GLA is better than placebo in treatment of cyclical mastalgia [18].

Lifestyle issues

Although the primary pathology in PMS is likely to be biochemical, there is little doubt that lifestyle factors can modify the effects. Explanation of this can allow some women to reduce their premenstrual symptoms to a manageable level without drug treatment.

Diet

There is great debate in the literature about whether dietary manipulation is of any benefit. Sweet craving is a common complaint in PMS. The subsequent fluctuation in blood sugar and insulin levels may explain some of the PMS symptoms. Others claim that the high phenylethylamine content of chocolate has a psychotrophic effect through dopamine stimulation or serotonin synthesis. Eating a low-fat, high-protein and high-complex-carbohydrate diet may ameliorate cyclical mastalgia.

It is commonly advised that there should be a regular intake of complex carbohydrates in order to keep the blood sugar stable and anecdotally this appears to be helpful in some women. The three main meals are supplemented by a mid-morning snack of high-fibre carbohydrate (biscuit, crispbread), a similar mid-afternoon snack and a bedtime snack.

Other workers recommend supplementation with magnesium, zinc, vitamin B_6, vitamin E and others. The basis for this is that deficiency of these can cause irritability, but there is no evidence of lower levels of these factors in women with PMS, nor is there evidence that supplementation is more effective than placebo treatment. Vitamin A was advocated for treatment of bloating, weight gain and breast tension, but no controlled trials are available to verify this effect.

Vitamin B_6 is a cofactor in the synthesis of serotonin from tryptophans, so potentially its deficiency could be implicated in the aetiology. However, supplementation has not been shown to be any more effective than placebo. It has been used in women with 'mood' dysphorias.

Doses of over 150 mg/day cause peripheral neuropathy and must be avoided.

Most dieticians advise a good varied diet, including fresh fruit and vegetables, pulses and cereals. It is also wise to advise regular meals including breakfast. Whether this has a specific effect on PMS or simply improves a woman's general well-being is a matter of academic debate.

Evening primrose oil is obtainable over the counter and most PMS sufferers will have used it before presenting to a specialist clinic. In placebo-controlled trials it was not consistently superior to placebo.

Caffeine

Caffeine is a stimulant, and can cause anxiety, palpitations and panic attacks if taken in excess. There is also some evidence that caffeine excess can cause headaches and exacerbate mastalgia. Many women with PMS symptoms do have a high intake, via either tea and coffee or carbonated drinks, and reduction of this intake can be effective in reducing superadded anxiety symptoms.

Alcohol

It is documented that many PMS sufferers consume more alcohol in the premenstrual phase of the cycle. There is no suggestion that this is the cause of symptoms, but it is a depressant, and may increase symptoms of lethargy and low mood.

Exercise

Many women pursue very little or no exercise. Exercise does increase endorphin levels, and thus may be helpful for women with PMS. It is important, however, that the exercise is regular, and not just in the relatively buoyant follicular phase. Exercise also generally improves well-being and self-esteem, and may provide a safe way of releasing aggression.

Stress

Many women find that their PMS symptoms are worse in times of stress. This could be due to the effect of stress on hypothalamic activity, or that stress reduces the ability to cope with cyclical mood changes which might otherwise be considered normal.

Psychological theories

Various workers have suggested that PMS is either purely or partly a psychological problem, and thus that a psychological intervention is an appropriate tool in its management. Ussher [19] suggests a multicomponent model of PMS (Figure 26.1), which accepts that there may be biological differences between women with and without PMS, but argues that the behaviour of the woman, in terms of self-diagnosis and help-seeking or coping behaviour, depends also on a number of psychological and social factors. Some studies suggest that women with PMS show higher neuroticism scores on personality scales (although others dispute this) and this could be considered a vulnerability factor.

The presence of psychosocial difficulty, and lack of social support, could result in a woman becoming depressed in the second half of the cycle, a time when she is naturally less buoyant. Factors that affect the woman's interpretation of this include her self-esteem, itself affected by past life events, and her attitude towards her menstrual cycle, which is affected by the culture within which she lives and by her education. Ussher argues that Western societies tend to view reproduction and thus menstruation negatively, and that this is instilled in adolescent girls. A woman who internalizes these symptoms, and does not develop coping strategies, is more likely to seek medical help.

This would certainly explain the variation in severity of symptoms from woman to woman, and month to month, and also allows for intervention on various different levels.

Diagnosis

It is most important that the diagnosis of PMS is made objectively before treatment is started. It has been estimated that only about half of the women attending specialist PMS clinics – often certain of the diagnosis themselves – actually fit into the definition of primary and secondary PMS. Treatment before diagnosis results in confusion for both patient and doctor, may not be successful, and can result in the true cause of distress being missed. Although this appears obvious in general practice, it is a rule that is very difficult to adhere to in the management of PMS.

Since there are no biological markers for PMS, and the

Figure 26.1 Multicomponent model of PMS – Ussher. Reproduced with permission of Jane Ussher, Womens Health Research Group, Department of Psychology, University College, London.

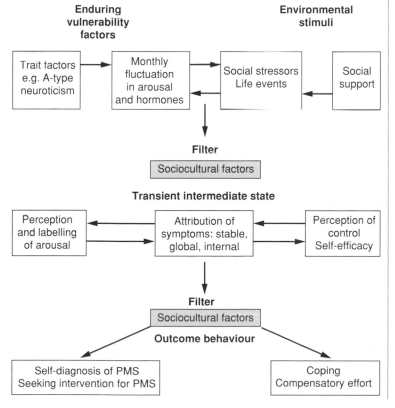

symptomatology of PMS is so varied and overlaps with the symptomatology of many other conditions, diagnosis depends on:

- demonstrating the cyclical nature of the symptoms prospectively; and

- excluding other pathologies such as premenstrual exacerbation of psychological syndromes or other non-cyclical pathologies such as relationship problems, anxiety, phobia, etc.

Symptom charts

The mainstay of diagnosis is the *prospective symptom record*. It has been clearly shown that retrospective recording of symptoms based on a woman's recall and perception of her symptoms is less accurate. Indeed the use of retrospective measures is a criticism of many of the published studies on the subject. The prospective measure can take many forms (Figures 26.2 and 26.3), the main difference being that some charts contain a list of the commonest symptoms of PMS, leaving the patient to score each one on a day of the cycle, while others are blank, allowing the patient to list her own most troublesome symptoms. The criticism of the former is that aspects of the cycle which are not originally troublesome may become so at the suggestion of the chart, and also that it encourages a negative view of the menstrual cycle, by only including its adverse features. The problem with the 'empty' chart is that it does not allow comparison of one woman with another and

thus cannot be used as a research tool. Most of the charts containing lists of symptoms are too lengthy for use in the everyday clinical setting.

The absence of any one accepted 'gold standard' chart makes interpretation of the literature on PMS extremely difficult as trials cannot be compared easily [20].

For everyday practice, the 'empty' chart may well be the simplest and most useful, but the practitioner must help the patient to complete her symptom list at the first visit, so that a useful record can be obtained. Whatever chart is used, the symptom recording must be over at least two and preferably three cycles.

Ovarian suppression

Some women find symptom charting extremely difficult, either because of the severity of the symptoms, or because of coexisting symptoms, stresses or psychosocial difficulties. In this case it may be appropriate to suppress the ovarian cycle completely for, say, 3 months, with a gonadotrophin releasing hormone agonist (GnRHa). This will reliably suppress all 'true' PMS symptoms, i.e. it has 100% response in 'true' PMS [21]. It must be stressed to the woman involved that this is a temporary measure, and it is not advisable to continue the treatment for more than 3 months because of bone mineral density loss. The other problem with this is that most women will suffer from oestrogen-deficiency symptoms after the second month of treatment, which may confuse

the picture, as well as causing distress. This can be overcome by a small dose of 'add-back' oestrogen such as a 25 μg transdermal oestrogen patch. It is certainly wise to perform this diagnostic test whenever such radical measures as hysterectomy and bilateral oophorectomy are considered.

Exclude other conditions

Whether a particular examination or investigation is necessary to exclude other conditions will depend on the assessment of the patient's history. The history should be detailed enough to give real insight into not only what the woman is suffering, but also her personality and her background. In practice, a first appointment for a woman complaining of PMS will need to be at least 20 min, but more likely 30 or more, so that a good initial assessment can be made (Box 26.1).

It is estimated that about 30% of women complaining of PMS will have other gynaecological problems, especially menorrhagia, dysmenorrhoea or dyspareunia. In some cases, elimination of these will reduce the distress to the extent that nothing else needs to be done.

It may be necessary to exclude thyroid disease, perimenopause and anaemia by appropriate tests.

Underlying psychological or psychiatric disorders, particularly depression, schizophrenia and organic brain disease, will need to be excluded. In routine clinical practice, this can be done during the initial history, but for research purposes, a full psychological assessment is

Calendar of Premenstrual Experiences

Name... Month/Year................................. Age....................Unit.................................

Begin your calendar on the first day of your menstrual cycle. Enter the calendar date below the cycle day. Day 1 is your first day of bleeding. Shade the box above the cycle day if you have bleeding. Put an X for spotting.

If more than one symptom is listed in a category, i.e. nausea, diarrhea, constipation, you do not need to experience all of these. Rate the most disturbing of the symptoms on the 1–3 scale.

Weight: Weigh yourself before breakfast. Record weight in the box below date.
Symptoms: Indicate the severity of your symptoms by using the scale below. Rate each symptom at about the same time each evening.

| 0=None (symptom not present) | 2=Moderate (interferes with normal activities) |
| 1=Mild (noticeable but not troublesome) | 3=Severe (intolerable, unable to perform normal activities) |

Other symptoms: If there are other symptoms you experience, list and indicate severity.
Medications: List any medications taken. Put an X on the corresponding day(s).

Bleeding																																								
Cycle day	1	2	3	4	5	6	7	8	9	10	11	12	13	14	15	16	17	18	19	20	21	22	23	24	25	26	27	28	29	30	31	32	33	34	35	36	37	38	39	40
Date																																								
Weight																																								
SYMPTOMS																																								
Acne																																								
Bloatedness																																								
Breast tenderness																																								
Dizziness																																								
Fatigue																																								
Headache																																								
Hot flushes																																								
Trauma, diarrhea, constipation																																								
Perspiration																																								
Swelling of hands, ankles, breasts																																								
Angry outbursts, arguments, violent tendencies																																								
Anxiety, tension, nervousness																																								
Confusion, difficulty concentrating																																								
Crying easily																																								
Depression																																								
Food cravings (sweets, smells)																																								
Forgetfulness																																								
Irritability																																								
Increased appetite																																								
Mood swings																																								
Overly sensitive																																								
Wish to be alone																																								
Other symptoms 1 _____ 2 _____																																								
Medication 1 _____ 2 _____																																								

Fig. 26.2 The calendar of premenstrual experiences (COPE). Reproduced with permission of Joseph Mortola, Harvard Medical School and Beth Israel Hospital, Boston, Massachusetts.

Date	10	11	12	13	14	15	16	17	18	19	20	21	22	23	24	25	26	27	28	29	30	1	2	3	4	5	6	7	8	9	10
Period	x	x	x	x	x																									x	x
Depressed	2	1		0	0	0	0	0	0	0	0	0	0	0	0	0	0	0	1	1	1	1	2	2	2	3	3	3	3	2	3	2	1
Irritable	2	1	1	0	0	0	0	0	1	0	1	0	1	0	0	0	2	1	1	2	3	2	3	3	2	2	3	2	2	2	1
Tired	1	3	1	0	0	0	0	0	0	0	1	0	0	1	0	0	1	1	1	1	1	2	2	1	1	2	2	3	3	2	1
Insomnia	2	2			0	0	0	1	0	0	0	1	0	0	0	0	1	1	2	2	1	2	1	1	1	2	2	3		2	2
Sweet cravings	2	0	0	0	0	0	0	0	0	0	0	0	0	0	0	0	0	0	1	1	2	2	1	1	2	3	3	3	3	3	2	1	0
·																															

(a)

Date	13	14	15	16	17	18	19	20	21	22	23	24	25	26	27	28	29	30	1	2	3	4	5	6	7	8	9	10	11	12	13
Period	x	x	x																							x	x	x	x	x	x
Insomnia	1	1	0	1	1	0	2	2	2	2	0	2	2	2	3	1	1	0	0	0	3	3	1	3	2	2	3	3	0	1	2
Anxious	0	0	0	3	3	2	3	2	1	2	0	1	1	2	1	1	1	2	2	1	3	1	1	1	3	0	1	2	3	3	3
Irritable	1	1	2	2	3	2	2	2	2	1	0	1	2	2	2	0	0	1	1	2	0	0	1	2	1	3	1	0	0	1	2
Depressed	2	3	2	1	1	3	1	0	1	1	1	2	0	1	1	2	0	1	1	2	1	3	2	1	2	1	3	2	2	1	0
Backache	1	0	1	2	1	0	0	0	2	2	2	3	3	3	1	1	0	0	0	0	2	1	2	1	1	1	1	0	0	0	0

(b)

Figure 26.3 Sample 'empty' charts demonstrating (a) PMS and (b) non-PMS symptoms.

desirable. The history may also reveal unresolved problems, such as bereavement or abuse in childhood, which should provoke a referral to a psychologist or counsellor before any medical therapy is instituted.

Treatment

Again, the literature regarding treatment of PMS is difficult to interpret. There are a huge number of papers looking at many different therapies, but there is no consensus of entry criteria, diagnostic methods or monitoring of improvement with treatment. This has resulted in confusion over the years as to how PMS should be treated. One practical result of this confusion is that the most commonly used treatments are not licensed for use in PMS, and those that are licensed are not the best therapies. This means that all treatments must be given with great care, thorough explanation and accurate documentation. All cautions and contraindications should be heeded and side effects taken seriously.

The major problem is that there is a large placebo effect with all treatment choices. Most studies put the placebo effect at between 60% and 90%, which means that any study which is not randomized and placebo controlled cannot be viewed as providing any dependable, usable information.

Once the various methods of treatment are discussed and understood, the next difficulty is deciding when to use each method. The most commonly recommended strategy is to divide the treatments into those appropriate for mild, moderate and severe PMS. Another way would be to categorize women by the predominant symptoms, e.g. anxiety and aggression, depression, mastalgia, physical symptoms, etc.

PMS can be treated in primary care. The indications for referral to a specialist PMS clinic are:

- if simple measures are ineffective;

- if symptoms are extremely severe;

- if there is evidence of violence to self or relations;

- if there are multiple symptoms with psychological components;

- for specialist investigations or treatment;

- if monitoring is required;

Box 26.1 Questions to be asked in the initial consultation

Symptoms
- Exactly what does she suffer?
- Exact timing of symptoms?
- How do symptoms affect life/relationships/work?
- How does she cope with them?
- How do others cope?
- Onset? any triggers or associated events?
- Remedies used to date?

Gynaecological history
- Cycle
- Other gynaecological symptoms, e.g. menorrhagia, abnormal bleeding, dysmenorrhoea, dyspareunia, lack of libido?
- Contraception issues

Medical history
- Other problems that could cause symptoms, e.g. diabetes, thyroid disease, autoimmune disease, epilepsy, migraine, irritable bowel syndrome?
- possible contraindications to hormonal therapies, e.g. thrombotic disease, focal migraine, breast disease?

Current medication

Allergies

Social history
- Relationships
- Work
- Family support and relationships
- Smoking habits
- Diet
- Alcohol intake
- Caffeine intake
- Exercise

Family history
- Any familial disorders?
- Memory of maternal PMS?
- Childhood experience

- if the aim is the 'placebo' effect of 'specialist' advice.

History and acceptance

The first step in treating PMS is probably the most important, that is, history taking, discussion of symptoms and acceptance that there is a problem. Whether or not the diagnosis is one of PMS after the charts have been completed, this initial consultation will inspire trust, and establish a relationship between patient and doctor that will be invaluable in the future. Education, empathy and continuing support are a cornerstone for successful treatment.

Charting is not only a useful diagnostic tool, but also allows the patient to understand the pattern of symptoms more clearly and thus begin to establish some control over the problem. It is not unusual for women to feel so much better after the first consultation in a PMS clinic and 3 months of charting that medical treatment becomes unnecessary. It may well be that this is responsible, at least in part, for the placebo effect noticed in so many studies.

Lifestyle measures

The multifactorial aetiology of PMS should be explained to the patient and it should be stressed that, although her lifestyle will not be causing her PMS, there may be some aspects of it that could be making the situation worse. A full dietary history should be taken, and the advantages of regular meals, a balanced diet, caffeine and alcohol reduction and regular exercise explained. A full social history should also be taken and areas of stress discussed. Sensitive exploration of stressful life events in the past may reveal unresolved issues which could be usefully explored with a psychologist or counsellor. Many women have

Box 26.2 Alternative therapies for PMS

- Acupuncture

Acupuncture has been used to treat other menstrual disorders and pain. The basis of therapies is the release of endogenous opioids. Acupuncture can complement orthodox short-term therapy and can be a confidence-building line of therapy. No randomized controlled trials are available on its value.

- Relaxation therapies

Yoga, aromatherapy, massage, reflexology and stress management may improve self-esteem and relieve mood deterioration. No objective evaluation has been conducted.

- Hypnotherapy

Hypnotherapy may be chosen to treat anxiety.

Table 26.3   Medical Treatment of PMS

Treatment	Dose	Useful for	Notes
Lifestyle advice		All sufferers	See text
Psychological methods Cognitive behavioural therapy (learning adaptive behaviour)		Possibly all sufferers	Helps reduce general stress May be a useful adjunct to psychotropic medication

Gonadotrophin-releasing
hormone agonists (GnRHa)
	Zoladex 3.6 g monthly
	Nafarelin and buserelin in
	ovarian-suppressing dose
	(dependent on preparation
	used)
		1. Diagnosis
		2. To confirm diagnosis
		   before total abdominal
		   hysterectomy and bilateral
		   salpingo-oophorectomy
		3. In extremely severe PMS
		4. To give a short respite
		   from symptoms
			Usually with add-back HRT or in
			courses of 6 months or less with
			assessment of bone density
			before repeating the course

Danazol
 	
or
 	
Gestrinone
	100–200 mg daily
	continuously. Consider
	400 mg if ovarian
	suppression required
	2.5 mg twice weekly
		1. Mastalgia
		2. Severe PMS with
		   predominantly physical
		   symptoms: coexisting
		   menorrhagia or
		   dysmenorrhoea
			Monitor bone density and lipids
			if used long term; beware
			androgenic side effects
			For mastalgia, can be used in
			luteal phase only

Oestrogen alone	25 μg oestradiol patch during symptoms (no more than 10 days per cycle, and only if ovulation confirmed Higher doses should not be used because of the risk of endometrial hyperplasia	Predominant oestrogen- deficiency-type symptoms; short duration symptoms; older women	
Progesterone alone: Cyclogest ® or Dydrogesterone	400 mg per vaginam or per rectum b.d. or t.d.s. in luteal phase only 10 mg b.d. in luteal phase	May be useful for predominantly anxiety/ aggressive PMS	Not proven in RCT Avoid 'androgenic' progestogens Cyclogest causes deterioration of latex rubber barriers
Continuous natural oestrogen and cyclical progestogen	100 μg transdermal oestradiol patch or gel with dydrogesterone, norethisterone or medroxyprogesterone for at least 7 days of cycle or longer every other month or LNG IUS	Moderate to severe PMS Predominantly physical symptoms or combined physical and psychological, coexisting medical problems	Cyclical progestin can activate PMS symptoms in 25–50% of cases
Synthetic oestrogen and progestogen	The combined oral contraceptive pill used continuously for 3–4 cycles followed by 7-day break (tricycling)	When contraception is required, if sufferer already on COCP but getting symptoms	No RCT evidence Usual contraindications to COC apply Variable response, may exacerbate symptoms
Prostaglandin synthetase inhibitors, e.g. mefenamic acid	250 mg q.d.s. in luteal phase	1. Headache 2. Fatigue 3. Dysmenorrhoea 4. Mood changes	Proven in RCT for limited number of symptoms
Selective serotonin reuptake inhibitors (fluoxetine, paroxetine)	20 mg daily throughout cycle (taken at night)	Moderate to severe PMS Predominant psychological symptoms Secondary PMS with underlying depression	Should be combined with psychotherapy Good tolerance, high efficacy in placebo-controlled trials (? first-line therapy)
Gammalinolenic acid (GLA) or GLA as Efamast®	100 mg once or twice daily 120–160 mg b.d. (POM)	Predominant mastalgia	Has not been shown to be useful in PMS in RCT Need to persevere for 3 months for therapeutic effect
Spironolactone	50–100 mg/day or less if effective Usually luteal phase only	Only if true fluid retention, i.e. increased weight premenstrually or if swelling of fingers/ankles	Monitor potassium

Table 26.3   *continued*

Table 26.3 *continued*

Treatment	Dose	Useful for	Notes
Benzodiazepines (alprazolam in literature)	Alprazolam 0.25 mg q.d.s. during luteal phase	Moderate PMS, predominant anxiety	Beware misuse and addiction; may be useful in short-term crises
Bromocriptine	5 mg/day	Mastalgia	Beware side effects
Propranolol	40 mg 1–3 times daily	Predominant migraine, headaches, anxiety	
Total abdominal hysterectomy and bilateral salpingo-oophorectomy		Severe intractable PMS	

RCT = randomized clinical trial; HRT = hormone replacement therapy; POM = prescription-only medicine; LNG-IUS = levonorgestrel-releasing intrauterine system; COCP = combined oral contraceptive pill.

found alternative therapies helpful (Box 26.2) and should not be discouraged from exploring relaxation techniques, aromatherapy, etc. There is, however, insufficient scientific evidence for the efficacy of alternative therapies.

Medical treatment

The medical treatment of PMS is detailed in Table 26.3. Figure 26.4 presents an algorithm for the management of PMS.

Fig. 26.4 An algorithm for the management of PMS. HRT = hormone replacement therapy; OEP = oil of evening primrose; COCP = combined oral contraceptive pill.

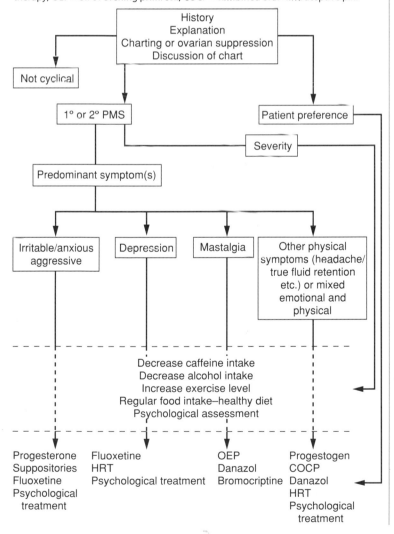

Conclusion

Although PMS is likely to remain a difficult problem to understand and manage, the recent increase in our understanding of its aetiology should allow the practitioner to approach it with less trepidation than in the past. Clear history taking and diagnosis, sympathetic explanation and logical treatments tailored to the patient's particular complaints will, in almost every case, result in some amelioration of her symptoms, and an improvement in her quality of life.

Tips for safe practice

- Diagnose by prospective daily charting.

- Provide empathy and support for all.

- Consider lifestyle measures initially.

- Use hormonal therapies if acceptable and safe.

- Use symptomatic therapies if predominant symptom identified.

- Discuss concerns about teratogenicity of any non-contraceptive regimen.

Resource list

- UK National Association for Premenstrual Syndrome (publish booklets on PMS and a newsletter). NAPS – PO Box 72, Sevenoaks, Kent TN13 1XQ (Tel. 01732 741709)

- Womens' Nutritional Advisory Service, PO Box 268, Lewes, East Sussex, BN7 2QN, UK (Tel. 01273 487366)

- Women's Health Concern, PO Box 1629, London W8 6AU, UK (Tel. 0207-938 3932)

- British Association for Counselling, 1 Regent Place, Rubgy, Warwicks CV21 2PJ, UK (Tel. 01788 578328)

- The Institute of Complementary Medicine, PO Box 194, London SE16 1QZ, UK (Tel. 0207 237 5165)

References

1. Frank RT. The hormonal causes of premenstrual tension. *Arch Neurol Psychiatr* 1931;26:1053–7.

2. Hamilton JA, Parry BA, Alagna S, Blumenthal S, Herz E. Premenstrual mood changes: a guide to evaluation and treatment. *Psychiatr Ann* 1984;14:406–20.

3. Dalton K. The premenstrual syndrome and progesterone therapy. London: William Heinemann, 1984.

4. Finak G, Sumner BE, Rosie R, Grace O, Quinn JP. Oestrogen control of central neurotransmission: effect on mood, mental state and memory. *Cell Mol Neurobiol* 1996;16:325–44.

5. Chuong CJ, Pearsall-Otey LR, Rosenfeld BL. Revising treatments for premenstrual syndrome. *Contemp Obstet Gynecol* 1994;Jan:66–76.

6. Rapkin AJ, Edelmuth E, Chang LC, Reading AE, McGuire MT, Su TP. Whole blood serotonin in premenstrual syndrome. *Am J Obstet Gynecol* 1987;70:533–7.

7. Taylor DL, Matthew RW, Ho BT, Weinman ML. Serotonin levels and platelet uptake during premenstrual tension. *Neuropsychobiology* 1984;12:16–18.

8. Dinan TG, O'Keane V. The premenstrual syndrome: a psychoneuroendocrine perspective. *Bailliere's Clin Endocrinol Metab* 1991;51:143–65.

9. Mortola JF. Assessment and management of premenstrual syndrome. *Curr Opin Obstet Gynaecol* 1992;4:877–85.

10. Wood SH, Mortola JF, Chan Y, Moossazadeh F, Yen SSC. Treatment of premenstrual syndrome with fluoxetine: a double blind, placebo-controlled crossover study. *Obstet Gynecol* 1992;80:339–44.

11. Stone AB, Pearlstein TB, Brown WA. Fluoxetine in the treatment of premenstrual syndrome. *Psychopharmacol Bull* 1991; 26:331–35.

12. Brzezinski AA, Wurtman JJ, Wurtman RJ, Gleason R, Greenfield J, Nadar T. D-Fenfluramine suppresses the increased calorie and carbohydrate intakes and improves the mood of women with premenstrual depression. *Obstet Gynecol* 1990;76:296–301.

13. Cohen MR, Cohen RM, Pickar D, Weingartner H, Murphy DL, Bunney WE. Behavioural effects after high dose naloxone administration to normal volunteers. *Lancet* 1981;2:1110.

14. Chihal HJ. Premenstrual syndrome: an update for the clinician. *Obstet Gynecol Clin North Am* 1990;17:457–79.

15. Chuong CJ, Coulam CB, Kao PC, Bergstalh EJ, Go VLW. Neuropeptide levels in premenstrual syndrome. *Fertil Steril* 1985;44:760–5.

16. Brush MG, Watson SJ, Horrobin DF, Manku MS. Abnormal essential fatty acid levels in plasma of women with premenstrual syndrome. *Am J Obstet Gynecol* 1984;10:363–6.

17. O'Brien PMS, Massil H. Premenstrual syndrome: clinical studies on essential fatty acids. In: Omega-6 essential fatty acids: pathophysiology and roles in clinical medicine. New York: Alan R Liss, Inc., 1990;523–45.

18. Pye JK, Mansel RE, Hughes LE. Clinical experience of the drug treatments for mastalgia. *Lancet* 1985;ii:373–7.

19. Ussher JM. Research and theory related to female reproduction: implications for clinical psychology. *Br J Clin Psychol* 1992;31:129–51.

20. Budieri DJ, Li Wan Po A, Dornan JC. Clinical trials of treatments of premenstrual syndrome: entry criteria and scales for measuring treatment outcomes. *Br J Obstet Gynaecol* 1994;101:689–95.

21. Muse K, Cetal N, Futterman L, Yen S. Premenstrual syndrome, effect of 'medical ovariectomy'. *N Engl J Med* 1984;311:1345–9.

The perimenopause, including disorders of menstruation, contraception and screening strategies

Margaret Rees MA DPhil MRCOG

Definition

Reproductive ageing is characterized by deterioration in ovarian function resulting in changes in menstrual pattern and reduction in fertility, culminating in the menopause: the last menstrual period. Overall the mean age of menopause is 51 years, but it occurs up to 2 years earlier in smokers than in non-smokers [1, 2]. A premature menopause is one that occurs before the age of 40, though many authorities would give the age as 45. The menopause can occur as early as 23. Premature menopause increases the risk of cardiovascular disease and osteoporosis [3] (Chapter 28). While it may occur naturally, premature menopause can follow surgery or radiation and chemotherapy. Surgical menopause occurs after bilateral oophorectomy. It can also occur after hysterectomy, even if the ovaries are conserved, when the age of menopause is advanced by about 4 years [4]. Radiation and chemotherapy when used to treat malignancy, e.g. Hodgkin's disease, can compromise ovarian function and induce the menopause.

Various definitions are used to describe the menopause, these are [2,5]:

1. The menopause is the permanent cessation of menstruation resulting from loss of ovarian follicular activity
2. The menopause transition includes the period immediately prior to the menopause with endocrinological, biological and clinical features of the approaching menopause. The length of this transition has been reported to be 4 years (onset of perimenopause 47.5 years) and to be shorter in smokers [2]. Furthermore, 10% of women in this study were found not to experience the transition, but to cease menstruation abruptly.
3. The postmenopause should be defined as dating from the menopause, although it cannot be determined until after a period of 12 months of spontaneous amenorrhoea has been observed.

Changes in ovarian function

The menopause is caused by ovarian failure. The ovary has a finite endowment of germ cells with maximal numbers at 20 weeks of intrauterine life. From mid-gestation onwards, there is a logarithmic reduction in germ cells until some 50 years later, when the oocyte reserve is exhausted. This results in a fall in oestrogen production and an increase in gonadotrophin levels. The ovary gradually becomes less responsive to gonadotrophins several years before menses cease. Thus there is a gradual increase in circulating levels of follicle-stimulating hormone (FSH) and later luteinizing hormone (LH), and a decrease in oestradiol and inhibin levels. A progressive increase of FSH levels has been documented from the age of 27 years, with wide ranges of values in population-based samples [5–7]. FSH levels fluctuate markedly from premenopausal to postmenopausal values virtually on a daily basis. These changes in circulating hormone levels frequently occur in the face of ovulatory menstrual cycles. As ovarian unresponsiveness becomes more marked, cycles tend to become anovulatory. Complete failure of follicular development eventually occurs and oestradiol production is no longer sufficient to stimulate the endometrium, amenorrhoea ensues and FSH and LH levels are persistently elevated.

Symptoms – the climacteric syndrome

Menstrual disruption

The pattern of menstrual cycle changes was best documented in the study by Treloar et al. of 2700 women [8]. Perimenopausal endocrine changes result in changes in menstrual cycle length, which are almost a mirror of those found in the immediate postmenarcheal years. Initially, the length of the menstrual cycle shortens from about 28 days to 21–24 days. This is mainly due to a reduction in the follicular phase. As anovulatory cycles predominate, cycle length can vary enormously with up to several months of amenorrhoea. The amount of menstrual blood loss changes at the perimenopause, tending to increase slightly. This is probably related to the increased likelihood of anovulation.

Hot flushes and sweats

Hot flushes and sweats are episodes of inappropriate heat loss which occur in about 40% of perimenopausal women [9]. The frequency of flushes varies within and between individual women from a few per week to several per hour. The pathophysiology of flushes is unclear. The occurrence is not related to absolute plasma oestradiol levels but their onset may be related to decreases in these levels. The sympathetic nervous system control of skin blood flow is impaired in women with menopausal flushes in that reflex vasoconstriction to cold stimulus cannot be elicited [10].

Psychosocial

A cluster of symptoms including nervousness, anxiety, irritability, depression, forgetfulness and difficulty in concentration have been associated with the menopause, and are described in perimenopausal women. The proportion of women with psychological complaints is uncertain and estimates vary between 25% and 50%. There appear to be cultural differences in attitudes towards the menopause; for example, menopausal complaints are fewer in Japanese women than in North American women [9]. The underlying reasons are unclear. Estrogen replacement therapy (ERT) is not a universal panacea for these symptoms, especially as factors such as lifestyle changes may also be involved.

Urinary and vaginal symptoms (see Chapter 28)

Gynaecological problems

The following gynaecological problems are encountered in women over 40 years old:

- climacteric symptoms;
- menorrhagia;
- premenstrual syndrome (PMS) (see Chapter 26);
- pelvic pain/dysmenorrhoea/dyspareunia;
- endometriosis;
- fibroids;
- endometrial cancer;
- ovarian cysts/cancer;
- contraceptive decisions/problems.

Menorrhagia

A menstrual blood loss (MBL) of over 80 ml per menses defines objective menorrhagia. Menorrhagia is a common perimenopausal complaint [11] presenting alone or with PMS, dysmenorrhoea or other symptoms of note. A total of 30% of women complain of menorrhagia and 5% consult their primary care physician. The postulated causes of menorrhagia are listed in Box 27.1. Few have been evaluated with objective measurement of menstrual blood loss. While various pathologies have been implicated in menorrhagia, in 50% of cases no pathology is found at hysterectomy. The commonest pathologies in the perimenopause are leiomyomas or endometrial polyps. However, it must also be

---

Box 27.1   Causes of menorrhagia

- Pelvic pathology, e.g. fibroids, adenomyosis, polyps, endometrial cancer
- Systemic disease, e.g. hypothyroidism
- Intrauterine contraceptive devices (IUDs)
- Dysfunctional uterine bleeding – defined as menorrhagia in the absence of anatomical conditions or pelvic pathology; it accounts for 50% of menorrhagia. Disorders of prostaglandin activity (such as excess production of prostacyclin and prostaglandin E_2) and local fibrinolysis are believed to be responsible in some cases
- Personal risk factors contribute in some women, e.g. genetics

noted that the incidence of endometrial hyperplasia and carcinoma increases over the age of 40. Box 27.2 outlines the management of menorrhagia.

Initial management involves pelvic examination and consideration of endometrial biopsy. It should certainly be performed if there is intermenstrual bleeding. The use of dilatation and curettage (D&C) has been seriously questioned since it is not a procedure without risk, has no therapeutic value and its diagnostic potential has been superseded by hysteroscopy; it is inappropriate for women under 40 years. It is therefore being replaced by outpatient biopsy techniques using various endometrial samplers (Pipelle de Cornier, Vabra, Endocell). A biopsy is unlikely to disturb an IUD *in situ*. Endometrial sampling using 'vacuum techniques' is considered to be a reliable way of identifying endometrial carcinoma because malignant tissue is friable. Comparative studies of D&C and aspiration techniques show that they are equally accurate. Techniques that aim at cytological diagnosis of endometrial disease are not recommended. Although endometrial biopsy allows the exclusion of endometrial cancer and hyperplasia, it is inferior to hysteroscopy in detecting endometrial polyps. Hysteroscopy allows direct visualization of the endometrial cavity. Vaginal ultrasound measures endometrial thickness but does not provide a histological diagnosis: it therefore complements endometrial biopsy. Endometrial assessment is difficult in women who have had a previous endometrial resection or ablation.

Treatment is either medical or surgical.

Drug therapy

The first-line treatment in the absence of pelvic pathology should be medical [12,13]. Medical treatments for menorrhagia can be divided into two main classes: non-hormonal and hormonal (Boxes 27.3 and 27.4).

Low-dose progestogens are ineffective for ovulatory menorrhagia, but reduce MBL in high dose. Intrauterine

---

Box 27.2   Management of menorrhagia

- Document duration and frequency of menses with menstrual chart
- Exclude pelvic pathology
- Exclude and correct anaemia
- Consider endometrial biopsy in > 40 years of age or if intermenstrual bleeding
- Ultrasound, if organic cause suspected
- Hysteroscopy if endometrial polyp suspected, or if intermenstrual bleeding < 40 years of age or symptoms persist in spite of medical treatment and having had a negative endometrial biopsy. At hysteroscopy, polyps and submucous fibroids can be dealt with. Hysteroscopy can be done in the 'office' with or without local anaesthetic
- Reassure/treat medically if no pathology found
- Discuss contraception
- Sex hormone assays are of no value

Box 27.3   Non-hormonal treatments for menorrhagia

Prostaglandin synthetase inhibitors

- Mefenamic acid (500 mg 6–8 hourly)
- Meclofenamic acid
- Naproxen (500 mg 8–12 hourly)
- Ibuprofen
- Flurbiprofen
- Diclofenac
- Prostaglandins synthetase inhibitors will deal with dysmenorrhoea. They are considered by many to be first-line treatment.

Antifibrinolytics

These counteract the fibrinolytic activity in the endometrium.

- Tranexamic acid (1 g 6 hourly until bleeding stops)

Used as first-line therapy in Scandinavia; preferred option if patient anaemic. Now licensed in UK without time limitation for use. Use with caution with a history of thromboembolism.

- Ethamsylate

250 mg b.d. until bleeding stops. Conflicting evidence about efficacy.

Non-hormonal treatment is taken during menstruation itself and is suitable for long-term therapy. For prostaglandin synthetase inhibitors, the percentage reduction in blood loss varies from 25% to 47% depending on the agent and the dose used. Tranexamic acid reduces blood loss by about 50%. The data regarding the efficacy of ethamsylate are conflicting. Recently, a randomized controlled trial of ethamsylate, mefenamic acid and tranexamic acid during menses showed no effect for ethamsylate, 20% reduction with mefenamic acid and 54% reduction with tranexamic acid [14].

Box 27.4 Hormonal treatments for menorrhagia (especially suitable for anovulatory bleeding)

Low dose oral progestogens

Least effective therapies for menorrhagia effecting only 20% reduction in MBL when used cyclically

- Norethisterone/norethindrone
- Medroxyprogesterone acetate
- Dydrogesterone

Low-dose luteal progestogens are of little use; higher dose regimens more effective.

Intrauterine progestogens

- Levonorgestrel IUS – a licence for treatment of menorrhagia is anticipated in UK in 1999/2000

Combined oestrogens/progestogens

- Hormone replacement therapy
- Combined oral contraceptive pill – 45% decrease in MBL, is a contraceptive and reduces dysmenorrhoea. 'Tricycling' reduces the numbers of bleeds per year, and protects against ovarian and endometrial cancer. Preferred option for younger women also requiring contraception, and for older women who have no arterial disease risks and do not smoke.

Other

- Danazol (200 mg o.d.) – an antioestrogen, mild androgen and a supressant of pituitary gonadotrophins
- Gestrinone (2.5 mg twice weekly)
- GnRH analogues (see section on endometriosis)

Only suitable for short-term use unless specialist monitoring.

progesterone, or more especially levonorgestrel is much more successful. With the levonorgestrel intrauterine system (IUS), reductions in MBL of 88% and 96% are found after 3 and 12 months, respectively. The levonorgestrel IUS also provides very effective contraception and can provide the progestogen component of hormone replacement therapy (HRT) regimen. Monthly cyclical oestrogen/progestogen hormone replacement therapy is also effective with measured withdrawal bleeds no heavier than normal periods [15]. Danazol, gestrinone or gonadotrophin–releasing hormone (GnRH) analogues are effective treatments but their side effects limit their use to 6 months.

Surgery

Surgical treatment may be necessary to deal with pelvic abnormalities and is also indicated when medical treatment has failed. The ultimate solution is hysterectomy. Recently, there has been increasing use of minimally invasive surgery options using laparoscopic or hysteroscopic approaches, which have the advantages of shorter hospital stay and recovery times. Endometrial destructive techniques include transcervical resection of the endometrium (TCRE), rollerball coagulation, the neodynium yttrium aluminium garnet (Nd.YAG) laser, radiofrequency-induced thermal endometrial ablation, microwaves and thermal balloons.

Endometrial ablative techniques result in amenorrhoea or oligomenorrhoea, but may also fail (in 20% of cases), requiring repeat surgery [12]. These procedures have the advantage of a shorter hospital stay and resumption of normal activities [12,13]. The woman should have completed her family but contraception must continue to be used. She will also need to continue with cervical smears. Treatment outcome/satisfaction rates are better in women over 40. Ablative techniques may be an option in managing unacceptable bleeding in HRT users.

Leiomyomata

Leiomyomata are detected in about 30% of perimenopausal women. While frequently asymptomatic, they may cause menorrhagia, pelvic pain or pressure symptoms. The management of women with uterine fibroids depends on size and associated symptoms. Small asymptomatic ones rarely require treatment. Women with leiomyomata and menorrhagia are usually treated by hysterectomy. The advent of new endoscopic techniques makes it possible to remove subserous and intramural leiomyomata by laparoscopy and submucous ones by hysteroscopy [17] (Box 27.5). There is considerable demand for an alternative to surgery in the management of fibroids. GnRH analogues are effective, but are limited to short-term use unless

Fibroids behave as oestrogen-dependent tumours; curative treatment is surgical. Medical treatment may moderate symptoms, reduce size before surgery or prevent further growth, while treatment is continued.

Medical options

- GnRH analogues – highly effective short-term (6 months) treatment, especially presurgery when fibroid is large
- Mifepristone – the antiprogesterone may have a role in reducing fibroid size presurgery
- Progestogens – unless used in high doses to induce amenorrhoea, progestogens are of doubtful effect (limited studies)
- Gestrinone – studies limited

Surgical options

Open surgery:
- Hysterectomy
- Myomectomy

Endoscopic surgery:
- Hysteroscopic resection of submucous fibroids
- Laparoscopic myomectomy – still being evaluated
- Laparoscopic myolysis – still experimental [16]

add-back therapy is used, and fibroid size will increase on stopping therapy. Alternatives are mifepristone, progestogens and gestrinone, but trial evidence is limited [18].

Endometriosis

Endometriosis can affect women at any time during their reproductive years. It is an important cause of pelvic pain which may occur premenstrually or postmenstrually, as well as during menstruation, as opposed to primary dysmenorrhoea, which is confined to menstruation. It can also cause deep dyspareunia. It has been associated with subfertility, but the mechanisms are poorly understood. The options are analgesics or ovarian suppression. It must be remembered that treatment is long term. Options for ovarian suppression are high-dose progestogens, Danazol, gestrinone or GnRH analogues,

which may be combined with add-back therapy to minimize adverse symptoms and effects on the skeleton. The use and type of surgery depend on the woman's fertility goals and the severity of disease. Table 27.1 discusses the indications for medical versus surgical management of endometriosis.

Fertility changes

Natural fecundity in women declines gradually after the age of 30, with an acceleration some

time between 35 and 40 years, reaching almost zero by 45 years [19]. The declining chance of pregnancy is further compounded by an exponential rise in the risk of spontaneous abortion, thereby reducing the probability of having a baby. Studies from *in vitro* fertilization (IVF) and egg donation programmes suggest that reduced oocyte quality is the major factor for both reduced fertility and increased miscarriage rates, with a less than 10% pregnancy rate over the age of 40. Concurrently, there is an increase in chromosome abnormalities which occurs exponentially and seems to be linked to acceleration in the rate of depletion of oocytes in the ovaries. The acceleration appears to happen when the complement of follicles remaining in each ovary has fallen to about 25 000, which occurs on average at age 37.

Contraception

The age-linked biological decline in fecundity has to be considered against the background of the serious implications of an unplanned pregnancy in this age group. Effective, acceptable contraception is therefore essential. Contraception should be

Table 27.1   Indications for medical versus surgical therapy for endometriosis

Presenting complaint	Medical therapy	Surgical therapy
Pain	• Mild to moderate disease + symptoms • Presurgery in severe disease	• Severe disease or failed medical therapy • Laparoscopic surgery preferred (excision/ablation/adhesiolysis) TAH/BSO is a last resort
Subfertility	• Limited scope after other causes of subfertility have been excluded, except for analgesia • Pre-assisted conception	• Laparoscopic excision/ablation of local disease • Division of adhesions

TAH/BSO = total abdominal hysterectomy and bilateral salpingo-oopherectomy.

used for at least 1 year after the menopause. In women who achieve menopause before age 50, contraception may be required for a longer period of time.

Approximately 50% of couples in this age group choose sterilization (about 50:50 for male and female). Sterilization has the advantage of no long-term sequelae. The high prevalence of divorce and second marriage in this age group should be kept in mind when counselling couples. Table 27.2 provides an overview of contraceptive choices in women over 40. Efficacy is assured as long as the chosen method is used correctly and consistently.

Clinical evaluation of the perimenopausal woman

Clinical evaluation involves taking a detailed medical and gynaecological history, which includes a family history principally to ascertain risk factors for breast cancer, cardiovascular disease and osteoporosis.

The best way of making the diagnosis of the perimenopause is from a detailed history. Recent onset of hot flushes and night sweats, vaginal dryness and infrequent menstruation in women aged over 40 is a classic

Table 27.2 Contraceptive options for women over 40 years

Method	Advantages	Disadvantages	Treatment for menopausal symptoms	Bone sparing?
COC	• Convenience • Regular 'menses' • Less menorrhagia • Protection against ovarian and endometrial cancer • Other non-contraceptive benefits • Unrelated to sexual intercourse	• As background risk of breast cancer and arterial disease are relatively high in this age group, the risk–benefit balance shifts away from COC • Not suitable for women who smoke or have arterial or venous disease risk factors • No protection against STIs • Masks menopause	Yes	Yes (based on a limited number of observational studies)
POP/implant	• No increased risk of arterial or venous disease or cancer • High efficacy (>99%) in this age group • Suitable alternatives if contraindications to oestrogen • Norplant an alternative to sterilization • Unrelated to sexual intercourse	• Irregular bleeding in some; amenorrhoea in about 10% • Prolonged amenorrhoea may reflect hypo-oestrogenaemia • 15–30% risk of functional ovarian cysts • No protection against STIs	In some women	No evidence
Injectables	• No increased risk of arterial or venous disease or cancer • High efficacy (>99%) • Suitable alternative if contraindications to oestrogen • Amenorrhoea in up to 70% • Unrelated to sexual intercourse	• Initial irregular bleeding in some • Prolonged amenorrhoea may reflect hypo-oestrogenaemia • No protection against STIs	No	No evidence
IUD	• Effective, convenient and safe • Allows use of HRT • Unrelated to sexual intercourse	• May increase MBL • Not ideal in women with fibroids • No protection against STIs	No	No
IUS	• Effective, convenient and safe • Reduces MBL • Would allow use of systemic oestrogen replacement • Unrelated to sexual intercourse • Alternative to sterilization	• No protection against STIs	No	No
Barriers	• Protection against STIs (particularly if new relationship) • HRT can be used in conjunction • Allows tests to diagnose the menopause • Effective and safe if already familiar with method	• May be difficult to use if not familiar with method • May affect sexual enjoyment	No	No

N.B. Age is not a restricting factor for the use of emergency hormonal or intrauterine contraception.
COC = combined oral contraceptive; STIs = sexually transmitted infections; POP = progestogen – only pill; IUD = intrauterine device;
IUS = intrauterine system; HRT = hormone replacement therapy; MBL = menstrual blood loss.

presentation. Laboratory investigation is not needed in such cases and may indeed be of minimal use because of the wide range of FSH levels found [7]. Thus a woman aged 46 with hot flushes should not be denied HRT on the basis of a normal FSH level. In this case, a therapeutic trial of HRT for 4–6 months is more helpful. However, it is prudent to perform serial FSH estimations in younger women when a diagnosis of premature menopause is suspected.

It must be noted that FSH is an unreliable indicator of potential fertility in individual women because of the wide range of levels found in perimenopausal women. Thus, a perimenopausal woman with an elevated FSH level cannot be told she is infertile and no longer needs contraception.

In hysterectomized women the parameter of amenorrhoea is absent and this can make it more difficult to diagnose ovarian failure. It is important to remember that ovarian function may be compromised in ovaries retained after hysterectomy [4]. The underlying mechanism is unknown. On average, it has been estimated that the age of menopause is brought forward by 4 years in hysterectomized women compared to non-hysterectomized women. Thus the onset of menopausal symptoms in young women after hysterectomy must not be ignored and the patient should not be dismissed as being too young.

Screening strategies

The most important screening strategy is to ensure that women with premature ovarian failure are detected in primary care. In non-hysterectomized women this can be undertaken at the time of cervical screening, but different strategies need to be employed for hysterectomized women. Mammography need not be undertaken routinely before starting HRT unless the woman is at high risk. Breast cancer screening programmes vary worldwide and in the UK mammography is offered every 3 years between the ages of 50 and 65. Breast cancer is a common malignancy affecting 1 in 9 women in the USA and 1 in 11 women in the UK. A woman's individual risk depends on a number of factors which include family history [20, 21]. Estimates of the number of women with a family history of breast cancer varies from 5% to 20% depending on the population surveyed. Many of these women will not have a family history that suggests the presence of a highly penetrant susceptibility gene; however, a small subset of such women will come from families with a striking incidence of breast and other cancers (e.g. ovarian) often associated with inherited gene mutations. In these families, susceptibility can be transmitted by either parent. The frequency of dominant breast-cancer-related mutations accounts for about 5% of breast cancers in the population. The discovery of BRCA1 and BRCA2 and the acknowledgement that additional breast cancer susceptibility genes must exist provide a molecular basis for counselling some high-risk women. However, this must only be undertaken in specialist centres because of the ethical and legal implications, as well as the liability deriving from testing or prediction inaccuracy; the consequence of this is that high-risk women may elect to have prophylactic mastectomies.

Similarly for ovarian cancer, family clustering has been noted for over a century. Many of these families also segregate for early-onset breast cancer (BRCA1 implicated) or other cancers [22]. The issue that a perimenopausal woman who has no fertility goals will address is the role of prophylactic oophorectomy. Again referral to a specialist centre is recommended (see Chapter 31).

Risks and benefits of hormone replacement therapy

In discussing treatment, the goals that the woman wishes to achieve must be established. She may wish no treatment, but simply wants to know that there is no pathology. The endpoints of HRT are symptom control, and reduction in the risk of cardiovascular disease and osteoporosis [23]. While vasomotor symptoms respond well to HRT, mood changes and lack of libido may not improve if there is another underlying cause. It must also be mentioned that there is an increasing body of evidence that HRT may delay the onset of Alzheimer's disease [24,25]. In Western societies, the major cause of death is cardiovascular disease where HRT has a major impact [26] (Table 27.3). A recent study of secondary prevention however has not shown a protective effect of HRT [27].

One of the commonest issues that women wish to discuss is

Table 27.3 Causes of death in women in England and Wales 1993–1994 (Mortality Statistics, HMSO, 1995)

Disease	Number of women
Ischaemic heart disease	66 922
Cerebrovascular disease	38 558
Breast cancer	13 026
Uterine cancer	1303
Ovarian cancer	3819
Osteoporosis	770

HRT and breast cancer. The disease is dependent on duration of exposure to oestradiol with early menarche and late menopause increasing the risk. Examination of meta-analyses is of more benefit than individual studies, which may suffer from bias [28, 29]. Oestrogen replacement therapy increases the risk of breast cancer by about 2% per annum. In North America and Europe the cumulative incidence of breast cancer between the ages of 50 and 70 in never-users of HRT is about 45 per 1000 women. The cumulative excess numbers of breast cancers diagnosed between these ages per 1000 women who begin HRT at age 50 and use it for 5, 10 and 15 years, respectively, are estimated to be 2 (95% CI 1–3), 6 (3–9) and 12 (5–20). Against this must be balanced the fact that HRT reduces mortality from cardiovascular disease by 50%. Furthermore, the prognosis of a woman who develops a breast tumour while taking HRT is improved compared to a non-HRT user. While it may be possible that the improved prognosis of tumours detected on HRT is due to increased surveillance, it may also be related to differences in the biology of these tumours.

It must be noted that most of the studies have examined oral unopposed estrogen replacement therapy (ERT) using conjugated equine oestrogens, although there have been a few with oestradiol-based oral compounds or combined HRT. To date there have been no studies with transdermal oestrogen. There does not seem to be any effect of the dose of HRT. With regard to combination oestrogen/progestogen HRT, which has to be given for endometrial protection, it appears that, overall, it neither increases nor reduces breast cancer risk compared to oestrogen alone.

Major risk factors for breast cancer are family history and benign breast disease, which shows evidence of proliferation with or without atypia. Overviews indicate no significant additional increased risk in women with a family history of breast cancer given HRT. In women with breast disease, there is again no increased risk, and one study of 3303 women followed up for 17 years showed a significantly reduced risk [30].

Premature menopause

Women with a premature menopause have increased mortality and are at increased risk of cardiovascular disease and osteoporosis [3]. They should be recommended to take HRT up to the average age of menopause, i.e. about 51 years. With regard to breast cancer risk, there is a paucity of data, but it would seem rather odd to consider a woman with an early menopause taking HRT as being any different from a woman with her own spontaneous ovarian cycles.

Treatment options (Box 27.6)

It must be emphasized that HRT is not contraceptive, and that contraception needs to be continued either using a barrier method or an IUD. This is especially important for women with early ovarian failure who may ovulate unpredictably many years after diagnosis. Use of the progestogen-only pill and HRT has not yet been examined in clinical trials.

HRT consists of natural oestrogens, combined with progestogens in non-hysterectomized women to prevent the development of endometrial carcinoma [31, 32].

Box 27.6 **Options for hormone replacement therapy (HRT) in perimenopausal women. These are indicated for symptoms in menstruating women or for osteoporosis prevention**

- Sequential combined HRT (including long-cycle HRT) with non-systemic contraception
- Oestrogen replacement and levonorgestrel-releasing intrauterine system
- Combined oral contraceptive pill if no contraindications
- HRT and progestogen-only pill (POP) (no data on contraceptive efficacy).

Progestogen must be given to women who have undergone endometrial ablative techniques, since it cannot be assumed that all the endometrium has been removed. Hysterectomized women can be given oestrogen alone. Different routes of administration are employed: oral, transdermal, subcutaneous and vaginal (see Chapter 28).

Preparations

The options available for perimenopausal women are monthly cyclic or 3-monthly cyclic regimens, and the number of prepacked oestrogen/progestogen combinations has markedly increased. Prepacked monthly therapies contain combinations of oestradiol valerate, micronized oestradiol or conjugated equine oestrogens; with levonorgestrel/norgestrel, norethisterone, dydrogesterone or medroxyprogesterone acetate. For women with infrequent menstruation or who are intolerant of progestogen, a 3-monthly preparation should be considered. One preparation containing oestradiol valerate and medroxyprogesterone acetate is available [33]. Continuous combined regimens should not be used in perimenopausal women because of the risk of irregular bleeding [34].

Intrauterine progestogen-releasing systems

The levonorgestrel-releasing IUS delivers intrauterine progestogen and can provide the progestogen component of HRT, whose oestrogen can then be given orally or transdermally [35]. It also provides a solution to the problem of contraception in the perimenopause. A principal mode of action is by rendering the endometrium atrophic. It is effective for 5 years. Timing its removal as 1 year after the last spontaneous menstrual period is difficult, as it renders women amenorrhoeic and therefore this parameter is impossible to ascertain. It is also the only way in which a 'no-bleed' regimen can be achieved in perimenopausal women.

Future developments

Several options are in development: use of third-generation gestagens in HRT, vaginal rings, and silastic implants [36]. Phytoestrogens, which are plant substance, that are structurally or functionally similar to oestradiol, may become the HRT of the 21st century, since these have the potential to improve menopausal symptoms, reduce cardiovascular disease, and prevent osteoporosis without having adverse effects on the breast or endometrium [37]. Populations whose diet is high in phyto-oestrogens, such as the Japanese, appear to have a lower incidence of menopausal symptoms, coronary heart disease and osteoporosis compared to their Western counterparts. Similarly, selective oestrogen receptor modulators, such as raloxifene and droloxifene, may be used [38]. These agents appear to have the same beneficial effects as oestrogen on the skeletal system without proliferative effects on the breast and endometrium but are currently licensed for postmenopausal use only.

Tips for safe practice

Safe practice in the management of the perimenopausal woman involves careful history taking and examination, with full discussion of the goals that can be achieved by a particular treatment, especially since women tend to take HRT for symptom control rather than for long term therapy [39,40]. Fertility issues must be addressed. Most importantly, the risk of pregnancy must be emphasized. Follow-up once HRT is started should be initially at 4 months to establish that it is successful; thereafter annual follow-up will suffice.

References

1. Morabia A, Costanza MC. International variability in ages at menarche, first live birth, and menopause. World Health Organisation Collaborative Study of Neoplasia and Steroid Contraceptives. *Am J Epidemiol* 1998;148:1195–1205.

2. McKinlay SM, Brambilla DJ, Posner JG. The normal menopause transition. *Maturitas* 1992;14:103–15.

3. van der Schouw YT, van der Graaf Y, Steyerberg EW, Eijkemans MJC, Banga JD. Age at menopause as a risk factor for cardiovascular mortality. *Lancet* 1996;347:714–8.

4. Siddle N, Sarrel P, Whitehead M. The effect of hysterectomy on the age at ovarian failure: identification of a subgroup of women with premature loss of ovarian function and literature review. *Fertil Steril* 1987;47:94–100.

5. Richardson SJ. The biological basis of the menopause. In:

Burger HG (ed.) The menopause. *Bailliere's Clin Endocrinol Metabol* 1993;7:1–16.

6. Ebbiary NA, Lenton EA, Cooke ID. Hypothalamic–pituitary ageing: progressive increase in FSH and LH concentrations throughout the reproductive life in regularly menstruating women. *Clin Endocrinol* 1994;41:199–206.

7. Burger HG, Dudley EC, Hopper JL, et al. The endocrinology of the menopause transition: a cross-sectional study of a population based sample. *J Clin Endocrinol Metab* 1995;80: 3537–45.

8. Treloar AE, Boynton RE, Behn BG, Brown BW. Variation of the human menstrual cycle through reproductive life. *Int J Fertil* 1967;12,77–126.

9. Avis PE, Kaufert PA, Lock M, Mckinlay SM, Vass K. The evolution of menopausal symptoms. In: Burger HG (ed.) The menopause. *Balliere's Clin Endocrinol Metabol* 1993;7:17–32.

10. Rees MAP and Barlow DH. Absence of sustained reflex vasoconstriction in women with menopausal flushes. *Hum Reprod* 1988;3,823–5.

11. Rees M. Medical management of menorrhagia. In: Cameron IT, Fraser IS, Smith SK (eds) Clinical disorders of the menstrual cycle. Oxford: Oxford University Press, 1998;155–66.

12. Coulter A, Kelland J, Long A, et al. The management of menorrhagia. In: Effective Health Care Bulletin, no. 9. Halifax: Stott Bros, 1995.

13. Rees M. Menstrual problems. In: McPherson A, Waller D (eds) Women's problems in general practice. Oxford: Oxford University Press, 1997:304–42.

14. Bonnar J, Sheppard BL. Treatment of menorrhagia during menstruation: randomised controlled trial of ethamsylate, mefenamic acid and tranexamic acid. *Br Med J* 1996;313:579–82.

15. Rees MCP, Barlow DH. Quantition of hormone replacement induced withdrawal bleeds. *Br J Obstet Gynaecol*; 1991;98,106–7.

16. Overton C, Hargreaves J and Maresh M. A national survey of the complications of endometrial destruction for menstrual disorders: the Mistletoe study. *Br J Obstet Gynaecol* 1997;104,1351–9.

17. Jourdain O, Descamps P, Abusada N, et al. Treatment of Fibromas. *Eur J Obstet Gynecol Reprod Biol* 1996;66, 99–107.

18. Vollenhoven BJ, Healy DL. Pathophysiology and medical treatment of uterine fibroids. In: Cameron IT, Fraser IS, Smith SK (eds) Clinical disorders of the endometrium and the menstrual cycle. Oxford: Oxford University Press, 1998:207–18.

19. Hull MRG. Female age and fecundity. In: Hedon B, Bringer J, Mares P (eds) Fertility and sterility – a current overview. New York: Parthenon Publishing Group, 1995:181–6.

20. Hoskins KF, Stopfer JE, Calzone KA, et al. Assessment and counselling for wonen with a family history of breast cancer. *JAMA* 1995;273:577–85.

21. Lucassen A. Genetic screening for breast cancer? *J Br Meno Soc* 1997;3(4):20–24.

22. Easton DF, Ford D, Matthews PE, Peto J. The genetic epidemiology of ovarian cancer. In: Sharp F, Mason P, Blackett T, Berek J (eds) Ovarian cancer, Vol. 3. London: Chapman and Hall, 1945:3–12.

23. Barrett-Connor E. Hormone replacement threapy. *Brit Med J* 1998;317:457–61.

24. Paganini-Hill and Henderson VW. Estrogen deficiency and risk of Alzheimer's disease in women. *Am J Epidemiol* 1994;140,256–61.

25. Honjo H, Iwasa K, Urabe M. Clinical studies of oestrogen threapy for dementia. *J Br Meno Soc* 1998;4:12–17.

26. Grodstein F, Stampfer J, Manson JE et al. Postmenopausal estrogen use and the risk of cardiovascular disease. *N Engl J Med* 1996; 335:453–61.

27. Hulley S, Grady D, Bush T, et al. Randomized trial of estrogen plus progestin for secondary prevention of coronary heart disease in postmenopausal women. Heart and Estrogen/progestin Replacement Study (HERS) Research Group. *JAMA* 1998;280:605–13.

28. Howell A, Baildam A, Bundred N, et al. 'Should I take HRT doctor?' Hormone replacement therapy in women at increased risk of breast cancer and in survivors of the disease. *J Br Med Men Soc* 1995;1:9–18.

29. Collaborative Group on Hormonal Factors in Breast Cancer. Breast cancer and hormone replacement therapy: collaborative reanalysis of data from 51 epidemiological studies of 52,705 women with breast cancer and 108,411 women without breast cancer. *Lancet* 1997;350:1047–52.

30. Dupont WD, Page DL, Rogers LW, et al. Influence of exogenous oestrogens, proliferative breast disease and other variables on breast cancer risk. *Cancer* 1989;63:948–957.

31. Woodruff JD, Pickar, JH for the Menopause Study Group. Incidence of endometrial hyperplasia in postmenopausal women taking conjugated oestrogens (Premarin) with medroxyprogesterone acetate or conjugated oestrogens alone. *Am J Obstet Gynecol* 1994;170:1213–23.

32. Rees M. The menopause and the uterus. In: Barlow DH, (ed.) The menopause, Vol. 10. London: Bailliere Tindall, 1996;419–32.

33. Hirvonen E, Salmi T, Puolakk J, et al. Can progestin be limited to every third month only in postmenopausal women taking oestrogen? *Maturitas* 1995; **21**, 39–44.

34. Uldoff L, Lngenberg P, Adashi Ey. Continuous combined hormone replacement therapy: a critical review. *Obstet Gynecol* 1995;86:306–16.

35. Andersson K, Mattson L-A, Rybo G and Stadberg G. Intrauterine release of levonorgestrel – a new way of adding progestogen in hormone replacement therapy. *Obstet Gynecol* 1992; **79**,963–7.

36. Suhonen SP, AllonenHO and Lahtenmaki P. Sustained release oestradiol implants and a levonorgestrel releasing intrauterine device in hormone replacement therapy. *Am J Obstet Gynecol* 1995;172,562–7.

37. Makey R, Eden J. Phyto-oestrogens. *J Br Menopause Soc* 1998;4:18–23.

38. Beardsworth SA, Purdie DW. Selective oestrogen receptor modulators. *J Br Menopause Soc* 1998;4:30–2.

39. Buist DS, LaCroix AZ, Newton KM, Keenan NL. Are long-term hormone replacement therapy users different from short-term and never users? *Am J Epidemiol* 1999; 149:275–81.

40. Andersson K, Pedersen AT, Mattsson LA, Milsom I. Swedish gynecologists' and general practitioners' views on the climacteric period: knowledge, attitudes and management strategies. *Acta Obstet Gynecol Scand* 1998; 77:909–16.

Management of the menopause

R Don Gambrell Jr MD FACOG

Introduction

After the menopause, the average woman still has one-third of her life span ahead. However, women's experiences of the menopause and its effects on their remaining years vary widely. The declining ovarian function can be rapid for some and slower for others. Some women may produce sufficient endogenous estrogens to remain asymptomatic, but others develop a variety of disturbances during the climacteric – a term in current use for the pre-menopausal, menopausal and postmenopausal period. Postmenopause is defined as 1 year without menstrual periods. A surgical menopause occurs when the ovaries must be removed while still functioning during the reproductive years. Menopause symptoms may include:

- hot flushes (or flashes)/palpitations;

- night sweats;

- headaches;

- vaginal irritation or dryness;

- insomnia;

- depression, irritability, inability to cope;

- poor concentration and poor memory.

More serious consequences of long-term estrogen deficiency include:

- osteoporosis;

- atherosclerotic heart disease/vascular disease;

- urogenital atrophy;

- Alzheimer's disease.

Pathophysiology of the menopause

As a woman approaches the menopause, a number of biologic changes take place. The number of oocytes declines progressively from several million before birth to critically low levels by the time of menopause. Primordial follicles become less responsive to follicle-stimulating hormone (FSH) and produce less estrogen, thereby accentuating the negative feedback to the pituitary. Menstrual cycles become irregular as FSH levels increase and ovarian steroids decrease. At birth, the number of oocytes is 1–2 million but this number falls to 400 000 at menarche. By the menopause, there are only a few hundred oocytes. This accounts for declining estrogen levels.

The age of menopause varies from the mid-40s to the mid-50s. In our studies of over 2000 women undergoing a natural menopause, the mean age was 49.1 years (Figure 28.1) [1]. Globally, the mean age of menopause is 51. Postmenopausally, serum FSH and luteining hormone (LH) values are markedly elevated with FSH in the range of 75–200

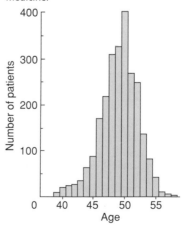

Fig. 28.1 The age of menopause in over 2000 women undergoing natural menopause (mean age = 49.1 years). Reproduced from Gambrell RD. The menopause: benefits and risks of estrogen–progestogen replacement therapy. *Fertil Steril* 1982:156:457–474. with permission of the publisher, The American Society for Reproductive Medicine.

mIU/ml and LH in the range of 60–90 mIU/ml. Postmenopausal women produce little, if any, progesterone. This deficiency of progesterone may lead to improper shedding of the endometrium, so that continuous unopposed exposure to estrogen may lead to hyperplasia and even endometrial cancer.

A wide variety of symptoms and physical changes are associated with menopause. Some patients may experience only a cessation of menses; others experience severe reactions that are occasionally disabling. Several factors influence development of symptoms during the climacteric years. The most important factor is the degree of estrogen deficiency and the rate at which estrogen levels decline. Very severe symptoms may occur with a surgical menopause because of the abrupt loss of circulating estrogens. Another factor may be the psychologic impact of aging and the women's ability to accept or deny the emotional changes of the menopause.

Consequences of the menopause

Osteoporosis

Estrogen deficiency contributes to the development of osteoporosis, a skeletal disorder primarily affecting trabecular bone, in which a reduction in the quality of bone predisposes to vertebral fractures. However, we are learning that estrogen deficiency is also related to type II, or age-related osteoporosis, affecting cortical bone which predisposes to hip fracture. As women become estrogen deficient, there is an increase in the frequency

with which new bone remodeling sites are activated [2]. As a result, the volume of bone undergoing remodeling at any time point is increased. Consequently, there is a net reduction in the mass of the skeleton and the balance between resorption and formation at each remodeling site alters in such a way that more bone is removed than synthesized. Calcium balance studies before and after menopause demonstrate a decrease in calcium economy, with increased urinary calcium loss and decreased intestinal calcium absorption. This calcium drain is dependent upon estrogen withdrawal and is reversed primarily with estrogen intervention, but not simply by increasing nutritional calcium supply. Bone loss after cessation of ovarian function occurs at an average rate of 2–3% per year. Although both sexes lose bone mass with aging, it is rare for men to develop symptomatic osteoporosis before age 70, since testosterone declines slowly in men after age 50.

Osteoporosis is a major public health problem affecting 20 million older Americans, of whom 90% are postmenopausal women [3]. It has been estimated that there are 1 700 000 fractures each year at an annual public health cost in excess of $6 billion. Approximately 25% of White women over age 60 have spinal compression fractures and this number increases to 50% by age 75. The incidence of hip fracture doubles every 5 years after the age of 60, so that by the time women reach age 90, 40% of White women have sustained a hip fracture. With increasing longevity, a woman now has a life expectancy of 80.4 years, at which

age the already serious morbidity and mortality associated with osteoporosis is accentuated. A total of 20–34% of all patients with hip fracture die within 6 months. Other fractures also occur, including those of the wrist and long bones, secondary to relatively minor trauma, and may be the first presenting sign of osteoporosis.

Cardiovascular disease

Myocardial infarction rarely occurs in women prior to menopause. Consequently, it has been suggested that endogenous estrogens provide a protective effect against atherosclerosis. Young women who have had a bilateral oophorectomy (surgical menopause) demonstrate a higher incidence of coronary artery disease unless estrogen replacement is begun soon after the ovaries are removed. Both surgical and natural menopause appear to be associated with changes in blood lipid profiles, development of atherosclerosis, increased hypertension and higher incidence of coronary artery disease. An increase in total cholesterol and low-density lipoprotein (LDL) is associated with coronary artery disease, while high-density lipoprotein (HDL) seems to have some protective effect. Although total cholesterol and LDL cholesterol tend to rise after menopause, HDL cholesterol begins its decline 12–18 months prior to the last menstrual period [4].

Only 25–50% of the protective effect of estrogen upon cardiovascular disease is mediated through improved lipid patterns. Estrogen also has direct vascular effects such as:

- interaction with estrogen and progesterone receptors in vessel walls;
- improved vascular blood flow;
- dilation of coronary arteries;
- increased endothelial-derived relaxing factor (EDRF);
- reduced vascular resistance;
- increased velocity of blood flow;
- increased cardiac output;
- inhibition of atherosclerotic progression;
- decreased platelet adhesiveness;
- inhibition of coronary thrombosis;
- effects on prostacyclin and thromboxane metabolism;
- peripheral vasodilation.

Urogenital atrophy

Declining estrogen levels result in atrophy of the urogenital epithelium within 1–3 years of menopause leading to a thin and easily traumatized vaginal mucosa, shortening and lessening of distensibility of the vagina, decreased secretions, changes in pH levels and a decrease in vaginal blood flow. This may lead to symptoms such as irritation, burning, pruritis, leukorrhea, dyspareunia, loss of sexual interest and physical discomfort. To a lesser extent, the vulvar epithelium also becomes thin and may be irritated or become more prone to infection. The integrity of the lower urinary tract mucosa is dependent upon estrogens. Estrogen deficiency may

therefore result in irritative symptoms such as:

- dysuria/burning on urination;
- cystitis;
- urethral caruncles;
- non-gonococcal urethritis.

The effects of estrogen on stress incontinence have been studied. While estrogen may be an adjunct to other medical or surgical therapies, it is not effective on its own.

Alzheimer's disease

There is considerable evidence that estrogen has an effect on the central nervous system (CNS). In addition to the vascular changes associated with atherosclerosis, estrogen deficiency may contribute to the neuro-degenerative changes of the aging CNS and increase the incidence of senile dementia of the Alzheimer's type. The incidence of Alzheimer's disease increases more in women than in men after age 65 so that age-specific rates vary from 1.5 to 3 times that of men [5]. One of the many findings in Alzheimer's disease is a decrease in dendritic spines and a deficiency of the cholinesterase enzymes necessary to reconvert the neurotransmitters to acetylcholine. Studies in oophorectomized animals indicate that axonal and/or dendritic concentrations of cholinergic enzymes increased in estrogen-treated animals, while in controls the acetylcholinesterase reaction was essentially localized only to cell bodies [6]. These cholinergic nuclei in the brain are

involved in most memory functions and this population of cells undergoes the most pronounced degenerative changes seen in Alzheimer's disease.

Some but not all clinical studies have observed that estrogen therapy improves cognitive function. In a study of 65-year-old women, estrogen users had significantly higher scores of short and long-term verbal memory tasks compared to women who had never used estrogen [7]. However, no differences were found between estrogen users and non-users in measures of visual/spatial memory. In a study of women with dementia, none of the 158 cases were currently using estrogens, whereas 15% of the matched controls were using estrogen [5]. The resulting relative risk (RR) of dementia in women taking estrogens was 0.7 ($P < 0.001$). The Leisure World studies observed a 30% reduction in Azheimer's disease in estrogen users [8].

Colon cancer

Sex steroid hormones modify hepatic cholesterol production and alter bile acid concentration. Increased concentrations of bile acids have long been thought to be important in human colon carcinogenesis. In animal studies, bile acids promote tumors. It has been suggested that exogenous estrogens and progestogens may reduce the secretion of bile acids [9]. Studies are now confirming that hormone replacement therapy, either estrogens alone or estrogen plus progestogen, significantly reduces the risk of colon cancer [10]. Overall, postmenopausal hormone use was associated with a 30% reduction in colon cancer for ever use and 46% for recent use.

In a recently published study of 422 373 postmenopausal women, the risk of colon cancer in estrogen users was reduced to RR = 0.71 (95% CI 0.61–0.83) [11]. With 11 or more years of estrogen use the RR = 0.54 (0.39–0.76) [11].

Criteria for diagnosis of menopause

The diagnosis of the menopause can be established based on symptoms, amenorrhea and, if required, confirmation of estrogen status by various parameters. Most women seek medical attention because of vasomotor symptoms manifested by hot flushes (flashes) or night sweats. Menstrual periods will at least be irregular or have ceased completely. Some patients may notice vaginal dryness or irritation, while a few will present with psychosomatic complaints. Late manifestations of postmenopause include osteoporosis and coronary artery disease. Confirmation of estrogen deficiency can be made with vaginal hormonal cytology, failure to respond to the progestogen challenge test (if uterus is intact) or an elevated serum FSH above 30 mIU/ml.

Physical findings

Atrophic vaginal mucosa will eventually be the principal physical finding in postmenopausal women; however, this may take 5–10 years to be manifest, and usually occurs after the onset of vasomotor and psychosomatic symptoms. The vaginal mucosa appears pale, is thinned and loses much of the rugae normally present throughout the reproductive years. Vaginitis is more frequent, evidenced by leukorrhea, but dryness may be the presenting finding. Urethral caruncles almost always indicate long-term estrogen deficiency. Even the vulvar skin may become thinned and lose some of its elasticity. Pubic hair may decrease due to decreased androgens associated with menopause.

Routine laboratory abnormalities

Estradiol and estrone levels fluctuate widely during the perimenopausal years and menopausal symptoms are almost always present before estradiol levels drop below the 50 pg/ml (100 pmol/l) diagnostic level. The most accurate laboratory test is the serum FSH and is diagnostic above 30 mIU/ml. During the reproductive years, serum FSH is 10 or below and begins to rise prior to menopause. HDL cholesterol declines 1–2 years prior to menopause while LDL cholesterol and total cholesterol may increase at menopause.

Vaginal hormonal cytology

The diagnosis of menopause can usually be made based on symptoms, physical findings and vaginal hormonal cytology. Papanicolaou smears usually report the cell-pattern reading. If they do not, a maturation index can be requested. This reports the percentage of superficial, intermediate and parabasal cells. High percentages of superficial and intermediate cells indicate normal endogenous estrogen production, while a predominance of parabasal cells predicts estrogen deficiency. If the patient has an intact uterus, cervical mucus can be examined for the presence or absence of the fern pattern. Ferning of the cervical mucus indicates normal estrogen levels; however, absence occurs after ovulation and during pregnancy, so a careful history must be taken.

Progestogen challenge test

Another good predictive test, if the patient still has her uterus and is not menstruating regularly, is the progestogen challenge test (PCT). This is performed by administering a progestogen, such as medroxyprogesterone acetate 10 mg or norethindrone acetate 5 mg for 5–13 days to the amenorrheic woman. If withdrawal bleeding occurs, this is predictive that normal endogenous estrogens are present. A negative response in the presence of menopausal symptoms diagnoses estrogen deficiency. Should vaginal hormonal cytology, cervical mucus testing and the progestogen challenge test not confirm the diagnosis of menopause, the best laboratory test is the serum FSH.

HRT regimens

Box 28.1 lists the indications for hormone replacement therapy.

Systemic regimens

Not all menopausal women need estrogen therapy, at least in the early postmenopausal years, since many produce sufficient endogenous estrogens through conversion of androgens in the subcutaneous fat and liver to remain asymptomatic. However, within this group are certain patients who may benefit from cyclic progestogen therapy to prevent endometrial hyperplasia (Table 28.1). If the patient has a positive response to the progestogen challenge test, manifested by withdrawal bleeding, after appropriate endometrial evaluation, the progestogen should be continued for 10–14 days each month or cycle for as long as withdrawal bleeding occurs (Table 28.2).

Patients with menopausal symptoms and without contraindications should be prescribed estrogens and cyclic progestogens. The cyclic sequential protocol is to give conjugated estrogens 0.625 mg or equivalent dosages of other estrogens (Table 28.3a), cyclically according to the calendar for the first 25 days of the month and the progestogen added during the last 13 days of estrogen therapy, from the 13th to the 25th days.

Continuous estrogen regimens are the norm in most centers. The regimen is to give estrogen continuously and add cyclical progestogen for 10–14 days of each month–cycle (continuous sequential). Estrogen–progestogen therapy for menopausal women with an intact uterus is not without consequence, since 97% experience withdrawal bleeding until age 60. Withdrawal bleeding from combination estrogen–progestogen therapy gradually declines from age 60 to age 65, at which time 60% continue with a bleeding response. Most women can accept these light 3–4-day menstrual periods, but for those who cannot, alternative methods are available (Tables 28.2b).

Several methods are available for treating menopausal symptoms and each has its advantages and disadvantages. Therapy should be individualized to fit each woman's need. The method preferred by the author for newly menopausal women with an intact uterus is the cyclic sequential method. This has the fewest side effects except for withdrawal bleeding. However, if

Table 28.1 Progestogens in hormone replacement therapy

Progestogen	Dosage available (mg)	Minimum effective dosage[a]
Medroxyprogesterone acetate	2.5, 5, 10	10 mg daily
Norethindrone acetate	5	2.5 mg daily
Norethindrone/norethisterone	1.0	1.0 mg daily
Megestrol acetate	20, 40	40 mg daily
Norgestrol	0.075	0.150 mg daily
Progesterone vaginal suppositories	25, 50	25 mg b.i.d.
Oral micronized progesterone	50, 100	300 mg in divided doses
Dydrogesterone[b]	10, 20	10–20 mg daily

Note: availability applies to USA.
[a]For prevention of endometrial hyperplasia with sequential HRT.
[b]Available in Europe.

Box 28.1   Indications for hormone replacement therapy (HRT)

Symptomatic women
- Postmenopause
- Menopause
- Perimenopause
- Premature menopause
- Post-hysterectomy

Prevention of osteoporosis
- Menopause and postmenopause
- Premature menopause
- Long-term steroid therapy
- Risk factors for osteoporosis

Prevention of arterial disease (coronary artery disease, cerebrovascular disease)
- Postmenopause and menopause
- ? risk factors
- ? personal history/syndrome X

Other indications – HRT may offer protection against the following, but ongoing research is awaited to confirm this further
- Alzheimer's disease
- Colorectal cancer
- Some rheumatic disorders
- Wrinkles
- Cataracts

Table 28.2a Methods of hormone administration

Regimen	Estrogen	Progestogen[a]
Progestogen only		13–25th/cycle
Cyclic sequential	1st–25th/month	13th–25th/month
Continuous sequential	Every day	1st–14th/month
Continuous combined	Every day	Every day
Cyclic combined	1st–25th/month	1st–25th/month

[a]Dose dependent.

women on this regimen have menopausal symptoms during the days off estrogen at the end of each month, the continuous sequential method should be used.

Some women object to resumption or continuation of menstruation, so the continuous combined and cyclic combined regimens have been devised to produce amenorrhea (Table 28.2a). With the continuous combined method, low dosages of estrogen such as 0.625 mg conjugated estrogens are given along with medroxyprogesterone acetate 2.5 mg every day for 365 days a year. For the first 4–6 months, spotting or breakthrough bleeding may occur, but by 6 months, 60–65% of women using continuous combined therapy become amenorrheic, rising to 80% at 12 months. Those who do not achieve amenorrhea will need to revert to one of the sequential combined methods. The continuous combined regimens are only advocated for women over 1 year postmenopause to minimize the chances of irregular bleeding.

After 2–3 years of amenorrhea with the continuous combined method, some women will start spotting or have breakthrough bleeding again; they must be investigated with pelvic ultrasound and/or endometrial biopsy. Until December 1992, all endometrial biopsies performed by this author on such cases showed atrophic endometrium. Another diagnostic tool is hysteroscopy, as some such women have endometrial pathology, especially polyps. These cases are difficult to manage in that increasing the dosage of progestogen to 5 mg, even 7.5 mg, rarely helps the breakthrough bleeding, so these patients usually need to change to one of the sequential regimens once endometrial pathology has been excluded.

Bleeding after a period of amenorrhea may also be due to endometrial carcinoma. There have been 73 reported cases [12–17] and the author is aware of 14 other cases, making a total of 87 cases of endometrial cancer with the continuous combined regimen. Although endometrial atrophy is the 'norm' with continuous combined therapy, sporadic cases of endometrial carcinoma do occur.

In the experience of the author, the cyclic combined regimen is clinically superior to continuous combined regimens, since 75% of patients will become amenorrheic by 4 months compared with 60–65% with the continuous combined method at 6 months. Low-dosage estrogen, along with the lower dosage of progestogen, is given by the calendar from the 1st to the 25th of each month (Table 28.2a). After a comparable amount of spotting during the first month of therapy, there is less breakthrough bleeding, usually only 1 or 2 days of spotting on the 25th or 26th of the month or both, which only occurs in 25% of women. Most patients can accept this minimal withdrawal bleeding when a full explanation and reassurance are

Table 28.2b 'No bleed' hormone replacement regimens[b]

Regimen	Preparation	Comment
Oral CCT	CEE + MPA	Compliance better with a single tablet
Transdermal CCT	E₂ + NET	Compliance enhanced as a single patch
Gonadomimetic	Tibolone	Less chance of bleeding in the early cycles No epidemiological data on cardioprotection
Unopposed estrogen	Any estrogen from Table 28.3	Annual endometrial biopsy and ultrasound mandatory
SERMs	Raloxifene	No protection against vasomotor symptoms
Systemic estrogen + LNG IUS	Any estrogen + LNG IUS	The only combination suitable for peri- and early menopausal women LNG IUS not yet licensed for this use

CCT = continuous combined therapy; CEE = conjugated equine estrogens;
MPA = medroxyprogesterone acetate; E₂ = estradiol; NET = norethisterone;
NETA = norethisterone acetate; SERMs = selective estrogen receptor modulators;
LNG = levonorgestrel; IUS = intrauterine system.
[b]Unless stated otherwise, these apply to use 1 year postmenopause.

Table 28.3a Currently recommended estrogens

Estrogen	Dosage available in USA (mg)	Minimum effective dosage[a]
Conjugated estrogens	0.3, 0.625[b], 0.9, 1.25[b], 2.5	0.625
Micronized	0.5, 1.0[b], 2.0[b]	2.0
Esterified estrogens	0.3, 0.625, 1.25[b], 2.5	0.625
Estropipate	0.625, 1.25[b], 2.5, 5.0	1.25
Transdermal estradiol	0.025, 0.05, 0.1	0.05
Estradiol valerate	1.0[b], 2.0[b]	2.0

[a]For bone protection.
[b]Available in Europe.

given. Whether the cyclic combined method will be more endometrially protective than the continuous combined regimen remains to be proven since there is only limited experience at this time. Most women will develop atrophic endometrium with continuous combined therapy but, for those who do not, interrupting the progestogen for a few days each month should allow shedding of any endometrium that has built up.

Estrogen vaginal preparations

Some estrogen vaginal creams are well absorbed through the vaginal mucosa so that good systemic levels are obtained as well as the local beneficial effects. Vaginal creams probably provide the quickest response and subsequent relief of symptoms of atrophic vaginitis, such as vaginal irritation, pruritus, vaginal dryness and dyspareunia.

One common course of treatment is to apply the estrogen vaginal cream (Table 28.3b) while starting oral estrogens simultaneously. After 2 weeks of dual therapy, the maintenance dosage of the vaginal cream can be reduced to three times weekly or can be entirely eliminated. However, some patients on oral estrogens may continue to require estrogen vaginal cream for maintenance of the vaginal mucosa. Also, some women may not respond adequately to oral estrogens alone, developing dryness or pruritus of the vagina. Instead of increasing the oral estrogen dosage, these women frequently benefit more from the addition of estrogen vaginal cream to the therapeutic regimen. That local estrogens are well absorbed through the vaginal mucosa and can produce endometrial effects was well demonstrated in the Wilford Hall studies in that two of the 31 endometrial cancers were observed in estrogen vaginal cream users (Table 28.4), although the risk was much lower than in the untreated population.

A vaginal ring containing 2 mg of estradiol has recently become available for treatment of atrophic vaginitis. There is little to no systemic absorption, so it is intended for local use only. One ring is effective for 90 days; there is improvement in vaginal mucosal epithelium after 12 weeks and the vaginal pH is restored to normal. Other estriol-based vaginal creams and pessaries also tend to have minimal systemic absorption. In Europe, estradiol vaginal tablets are available and fall into the same category.

Endometrial cancer

Unopposed estrogens have a role in the development of endometrial hyperplasia which may lead to adenocarcinoma. Numerous studies have shown that estrogen-only replacement therapy increases the risk of endometrial cancer from 5- to 8-fold [18–20]. This is primarily because of unopposed estrogen stimulation and incomplete shedding of the endometrium. Added progestogen for 10–14 days opposes proliferation and ensures more complete shedding of the endometrium. In fact, progestogen therapy can reverse 98.4% of endometrial hyperplasia to normal proliferative or secretory endometrium [21]. The protective action of progestogens on the endometrium is partly physical in that more cells and glands are shed, thus leaving behind fewer glands for continued proliferation. This is the perceived mechanism through which the cyclic combined regimen provides endometrial protection. Stopping the progestogen allows

Table 28.3b Estrogen vaginal creams and ring

Estrogen	Dose (mg/g)
Conjugated estrogens vaginal cream	0.625 mg
17β-Estradiol vaginal cream	0.1 mg
Estropipate vaginal cream	1.5 mg
Diethylstilbestrol vaginal cream	0.01%
Estradiol vaginal ring	2 mg total

Table 28.4 Incidence of endometrial cancer at Wilford Hall USAF Medical Center 1975–1983

Therapy group	Patient-years of observation	Patients with cancer	Incidence (per 100 000)
Estrogen–progestogen users	16 327	8	49.0
Unopposed estrogen users	2560	10	390.6
Estrogen vaginal cream (EVC) users	2716	2[a]	73.6
Progestogen or androgen users	1160	0	—
Untreated women	4480	11	245.5
Total	27 243	31	113.8

[a]Includes past users.
Modified from Gambrell RD Jr. Use of progestogen therapy. *Am J Obstet Gynecol* 1987;156:1304.

proliferating endometrium to be shed.

Many studies of sequential estrogen/progestogen therapy indicate that the risk of endometrial cancer is less than that for untreated postmenopausal women [21–27]. In the Wilford Hall USAF Medical Center studies [21], the incidence of endometrial cancer was significantly lower in the estrogen-progestogen users (49.0:100 000) when compared to both the unopposed estrogen users (390.6:100 000) and the untreated women (245.5:100 000) with $P <$ 0.005 (Table 28.4). Another study reported no endometrial cancers in 72 estrogen–progestogen users, but 11 cancers in 207 patients treated with unopposed estrogen [22]. In a double-blind study, no adenocarcinomas were diagnosed in the 84 patients using estrogen–progestogen for 10 years, but one endometrial cancer occurred in the 84 placebo users [23]. Studies from England have not uncovered any increased risk for endometrial malignancy in estrogen-treated postmenopausal women because they routinely add a progestogen [24,25]. However, a 15% endometrial hyperplasia rate was observed in the unopposed estrogen users before progestogens were added [24]. Even the epidemiologic studies find decreased risk with estrogen–progestogen use [26, 27].

Endometrial evaluation

Progestogen challenge test

The progestogen challenge test (PCT) was devised to identfy women at increased risk for endometrial cancer [28]. It is performed by prescribing a 13-day course of progestogen, either medroxyprogesterone acetate 10 mg or norethindrone acetate 2.5–5 mg. It should be considered in all postmenopausal women with an intact uterus, including those on unopposed estrogen therapy, women being evaluated for potential hormone replacement and asymptomatic postmenopausal women. If there is a positive response, as manifested by withdrawal bleeding, the endometrium may be sampled and the progestogen continued for 12–14 days each month–cycle. Ever increasing usage of the progestogen challenge test at Wilford Hall USAF Medical Center decreased the incidence of endometrial cancer from 257.3 per 100 000 women in 1975 down to 29.1 per 100 000 during 1983 [21].

Our original work with the

PCT has been confirmed by several other studies [29–34]. In a prospective study utilizing 100 mg of progesterone in oil given intramuscularly to 30 asymptomatic postmenopausal women, five had withdrawal bleeding with the PCT, and three of the five had either adenomatous or a typical adenomatous hyperplasia [29]. In the 25 subjects with no withdrawal bleeding, the endometrial histology was entirely normal, mostly atrophic or inactive endometrium.

Since tamoxifen can increase the risk of endometrial hyperplasia and possibly carcinoma, the PCT has been used to evaluate asymptomatic postmenopausal breast cancer patients receiving this hormone. In 60 tamoxifen-treated women given the PCT, there were three positive bleeding responses and all three had endometrial hyperplasia at endometrial biopsy. In the 57 non-responders, endometrial sampling was atrophic or hypoplastic. A study from Japan compared sonographic endometrial thickness to estradiol levels and response to the PCT [34]. In 44 patients with secondary amenorrhea, the endometrium was significantly thicker in the 32 women who had withdrawal bleeding (10.3 ± 1.3 mm) than in the 12 who did not bleed (5.0 ± 1.3 mm) from the PCT. The serum estradiol levels were significantly higher in the positive group (45.3 ± 19.4 pg/ml) than in the negative group (18.6 ± 8.0 pg/ml). Endometrial thickness of 6.0 mm or more predicted the occurrence of withdrawal bleeding from the PCT with an accuracy of 95.5%.

Endometrial biopsy

The traditional method for evaluating the endometrium in postmenopausal bleeding has been a diagnostic D&C. However, hospitalization for a D&C (even on an outpatient basis) has disadvantages, including the anesthetic risk, the additional expense and the delay in diagnosis. These problems can be avoided by a clinic or office endometrial biopsy, utilizing a small instrument such as the Pipelle endometrial suction sampler. The cavity may be sampled more than once if not much tissue is extracted. Frequently, the endometrial Pipelle can be utilized without a tenaculum or sounding the uterus. This process will yield as much information as a traditional D&C.

Although there is patient discomfort with this office procedure, it may be minimized with a gentle approach and a careful explanation of each step. Discomfort can also be reduced by placing 4% Xylocaine viscous on a small cotton-tipped applicator in the endocervical canal for 3–5 min. Paracervical blocks can also be performed; however, these may be more painful than the procedure itself. Other satisfactory endometrial evaluation methods include:

- Curity Isaacs endometrial cell sampler;
- Vabra aspirator;
- Milex endometrial cannula;
- Randall or Novak suction biopsy.

Some authorities feel that endometrial biopsies are desirable before beginning estrogen replacement therapy to assess the endometrium prior to treatment. Others restrict their use to those who respond by bleeding to the PCT. A practical point to note is that the postmenopausal cervix may be stenotic and difficult to sound or insert even a small instrument through. After the PCT if the patient bleeds and she comes in on the first or second day of withdrawal bleeding, this may dilate the cervix sufficiently to facilitate instrumentation.

Ultrasound of the endometrium

Pelvic anatomy can be more thoroughly evaluated with transvaginal sonography. Ovarian masses can be determined to be either cystic or solid, and their size measured. Intramural and subserous myomas may be detected. Endometrial evaluation is one of the most important uses of transvaginal ultrasound. In patients with postmenopausal bleeding, the vaginal probe can be used to delineate the endometrium and measure its thickness. For transvaginal ultrasonography, an empty bladder is preferred but not essential [35]. The endometrial cavity is normally seen as a bright line or stripe in the center of the uterus. It is recommended that the thickness of the endometrium be measured on a long axis image of the uterus rather than on an axial scan because of more reliable and reproducible plane sections. In postmenopausal patients, the normal unstimulated endometrium should be quite thin. The endometrium may be 2–3 mm thicker in women on hormone replacement. A linear

'pencil line' endometrium is uniformly associated with scant cellular material. An echogenic endometrium greater than 5 mm indicates the presence of tissue and would be an indication for hysteroscopy and/or biopsy [36].

Examination of the thickness of the endometrial stripe has been proposed as an adjunct in screening for endometrial cancer. The incidence of endometrial neoplasia is quite low in postmenopausal women when the endometrial stripe measures 3–5 mm, whereas a patient with a stripe greater than 10 mm has a 10–20% incidence of endometrial hyperplasia or neoplasia [37]. Ultrasound examination remains expensive and such costs prohibit its use in a screening study [38]. By separating the endometrial stripe with injection of some type of medium, such as saline hysterosonography, endometrial evaluation by transvaginal ultrasonography may be enhanced.

Hysteroscopy

With postmenopausal bleeding, uterine and cervical neoplasia must be excluded. D&C or an endometrial biopsy are likely to diagnose endometrial neoplasia. Hysteroscopy can serve as an adjunct to other diagnostic methods in patients in whom abnormal bleeding persists and endometrial biopsy is inadequate or suspicious. Atrophic endometrium, another common cause for postmenopausal bleeding, can easily be diagnosed on hysteroscopy [39]. Pale, thin and friable endometrial lining with an area of superficial bleeding can be seen throughout the cavity. The diagnosis of

submucous fibroids and
endometrial polyps, which may
be missed by endometrial biopsy
or even D&C, is best made by
hysteroscopy, along with ensuring
that no endometrial pathology is
missed [40].

Breast cancer

Risk factors (see Chapter 24)

Carcinoma of the breast is not
primarily a hormone disorder but
more related to family history, diet
and alcohol. The greatest risk
factor is age. Other factors
include:

- nulliparity;

- infertility;

- obesity;

- late age of first term birth;

- early menarche–late
  menopause.

Hormones or hormonal
imbalance may serve as cofactors,
predisposing factors or perhaps
promoting agents. Several studies
have shown an increased risk of
breast cancer with long-term
progesterone deficiency [41–44]
and with long-term HRT [45].
The latter study found a small
increased risk of breast cancer of
2.3% for each year of HRT use,
mirroring the risk accrued when
a woman has a late menopause
(i.e. stays premenopausal); the
latter risk is 2.8%. Use of HRT
over age 50 for 5, 10 and 20 years
produces an excess risk of breast
cancer of 2, 6 and 12 per 1000
women/year. The risk disappears
within 5 years of stopping HRT.
See Chapter 24 for additional
information on risk factors.

Results of epidemiologic studies

Figure 28.2 [46] illustrates the
more than 55 studies regarding
estrogen replacement and breast
cancer, including six meta-
analyses. The relative risk (RR)
for each study is shown in relation
to 1.0 (no risk) along with the 95%
confidence interval (CI) when
calculated or calculable. Most of
the risk estimates hover around
1.0, with almost as many studies
indicating non-significantly
decreased risk of breast cancer
from estrogen use as those
indicating a non-significantly
increased risk. When significantly
increased risk occurred, it was in
subgroups of estrogen users. No
study observed any significantly
increased risk of breast cancer in
its total patient population until
the recently widely publicized
Nurses' Health Study [47]. This
16-year questionnaire study
observed an overall RR of 1.32
(95% CI, 1.14–1.54). However,
there are some problems with this
study. Detection bias may be
present in that the estrogen users
had a 14% higher rate of screening
mammograms than non-users.
This study excluded *in situ* cancers
but, since 1988, *in situ* cancers
have been increasing while
invasive lesions have been
declining. Although the study
included most risk factors, such as
age, family history, type of
menopause, parity and age at first
term birth, it excluded two
important risk factors: alcohol use
(RR = 2.0) and body mass (RR =
1.5). Either one of these could
have accounted for the RR of
1.32 in the Nurses' Health Study.
In studies that showed
increased risk in subgroups, the
type of subgroup was different

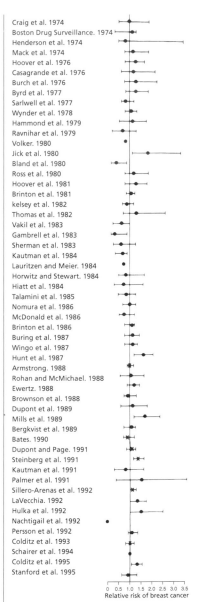

Fig. 28.2 Fifty-five studies of estrogen
therapy and breast cancer. Dots = risks;
horizontal lines = 95% confidence
intervals; X, meta-analysis. Reproduced
from Gambrell RD Jr. Hormone
replacement therapy and breast cancer
risk. *Arch Fam Med* 1996;5:34. with
permission. Copyright, The American
Medical Association.

across the studies with no
consistency observed. Conflicting
results have been reported in
estrogen users among similar
subgroups. While two studies
reported a significantly increased

risk of breast cancer in estrogen users undergoing a natural menopause, both of these observed either a non-significant decrease (RR = 0.8) or a non-significant increase (RR = 1.3) in estrogen users with a surgical menopause [48,49]. To the contrary, the study from the Centers for Disease Control observed non-significantly increased risk in estrogen users with a surgical menopause (RR = 1.3), while estrogen users undergoing a natural menopause had a non-significantly decreased risk (RR = 0.8) [50]. The most recent study observed no increased risk of breast cancer with any measure of estrogen use (RR = 0.9; 95% CI 0.7–1.3) [51].

Effects of progestogens

There is increasing evidence that added progestogen will significantly reduce the risk of breast cancer for some women. In the Wilford Hall USAF Medical Center studies, the incidence of breast cancer in the unopposed estrogen users (143.3: 100 000) was actually a little lower than that expected for this age group according to both the Third National Cancer Survey (188.3: 100 000) [52] and the National Cancer Institute (NCI) SEER data (273.9: 100 000) [53]. Table 28.5 indicates that the incidence of breast cancer in the oestrogen–progestogen users (66.8: 100 000) was significantly lower than that of the non-users (343.5: 100 000) and than that expected from both the Third National Cancer Survey and the NCI SEER data [21]. In the longest prospective and follow-up study to date, there were no breast cancers during 22

Table 28.5 Incidence of breast cancer at Wilford Hall USAF Medical Center 1975–1983

Therapy group	Patient-years of observation	Patients with cancer	Incidence (per 100 000)
Estrogen–progestogen users	16 466	11[a]	66.8
Unopposed estrogen users	19 676	28[a]	142.3
Estrogen vaginal cream users	4298	5[a]	116.3
Progestogen or androgen users	1825	3[a]	164.4
Non-users	6404	22	343.5
Total patients	48 669	69	141.8

[a]Includes past users.

years in the 116 estrogen–progestogen users, while six cancers developed in the 52 never-users, which was statistically significant with $P < 0.01$ [54]. In the 20-year prospective study from Germany, the incidence of breast cancer in the estrogen–progestogen users was 123.4:100 000, compared with 154.6:100 000 in the never-users, which was statistically significant with $P < 0.05$ [55].

Of the four epidemiologic studies of estrogen–progestogen use, one observed a 60% reduction after 8 years of added progestogen (RR = 0.4, 95% CI 0.2–1.0) [51] and the other three observed non-significant increased risks [47,56–58]. The Swedish study was based on only 10 patients with 6 years of hormone use (RR = 4.4; 95% CI 0.9–22.4) [56]. In a subsequent letter update in which the investigators added six more patients for a total of 16, and four more years of follow-up for a total of 10, the RR dropped from 4.4 to 1.3 [57]. The Danish study involved only 5 years of observation and the RR was 1.36 (95% CI 0.98–1.87) [58]. 'The Nurses' Health study did not show any decreased risk because only 18% of the estrogen users

were using progestogens by 1986, and this proportion rose to only 30% by 1990 [47].

Prognosis of breast cancer developing with estrogen replacement therapy

When women develop breast cancer while using estrogen replacement, they have a better survival rate. All but one of the nine studies that have looked at prognosis when breast cancer developed in estrogen users have observed a reduction in mortality of 16–44% (Table 28.6). Burch et al. in 1976 were the first to observe a 25% reduction in mortality when breast cancer developed in estrogen users [59]. In 1984, Gambrell reported a study with 2–8 years follow-up: the mortality was 22.2% in the 63 hormone users, compared with a death rate of 45.5% in the 165 non-users, which was statistically significant with $P < 0.005$ [60]. In a study of 4544 hormone users in England, the mortality from mammary malignancy was likewise reduced (RR = 0.76; 95% CI 0.45–1.06) [61].

In the study from Wilford Hall USAF Medical Center with 8–18 years of follow-up, life-table analysis revealed median survival

Table 28.6 Prognosis of breast cancer in estrogen users

Study	Patients with breast cancer	Relative risk	95% confidence interval (CI)/P value
Burch et al. (1976) [59]	33	0.75	—
Gambrell (1984) [60]	256	0.59	$P < 0.005$
Hunt et al. (1990) [61]	50	0.76	CI 0.45–1.06
Colditz et al. (1995) [47]	359	1.14	CI 0.85–1.51
Willis et al. (1996) [63]	1469	0.84	CI 0.75–0.94

times after diagnosis of breast cancer of 84 months for never-users, 80 months for past users, and more than 143 months for current users of estrogen ($P < 0.01$) [62]. Earlier diagnosis was one factor in the improved prognosis in estrogen users; however, there was an additional factor in that more of the current users had significantly higher positive progesterone receptors in their tumors (64.7%) than the non-users (34.8%) with $P < 0.05$. This has been a known protective factor. The Nurses' Health Study was the only study that failed to find improved prognosis (RR = 1.14; 95% CI 0.85–1.51) [47]. In the large American Cancer study of 422 373 women, there were 1469 breast cancer deaths during the 9 years of follow-up [63]. Fatal breast cancer was significantly reduced in the estrogen users (RR = 0.84; 95% CI 0.75–0.94).

Use of hormone replacement in breast cancer survivors

If estrogens do not increase the risk of mammary malignancy significantly, added progestogens may decrease the risk and survival is improved when the cancer develops in hormone users. Therefore, why cannot estrogens be given to breast cancer survivors? Breast cancer has always been considered a

contraindication, with the suspicion that estrogen therapy would hasten recurrences and increase mortality. However, there are no data to support this belief. Moreover, there are limited data to suggest that estrogen therapy is safe.

Several physicians, particularly gynecologic oncologists, have been advocating estrogen replacement therapy in women with previous breast cancer. Now the medical oncologists are joining in this recommendation [64]. A recent review concluded that the era of dogmatically denying estrogen replacement to women who previously had breast cancer is over, and recommended prospective trials to look at the benefits and risks of HRT in these women [65]. While awaiting definitive prospective study results which may take 10–20 years, we need to work with currently available data (Table 28.7). An Australian study showed no deaths and

significantly fewer recurrences in estrogen–progestogen users (7%) than controls (17%) (RR = 0.40; 95% CI 0.17–0.93) [66]. Surgeons from Southern California reported their experience with 25 women previously treated for breast cancer who subsequently received hormone replacement therapy for 24–82 months [67]. There were three recurrences and one death but the overall survival in this short-term study was 96%. In 77 breast cancer survivors given hormone replacement therapy by gynecologic oncologists for up to 15 years, there were seven recurrences and three deaths [68]. Therefore, HRT should be discussed with breast cancer survivors since the benefits appear to outweigh the risks; nevertheless, liaison with the attending breast oncologist is always a good idea.

Benign breast disease/fibroadenosis does not predispose to breast cancer, but women with lumpy, tender breasts may experience worsening of these symptoms in the initial months of HRT use. The postmenopausal breast responds to estrogen by becoming full and slightly tense, with tingling in the nipples. Progestogens increase this fullness and can cause severe mastalgia.

Table 28.7 Hormone replacement therapy (HRT) in women with breast cancer

Study	Number of patients	Duration of HRT (range)	Recurrences	Deaths
Stoll and Parbhoo (1988) [69]	50	24+ months	0	0
DiSaia et al. (1993) [68]	77	27 months (1–233)	6	3
Wile et al. (1993) [67]	25	35.2 months (24–82)	3	1
Powles et al. (1993) [70]	35	43 months	2	0
Bluming et al. (1994) [71]	70	8 months (1–18+)	2	0
Eden et al. (1995) [66]	90	18 months (4–144)	6 (7%)[a]	0[a]

[a]17% of controls had recurrences and 9.9% died from breast cancer.

The tender lumpy 'cystic' breasts are dense on mammography and difficult to examine, which may delay the diagnosis of a neoplastic tumor.

Cervical cancer

There is no increase in cervical cancer risk in HRT users.

Venous thromboembolism

Deep vein thrombosis and pulmonary embolism are rare. Estrogen use increases this risk, mainly in predisposed women, many of whom have a genetic predisposition that is unknown to them or their practitioners. Women using HRT have a threefold increase in risk of thromboembolism compared to non-users [72–74]. The risk is not influenced by the type of delivery system or the addition of progestins. The absolute risk remains small with an excess risk of two in 10 000 users per year and an excess mortality of two per million. The same studies found that obesity was a major risk factor for pulmonary embolism and increased the risk

of venous thromboembolism 12-fold. Women with a family history of idiopathic thrombosis or a personal history of venous thromboembolisms should be screened for thrombophilia before being prescribed HRT.

The risk–benefit ratio remains strongly in favor of HRT.

HRT for how long?

HRT is effective in relieving menopausal symptoms. Traditionally, women using HRT for symptomatic relief are advised to do so for 2–3 years, after which it is anticipated that symptoms would abate in three out of four women. For osteoporosis protection 5–10 years' use 'buys time' for the skeleton and halves the risk of osteoporotic fractures. This protection disappears 5–10 years after stopping therapy. However, there is a growing feeling among experts that lifelong use of HRT is necessary for maximum and continuing protection. Mechanisms of estrogen-dependent arterial disease protection also suggest that the advantage applies to current and recent users only.

Role of androgens in HRT

Androgen levels decline with age in women as well as men. Estrogen replacement therapy decreases bioavailable testosterone by its effect on sex hormone-binding globulin. Testosterone does improve energy level, libido and possibly cognitive function. Androgens may stimulate bone osteoblasts and, if given parenterally, do not depress high-density lipoprotein.

Selective estrogen receptor modulators (SERMS)

Tamoxifen exhibits a tissue-selective effect on estrogen receptors in 'target' organs. It is an antiestrogen at breast level, but acts like estrogen on bones and endometrium. A new breed of non-steroidal compounds (SERMS) is emerging with an estrogen-like effect on bone and arterial disease markers, and an antiestrogenic effect on breast and endometrium (hence bleed free) [75]. A total of 20–30% of SERM users experience mild vasomotor symptoms.

References

1. Gambrell RD Jr. The menopause: benefits and risks of estrogen–progestogen replacement therapy. *Fertil Steril* 1982;156:457–474.

2. Lindsay R. Pathophysiology of bone loss. In: Lobo RA (ed.) Treatment of the post-menopausal woman. New York: Raven Press, 1994:175–82.

3. Peck WA, Barrett-Conner E, Buckwalter JA, et al. Consensus conference: osteoporosis. *JAMA* 1984;252:799–802.

4. Jensen J, Nilas L, Christiansen C. Influence of menopause on serum lipids and lipoproteins. *Maturitas* 1990;12:321–331.

5. Birge SJ. The role of estrogen deficiency in the aging central nervous system. In: Lobo RA (ed.) Treatment of the postmenopausal woman. New York: Raven Press, 1994:153–7.

6. Honjo H, Tamura T, Matsumoto Y, et al. Estrogen as a growth factor to central nervous cells: estrogen treatment promotes development of acetylcholine

transferase – positive basal forebrain neurons transplanted in anterior eye chamber. *J Steroid Biochem Molec Biol* 1992;41:633.

7. Kampen DL, Sherwin BB. Estrogen use and verbal memory in healthy postmenopausal women. *Obstet Gynecol* 1994;83:979–983.

8. Paganini-Hill A, Henderson VW: Estrogen deficiency and risk of Alzheimer's disease in women. *Am J Epidemiol* 1994;140:256–261.

9. McMichael AJ, Potter JD: Host factors in carcinogenesis: certain

bile-acid metabolic profiles that selectively increase the risk of proximal colon cancer. *J Natl Cancer Inst* 1985;75:185–191.

10. Newcomb PA, Storer BE: Postmenopausal hormone use and risk of large-bowel cancer. *J Natl Cancer Inst* 1995;87: 1067–1071.

11. Kampman E, Potter JD, Slattery ML, et al. Hormone replacement therapy, reproductive history and colon cancer. A multi-center, case-control study in the United States. *Cancer Causes & Controls* 1997;8:146–58.

12. Gambrell RD Jr, McDonough PG: The 'Red Queen' and endometrial hyperplasia (letter). *Fertil Steril* 1994;61:401.

13. Leather AT, Savvas M, Studd JWW: Endometrial histology and bleeding patterns after 8 years of continuous combined estrogen and progestogen therapy in postmenopausal women. *Obstet Gynecol* 1991;1991;78:1008–1010.

14. Goodman L, Awwad J, Marc K, Schiff I. Continuous combined hormonal replacement therapy and the risk for endometrial cancer. Preliminary report. *Menopause J North Am Menopause Soc* 1994;1:57.

15. McGonigle KF, Karlan BY, Barbuto DA, et al. Development of endometrial cancer in women on estrogen and progestin hormone replacement therapy. *Gynecol Oncol* 1994;55:126–132.

16. Comerci JT Jr, Fields AL, Runowicz CD, et al. Continuous low-dose combined hormone replacement therapy and the risk of endometrial cancer. *Gynecol Oncol* 1997;64:425–430.

17. Gambrell RD, Jr. Strategies to reduce the incidence of endometrial cancer in postmenopausal women. *Am J Obstet Gynecol* 1997;177: 1196–1207.

18. Ziel HK, Finkle WD. Increased risk of endometrial carcinoma among users of conjugated estrogens. *N Engl J Med* 1975;293:1167–1170.

19. Shapiro S, Kelly JP, Rosenberg L, et al. Risk of localized and widespread endometrial cancer in relation to recent and discontinued use of conjugated estrogens. *N Engl J Med* 1985;313:969–972.

20. Grady D, Gebretsadik T, Kerlikowske K, et al. Hormone replacement therapy and endometrial cancer risk: a meta-analysis. *Obstet Gynecol* 1995;85:304–313.

21. Gambrell RD Jr. Use of progestogen therapy. *Am J Obstet Gynecol* 1987;156:1304.

22. Hammond CB, Jelovsek FR, Lee KL, et al. Effects of long term estrogen replacement therapy. II-Neoplasia. *Am J Obstet Gynecol* 1979;133:537–547.

23. Nachtigall LE, Nachtigall RH, Nachtigall RB, et al. Estrogen replacement therapy II: a prospective study in the relationship to carcinoma and cardiovascular and metabolic problems. *Obstet Gynecol* 1979;54:74–79.

24. Thom MH, White PJ, Williams RM, et al. Prevention and treatment of endometrial disease in climacteric women receiving oestrogen therapy. *Lancet* 1979;2:455–457.

25. Whitehead MI, Townsend PT, Pryse-Davies J., et al. Effects of estrogens and progestins on the biochemistry and morphology of the postmenopausal endometrium. *N Engl J Med* 1981;305:1599–1605.

26. Persson I, Adami H-O, Bergkvist L, et al. Risk of endometrial cancer after treatment with oestrogens alone or in conjunction with progestogens: results of a prospective study. *Br Med J* 1989;298:147–151.

27. Voight L, Weiss N, Chu J, et al. Progestogen supplementation of exogenous oestrogens and risk of endometrial cancer. *Lancet* 1991;338:274–277.

28. Gambrell RD Jr, Massey FM, Castaneda TA, et al. Use of the progestogen challenge test to reduce the risk of endometrial cancer. *Obstet Gynecol* 1980;55:732–738.

29. Hanna JH, Brady WK, Hill JM, et al. Detection of postmenopausal women at risk for endometrial carcinoma by a progesterone challenge test. *Am J Obstet Gynecol* 1983;147:872–873.

30. El-Maraghy MA, El-Badawy N, Wafa GA, et al. Progesterone challenge test in postmenopausal women at high risk. *Maturitas* 1994;19:53–57.

31. Petranik K, Kable WT, Bewtra C, et al. Use of progestin challenge test in elderly women (abstract). *Menopause J North Am Menopause Soc* 1995;2:278.

32. Guerrieri JP, Elkas JC, Nash JD: Evaluating the endometrium in women on tamoxifen: a pilot study to compare a 'gold standard' with an 'old standard'. *Menopause J North Am Menopause Soc* 1997;4:6.

33. Toppozada MK, Ismail AA, Hamed RSM, et al. Progesterone challenge test and estrogen assays in menopausal women with endometrial hyperplasia. *Int J Gynaecol Obstet* 26:115.

34. Nakamura S, Douchi T, Oki T, et al. Relationship between sonographic endometrial thickness and progestin-induced withdrawal bleeding. *Obstet Gynecol* 1996;87:722.

35. Gratton D, Harrington C, Holt SC, et al. Normal pelvic anatomy using transvaginal scanning. *Obstet Gynecol Clin North Am* 1991;18:693–711.

36. Goldstein SR: Use of endometrial ultrasound in the overall gynaecologic examination. *Obstet Gynecol Clin North Am* 1991;18:779–796.

37. Granberg S, Wikland M, Karisson B, et al. Endometrial thickness as measured by endovaginal ultrasonography for identifying endometrial abnormality. *Am J Obstet Gynecol* 1991;164:47–52.

38. Burke TW, Tortolero-Luna G, Malpica A, et al. Endometrial hyperplasia and endometrial

cancer. *Obstet Gynecol Clin North Am* 1996;23:411–456.

39. Lavy G: Hysteroscopy as a diagnostic aid. *Obstet Gynecol Clin North Am* 1988;15:61–72.

40. Nagele F, O'Connor H, Davies A, et al. 2500 outpatient diagnostic hysteroscopies. *Obstet Gynecol* 1996;88:87–92.

41. Coulan CB, Annegers JF: Chronic anovulation may increase postmenopausal breast cancer risk. *JAMA* 1983; 249:445–446.

42. Cowan LD, Gordis L, Tonascia JA, et al. Breast cancer incidence in women with a history of progesterone dificiency. *Am J Epidemiol* 1981;114:209–217.

43. Mauvais-Jarvis P, Sitruk-Ware R, Kuttenn F: Luteal phase defect and breast cancer genesis. *Breast Cancer Res Treat* 1982;2:139.

44. Ron E, Lunenfeld B, Menczer J, et al. Cancer incidence in a cohort of infertile women. *Am J Epidemiol* 1987;125:780–790.

45. Collaborative Group on Hormonal Factors in Breast Cancer. Breast cancer and hormone replacement therapy: collaborative re-analysis of data from 51 epidemiological studies of 52 705 women with breast cancer and 108 411 women without breast cancer. *Lancet* 1997;350:1547–59.

46. Gambrell RD Jr. Hormone replacement therapy and breast cancer risk. *Arch Fam Med* 1996;5:341.

47. Colditz GA, Hankinson SE, Hunter DJ, et al. The use of estrogens and progestins and the risk of breast cancer in postmenopausal women. *N Engl J Med* 1995;332:1589–1593.

48. Jick H, Walker AM, Watkins RN, et al. Replacement estrogens and breast cancer. *Am J Epidemiol* 1980:112:586–594.

49. Mills PK, Beeson WL, Phillips RL, et al. Prospective study of exogenous hormone use and breast cancer in Seventh-Day Adventists. *Cancer* 1989;64:591–597.

50. Wingo PA, Layde PM, Lee NC, et al. The risk of breast cancer in postmenopausal women who have used estrogen replacement therapy. *JAMA* 1987;257: 209–215.

51. Stanford JL, Weiss NS, Voight LF, et al. Combined estrogen and progestin hormone replacement therapy in relation to the risk of breast cancer in middle-aged women. *JAMA* 1995;274: 137–142.

52. Cutler SJ, Young JL Jr. Third national cancer survey: incidence data. *Natl Cancer Inst Monograph* 1975;41:110.

53. Miller BA, Ries LAG, Hankey BF, et al. SEER Cancer Statistics Review: 1973–1991 (NIH Publication 94-2789). Bethesda, Maryland: National Cancer Institute, 1994:IV.6.

54. Nachtigall MJ, Smilen SW, Nachtigall RD, et al. Incidence of breast cancer in a 22-year study of women receiving estrogen–progestin replacement therapy. *Obstet Gynecol* 1992;80:827–830.

55. Lauritzen C: Ostrogen-substitution in der postmenopause vor und nach bchandeltem genital und mammakar zinom. Menopause Lauritzen C. (ed) Basel: Aesopus 1993;6:76–88.

56. Bergkvist L, Adami H-O Persson I, et al. The risk of breast cancer after estrogen and estrogen–progestin replacement. *N Engl J Med* 1989;321:293–297.

57. Persson I, Yuen J, Bergkvist, et al. Combined oestrogen–progestogen replacement and breast cancer risk (letter). *Lancet* 1992;340–1044.

58. Ewertz M: Influence of noncontraceptive exogenous and endogenous sex hormones on breast cancer risk in Denmark. *Int J Cancer* 1988;52:832–838.

59. Burch JC, Byrd BF Jr, Vaughn WK: Results of estrogen treatment in one thousand hysterectomized women for 14 318 years. In: Van Keep PA, Greenblatt RD, Albeaux-Femet M (eds) Consensus on memopause research. Lancaster, UK: MTP Press, 1976:164–9.

60. Gambrell RD Jr. Proposal to decrease the risk and improve the prognosis of breast cancer. *Am J Obstet Gynecol* 1984; 150:119–128.

61. Hunt K, Vessey M, McPherson K: Mortality in a cohort of long-term users of hormone replacement therapy: an updated analysis. *Br J Obstet Gynaecol* 1990;97:1080–1086.

62. Strickland DM, Gambrell RD, Jr, Butzin CA, et al. The relationship between breast cancer survival and prior postmenopausal estrogen use. *Obstet Gynecol* 1992;80: 400–404.

63. Willis DB, Calle EE, Miracle-McMahill HL, et al. Estrogen replacement therapy and risk of fetal breast cancer in a prospective cohort of postmenopausal women in the United States. *Cancer Causes and Controls* 1996;7:449–457.

64. Cobleigh MA, Berris RF, Bush T, et al. Estrogen replacement therapy in breast cancer survivors: a time of change. *JAMA* 1994;272:540–547.

65. Sands R, Boshoff C, Junes A, Studd J: Current opinion: hormone replacement therapy after a diagnosis of breast cancer. *Menopause J N Am Menopause Soc* 1995;2:73.

66. Eden JA, Bush T, Nand S, et al. A case-controlled study of combined continuous estrogen–progestin replacement amongst women with a personal history of breast cancer. *J N Am Menopause Soc* 1995;2:67–72.

67. Wile AG, Opfell RW, Margileth DA: Hormone replacement therapy in previously treated breast cancer patients. *Am J Surg* 1993;165:372–375.

68. DiSaia PJ, Grosen EA, Odicino F, et al. Hormone replacement therapy in breast cancer. *Lancet* 1993;342:1232.

69. Stoll BA, Parbhoo S: Treatment of menopausal symptoms in breast cancer patients. *Lancet* 1988;1:1278–9.

70. Powles TJ, Hickish T, Casey S, et al. Hormone replacement after breast cancer. *Lancet* 1993;342:60–61.

71. Bluming AZ, Wile AG, Schain JR, et al. Hormone replacement therapy in women with previously treated primary breast cancer (abstract). Proceedings of the 32nd Annual Meeting of the American Society of Clinical Oncologists. 1996;65:136.

72. Daly E, Vessey MP, Hawkins MM, et al. Risk of venous thromboembolism in users of hormone replacement therapy. *Lancet* 1996;348:977–80.

73. Jick H, Derby LE, Wald Myers M, et al. Risk of hospital admission for idiopathic venous thromboembolism among users of postmenopausal oestrogens. *Lancet* 1996;348:981–3.

74. Grodstein F, Stampfer MJ, Goldhaber SZ, et al. Prospective study of exogenous hormones and risk of pulmonary embolisms in women. *Lancet* 1996;348:983–7.

75. Compston JE. Designer oestrogens: fact or fantasy? *Lancet* 1997;350:676–77.

Suggested reading

• Sitruk-Ware R, Utian WH (eds). The menopause and hormonal replacement therapy. New York: Marcel Dekker, 1991:1–296.

• Dusitsin N, Notelovitz M (eds). Physiological hormone replacement therapy. Carnforth: Parthenon★ 1991:1–112.

• Studd JWW, Whitehead MI, (eds). The menopause.

London: Blackwell Scientific Publications, 1988:1–312.

• Mann RD (ed.). Hormone replacement therapy and breast cancer risk. Carnforth: Parthenon, 1992:1–321.

• Gambrell RD Jr. Hormone replacement therapy, 5th edn. Dallas: Essential Medical Information Systems, 1997:1–167.

• Lobo RA (ed.). Treatment of the postmenopausal woman. New York: Raven Press, 1994:1–443.

★ Full address: Casterton Hall, Casterton, Carnforth, Lancs LA6 2LA, UK.

Osteoporosis

David W Purdie MD FRCOG FRCP(Ed)
Kate A Guthrie BSC MB FRCOG MFFP

Introduction

The term 'osteoporosis' derives from the Greek prefix *osteo* (bone) and the suffix *porosis* (full of pores). Thus, the original description depicted bones which, on sectioning, simply seemed to be full of holes due to the absence of bone tissue. The term remains accurate and serviceable today because the physical problems imposed by osteoporosis upon the individual ultimately relate to there being simply less bone than normal per unit area at key skeletal sites, such as the spine, the femoral neck and the distal radius. The World Health Organization (WHO) has accepted the definition proposed by a consensus development conference in 1991 [1] that the condition be defined as:

A disease characterised by low bone mass and microarchitectural deterioration of bone tissue, leading to enhanced bone fragility and a consequent increase in fracture risk.

The acceptance by the patient and indeed by the medical profession that osteoporosis is a true disease is relatively recent. Long recognized as being a concomitant of ageing, bone fragility, which manifests itself as height loss, kyphosis and low trauma fracture, was thought simply to be a function of senescence, hence the older term 'senile osteoporosis'. It was only with elucidation of the pathophysiology of the disease over the past 25 years that its true natural history has come to light. This chapter will concentrate upon the behaviour of bone in women and will examine those factors which promote bone gain in childhood and adolescence, and those which promote bone loss at any age. The relevance of the endogenous oestrogenic hormones will be emphasized together with the potentiality for their exogenous use in the prevention and treatment of osteoporosis. Given that the treatment of the established disease lies within the province of the rheumatologist and the orthopaedic surgeon, this chapter will concentrate on the origins and prevention of the condition in so far as this falls within the clinical activities of the gynaecologist and other doctors involved in primary and community reproductive health.

Background

The WHO has chosen to define osteoporosis and osteopenia quantitatively in addition to the qualitative definition described above. The definitions are given in Table 29.1.

The origin of osteoporosis as a pathological condition is certainly partly related to present longevity. Life expectancy for a British female is currently 81 years and for an American female is 78 years; with the age of menopause steady at a median of 51 years, this means that, on average, some 30 years will be spent in a state of oestrogen deficiency (Figure 29.1).

When we consider that there is

Table 29.1 Quantitative definitions of osteoporosis and osteopenia

Definition	Bone mineral density (g/cm²) (BMD)
Normal	<1.0 standard deviation below young normal mean
Osteopenia	1–2.5 standard deviations below young normal mean
Osteoporosis	> 2.5 standard deviations below young normal mean
Established osteoporosis	>2.5 standard deviations below young normal mean, and one or more fragility fractures

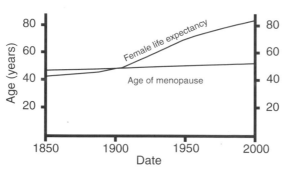

Fig. 29.1 The relationship of age at menopause to female life expectancy.

a background age-related bone loss from the skeleton and that oestrogen-related losses appear to be superimposed upon this, then it is perhaps not surprising that the prevalence of osteoporosis and the incidence of related fracture is substantial and increasing. In addition, the general lifestyle of the industrialized Western societies may not be helpful to the preservation of bone mass. For example, the physical pull of muscle upon bone, exemplified by the performance of hard physical exercise, is helpful to the maintenance of bone mass. In the developed countries, the availability of disposable capital has allowed the daily performance of hard physical exercise to be sequestered to a relatively small sector of the population. Women perform just as much work as ever in the past – indeed they do more – but they now use machines to help them to the extent that personal expenditure of energy is relatively low compared with the past. The skeleton, unless physically stressed, tends to lose tissue – most acutely observed in the osteoporosis of prolonged space flight – and thus the labour-saving domestic and transportation devices of our society may also be bone-losing devices.

Similarly, the diet of developed societies has been criticized for containing too little calcium to maintain the balance between intake and output, which is essential for skeletal health. In childhood, it has been shown that calcium supplementation can enhance the bone gain [2] and a daily intake of 1500 mg/day in adolescence is recommended in order to achieve that peak bone mass of which the individual is genetically capable. After menopause, the amount of calcium required for balance is also 1500 mg/day, a value which falls to 1000 mg/day in women receiving oestrogen replacement. Dietary intake studies particularly show that intakes are suboptimal, a fact compounded by the additional frequent presence of hypovitaminosis D, particularly during the winter months and among the house-bound or institutionalized elderly [3]. Box 29.1 shows calcium content of certain specific foods.

Another constitutional factor which may influence the prevalence of osteoporosis is race. In general, Black women have a higher bone mineral density, site for site, than Caucasian women of the same age and hormonal status [4]. It appears that this advantage begins to accrue at puberty, since Black and White children have similar prepubertal bone densities. However, risk of fracture is not determined by BMD alone but also by the geometry of bone, propensity to fall, presence of adipose tissue and many other factors (Box 29.2). The relative freedom of Black women from osteoporotic fractures, therefore, remains an observation whose investigation is likely to be highly productive in terms of an understanding of the history of bone behaviour. It has recently been shown that the origin of *Homo sapiens* lies in Africa and it has been hypothesized that the later rapid migration of humans into the northern latitudes applied selection pressure which included a lighter skin coloration [5]. The latter may be associated in certain circumstances with low bone mass density and, hence, the European skeleton may be a lighter evolved variant of the African original. It is certainly the case that the highest presence of osteoporosis-related fractures is found in Scandinavia, with the UK and USA exhibiting a

Box 29.1 Calcium content of foods	
2 slices of bread	66 mg
8 oz of semi-skimmed milk	350 mg
Baked beans serving	105 mg
Fruit yogurt pot	240 mg
100 g of cheddar cheese	800 mg
100 g of canned sardines	550 mg
100 g of raw broccoli	100 mg
100 g of dried figs	280 mg

> **Box 29.2   Causes of secondary osteoporosis** (accounts for 20% of total osteoporosis)
>
> - Endocrine – anorexia nervosa, hyperprolactinaemia, thyrotoxicosis, primary hyperparathyroidism, Cushing's syndrome, hypogonadism
> - Gastrointestinal – malabsorption (coeliac disease), liver disease (primary biliary cirrhosis), gastric surgery
> - Rheumatological – rheumatoid arthritis, ankylosing spondylitis
> - Malignancy – multiple myeloma, metastatic cancer
> - Drugs – steroids, heparin
> - Prolonged immobilization

prevalence below that of the Nordic countries and well above that seen in, for example, Afro-Americans. A comprehensive review of geographic variation in osteoporosis using precise equipment remains to be published.

In summary, osteoporosis is very much a contemporary disease in that the decline in physical activity and nutritional support for the skeleton is compounded by current longevity, imposing, on average, some 30 years of oestrogen deficiency.

The causes of secondary osteoporosis are shown in Box 29.2.

Scope of the problem

Osteoporosis is a major and increasingly recognized public health problem in developed countries: one in two women and one in six men will sustain an osteoporotic fracture by age 90. It is estimated that National Health Service expenditure of £750 million is required to deal with the acute and aftercare of osteoporosis-related fractures in the UK; similar data are available in the USA. In 1995, in UK, there were some 50 000 femoral neck fractures, some 60 000 fractures of the distal radius and an estimated 100 000 vertebral

fractures arising *de novo* [6]. The global load of hip fractures is expected to treble to 6 million by 2050. The disease is largely, but not exclusively, one of the female sex, the ratio of femoral neck fracture between females and males being 8:1. The prevalence of osteoporosis in women aged 50–54 is 3.5% and 2% for spine and hip, respectively, rising to 15% and 20% in women aged 70–74. Prevalence of osteopenia in perimenopausal women is 15% rising to 90% at age 80. The prevalence of osteoporosis may be rising even after allowance is made for ageing of the population, a fact which has major implications for expenditure and service planning, and which provides an insight into the basic causes of

bone loss. It has been calculated in the USA that, if the present rate of increase in fracture is maintained, then it will become progressively difficult for the health services to fund the cost implication.

The social cost to osteoporosis-affected women is also high. The occurrence of non-traumatic vertebral fractures – only one in three of which comes to medical attention – may result in chronic backache, height loss and the classic accentuations of the dorsal kyphus, known technically as kyphosis and, to the public, as the 'dowager's hump'. A vicious cycle is established with progressive deformity (Figure 29.2) and loss of self-esteem leading to further immobility, fear of trauma and reactive depression.

Most serious of all the consequences of osteoporosis is the femoral neck fracture which is often the result of a fall by an elderly, perhaps neuromuscular incoordinated patient, upon a fragile hip. It is likely that many falls, which in a younger person would result in a Colles' distal radial fracture due to

Fig. 29.2   Severe spinal osteoporosis. Only symptomatic treatment is available at this stage. Lost height cannot be regained.

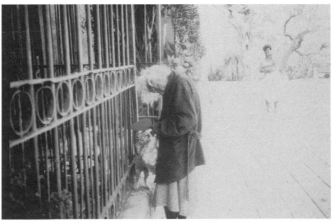

interposition of the hand between the falling body and the ground, are converted in older patients into femoral neck fractures by neuromuscular incoordination, with the patient consequently falling on the head of femur. The factors contributing to the occurrence of fractures are summarized in Figure 29.3.

Femoral neck fractures are highly morbid and may be associated with mortality. It is estimated that the fracture imposes an approximate 25% excess mortality within 6 months. It should be emphasized that this excess is present even when allowance is made for the underlying mortality among this elderly cohort. Of survivors, some 50% will fail to regain a fully independent life. In other words, they will become dependent upon their families or upon private health agencies, or upon the State. Such dependency with its consequent physical and emotional trauma is itself debilitating.

To account for the present clinical and social problem of osteoporosis, we will now turn to the behaviour of human bone itself and to the factors which govern its density and strength.

Physiology of bone

The skeleton is alive. It is just as active and dynamic an organ system as the brain or bowel. In common with all systems, the skeleton requires to constantly maintain and restore itself and thus to replace old bone with new. The process, known as remodelling, is at the very heart of bone physiology and one of the agents which holds the key to bone balance and maintenance of skeletal integrity and health is oestrogen. Before looking at bone turnover in greater detail, it would be prudent to sketch the overall changes in bone density which occur throughout a human life.

Bone mass accretion begins before birth when the fetal skeleton begins to receive, through the placenta, substantial amounts of maternal calcium. This process is promoted by the parathyroid hormone-related peptide (PTHrP), which is produced in the placenta and literally drives the high-energy calcium pump, which maintains fetal plasma calcium at a substantially higher level than that which is normal in the adult. In all, some 30 000 mg of calcium are transferred to the fetus, largely during the last 12 weeks of pregnancy. The newborn thus has at its disposal a skeleton that is adequately robust, which has, of course, a great potential to grow, both in size and density, and which will arrive at full size at around age 20 and at full densiometric growth a decade later.

Peak bone mass

Growth of the young skeleton is non-linear. In young children, the appendicular skeleton (the limb bones) grows relatively more rapidly than the axial skeleton – principally the spine – which grows more quickly under the growth spurt of puberty. The latter also heralds the time when the growth in bone mineral density in boys begins to advance in relation to girls. Site for site male bone density is usually 15–20% greater than female. The attainment of peak bone mass (PBM) is a key concept, which is directly related to osteoporosis risk later, since, essentially, the achieved PBM is the bone strength which the female individual will bring to her menopause 20 years later and from which the inevitable losses of older age will occur. The three central variables which contribute to a woman's risk of osteoporosis are her peak bone density, the rate of postmenopausal bone loss and longevity.

Peak bone mass is largely determined by heredity with the

Fig. 29.3 Factors intrinsic (left) and extrinsic (right) to bone which influence the likelihood of fracture.

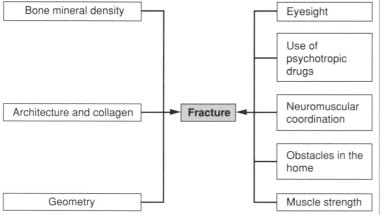

genetic component accounting for some 80% of the variance in density. Other factors which contribute include dietary calcium content, exercise profile and sex-hormone status.

Postmenopausal bone loss

The relationship between the loss of oestrogen and the menopause was first described by Albright in 1941 [7] and is now universally accepted. The progressive fall in plasma oestradiol which attends the climacteric is accompanied by increases in the gonadotrophins, follicle-stimulating hormone and luteinizing hormone, as the ovary, now producing less inhibin and containing few responsive follicles, is subjected unsuccessfully to high gonadotrophin drive. Eventual ovarian failure, when the organ is incapable of maintaining a menstrual cycle, is a key event in the climacteric era and is attended by an acceleration of bone loss. For the following 10 years, a relatively rapid bone loss occurs after which rates of loss decline and blend with the lower background and age-related bone loss which applies to both sexes in older age. The absolute risk of fracture doubles for each decade after 50 (Figure 29.4). The relative risk of fractures increases 1.5–2-fold for each standard deviation decrease in bone mass (equivalent to 10% loss).

This oestrogen-related bone loss of the menopause is seen most dramatically after bilateral oophorectomy, when the loss of trabecular bone at spine, hip and distal radius – the key sites of later fracture – can reach 20% in 18

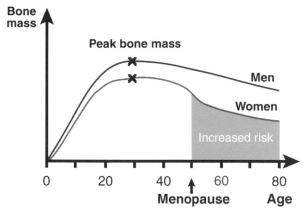

Fig. 29.4 Pattern of bone loss with age.

months, postoperatively. In contrast, the less oestrogen-sensitive cortical bone exhibits losses in the order of 2–3% [8]. It can be seen immediately that, if the peak bone mass has been suboptimal, then the losses consequent upon oestrogen withdrawal may take the BMD down into the range of osteopenia or osteoporosis.

The dynamic maintenance of bone mass and architecture is a key area of skeletal physiology, and is achieved through regular removal of old bone and its replacement with new. This process, which is accomplished in an orderly sequence of events, is summarized in Figure 29.5. Responding to an as yet unidentified signal, bone resorbing cells, osteoclasts, assemble at an area of bone surface and proceed to excavate a cavity in bone by proteolytic digestion. This is the resorption

Fig. 29.5 Bone dynamics coupling.

Bone Dynamics

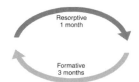

phase. The osteoclasts then disperse and, after a defined pause of 2 weeks, the formation phase commences with the cavity being invaded by bone-forming cells, osteoblasts, which proceed to lay down new osteoid. The mineralization of the osteoid completes the process with the refilled cavity being levelled off with the surrounding bone and covered by a thin cellular layer of restoring osteocytes.

The factors which influence this central bone housekeeping are many and complex, and have been well summarized by Einhorn [9]. One of the most important endocrine agents that modulate bone turnover is oestrogen. In summary, the oestrogens operate by restraining the activity of the osteoclasts (thereby protecting bone from the loss of bone tissue and hence bone density), which begin to accrue if bone resorption is unrestrained. Oestrogens operate through a series of cytokines, a principal example of which is interleukin-6. This agent promotes the differentiation, activity and life span of the osteoclast and is inhibited by oestrogen. Hence, lack of oestrogen, the postmenopausal unfettered osteoclasts proceed to create deeper and more frequent cavities, which tend to be incompletely refilled by subsequent osteoblast activity. The real loss at each of the 600 000 or so concurrent turnover sites is small but, given that the effect is most pronounced in the trabecular bone of hip, spine and radius, the prolonged excess of resorption over formation results eventually in a bone loss which is clinically significant and productive of fracture after minimal or moderate trauma. The loss of trabecular number, thickness and cohesiveness, as displayed in the loss of normal bone framework (Figure 29.6), deprives the remaining bone of its key ability to absorb shock, with the consequent likelihood of fracture after moderate or minimal trauma. The 20% of the human skeleton charged with shock absorption is located, as expected, in the calcaneus, the metaphyses of long bones, the femoral neck and the spine. Its integrity is literally central to healthy bone activity.

Premenopausal conditions influencing bone mineral density

Essentially, the period between attainment of peak bone mass and the climacteric is one of stability.

Given that an individual has a normal menstrual cycle, a diet reasonably replete with calcium and a normal amount of weight-bearing physical exercise, the BMD of the skeleton is unlikely to undergo significant change. However, the onset of oestrogen deficiency, whether spontaneous or iatrogenic, medical or surgical, may be attended by onset of bone loss which is of long-term clinical significance.

In gonadal dysgenesis, marked osteopenia is commonly found and the use of hormone replacement therapy (HRT) from the mid-second decade has been advocated to complete pubertal development and promote tissue acquisition [10]. In highly trained young female athletes, a problem may develop in response to the reduction in fat mass, being associated with a low plasma oestradiol and oligomenorrhoea or amenorrhoea. In fact, such individuals are a good example of the primacy of oestrogen in the maintenance of BMD in the female skeleton. These women are karyotypically normal, have diets replete with calcium and have abundant physical exercise, yet they lose bone if the plasma oestradiol declines into the postmenopausal range of <150 pmol/l. Low bone density may be found in the spine, femoral neck and in the total body [11]

but, even if detected and adequately treated by the combined oral contraceptive (COC) pill or an HRT preparation, a full restoration of bone mass may not be achieved [12]. Other relatively common conditions which may result in bone loss in young women include hyperprolactinaemia, where the high prolactin (PRL) levels suppress gonadotrophin output from the anterior pituitary and hence depress circulating oestradiol. Patients with the condition, regardless of its cause, may fail to respond to the re-establishment of normal plasma PRL levels [13]. Nevertheless, treatment aimed at restoring plasma oestradiol to a normal level through the re-establishment of ovarian cycling should be offered, even if the patient does not wish to conceive.

In anorexia nervosa, a psychiatric disorder associated with low body weight, distorted body image and amenorrhoea, the low circulating oestradiol may trigger accelerated bone loss. There is disagreement over the precise cause of osteoporosis in these patients who are affected by low lean body mass, amenorrhoea, calcium malnutrition and, in some cases, glucocorticoid excess. Treatment should be aimed at restoring body weight and composition, which will permit normal ovarian function. However, if the endogenous oestrogen remains low, it should be restored by exogenous replacement to protect the skeleton from further losses.

The gynaecologist is often asked if use of the combined oral contraceptive has a bearing on

Fig. 29.6 The normal spinal bone architecture is shown on the left. The osteoporotic segment on the right displays loss of trabecular bone number, thickness and cohesiveness.

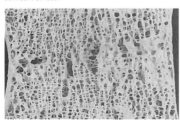
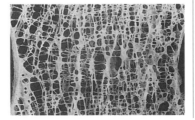

BMD and later risk of fracture. The best evidence to date indicates that patients receiving COC exhibit a slightly higher spinal BMD than controls and, in the key fifth decade, as the menopause approaches, there is biochemical and densitometric evidence for maintenance of bone health [14]. This constitutes a further reason for the use of COC right up to the time of menopause in selected women of low cardiovascular risk.

Pregnancy and lactation have been extensively studied in relation to bone strength and the risk of future osteoporosis. Bone is lost during early pregnancy as skeletal calcium is mobilized to maintain the key variable of ionized plasma calcium in an expanding plasma volume. These bone losses are, however, restored at term, owing to an enhanced calcium absorption by the gut and retention by the renal system. Overall, the reproductive cycle of pregnancy and lactation is neutral in its effects on BMD [15].

During normal lactation, a biphasic pattern of bone loss and regain, similar to that of pregnancy, has been described. Lactation is, in effect, a physiological hyper-prolactinaemic state and, as in other such conditions, is attended by a lower plasma oestradiol level. The latter, which may manifest itself by vasomotor symptoms and vaginal dryness, is associated with skeletal calcium loss amounting over 3 months to a 5% decline in spinal and femoral neck bone mass [16]. However, by a mechanism yet to be fully elucidated, the process of weaning, with its concomitant re-establishment of a menstrual cycle, results in regaining of bone mass such that the lactational episode is not to the long-term detriment of the skeleton. This is confirmed by longer range studies which have failed to show an association between lactational history and fracture [17].

In general, the minimal value of circulating oestradiol necessary to maintain bone health would appear to be around 150 pmol/l. This is achievable therapeutically with the use of the regimens shown in Table 29.2. Whether the oestrogen-driven anti-resorptive activity would halt bone loss. However, current evidence does not confirm that standard oestrogen replacement therapy (ERT) produces further new bone formation, i.e. there is a plateau in bone mass gain. Whether higher doses of ERT or high-dose continuous combined therapy should change this view awaits research confirmation. Table 29.3 shows other therapeutic options for osteopenia/osteoporosis.

The measurement of bone mass

In general, it has not proved possible to measure bone mass indirectly, by means of history taking, biochemical

Table 29.2 Osteoprotective HRT Regimens (per day)[a]

Agent	Dose
Oral 17 β-estradiol– or estradiol esters	2 mg
Conjugated equine estrogens	0.625 mg
Percutaneous/transdermal 17 β-estradiol	50 µg
Subcutaneous 17 β-estradiol	50 mg (6 monthly)
Tibolone	2.5 mg
Raloxifene[b]	60 mg

[a]Adequate for prevention and treatment in perimenopausal and postmenopausal women.
[b] Not strictly HRT.

Table 29.3 Other therapeutic options for osteopenia/osteoporosis

Agent	Main use/action	Points to consider
Calcitonin (25–100 IU s.c. or i.m. thrice weekly)	Antiresorptive peptide hormone beneficial postfracture as has analgesic effect	Available as s.c.injection or nasal spray High cost; less side effects with nasal spray
Calcium 0.7–1.2 g/day/+ vitamin D (400 IU)	Older postmenopausal women (e.g. >75)	Safe as long as dose not exceeded No consensus on efficacy in reducing fractures
Fluoride	Stimulates bone formation No concrete evidence that it reduces fracture risk	Currently not advocated for the management of osteoporosis, although slow-release fluoride and calcium are being assessed
Cyclical sodium etidronate (400 mg/ day for 14 days with calcium carbonate 1250 mg for 74 days)	Effective for vertebral osteoporosis, mainly antiresorptive (ideal of >65 with vertebral disease)	Low incidence of side effects Licensed for corticosteroid induced osteoporosis
Alendronate sodium (10 mg/day)	Effective at all fracture sites	Need to take supplementary calcium Risk of oesophageal ulcers, if not taken according to instructions

measurements or epidemiological characteristics. Although each of these procedures is capable of telling us about the behaviour of osteoporosis in populations, they do not allow us to specify the BMD of an individual in an outpatient clinic or a health centre. Indeed, it is a common and major error in clinical medicine to extrapolate an individual risk from the existence of a population risk factor. Thus, the population risk factors shown in Box 29.3 can only act as a guide to the presence of risk in an individual patient which requires to be determined precisely by densitometry.

Radiology

Standard radiological views are not a precise means of measuring bone strength. The skeleton has to be highly demineralized before this becomes quantitatively apparent to the radiologist, and hence a substantial amount of early or moderate osteoporosis will not be diagnosed radiologically. However, the practice of radiologists commenting upon an apparently

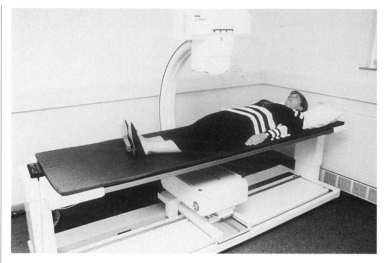

Fig. 29.7   DEXA scanning. The procedure is rapid, non-invasive and safe.

osteoporotic skeleton noted in the course of any X-ray examination is valuable, as the patient may thus be referred for bone densitometry to settle the issue.

Densitometry

The standard technique for precise measurement of BMD is dual-energy X-ray absorptiometry (DEXA). In this process, a pencil beam of dual-energy X-rays is directed at the target bone – usually femoral

neck or spine – while, on the distal side of the bone, a collector records the photons which have passed through (Figure 29.7). The basis of the test is that, if the bone is hard, dense and healthy, relatively fewer photons will emerge compared with the higher number which will pass through if the bone is thin and porous. Thus, measurement of the amount of X-ray energy absorbed (absorptiometry) is the key to the procedure. The technique of DEXA is painless, safe, non-invasive and requires approximately 25–30 min of the patient's time, although modern machines will take less time. The results of the examination are expressed as an 'area density' of bone in grams per square centimetre and are compared to normal populations.

When a specific result is compared to the mean value for that site among young normal persons in the population, the number of standard deviations by which the patient deviates is known as the T score. Similarly, when a patient is compared to age-matched controls the result

---

Box 29.3   Risk factors for osteoporosis

Innate
- Female sex
- Ethnic origin (Caucasians and Asians at risk)
- Increasing age
- Family history
- Nulliparity

Preventable
- Low body mass (thin body type)
- Smoking (5% reduction in bone mass – associated with low body mass, early menopause and hypo-oestrogenism)
- High caffeine intake
- High alcohol intake – direct effect on bone
- Sedentary lifestyle
- Low dietary vitamin D/calcium
- Prolonged immobilization
- Susceptibility to falls
- Glucocorticoid (≥7.5 mg/day of prednisolone) or heparin therapy

is known as a Z score. The WHO has stated that, for international comparisons, osteoporosis is present when the T score is greater than 2.5 standard deviations (SD) below the young normal mean. The milder condition of osteopenia is diagnosed when the value falls at 1–2.5 SD below this mean. The standard values for osteopenia and osteoporosis at hip and spine are shown in Table 29.4.

Recently, data have begun to accumulate which indicate that the use of ultrasound may play a role in the determination of bone density, architecture and the likelihood of fracture, using ultrasound velocity and attenuation. Applied to the calcaneus, ultrasound, a non-ionizing and entirely safe propagation of high-energy 1 MHz sound, produces data on the attenuation of the sound beam by the intervening bone, together with the effect of the latter upon its velocity (Figure 29.8). This technique has begun to demonstrate its clinical application through an ability, in a prospective trial, to delineate the population at risk of femoral neck fracture in individuals over the age of 75, the sector of the population at greatest risk [18].

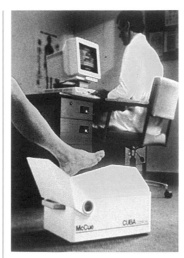

Fig. 29.8 Ultrasonic measurement of the calcaneus. This technique is rapid, painless and avoids ionizing radiation. (Courtesy of McCue Ultrasonics.)

The ability of the technique to predict spinal fracture and its applicability to the perimenopausal population is being determined. The combined use of DEXA and ultrasound may identify women at very high or very low risk. In contrast to DEXA, ultrasound may be of lower cost and has the advantage of using portable machines. Ultrasound of the tibia and patella is also being assessed.

Box 29.4 shows the biochemical markers of bone turnover.

Indications for densitometry

The indications for densitometry are shown in Box 29.5.

It is essential that good and understandable reports flow from the densitometry laboratory to the referring physician. These should be a matter of joint negotiation between the densitometry laboratory and the medical community, and should be clearly unambiguous, carrying recommendation for treatment where indicated.

For these indications it is likely that 175 bone scans will be needed per 100 000 of population per year. Priority should be given to bone scans that are likely to influence the clinical decision to treat.

Selective oestrogen receptor modulators (SERMs)

Hormone replacement therapy is now recognized as the favoured option for the prevention of osteoporosis; it has a dual protective effect in substantially reducing the risk of ischaemic heart disease. Uptake of HRT should understandably be increasing. However, continuation of use and compliance with the regimens is hampered by two problems: the return of cyclic bleeding and the fear of breast cancer. SERMs are tissue-specific compounds that act as oestrogen agonists on bone and the surrogate biochemical markers for arterial disease, while also acting as antagonists on the breast and endometrium. They are, therefore, bone protective

Table 29.4 Bone mineral densitometry (BMD) – young normal range (female, age 20–45 years)

BMD L2–L4 (g/cm²)		BMD femoral neck (g/cm²)
1.440	+2 SD	1.220
1.320	+1 SD	1.100
1.200	Mean	0.980
1.080 Osteopenic	−1 SD	0.860
0.960	−2 SD	0.740
0.900 Osteoporotic	−2.5 SD	0.680
0.840	−3 SD	0.620

Most bone mass studies are based on women in their 60s. Further work is needed on the relation between the perimenopausal bone mass and the risk of fracture.

Box 29.4 Biochemical markers of bone turnover

Bone formation markers
- Bone specific serum alkaline phosphatase
- Serum osteocalcin
- Serum procollagen I extension peptides

Bone resorption markers
- Urinary calcium levels
- Urinary hydroxyproline – not specific for bone
- Urinary pyrodinoline
- Urinary N-telopeptides – more specific to bone
- Urinary collagen 1 c-telopeptides – bone specific
- Urinary collagen 1 μ-telopeptides – bone specific

while at the same time not increasing the risk of breast cancer or causing endometrial stimulation. They should have an important role in women who seek the prophylactic advantages of HRT without the anxiety about breast cancer or the inconvenience of cyclic bleeding. The absence of endometrial stimulation by an oestrogen agonist would alleviate the need for concomitant progestogen use with its recognized side effects [19].

Raloxifene is the first such compound licensed in the USA and UK for the prevention/treatment of vertebral osteoporosis.

Conclusion

Osteoporosis is a prevalent and morbid condition with profound implications both for the personal welfare of patients and for the public health. The disease is difficult to treat once established, but is capable of prevention given that resources and facilities are available to measure the mineral density of bone and to intervene therapeutically where necessary. Bone protective regimens

involving lifestyle alterations, oestrogen and bisphosphonates are generally available for use, but the overall quality of osteoporosis care remains a concern. There is a need for health authorities across the world to take cognisance of the recent advances in understanding the natural history of osteoporosis and to make available services for its prevention. Specifically, every general hospital should have a densitometric capability where patients exhibiting high–risk factors, such as premature menopause, early height loss, steroid ingestion or family history, can be assessed and treated. Women should be reassured that the radiation dose is less than the daily background radiation exposure.

Doctors and nurses involved in reproductive health care can play a vital role in the prevention of osteoporosis by being alert to such risk factors as primary or secondary amenorrhoea and premature menopause, whether spontaneous or after surgery. Women should be encouraged to adopt lifestyles conducive to strong bones. Equally, at natural menopause, those responsible for providing HRT should be aware of the need to tailor the route, dose and duration of therapy for those patients known to be at risk of osteoporosis.

The health of women does not automatically improve with cessation of fertility. The 30 or so years spent on average in the postmenopause may generate clinical problems related to osteoporosis whose prevention is technically possible and whose treatment is clinically necessary.

Box 29.5 Indications for densitometry

- Any oestrogen-deficient woman who would want to be treated or would want to continue treatment only if found to be osteopenic or osteoporotic.
- Patients suspected to be osteoporotic from radiological and clinical findings, such as low-energy trauma fracture.
- Patients who have a medical condition predisposing to osteoporosis if effective treatment is available, e.g. metabolic bone disease, liver disease, anorexia nervosa, malabsorption syndromes and other rarer causes of osteoporosis.
- Patients prior to starting management with oral corticosteroids of a prolonged duration of 6 months or greater.
- Patients receiving corticosteroids at a dose of ≥5 mg prednisolone or equivalent.
- To monitor response to treatment in patients with established osteopenia or osteoporosis. As the margin of error for DEXA is 1% for spine and 2–3% for hip, monitoring of bone loss or gain is best done by repeating the test every 2–3 years.
- Women who experience primary amenorrhoea or secondary amenorrhoea (including hysterectomy) below the age of 45 years (premature menopause).
- Patients with a positive family history of osteoporosis in at least one first-degree relative.

References

1. Consensus Development Conference. Prophylaxis and treatment of osteoporosis. *Am J Med* 1991;90:107–10.

2. Lloyd T. Calcium supplementation and bone mineral density in children. *JAMA* 1993;270:841–4.

3. Villareal DT, Civitelli R, Chines A, Avioli LV. Subclinical vitamin D deficiency in postmenopausal women with low vertebral bone bass. *J Clin Endocrinol Metabol* 1991;72:628–34.

4. Liel Y, Edwards J, Shary J, et al. The effects of race and body habitus on bone mineral density of the radius, hip and spine in premenopausal women. *J Clin Endocrinol Metab* 1988; 66:1247–50.

5. Purdie DW. Evolution of osteoporosis. *Ann Rheum Dis* 1996;55:335–7.

6. Cooper C. Epidemiology and public health impact of osteoporosis. *Baillieres Clin Rheumatol* 1993;7:459–77.

7. Albright F, Smith PH, Richardson AM. Postmenopausal osteoporosis. *JAMA* 1941;116:2465–74.

8. Cann CE, Genant HK, Ettinger B, Gordon GS. Spinal mineral loss in oophorectomized women. Determination by quantitative computed tomography. *JAMA* 1980; 244:2056–2059.

9. Einhorn TA. Bone metabolism and metabolic bone disease. In: Frymoyer JW (ed.) Orthopaedic knowledge update 4, home study syllabus. Rosemont: American Academy of Orthopedic Surgeons, 1994:69–89.

10. Neely EK, Marcus R, Rosenfeld RG & Bachrach LK. Turner syndrome adolescents receiving growth hormone are not osteopenic. *J Clin Endocrinol Metab* 1993;76:861–66.

11. Myburgh KH, Bachrach LK, Lewis B, et al. Low bone mineral density at axial and appendicular sites in amenorrheic athletes. *Med Sci Sports Exercise* 1993;25:1197–202.

12. Drinkwater BL, Nilson K, Ott S & Chestnut III CH. Bone mineral density after resumption of menses in amenorrheic athletes. *JAMA* 1986;256:380–2.

13. Schlechte J, Walkner L, Kathol M. A longitudinal analysis of premenopausal bone loss in healthy women and women with hyperprolactinemia. *J Clin Endocrinol Metab* 1992; 75:698–703.

14. Gambacciani M, Spinetti A, Cappagli B, et al. Hormone replacement therapy in perimenopausal women with a low dose oral contraceptive preparation: effects on bone mineral density and metabolism. *Maturitas* 1994;119:125–31.

15. Purdie DW, Aaron J, Selby PL. Bone histology and homeostasis in human pregnancy. *Br J Obstet Gynaecol* 1988;95:849–54.

16. Sowers MF, Corton G, Shapiro B, et al. Changes in bone density with lactation. *JAMA* 1993; 269:3130–5.

17. Ribot C, Tremollieres F, Pouilles JM, et al. Risk factors for hip fracture. *Bone* 1993;14:S77–S80.

18. Hans D, D'argent-Molina P, Schott A, et al. Ultrasonographic heel measurement to predict hip fracture in elderly women: the EPIDOS Study. *Lancet* 1996; 348:511–4.

19. Purdie DW. Selective oestrogen receptor modulation: HRT replacement therapy? *Br J Obstet Gynaecol* 1997;104:1103–5.

Resources

Further reading for clinicians

- Marcus R, Feldman D, Kelsey J (eds). Osteoporosis. London: Academic Press, 1996. (ISBN 0–12–470860–9)

- UK Department of Health. Quick Reference Primary Care Guide on the Prevention and Treatment of Osteoporosis. London: DOH, 1998.

Resources for clinicians

- The British Menopause Society, 36 West Street, Marlow, Bucks SL7 1AB, UK.

Resources for patients

- The National Osteoporosis Society, PO Box 10, Radstock, Bath, BA3 3YB, UK. Helpline (UK) 01761 472 721

- The North American Menopause Society (NAMS), c/o University Hospitals, 11100 Euclid Avenue, Cleveland, Ohio 44106, USA. (Tel. 216–844–8748; Fax 216–844–8708)

- MenoTimes, 1108 Irwin Street, San Rafael, CA 94901, USA.

The prevention of cervical cancer

Walter Prendiville MAO FRCOG FRACOG

Introduction

Cervical cancer is a preventable disease. As a result of systematic screening programmes, the incidence of and mortality from cervical cancer are falling in many developed parts of the world. The treatment of the preinvasive stage is simple, effective and associated with minimal morbidity. It is a tragedy of modern medicine in the developing world that the disease is still a major killer of women in their prime. A total of 500 000 women die from the disease each year. Outside pregnancy it kills more women than any other gynaecological disease. The prevention of this catastrophe should be a primary aim of health decision makers throughout the world.

Aetiology of cervical cancer

The precise cause of cervical cancer is not known. It is a complex phenomenon whereby some women, in certain circumstances, are predisposed to the initiation of intraepithelial dysplastic changes which will develop into invasive disease in a proportion of cases. Genetic factors may operate through a deficiency of detoxifying enzymes of the P450 cytochrome system. These may interact with such environmental factors as smoking. Although there is no simple single causative agent, there is good evidence for the following statements:

- Squamous cervical cancer is preceded by a non-invasive intraepithelial phase which lasts approximately 10 years (see 'Natural history of cervical precancer lesions')

- Initiation of the disease process involves a sexually transmissible agent. Almost certainly specific types of the human papilloma virus (HPV). HPV16 and 18 are thought to be oncogenic. The former is associated with squamous neoplasia and the latter possibly with adenocarcinoma.

- The transformation zone of epithelium between the squamous (vaginal) and columnar (endocervical) epithelia is the site of origin for neoplasia in 95% of cases. It is most susceptible to oncogenesis during early reproductive life.

- A small proportion of women with cervical intraepithelial neoplasia (CIN) will develop cervical cancer. This proportion increases according to the severity of dysplasia present. In a proportion of women with mild cytological abnormality, regression to normal will occur.

The changes which may occur in the cervical transformation zone are represented in simplified form in Figure 30.1.

Risk factors for cervical cancer

The common denominator in the development of squamous carcinoma of the cervix is sexual intercourse. Cervical cancer is rare in virgins. It is more common in women who become sexually active during adolescence, who have multiple partners, and in those who have had sexually transmitted diseases. The risk of developing cervical cancer is not related to the frequency of intercourse, racial origin or male circumcision. The sexual history of a woman's partner is probably as important as her own in terms of the risk of developing cancer.

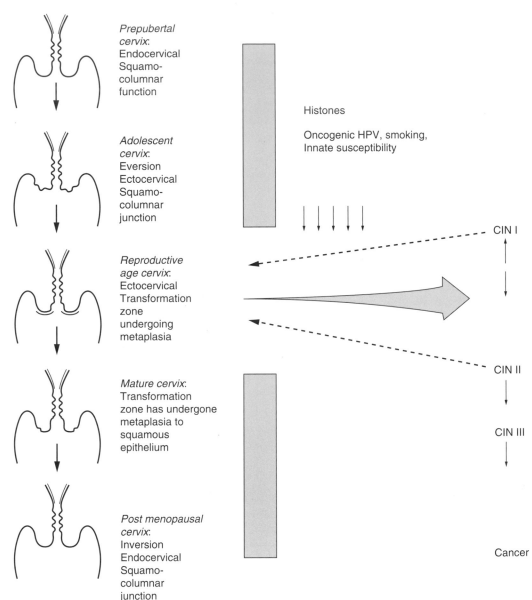

Morphological changes occurring in response
to influence of oestrogen and resultant acidity
of vaginal environment

Oncogenic changes

Prepubertal cervix: Endocervical Squamo-columnar function

Adolescent cervix: Eversion Ectocervical Squamo-columnar junction

Reproductive age cervix: Ectocervical Transformation zone undergoing metaplasia

Mature cervix: Transformation zone has undergone metaplasia to squamous epithelium

Post menopausal cervix: Inversion Endocervical Squamo-columnar junction

Histones

Oncogenic HPV, smoking, Innate susceptibility

CIN I

CIN II

CIN III

Cancer

Fig. 30.1 A crude representation of the natural history of the transformation zone and cervical intraepithelial neoplasia. HPV = human papilloma virus; CIN = cervical intraepithelial neoplasm.

Whilst there is little doubt that a woman can increase her risk of developing cervical cancer by having many partners (especially as an adolescent), it is also true that one does not have to fall into this category in order to develop CIN or cervical cancer. Indeed, the majority of women who attend colposcopy clinics with cytological abnormality are not promiscuous and have standard sexual mores. Being the partner of a 'high-risk male' is equally important.

Furthermore, having a normal sexual history is no protection against the development of CIN and cervical cancer. To date, the ability to lower the incidence is only afforded by either virginity or by entering a systematic cervical cytological screening programme.

Finally, whilst it is of undoubted academic importance to the understanding of how cancer occurs, there is little value in emphasizing the relationship between cervical cancer and coitus. For the individual woman attending a gynaecologist with CIN or cancer, there is no value in pointing out this epidemiological association. She cannot change her sexual history. Documenting it merely embarrasses her and is likely to inflict psychosexual morbidity upon her and her partner. Taking a sexual history from a patient in these circumstances is simply voyeuristic. Finally, emphasizing the increased risk for promiscuous women is likely to offend women, induce guilt and reduce the likelihood of attendance for cytological screening. It also confers a very false sense of immunity in so-called normal women. It is salutary to consider that a woman's lifetime risk of acquiring HPV (as a crude risk marker for CIN and cancer) from a single lifetime partner is still 20%.

Adenocarcinoma of the cervix (ACC) is less common but its incidence is increasing, especially in young women. An association between ACC and oral contraception has been hypothesized (relative risk, RR = 2), although epidemiological evidence is not totally convincing. Cervical cytology is not very effective in screening for ACC. HPV18 may be associated with glandular atypia/ adenocarcinoma.

Natural history of cervical precancer lesions: progression from preinvasive to invasive disease

The interested reader is referred to comprehensive reviews of this subject by Syrjanen [1] and Ostor [2]. It is widely accepted that the great majority of cervical cancers have progressed from precursor intraepithelial stages: the following observations support this contention.

- The mean age for the development of cervical cancer is approximately a decade later than the mean age for the development of cervical intraepithelial neoplasia.

- Women with cervical intraepithelial neoplasia develop invasive cancer far more frequently than do those without CIN.

- Microinvasive disease usually arises from areas of CIN, whether this be on the surface or in a gland crypt. Early invasive disease is almost always surrounded by CIN.

- A wide range of parameters have been used to compare the characteristics of CIN and cervical cancer. The evidence from electron microscopy studies, molecular biology and tissue culture studies, autoradiography and quantitative morphometric measurement studies reveals important similarities between high-grade CIN and cervical cancer.

- In two 1950s studies of women with CIN who did not receive treatment, 65–70%

developed invasive cancer [3]. In a more recent and infamous experiment in New Zealand, 36% of women incompletely treated for CIN III developed invasive cancer after 20 years, whilst 18% had developed it after 10 years [4].

- There is currently a debate about whether adenocarcinoma of the cervix is preceded by a preinvasive stage. Indeed, it is not clear whether interval cancers are preceded by a preinvasive phase.

Cervical screening: the prevention of cancer

The immediate appeal of prevention has led to the implementation of many national screening programmes. Because screening tests are interventions which are applied to asymptomatic people, it is even more important than for treatments of known disease that they are of proven value. Value in this context should include effectiveness, efficiency and freedom from serious disadvantage. In trying to create some sort of balance for screening programmes, Wilson and Jungner [5] laid down ten guiding principles for screening programmes. These World Health Organization (WHO) guidelines are listed below and appear as valid today as when they were published 30 years ago.

- The condition should pose an important health problem.

- The natural history of the disease should be well understood.

- There should be a recognizable early stage.

- Treatment of the disease at an early stage should be of more benefit than treatment started at a later stage.

- There should be a suitable test.

- Tests should be acceptable to the population.

- There should be adequate facilities for the diagnosis and treatment of abnormalities detected.

- For diseases of insidious onset, screening should be repeated at intervals determined by the natural history of the disease.

- The chance of physical or psychological harm to those screened should be less than the chance of benefit.

- The cost of the screening programme should be balanced against the benefit it provides.

A perfect screening tool for cervical cancer does not exist. Such a tool would, for example, detect cancer in its precancerous stage without morbidity, expense or specificity problems. Indeed, the perfect screening test may not be available for any serious human disease. However, cervical cytology does satisfy most of Wilson and Jungner's principles.

The perfect screening test would be highly effective in preventing cancer of the cervix, and its associated morbidity and mortality. Is cytology so effective? It is unfortunately not possible to state categorically whether it is effective or how effective it is by virtue of the lack of 'gold-standard' evidence. In other words, the definitive randomized controlled trial (RCT) has not been done. It is doubtful if such a RCT is ever likely to be done.

In the absence of such 'gold-standard' evidence, a variety of epidemiological methods have been employed to assess the merit of cervical cytological screening where such programmes have been introduced. These techniques may be divided into four main categories:

- temporal studies;

- geographic studies;

- cohort studies;

- case-control studies.

Temporal studies

There are many factors which influence the incidence of and/or mortality from cervical cancer, such as lifestyle and behaviour of the population, the structure and process of the screening programme and the availability of health services to manage those who have been detected by the programme.

In Finland, the incidence of CIN III and cervical cancer was documented from 1953 to 1984, predating the introduction of a systematic screening programme. Following its introduction, the number of cases of CIN III (Figure 30.2) increased, as would be expected, and mortality from the disease and the incidence of cervical cancer fell. Eventually, the number of cases of CIN III also fell.

Whilst there are variations in data from different studies, it is nevertheless possible to give general estimates of the effectiveness of cervical screening programmes. The detection of preinvasive lesions increases initially by the order of 60%. It is more difficult to interpret the mortality and incidence trends because mortality rates were declining in some countries before the introduction of screening. The overall data, however, indicate that incidence and mortality from invasive cervical cancer are reduced by 65% and 55%, respectively, once the programme is well established (such as after a 10-year interval).

Fig. 30.2 Annual age-adjusted incidence and mortality rates of invasive cervical cancer and detection rates of carcinoma *in situ* (Finland, 1953–1984). From Finnish Cancer Registry.

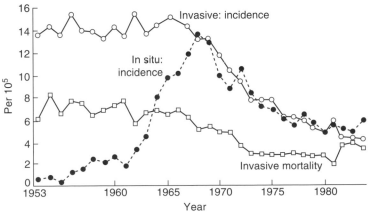

Geographic factors

Mortality and incidence rates have fallen very substantially in those countries in Scandinavia with a systematic screening programme when compared to those countries with opportunistic programmes (Figures 30.3 and 30.4). These show that Denmark, Finland, Iceland and Sweden achieved a more marked reduction in incidence and mortality than did Norway. Norway did not have a systematic screening programme.

However, global data would suggest a slight fall in the rates anyway. Within individual countries, some regions have implemented more comprehensive programmes than others, and this has been associated with significantly lower mortality and incidence rates than either national or other regional rates.

However, the cohort effect confounds evaluation of geographical trend comparison. In other words, the risk of cervical cancer may actually be very low in some societies and,

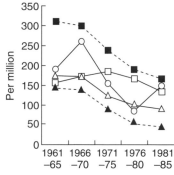

Fig. 30.4 Trends in the age-adjusted (world standard) incidence rates of invasive cancer in 1961–1985 in Denmark (■), Finland (▲), Iceland (◇), Norway (□) and Sweden (△). Reproduced from Hakama M, Magnus K, Pettersson F, Storm H, and Tilinius H.

therefore, the need for and impact of a screening programme may also be low (e.g. Middle Eastern countries).

Cohort studies

There are several such studies in the literature. They reveal a reduction in risk (as measured by odds ratios or relative risk models) for those who have been screened compared to those who have not (Tables 30.1–30.3).

One of the problems with cohort studies is that, as with all observational studies, the exposure (in this case screening) is self-selected; this means that those who elect to go for screening may differ from those who refuse. Those who refuse are almost invariably at higher risk

even in the absence of screening. The result of this is that cohort studies, as well as case control studies, tend to overestimate the benefit of screening. Data from the Finnish mass screening programme [6] support this. Table 30.1 shows that the relative risk of cervical cancer for the 15% of women who did not attend screening was 1.6 that of the unit risk of the total Finnish population just prior to the period of intensive screening. The relative risk for attendees, compared to the same population, was 0.2. The incidence rate for attendees was one-eighth that of non-attendees.

Screening intervals

A number of cohort and case-control studies estimate the risk of invasive cervical cancer in women who have been screened and relate this risk to the time interval since their last negative smear [6]. An approximation of relative protection is detailed in Table 30.2 [6].

Table 30.2 demonstrates that there is a protective effect from screening and that this is linked to the time interval since the last negative smear. If a woman has had a negative smear within 1 year, the relative risk of her developing cervical cancer is 0.1 (one-tenth) that of a woman who has never had a smear. The period of relative protection (inverse of relative risk) reduces with the

Fig. 30.3 Trends in the age-adjusted (world standard) mortality rates from cervical cancer in 1966–1985 in Denmark (●), Finland (■) and Norway (○). Reproduced from Hakama M, Magnus K, Pettersson F, Storm H, and Tilinius H.

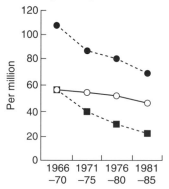

Table 30.1 Finnish mass screening programme – risk of cervical cancer

Population group	P (30–59)
Control	0.010[a]
Target population total	0.004
Attendee after first negative smear	0.002
Non-attendee after first invitation	0.016

[a]Total Finnish population prior to period of intensive screening.
Reproduced from Hakama M, Rasanan-Virtanen U. Effect of a mass screening programme on the risk of cervical cancer. *Am J Epidemiol* 1976;103:512–7.

Table 30.2 Screening intervals and risk of cervical cancer

Years since last negative smear	Relative risk	Relative protection (years)
1	0.1	10
2	0.15	7
3	0.2	5
4	0.3	3
5	0.4	3
6	0.5	2
7	0.6	2
10	0.7	1
>10	1.0	1

time interval since the smear was taken and there is no protective effect after 10 years. In general, these studies indicate a significant duration of relative protection of approximately 5 years, whilst there is some residual protection up to 10 years since the smear was taken.

The International Agency for Research in Cancer (IARC) Working Group [7] examined the relationship between screening schedules and the reduction in cervical cancer rates (Table 30.3). It is clear that intensive screening such as that performed annually offers the greatest reduction in cervical cancer rates (93%); however, the number of smear tests rises to 45 per woman per screening 'lifetime' and the efficiency of the screening programme reduces considerably. On the other hand, screening every 10 years is efficient, but the reduction in cervical cancer is of the order of 61%.

These data would suggest impressive protection from cancer afforded to those who are screened when compared to those who have not been screened. However, a cervical smear does not actually protect a woman from contracting cervical cancer. The actual test merely reveals or rules out a potentially cancerous or precancerous lesion. It is the treatment of this lesion which is protective for the few who actually have an abnormality.

Case-control studies

These studies compare cases with controls (women without cervical cancer) with respect to their prior history of screening for cervical cancer. Such studies have merits in that they are inexpensive, can be performed rapidly, and there is an explicit comparison group. However, they have many disadvantages, such as the selection of control groups, and recall bias by participating women. Case-control studies cannot determine the absolute risk of a woman developing cervical cancer and cannot control for the natural history of the disease being affected by the screening test. These studies may overestimate the benefit of screening in situations where (1) cases of invasive disease detected by screening are excluded because this results in a deficit of screen-detected cases, and (2) the effect of a possible selection bias because women at highest risk of developing cervical cancer are least likely to attend for screening. In spite of these difficulties and the fact that cervical screening has already been introduced in many countries, case-control studies are used in the evaluation process because randomized controlled trials have not been conducted.

In general, case-control studies demonstrate that women who develop cervical cancer (cases) are less likely to have had a smear test than those women without cervical cancer (controls). Approximately two-thirds of controls have had at least one screen compared to only 40% of cases. The overall relative risk of a woman who has had a smear developing cervical cancer is only 39% that of a woman who has never had a smear. Relative risk is also dependent on the time interval since the smear was taken (as demonstrated in Table 30.3).

Table 30.3 Screening for cervical cancer in developing countries: effect on cervical cancer incidence of different screening policies, starting at age 20[a]

Screening schedule	Cumulative rate, 20–64 per 10⁵	Reduction in rate (%)	Number of tests	Number of cases prevented per 10⁵ tests
None	3311.5			
Every 10 years, 25–64	1298	61	4	503
Every 10 years, 35–64	1476	55	3	612
Every 10 years, 45–64	1895	43	2	708
Every 5 years, 20–64	544	84	9	308
Every 5 years, 30–64	630	81	7	383
Every 3 years, 20–64	303	91	15	201
Every year, 20–64	216	93	45	69

[a]From IARC Working Group (1986) [7]; assuming incidence rates from Cali, Colombia. The first screening test is assumed to be 70% sensitive. DM Parkin, Cancer Screening, UICC 1991.

The question of the validity and effectiveness of cervical cytology has been addressed by a number of august bodies during the last 20 years, most notably by the IARC Working Group on Cervical Screening [8]. They concluded that systematic cervical screening is an appropriate and worthwhile preventive health policy.

Ensuring effectiveness in screening programmes

The general aim of any medical intervention is to achieve maximum benefit and minimum harm. This is even more important when considering preventive healthcare. In order to satisfy these general aims, specific ambitions and monitors should be instituted in association with any cervical screening programme, whether it be cytology, speculoscopy, cervicography or colposcopy. There may be good arguments for employing each of these in individual circumstances, but there is as yet very little hard evidence to support (or refute) the value of any of these in terms of effectiveness with the single exception of cervical cytology (Box 30.1). A number of countries have implemented systematic programmes. In the UK, a number of local or regional cervical cytology screening programmes were instituted on an *ad hoc* basis with varying degrees of success. In 1988, each health authority was instructed to introduce a cervical screening programme for women between 20 and 64 on a 5-yearly basis, to establish a computerized call and recall system, and to nominate a manager responsible for the organization and effectiveness of the programme. Later that year, a national co-ordinating network for the National Health Service Cervical Screening Programme (NHS CSP) was established. It comprised the UK Health Departments, health authorities, representatives/nominees of professional bodies and others. This body facilitated the adoption of common standards and working practices throughout the UK. Because of the considerable investments involved in the implementation of a systematic cytology screening programme, it is of crucial importance that the programme is both efficient and effective in achieving specific targets. A specific goal of the UK CSP is *to reduce the incidence of invasive cervical cancer by at least 20% before the year 2000* (i.e. from 15 per 100 000 population in 1986 to no more than 12 per 100 000).

In January 1996, this group reported the deliberations of a working party entitled 'Quality assurance guidelines for the cervical screening programme' [9]. Its recommendations are detailed in Box 30.2. The individual recommendations may vary according to local circumstances and available resources and as knowledge of the natural history of precancer evolves. However, as a template for quality assurance, they represent a sensible approach to achieving an effective, value for money investment for any community which has implemented a systematic cervical screening programme.

Precancerous lesions of the cervix: nomenclature

By any standards, the nomenclature of cervical precancer has had a confusing evolution. The traditional WHO classification discriminated between dysplasia and carcinoma *in situ* (the latter always expected to progress to invasion; the former sometimes). This system was then almost universally replaced by the cervical intraepithelial neoplasia (CIN) classification. Unfortunately, in the late 1980s, two further classification systems were introduced and these compete with each other. Table 30.4 relates these systems to each other.

Referral threshold for colposcopy

Where colposcopic facilities are available, it is mandatory to perform, or refer patients for, a colposcopic examination prior to treatment of cervical dysplasia (see Appendix).

Box 30.1   The smear (pap) test

Sampling the cervix is done using the appropriate sampler, preferably an extended tip spatula, either wooden (Aylesbury) or plastic (Rolon).

The endocervix can be specifically sampled using the Cytobrush. The special indications for use of the Cytobrush are:
- Squamocolumnar junction not visible
- After ablation of the cervical transformation zone
- In women over 45 years
- When a previous smear was inadequate

Box 30.2   Quality standards for cervical screening in the UK (From NHSCSP Publication No. 3 January 1996, with permission of NHSCSP)

OBJECTIVE	MEASUREMENT	ACCEPTABLE VALUE
1. To minimise the incidence of invasive cancer of the cervix.	Women aged 20–64 should be screened at least once every 5 years. Ascertainment of screening history of all women with cancer of the cervix.	>80% coverage of women aged 25–64. 100% of women with invasive cancer of the cervix audited.
2. To ensure effective sampling of the Transformation Zone.	Cytological evidence of sampling from the Transformation Zone in women aged 20–50 years.	>80% of smears contain metaplastic and/or endocervical cells.
3. All women to receive result in writing.	Proportion of women to receive result in 4 weeks from the date of smear taking. Proportion of women to receive result in 6 weeks.	>80% 100%
4. To ensure accuracy of smear reporting.	1. Sensitivity of primary screening with respect to final report after rapid review of all negative and inadequate smears. 2. Laboratory Report Profile: a) moderate/severe b) mild/borderline c) inadequate 3. PPV for moderate/severely dyskaryotic smears.	85–95% a) 1.6% ± 0.4 b) 5.5% ± 1.5 c) 7.0% ± 2.0 65–85% CIN2 or worse.
5. To ensure that all staff screening or reporting smears are competent.	Participation in UK proficiency testing scheme.	100% of staff to have acceptable performance.
6. To maintain and improve recommended standards and skills.	Number of screening programme slides processed/reviewed annually by: 1. Laboratory 2. Individual screeners (incl checkers) 3. Individual medical staff	>15 000 slides >3 000 per primary screener (not WTE) 7500 per WTE maximum >750 cases reported
7. To ensure that appropriate action is taken for all women with other than routine recall schedule.	Proportion of women with unknown outcome within 12 months.	<5%
8. To ensure prompt colposcopic assessment for women referred.	Waiting time for colposcopic assessment for all referrals. Waiting time for colposcopic assessment for women with moderately/severely dyskaryotic smears.	≥90% seen in < 8 weeks. ≥90% seen in <4 weeks.
9. To ensure the colposcopy service is of high quality.	1. No dyskaryosis on cytology in treated women at 6 months. 2. Number of women managed by each colposcopist.	≥90% >100 new cases per year
10. To minimise unnecessary treatment of women referred for colposcopy.	Proportion of women treated at the first visit who have evidence of CIN on histology.	≥90%

The usual indication for colposcopy will be the presence of an abnormal smear, suggesting a significant potential for progression to cervical cancer (i.e. ≥ moderate dyskaryosis; ≥ CIN II; high-grade squamous intraepithelial lesion).

The management of the mildly abnormal smear (low grade SIL) pap test

This is a common problem. An agreed and appropriate policy has not yet emerged. Authorities differ as to the optimal advice to offer these women. Some authorities advocate immediate referral in women with a smear reporting mild dyskaryosis (≤ CIN I or low-grade SIL), whilst others recommend continued cytological surveillance for 6, 12 or 18 months, and referral if the

Table 30.4 Cervical precancer classifications

BSCC systems	CIN system	Bethesda system
Negative	Normal	Within normal limits, benign cellular changes, infection, reactive and reparative changes
Action Line 1: repeat cytology/refer if auxiliary indication		
Borderline nuclear abnormalities (BNA)	BNA	Atypical squamous cells of undetermined significance (ASCUS)
Mild dyskaryosis	CIN I	Low-grade squamous intraepithelial lesion
Action Line 2: Always refer for colposcopy		
Moderate dyskaryosis	CIN II	High-grade squamous intraepithelial lesion
Severe dyskaryosis	CIN III	
Malignant		Squamous cell carcinoma
Glandular cell abnormality		Glandular cell abnormalities

BSCC = British Society of Clinical Cytology; CIN = cervical intraepithelial neoplasia.

cytological abnormality persists and progresses. Several factors prevent unequivocal and universal advice. Firstly, cytology laboratories have variable criteria for discriminating between borderline nuclear abnormality and mild cytological abnormality and normal cytology. The percentage of women harbouring moderate or severe dyskaryosis in the presence of mild cytological abnormality also varies from one study to another [10,11]. For example, in Flannelly's study in 1994, 57 of 174 women (33%) not treated for cytological evidence of CIN I or CIN II had normal cytology after 24 months of surveillance [11]. Furthermore, only 40 women who started the 2-year surveillance ($n = 158$) finished with a normal smear and were not treated, or did not default. In Kirby's 1992 study [10] on the other hand, 60% of 500 women with an abnormal smear reverted to cytological normality over a 7-year (median) follow-up surveillance. Similar studies arrive at different conclusions concerning the natural history of mild cytological abnormality. This can be partly explained by

the fact that these studies did not use the same entry criteria, methodology or outcome measures. The fact remains, however, that we have a poor understanding of the natural history of mild cytological abnormality. In the presence of such uncertainty, the management of women with CIN I or a borderline nuclear abnormality/low grade SIL, remains a conundrum. Secondary indications for colposcopy referral in the presence of a mild cytological abnormality might include patient anxiety, the risk of subsequent default at follow-up attendance, a clinically suspicious cervix, perhaps heavy smoking and, finally, the presence of oncogenic HPV types. None of these secondary screening tools have yet been properly evaluated.

The following suggestions are loose guidelines which are appropriate at this time and are likely to change as we learn more about CIN.

1. Women with a smear report suggesting the possibility of CIN II or worse should be referred for colposcopy.
2. Women with a smear

suggesting CIN I may be referred for colposcopy or kept under close cytological surveillance. Persistence or progression over a year to 18 months should precipitate referral.
3. The classification of smears should be based on the degree of *nuclear* abnormality which should take preference over comments on HPV. *Smears showing viral changes, but no nuclear abnormality, should be considered normal and the women recalled accordingly.*

Finally, counselling women *before* taking a routine smear will almost certainly reduce unnecessary anxiety for those women with a mild cytological abnormality for whom referral is not immediately indicated.

Other indications for colposcopy

Apart from cytological abnormality, there are several circumstances where colposcopy may be helpful. These include a symptomatic ectropion, a cervical polyp (both of which are very amenable to ablation or loop-diathermy excision), postcoital bleeding and a clinically suspicious looking cervix. Women with more than three inadequate smears also benefit from referral for colposcopy.

The colposcopic examination

Aims of colposcopy

Colposcopy facilitates low-powered light-illuminated

examination of the cervix and lower genital tract. The particular focus of attention in the context of CIN is the transformation zone of the cervix. The primary ambitions of a colposcopic examination are as follows:

- to delineate the transformation zone;

- to confirm (or refute) the cytological suspicion of dysplasia;

- to rule out (or recognize) microinvasive disease;

- to facilitate/plan treatment.

The transformation zone (T-Z)

The transformation zone is that area of epithelium which lies on the cervical surface between normal mature squamous epithelium and normal mature columnar epithelium. It comprises a number of cell types including squamous epithelium, metaplastic epithelium and columnar epithelium. The transformation zone derives its epithelium from original columnar epithelium which is undergoing metaplastic change to squamous epithelium in response to the vaginal environment (see Figure 30.1). This occurs because of the natural eversion associated with oestrogen during reproductive life. In normal circumstances, the T-Z is to be found on the ectocervix in the majority of women under 40 and in the endocervical canal in most postmenopausal women. It may be quite small, occupying only a few millimetres' diameter, or be

quite large, extending from the cervical os right out to the vaginal epithelium. For a further description of the transformation zone, the reader is referred to Cartier's *Atlas of Colposcopy* [12].

The T-Z is crucial to an understanding of colposcopy. Without being able to visualize its entire geography, colposcopy is unsatisfactory and, if treatment is indicated, a cone biopsy will be necessary. A total of 95% of cervical cancers are squamous and arise from the T-Z. The remaining 5% or less arise from just above and adjacent to the T-Z. Complete excision, or destruction of the T-Z is the objective of treatment for CIN in order to prevent cervical carcinoma.

Space does not allow for a comprehensive description of the colposcopic features of CIN and microinvasive carcinoma. A number of reference textbooks and atlases are available (see recommended reading). Colposcopic practice varies enormously throughout the world. In some European countries and in some parts of the USA colposcopic examination may be an integral part of the routine gynaecological examination. In the UK and other Commonwealth countries, on the other hand, colposcopy is usually confined to specialty colposcopy clinics run by clinicians with a special interest in lower genital tract neoplasia. Both these approaches have their advantages and disadvantages. The value of recognizing colposcopically evident pathology not revealed by cytology needs to be weighed against the inconvenience of the procedure, the dilution of

expertise which routine colposcopy entails and the risk of overtreatment or unnecessary treatment.

The emphasis of the colposcopic examination has changed over the last decade. Traditionally, the expert colposcopist would be particularly skilled at recognizing the difference between CIN II and CIN III, and between CIN III and microinvasive disease. To this end, the trainee colposcopist was encouraged to familiarize himself or herself with the subtle variations of acetic acid uptake and epithelial vascular patterns. Today, however, the treatment of CIN II, CIN III and microinvasive disease may be achieved by similar means (large loop excision of the transformation zone or LLETZ). The emphasis has perhaps shifted towards assessment of the milder intraepithelial abnormalities. In other words, today's colposcopist may be more concerned, *at a diagnostic level*, with the difficulty recognizing those mild lesions which have a significant chance of progressing to cancer. One skill which has not changed is the ability to demarcate the geography of the T-Z. Without the ability to do this, the colposcopist will have a high rate of overtreatment and/or undertreatment.

Treatment of cervical intraepithelial neoplasia

There are essentially two modalities of treatment for women with CIN – destruction or excision of the transformation zone. Hysterectomy is nearly always overtreatment and it risks leaving potentially dysplastic epithelium in the 4% of cases where the T-Z extends on to the vaginal epithelium. Also, if invasive disease is revealed in the hysterectomy specimen, appropriate treatment would have been compromised, whether this be radiotherapy or radical hysterectomy.

The incompletely visible transformation zone

Cone biopsy still has a crucial place in the armentarium of treatment. The indications for cone biopsy are as follows:

- an incompletely visible transformation zone in the presence of CIN II or worse;

- any suspicion of microinvasive squamous carcinoma;

- any suspicion of adenocarcinoma *in situ* or adenocarcinoma of the cervix;

- an unsatisfactory colposcopic examination in the presence of a significant cytological abnormality;

- significant disparity between cytology and colposcopy (i.e. cytology worse).

Whether the cone biopsy be performed by laser beam, LLETZ or straight wire excision of the transformation zone (SWETZ) is currently down to personal preference. Most cone biopsies may be performed under local anaesthesia. Cold knife cone biopsy has little to recommend it over laser or SWETZ cone.

When performing a cone biopsy, *it is important to remember* that:

1. when the transformation zone is not completely visible, its upper limit is likely to be ≥ 2 cm up the endocervical canal;
2. transecting the T-Z which contains microinvasive disease leaves the clinician with a difficult management dilemma;
3. a second cone biopsy is technically a more difficult procedure.

For these reasons it is *usually* preferable to remove 2–3 cm of cervical canal when performing a cone biopsy. This advice should of course be tempered by the patient's age, the cervical morphology and the particular indication.

Management of the fully visible transformation zone

In the majority of circumstances where treatment is indicated, the transformation zone will be fully visible and a simple choice may be made between excision (LLETZ/LEEP or laser excision) and destruction. Providing that certain conditions have been met, ablating the T-Z by any of the destructive techniques is entirely reasonable. The success/failure rate and complications associated with each of them do not differ significantly with the possible exception that radical diathermy may have a higher risk of cervical stenosis.

However, the ease, flexibility and security of local excision (LLETZ) has led to this method becoming the most popular modality of treatment in UK colposcopy clinics [13].

Finally, any differences in success rates which exist between the treatment methods described below are very much more likely to be operator-dependent rather than method-dependent.

A competent colposcopic assessment is the key to optimizing individual patient management.

Local destructive treatment

Before considering a local destructive method of treatment, certain criteria must be satisfied. These are detailed below.

- a competent colposcopic examination;

- a fully visible T-Z;

- histopathological examination of the most dysplastic epithelium within the T-Z;

- no cytological, colposcopic or histological suspicion of invasive disease;

- no cytological, colposcopic or histological suspicion of glandular disease;

- assurance of follow-up compliance.

A problem with these criteria is immediately apparent. They expect that it is always, or even usually, possible for a competent colposcopist to recognize the most dysplastic epithelium within the T-Z and to recognize the difference between CIN and microinvasive disease. Also they expect the colposcopist always to procure a biopsy of adequate size and quality that will allow the pathologist to make a definitive diagnosis. Unfortunately, none of these expectations is valid [14–16].

However, despite these concerns, locally destructive techniques continue to be employed successfully in many centres throughout the world. In competent hands, they have the specific advantages over conization of being highly effective office procedures for selective cases. Again, it should be stressed that the chance of inadequate treatment (or overtreatment) is more operator-dependent than method-dependent.

Radical diathermy

Usually performed under general anaesthesia, this electro-coagulation method was developed by Chanen [17] in Melbourne, who advocates a concurrent cervical dilation to prevent subsequent cervical stenosis. After outlining the transformation zone with Lugol's iodine, the T-Z is destroyed using needle diathermy destruction with multiple insertions 2 mm apart and 7 mm deep. After this, the surface epithelium is further coagulated using dessicative ball electrode coagulation. Some authorities advocate cold saline douching intermittently throughout the procedure in order to minimize heat artefactual damage.

Cryocautery

Popularized by Townsend [18] and others in the USA, cryocautery is an office procedure performed without analgesia. Using a variety of cryoprobes, the T-Z is destroyed using one or more applications for 3 min twice with a 5-min cooling

interval. The technique is now relatively uncommon because of concerns of temperature reduction consistency, depth of tissue destruction and the problem of post-cryocautery wound discharge.

Laser vaporization

This exceptionally expensive modality of destroying the T-Z has some advantages over other destructive methods in that laser may also be used to excise the T-Z, it may be used to treat vulval and vaginal lesions, and it is very exact in terms of depth. Its expense also means that it is usually only available in large devoted colposcopy clinics run by experienced colposcopists, where the level of expertise is likely to be high. The T-Z is usually vaporized to a depth of 8–10 mm as a cylindrical crater. It is usually performed under local analgesia [19].

Cold coagulation

Introduced by Semm, and popularized by himself and Duncan [20], cold coagulation is a misnomer as it achieves a temperature of 100°C. It has been called 'cold' to distinguish it from hot cautery (300°C). Treatment involves several overlapping applications of heated probes throughout the T-Z for approximately 20 s each. Depth of destruction is, like cryocautery, difficult to ascertain and, like cryocautery, the procedure may be associated with a subsequent post-treatment discharge from the cervical wound as the destroyed epithelium sloughs off. However, in protagonists' hands the results of treatment by cold coagulation – or any of the destructive methods – are excellent.

Large loop excision of the transformation zone (LLETZ/LEEP)

LLETZ is a simple technique whereby the T-Z is resected using a very thin wire loop and low-voltage fulgurative diathermy (Figure 30.5). The technique has been described in detail elsewhere [21,22]. The method is office-based, uses local infiltration and may be adopted for any transformation zone, including that requiring a cone biopsy. The advantages over destructive methods of treatment have been described by several authors [23–28].

The advantages of LLETZ, which is also known as loop excision, loop diathermy excision and (in the USA) loop electrosurgical excision procedure (LEEP), are summarized below.

1. It allows a comprehensive histological examination of the excised transformation zone such that:
   - microinvasive disease may be comprehensively ruled out;
   - excision of the entire T-Z may be confirmed or incomplete excision recognized;
   - colposcopic practice may be audited.
2. It may be performed at the first colposcopic visit.
3. It is adaptable to any circumstance where the T-Z needs to be treated, including cone biopsy.
4. It is an easily learned technique.
5. It uses inexpensive equipment with low operating costs.
6. It is an office procedure using local anaesthesia.

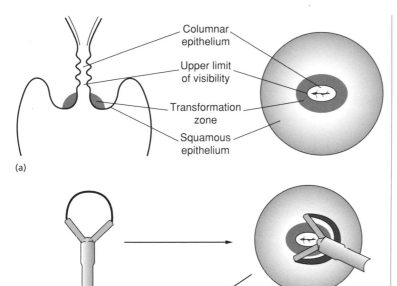

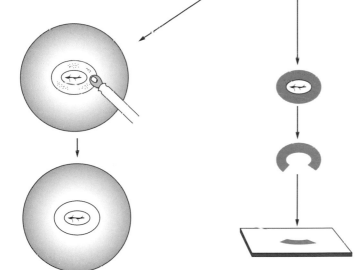

Fig. 30.5 Large loop excision of the transformation zone (LLETZ). (a) A fully visible transformation zone that is situated on the ectocervix or has an upper limit which lies just (< 0.5 mm) inside the ectocervical canal. Evidence of CIN with suspicion of microinvasion or glandular abnormality. Widest diameter not greater than 18 mm. (b) LLETZ excision of a small, fully visible ectocervical transformation zone. A medium loop is used for the procedure.

sufficient flexibility to accommodate transformation zones of every site and dimension, it is inevitable that women who would otherwise have had a cone biopsy will now have a LLETZ procedure. The morbidity of a cone biopsy (LLETZ, laser or cold knife) is related to the volume and also the amount of endocervical tissue excised. It is important that the morbidity associated with removal of a long endocervical transformation zone be recognized as a consequence of the size and site of the transformation zone, rather than of the choice of the excisional technique. Studies of fertility and pregnancy outcome following LLETZ have failed to show an adverse effect.

Ease of use

The method is technically straightforward and undemanding to an experienced and relatively dextrous colposcopist.

Cost

When compared with laser treatment, the method is less expensive. However, the other destructive modalities are equally inexpensive (cold coagulation, cryocautery and radical diathermy). Many of the electrosurgical units that are used for LLETZ may also be used for a variety of other gynaeco-logical procedures in the operating theatre.

Effectiveness

It is evident that a method of excising the transformation zone will have the same likelihood of successfully treating women with CIN as do the destructive techniques, and this has been

The last five of these advantages are also potential disadvantages of the technique that may actually combine to increase the morbidity of the procedure. Women may be treated more easily and at a lower threshold of abnormality in the office with local anaesthesia and with transformation zones of almost any dimension, situated on the ectocervix, in the endocervical canal or both. If more women are treated (at a lower threshold of suspected abnormality), then procedure-related morbidity will increase.

Because the technique allows

supported by the published series of patients treated with LLETZ. It is also true that LLETZ is unlikely to significantly improve on the success/failure rates of treatment achieved by the protagonists of each other destructive method of treatment. This is because the success/failure rates of destructive methods are high when performed by experts. However, women with CIN cannot always be treated by experts of individual destructive techniques. Perhaps a more clinically important question is whether LLETZ is associated with a superior success/failure rate compared with destructive methods, where each is performed by the non-specialized practising gynaecologist.

Follow-up after treatment

Colposcopy is a more sensitive follow-up tool than cytology alone; the latter has a higher specificity. Follow-up policies tend to be influenced by logistic considerations, pragmatism, fear of litigation and patient preference. The 'gold standard' is to have at least one colposcopic assessment 4–6 months post-treatment followed by cytological follow-up for 5 years in low-grade disease and 10 years for high-grade disease. Some protocols interpose a 'cytology' visit at 4 months followed by colposcopy at 8 months.

Treatment failure

The rate of margin involvement with CIN is influenced by the size of the lesion among other factors. Rates vary widely from 5% to 50%. However, around 20% of such patients prove to have histologically proven residual disease and are true treatment failures. This has to be balanced against the disadvantages of deep excision where cervical stenosis is a rare but important complication in 1–2% of cases.

Future developments

Automated screening

Computer-assisted automated screening of cervical cytology slides using so-called neural network technology (PaPnet) has been developed recently in the USA. The idea is to use a computer to sift through the 250 000 or so cells in a smear and identify the 128 most 'abnormal cells,' which are selected for video display to the screener, thus facilitating the task for cytotechnologists and reducing their 'boredom factor'. More importantly, the system may reduce the false-negative rate of screened cytology slides. Used for quality assurance in cytopathology units, automated screening may be cost-effective. It is recognized that the main cause of false negatives is sampling failure (in two-thirds of cases). The system itself has a false-negative rate of 4% and a false-positive rate of 10% [29].

Thin-layer technique

The procedure is to sample the cervix in the standard way, but to place the spatula/sampler material into a liquid preservative by agitating the sampler into the fluid. The preserving liquid destroys red blood cells, but preserves all other cells. The fluid is spun, thus separating the epithelial cells from white cells and other contaminants. The epithelial cells are transferred to a slide and fixed in the usual way and examined. Thus the cellular material should have a higher percentage of epithelial cells free of debris spread over a smaller area of the slide.

Features of thin-layer preparations are as follows.

- They reduce sampling error believed to be responsible for over half of false-negative cytology results.

- They reduce fixation errors as the slide is prepared and fixed in the laboratory.

- They reduce 'screening time' as a smaller 'spread' of cells needs to be examined.

- The liquid suspended sample can be used for HPV typing, immunofluorescent microbiological testing and other investigative purposes.

- They are expected to reduce false-positive and false-negative rates of cytology and eliminate operator factors.

The cost of consumables and requirements for training cytotechnicians may prohibit the routine use of this technique.

HPV detection and typing

Again this may be an adjunct to cervical cytology, although it is unlikely to have a primary role in screening. It may be useful in triaging patients with low-grade disease, to identify those to refer early for further assessment. With polymerase chain reaction and hybrid culture technology, the test achieves high sensitivity. HPV prevalence rates in young women (under 30) are very high. Therefore, the predictive value of oncogenic HPV typing becomes clinically useful only in women over 30 years. In these women, oncogenic HPV recognition should prove valuable.

Development of HPV vaccines

Two types of vaccine are being developed:

- vaccines for primary prevention of cervical neoplasia and HPV-generated abnormalities;

- vaccines to aid regression of CIN or to treat advanced cancer.

The potential of vaccines is immense, especially in preventing cancer in developing countries, but the technique is still in the early stages of development.

Tips for safe practice

- Any cervical screening programme is as good as its components. A 'failsafe' and quality assurance element should be incorporated within each component (primary care/community/ cytopathology units/ colposcopy/oncology).

- Communication between the various tiers of the programme should be such that women receive the same message and are informed about the expectations and aims of their screening.

- A prerequisite for ablating the cervical T-Z is a colposcopic assessment and histological confirmation of any abnormality.

References

1. Syrajnen K. Natural history of low grade SIL lesions. In: Monsonega J (ed.) Eurogin experts consensus conference. Paris: Eurogin Scientific Publications, 1995:10–17.

2. Ostor AG. Natural history of cervical intraepithelial neoplasia: a critical review. *Int J Gynecol Pathol* 1993;12:186–91.

3. Anderson M. Aetiology and natural history of cervical carcinoma. In: Anderson M, Jordan J, Morse A, Sharpe F (eds) Integrated colposcopy. London: Chapman & Hall, 1992.

4. McIndoe W, McLean MR, Jones RW, Mullins PR. The invasive potential of carcinoma in situ of the cervix. *Obstet Gynecol* 1984;64:451–8.

5. Wilson JMG, Jungner YG. Principles and practice of mass screening for disease. *Public Health Papers* No. 34. Geneva: World Health Organization, 1968.

6. Hakama M, Rasanen–Virtanen U. Effect of a mass screening programme on the risk of cervical cancer. *Am J Epidemiol* 1976;103:512–7.

7. IARC Working Group on Cervical Cancer Screening. Cancer occurrence in developing countries. Parkin DM (ed.). IARC Scientific Publications no. 75. Lyons: International Agency for Research on Cancer, 1986.

8. IARC Working Group on Cervical Cancer Screening. Summary chapter. In: Screening for cancer of the uterine cervix. IARC Scientific Publications no. 76. Lyons: IARC, 1986:133.

9. Report of a Working Party Convened by the NHS Cervical Screening Programme. Pritchard J (Chairman). Sheffield: NHSCSP Publication no. 3, January, 1996.

10. Kirby AJ, Spiegelhalter DJ, Day NE, Fenton L, Swanson K, Mann EMF, McGregor JE. Conservative treatment of mild/moderate dyskaryosis: long term outcome. *Lancet* 1992;339:828–31.

11. Flannelly G, Anderson D, Kitchener HC, Mann EMF, Campbell M, Fisher P, Walker F, Templeton AA. The management of women with mild and moderate cervical dyskaryosis. *Br Med J* 1994; 308:1399–403.

12. Cartier R, Cartier I. Practical colposcopy. Laboratoire Cartier, 20 rue des Condelieres, F 75013 Paris, 1993.

13. Kitchener HC, Cruickshank ME & Farmery E. The 1993 British Society for Colposcopy and Cervical Pathology/National Co-ordinating Network United Kingdom Colposcopy Survey. *Br J Obstet Gynaecol* 1995;102:549.

14. Benedet JL, Anderson GH and Boyes DA Colposcopic accuracy in the diagnosis of microinvasive and occult invasive carcinoma of the cervix. *Obstet Gynecol* 1985;65:557–62.

15. Howell R, Hammond R and Pryse-Davies J The histologic reliability of laser cone biopsy of the cervix. *Obstet Gynecol* 1991;29:410–412.

16. Cartier I, Richart R, Wright T. The evolution of loop diathermy in cervical disease. In: Prendiville W (ed.) Large loop excision of the transformation zone: a practical guide to LLETZ. London: Chapman and Hall Medical, 1993;25–33.

17. Chanen W and Rome RM Electrocoagulation diathermy for cervical dysplasia and carcinoma in situ: a 15 year survey. *Obstet Gynecol*; (1983) 61:673–679.

18. Townsend DE, Richart RM. Cryotherapy and carbon dioxide laser management of cervical intraepithelial neoplasia: a controlled comparison. *Obstet Gynecol* 1983; 61:75–8.

19. Anderson MC. Treatment of cervical intraepithelial neoplasia with the carbon dioxide laser: report of 543 patients. *Obstet Gynecol* 1982: 59;720–725.

20. Duncan ID. The Semm cold coagulator in the management of cervical intraepithelial neoplasia. *Clin Obstet Gynecol* 1983; 26:996–1006.

21. Prendiville W, Cullimore J, Norman S. Large loop excision of the transformation zone (LLETZ). A new method of management for women with cervical intraepithehal neoplasia. *Br J Obstet Gynaecol* 1989; 93:773–776.

22. Prendiville W. Large loop excision of the transformation zone. In: Prendiville W (ed.) Large loop excision of the transfonnafion zone: a practical guide to LLETZ. London: Chapman and Hall Medical, 1993;42.

23. Murdoch JB, Grimshaw RN, Monaghan JM. Loop diathermy excision of the abnormal cervical transformation zone. *Gynecol Cancer* 1991;1:105–11.

24. Whiteley PF, Olah KS. Treatment of cervical intraepithelial neoplasia: experience with low voltage diathermy loop. *J Obstet Gynecol* 1990;162:1272–7.

25. Luesley DM, Cullimore J, Redman CWE, et al. Loop diathermy excision of the cervical transformation zone in patients with abnormal cervical smears. *Br Med J* 1990;300:1690–3.

26. Anderson M. Selection of patients for treatment – the British view. In: Prendiville W (ed.) Large loop excision of the transformation zone: a practical guide to LLETZ. London: Chapman and Hall Medical, 1993:83.

27. Bigrigg MA, Codling BW, Pearson P, Read NM, Swingler GR. Colposcopic diagnosis and treatment of cervical dysplasia at a single clinic visit: experience of low-voltage diathermy loop in 1000 patients. *Lancet* 1991; 336:229–31.

28. Carter PG, Harris VG, Wilson POG. The management of the abnormal cervical smear: a comparative study between loop diathermy alone and laser ablation preceded by colposcopically directed punch biopsy. *J Obstet Gynecol* 1993;13:59–6.

29. Hussain NA, Butler B, Nayagam M, et al. An analysis of the variation of human interpretation; PaPnet – a mini challenge. *Analyt Cell Pathol* 1994;6:157–63.

Further reading

- Cartier R, Cartier I. Practical colposcopy, 3rd edn. Laboratoire Cartier, 20 rue des Cordelieres, F 75013 Paris, 1993.

- Anderson M, Jordon J, Morse A, Sharp F. A text and atlas of integrated colposcopy. London: Chapman and Hall Medical, 1992.

UK NHSCSP publications

- No. 1: Achievable standards, benchmarks for reporting and criteria for evaluating cervical cytopathology. Report of a Working Party set up by RCPath, BSCC and NHSCSP, Sheffield, October 1995

- No. 2: Standards and quality in colposcopy. Luesley, D (ed.). January 1996.

- No. 3: Quality assurance guidelines for the cervical screening programme. Report of a Working Party Convened by the NHS Cervical Screening Programme. Pritchard J (Chairman). January 1996.

- No. 5: Improving the quality of the written information sent to women about cervical screening. Guidelines on the presentation and content of letters and leaflets. Austoker et al.

UK NHS Cervical Screening Programme

- Report of the first five years of the NHS Cervical Screening Programme. National Co-ordinating Network, October 1994.

- Assuring the quality and measuring the effectivenes of cervical screening. National Co-ordinating Network, October 1994.

- The role of genitourinary medicine cytology and colposcopy in cervical screening: does the GU female population merit a different cytology/colposcopy strategy? August 1994.

Other publications/resources

- Burghardt E. Colposcopy – cervical pathology. Textbook and atlas. (2nd revised and enlarged edition). Stuttgart: Georg Thieme, 1991.

- Prendiville W (ed.) Large loop excision of the transformation zone: a practical guide to LLETZ. London: Chapman and Hall Medical, 1993.

- Clinical Obstetrics and Gynecology. Volume 38, Number 3, September 1995. New York: Lippincott–Raven.

- The American College of Obstetricians and

Gynecologists publishes patient education leaflets. Contact ACOG at 409 12th Street SW, Washington, DC 20024–2188, USA.

- The American Society of

Colposcopy and Cervical Pathology publishes The Colposcopist. Contact the national office at 6900 Grove Road, Thorofare, New Jersey 08086, USA.

Appendix

Colposcopy ± biopsy **Management options**

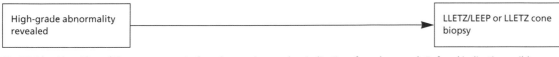

Fig. 30.A1 Algorithm of the management of an abnormal smear (see indications for colposcopy). Referral indication: mild cytological abnormality (≤ CIN I/low grade SIL). NAD = no abnormality detected; LLETZ = Large loop excision of the transformation zone; T-Z = transformation zone.

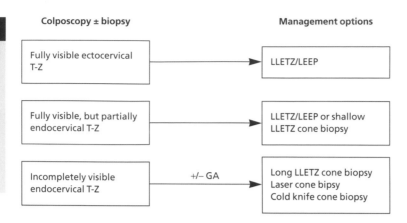

Colposcopy ± biopsy

Fully visible ectocervical T-Z	→ LLETZ/LEEP
Fully visible, but partially endocervical T-Z	→ LLETZ/LEEP or shallow LLETZ cone biopsy
Incompletely visible endocervical T-Z	+/– GA → Long LLETZ cone biopsy / Laser cone bipsy / Cold knife cone biopsy

Management options

Fig. 30.A2 Algorithm of the management of an abnormal smear (see indications for colposcopy). Referral indication: a high-grade lesion suspected cytologically, i.e. ≥ CIN II. High grade SIL. GA = glandular atypia; T-Z = transformation zone; LLETZ = large loop excision of the transformation zone.

These algorithms accommodate the usual circumstances of women presenting to the colposcopist. They do not accommodate every eventuality and are not cast in stone. They are useful as a guide.

Screening for ovarian and endometrial cancers

David Oram FRCOG

Arjun Jeyarajah MA MRCOG

Introduction

The World Health Organization (WHO) has established requirements for prospective screening programmes [1]. A modified version of these requirements is given below.

- Is the condition an important health problem?

- Is there a recognizable early stage?

- Is treatment at an early stage more beneficial than at a later stage?

- Is there a suitable test?

- How often should screening take place?

- Which subgroups should be screened?

- Is the test acceptable to the population?

- Are there adequate facilities for diagnosis and treatment?

- What are the costs and benefits?

These recommendations form the basis of guidelines on cancer screening of the UK Co-ordinating Committee on Cancer Research. This chapter examines how these criteria can be applied to ovarian and endometrial malignancies.

Ovarian cancer

The concept of earlier diagnosis of epithelial ovarian cancer has become a real possibility during the last decade. Towards the end of the 1990s, we hope to be in a position to assess whether screening for epithelial ovarian cancer should be offered as a routine service, along the lines of cervical and breast cancer screening. Ovarian cancer screening programmes are still in their relative infancy and further research is needed to ensure that such programmes can fulfil these criteria prior to their widespread implementation.

Is the condition an important health problem?

In the UK and the USA ovarian cancer is the fourth most common cause of cancer mortality in women. Worldwide approximately 140 000 women develop ovarian cancer each year. In the USA the annual incidence is 26 000 and over 12 000 die every year of the disease. Ovarian cancer is the most common cause of death from genital tract malignancies in the Western world.

The most recent data indicate that over 5800 women develop the disease in the UK each year, with more than 4000 deaths [2]. These data confirm that it is the commonest gynaecological cancer in the UK and it kills more women each year than all of the other gynaecological malignancies combined. Furthermore, in spite of improvements in surgical and chemotherapeutic techniques which may give rise to longer periods of remission, the overall 5-year survival is variously quoted between 20% and at best 30%, a figure that has changed little during the past 30 years.

The risk factors for ovarian cancer are as follows:

- nulliparity and delayed childbearing (oral contraception and breast feeding are protective);

- early menarche;

- family history/autosomal dominant inheritance;

- possibly the use of fertility drugs.

The poor survival rates for women with epithelial ovarian

cancer can be directly correlated with the stage of the disease at presentation. Figure 31.1 illustrates the frequency with which the disease presents in each stage and the associated 5-year survival rate. It is particularly noteworthy that the most significant factor associated with good outcome is presentation, whilst the disease is still confined to the ovary (FIGO stage 1). In such patients when a thorough histological search has been made to exclude metastatic disease, survival rates in excess of 90% have been reported [3]. Conversely, once metastases have occurred, the chance of success for therapy decreases proportionately. These observations form the basic rationale for the quest to develop a screening programme which would effect a stage shift in the yet to be proven belief that earlier diagnosis and intervention may have a positive impact on survival.

Is there a recognizable early stage?

Figure 31.2 shows a model which illustrates the progression that is universal to epithelial tumours and it is logical to apply this to ovarian cancer. However, the biological behaviour of ovarian cancer in its early stages remains a mystery and the natural history of preclinical disease is poorly documented. A preinvasive condition has not been identified and the malignant potential of benign ovarian cysts remains uncertain. Methods of screening for ovarian cancer must, therefore, necessarily be directed at the detection of asymptomatic but invasive disease. The situation is further compounded by the fact that the duration of this preclinical screen-detectable stage of ovarian cancer is unknown but in all probability is highly variable.

Is treatment at an early stage more beneficial than at a later stage?

Although data exist which confirm the ability to detect certain ovarian cancers as much as 2 years prior to their clinical presentation [4], whether this knowledge can be translated into an improvement in survival figures is unknown. The question of whether early detection and intervention confers a survival benefit or merely highlights the effects of lead time and length bias can only be answered by the performance of a randomized controlled trial. Until such a study has reported its findings, all evidence concerning the efficacy of potential screening tests and programmes is indirect.

Is there a suitable test?

The reason that such a randomized controlled study has not yet been performed is because doubts exist as to the adequacy of the currently available tests. The requirements of a screening test for ovarian cancer are necessarily rigorous because the consequence of a positive test is surgical investigation. Such invasive procedures are inevitably associated with psychological and occasionally physical morbidity. Consequently, the primary requirement of any screening procedure for ovarian cancer is extremely high specificity in order to ensure an acceptable positive predictive value

PPV = true positives/true positives + false positives × 100%.

The definition of an acceptable positive predictive value is arbitrary but a working definition is a minimum level of 10% (i.e. nine false-positive procedures for each case of ovarian cancer detected). It is unlikely that a test with a positive predictive value of less than 10% would be acceptable to clinicians, patients or indeed, the state.

The demand for very high specificity is compounded by the relatively low incidence of ovarian cancer in the general population. This requires that any screening test should have an adequate detection rate for preclinical disease. The sensitivity required to have an impact on survival, however, is difficult to estimate and again can only be

Fig. 31.1 The rationale for screening for ovarian cancer.

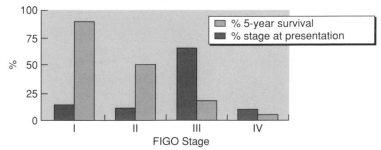

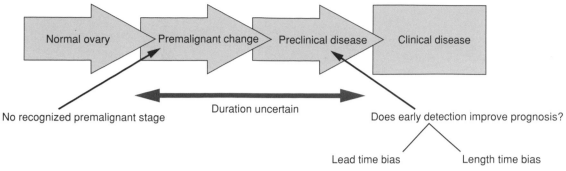

Fig. 31.2   Is ovarian cancer a suitable disease for screening?

determined by a randomized controlled trial. Nevertheless, it is reasonable to assume that an effective screening test will detect at least 50% of ovarian cancers at least 1 year prior to clinical presentation.

The tests

Bimanual pelvic examination

The main advantages of pelvic examination as a screening test for ovarian cancer are its relatively low cost, the ease with which it may be performed, and that it does not require specialist equipment. Although at the time of clinical presentation ovarian cancer is almost invariably associated with abnormal findings on pelvic examination, it is unlikely that palpable abnormalities will be detectable sufficiently in advance of clinical presentation for treatment to influence outcome. The specificity of pelvic examination for ovarian cancer varies with a woman's age and menopausal status. An enlarged ovary in a postmenopausal woman must be considered pathological but the ability of the assessment to distinguish benign from malignant disease is extremely limited. Equally, although studies

to assess the sensitivity of pelvic examination as a screening test for ovarian cancer are few, it is unlikely that the detection rate of early stage, small volume disease is sufficient to make it suitable for use in the general population.

Ultrasound

There is no doubt that ultrasound is capable of diagnosing ovarian cancer prior to its clinical presentation. The first ultrasound screening study reported by the King's College Hospital group [5] recruited 5479 volunteers and undertook 15 977 transabdominal scans. Five ovarian cancers, all stage 1, were identified, two in the first and three in the second year of screening. The sensitivity of the modality was reported as 100%. However, the positive predictive value for primary ovarian cancer at laparotomy following an abnormal scan was only 1.5%.

The advent of the transvaginal probe has improved the resolution of morphological imaging. Transvaginal ultrasound is an acceptable examination that takes 5–10 minutes to perform. It can be placed closer to the organs being studied, higher frequency ultrasound can be used and clearer images produced. It has been employed in combination

with pulsed colour-flow Doppler and also with morphological scoring indices in an attempt to improve the specificity of ultrasound screening. Specificity remains a real problem. A review of the most significant studies [5–7], reveals that over 300 laparotomies have been performed in order to detect 13 cancers. Furthermore, 50% of the ovarian cancers detected in these studies were of the borderline variety, which in all probability is a reflection of length bias, as these are indolent tumours with an associated excellent prognosis. Their identification prior to clinical presentation consequently will have little impact on overall mortality.

The quest to improve the positive predictive value of ultrasound screening has led to the use of colour Doppler and morphological scoring systems. Whilst specificity can be increased with these secondary techniques, the sophistication in terms of expertise, equipment, time and expense that would be necessary to reproduce acceptable results on a wider scale would require a massive investment in training and technology. Also it begs the question of what really should be advised in the case of postmenopausal women who are found to have cystic ovarian enlargement which does not demonstrate an abnormal blood flow pattern.

For all these reasons, whereas ultrasound screening may be ideal for high-risk individuals from ovarian cancer families, when high sensitivity is desirable and lower specificity is acceptable, for the general population its ideal use in any screening strategy is as a second-line test.

Serum tumour markers

The concept of performing serum assays to detect circulating marker substances produced by the tumour is attractive because such an approach is simple and reproducible. With second-line ultrasound examination being required in only a small proportion of cases, the economic implications are also potentially favourable. The most important and extensively studied serum marker for ovarian cancer is the CA 125 antigen. CA 125 is a high molecular weight glycoprotein recognized by a murine monoclonal antibody OC 125; it was first described in 1983 [8]. Serum levels in excess of 35 U/ml are recorded in over 80% of patients with surgically proven ovarian cancer in contrast to 1% of healthy blood donors.

CA 125 levels in the serum have been used to monitor disease status in terms of response to chemotherapy [9] and as a predictor of relapse [10] (Box 31.1). CA125 status has also been incorporated into a Risk of Malignancy Index in association with an ultrasound score and menopausal status [11] in order to predict the nature of an adnexal mass in the preoperative period

> **Box 31.1 Uses of CA 125 screening**
>
> - Identification of early ovarian cancer in asymptomatic women (only cost effective in postmenopausal women)
> - Investigation of an ovarian mass
> - Monitoring therapy
> - Predicting relapse

(see Appendix also). The use of CA 125 as a screening test for preclinical ovarian cancer is supported by the findings of a retrospective study of the Janus serum bank, which has demonstrated that approximately 50% of cases have elevated levels of the marker (>30 U/ml) as much as 18 months before clinical diagnosis [4]. Against this is the observation that only approximately 50% of cases of stage 1 ovarian cancer have elevated serum CA 125 levels at the time of diagnosis [12]. This apparently restricted sensitivity of CA 125 in early-stage small-volume disease would appear to limit its potential usefulness in a screening context.

The stepwise combination of CA 125 and ultrasound in a prospective multimodal study of 22 000 postmenopausal volunteers has been reported by Jacobs et al. [13]. The design of the Royal London Hospital study is shown in Figure 31.3. The details of the CA 125 assay (CA 125 radioimmunoassay; Abbott Laboratories, Chicago, USA) used in this study are as follows: the detection limit of the assay was 7 U/ml, and the intra-assay and interassay coefficients of variation at 30 U/ml were 8.5% and 9.1%, respectively.

This very large study confirms the exceptionally high specificity of this combination of tests (99.8%), consequently the positive predictive value for ovarian cancer at laparotomy was 26%.

However, the apparent sensitivity for the detection of preclinical ovarian cancer at 1 year was only 78%, and this fell to around 50% at 2 years (Figure 31.4).

These data highlighted the need to improve the sensitivity of tumour marker screening. This can be achieved by reducing the assay threshold, by serial screening with a shorter screening interval, or by the use of multiple, complementary markers. Reducing the assay threshold inevitably compromises specificity and is therefore an unacceptable option. The enormous serum bank accumulated during the last 10 years of screening at the Royal London Hospital (RLH) is a valuable resource which permits ready and rapid evaluation of new tumour markers as they emerge. Unpublished data generated by this resource have demonstrated that the most useful of these is a combination of CA 125 and OVXI. Data from Woolas et al. [14] suggest that OVXI is complementary to CA125, being raised in approximately 50% of cases of ovarian cancer that are CA 125 negative.

The observation that CA 125 levels increase with time in screen-detected ovarian cancer patients has led to the development of a mathematical algorithm [15] which is able to discriminate between ovarian cancer and non-ovarian cancer patients. The risk of ovarian cancer (ROC) is calculated from absolute and serial values of CA

Objectives

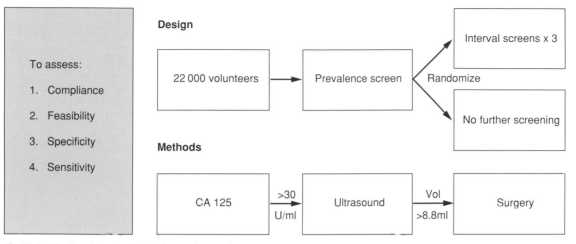

To assess:

1. Compliance
2. Feasibility
3. Specificity
4. Sensitivity

Design

22 000 volunteers → Prevalence screen → Interval screens x 3

Randomize → No further screening

Methods

CA 125 → >30 U/ml → Ultrasound → Vol >8.8ml → Surgery

Fig. 31.3 The Royal London Hospital screening study.

125, and is valid even within the normal range, thereby improving the sensitivity of primary tumour marker screening even further.

The combined use of serum CA 125, with transvaginal ultrasound as a secondary test for use as dictated by the ROC algorithm, is a formula which achieves the required specificity and sensitivity to permit its use as a screening strategy.

How often should screening take place?

The frequency of screening in this disease is unknown, but a screening interval of more than 1 year is unlikely to be effective. Data (as yet unpublished) of 19 false-negative cases in the RLH study demonstrate that only three cases occurred within 1 year of a negative screening test using CA 125 alone.

Which subgroups should be screened?

The objectives of screening are twofold: to have a positive impact on mortality in the general population; and to protect individuals who are at particularly high risk. In the general population, in women over the age of 45, the incidence of

ovarian cancer is 1 in 2500 women per year. The relative risk increases with increasing age and this fact, together with the knowledge that both tumour markers and ultrasound are less open to misinterpretation in the postmenopausal period, dictates that, in the general population, screening should be targeted at women over the age of 50. The benefits of screening the general population are, however, as yet unproven, and for as long as this is the case, screening should only be offered as part of a research protocol.

Familial ovarian cancer accounts for about 3% of cases. Individuals with one first-degree relative with the disease have a risk of developing ovarian cancer themselves which is increased 2–3 times over the general population. This risk may be even greater when the index case was diagnosed before the age of 50. Within this group there is an even smaller cohort who belong to families where a striking pattern of hereditary cancer exists. In these rare hereditary ovarian cancer syndromes (see

Fig. 31.4 Performance of the screening strategy utilizing CA 125 and ultrasound in a sequential fashion.

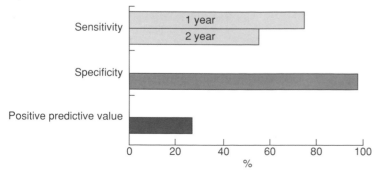

Box 31.2), the inheritance of an autosomal dominant gene of variable penetrance might increase the lifetime risk to 50–80% with the disease appearing at a much younger age. The siblings and children of an affected individual have a 50% risk of inheriting the disease trait.

In populations with this level of risk, most screening options can achieve an acceptable PPV. The most sensitive options are vaginal ultrasonography or the combination of CA 125 and OVXI. It should be regarded as unethical to include women with this level of risk in a randomized controlled trial. They should, therefore, be offered screening with either ultrasound or tumour markers, and trials comparing the performance of these two screening strategies in this high-risk group are required. Screening should not employ both ultrasound and tumour markers as first-line tests because the combined false-positive rates of both tests are likely to reduce the PPV below 10%, even in a population with a high incidence of ovarian cancer.

In women with a family history which does not constitute an ovarian cancer syndrome, the incidence of ovarian cancer may be in the region of 200 per 100 000 per year. At this level of risk a satisfactory PPV may be achieved by either vaginal ultrasonography and Doppler imaging, or the sequential use of

tumour markers and ultrasound. It would be reasonable to include this group of women in randomized controlled trials to assess the impact of screening on ovarian cancer mortality.

Is the test acceptable to the population?

Following the prevalence screen of 22 000 women, the design of the Royal London Hospital screening study required that a pilot randomization was performed which recalled 11 000 women for annual incidence screening for 3 years, while the remaining 11 000 were followed up with postal questionnaires.

Unpublished data, including a detailed analysis of the last study, demonstrate that the overwhelming majority of women attended all three screening episodes with a further significant number attending for at least two out of the three screens. It was felt that this high compliance rate demonstrated the widescale acceptability of this screening strategy.

Are there adequate facilities for diagnosis and treatment?

The initial venepuncture for tumour marker measurement is a simple and easily accepted procedure. With the standardization of modern

radioimmunoassays, tumour marker measurement may be carried out in most modern laboratories. Following the initial tumour marker screen, approximately 1.5% of patients will be recalled for transvaginal ultrasound. Of these, only a small proportion require surgical intervention. In the RLH study, of the 22 000 women screened 341 were recalled for ultrasound examination following the prevalence screen and, of these, only 42 required surgery. These cases were diffused by time and geography and, with a disease of this prevalence, the implications of screening should not add undue burdens to any individual hospital department or facility.

What are the costs and benefits?

The precise costs of any given screening strategy are not known and ultimately will be affected by final assay costs. However, Box 31.3 provides an example of the approximate costs involved and, although these appear to be expensive per case of ovarian cancer diagnosed, they are comparable to the costs involved in breast cancer screening.

The benefits of ovarian cancer screening in the general population are unproven and require a prospective randomized controlled trial to be performed on a large scale. The performance of the screening tests currently available is now of sufficient standard both in terms of sensitivity and PPV to justify such a trial being undertaken. At St Bartholomew's Hospital, London, last year, the trial outlined in Figure 31.5 was launched. It is

---

Box 31.2 Inherited ovarian cancer syndromes

- Breast/ovarian cancer syndrome – the most common
- Lynch type II – proximal colon carcinoma + ovarian carcinoma + endometrial carcinoma
- Site-specific ovarian cancer syndrome – least common; the risk is confined to ovarian carcinoma

Box 31.3 The economic feasibility of screening for ovarian cancer

Annual cost of screening (£– postmenopausal women)

Cost per primary screen £10 × 100 000	1 000 000
Cost per secondary screen £30 × 3000	90 000
Cost of false-positive surgery £1000 × 200	200 000
Total cost of screening	*1 290 000*
Cost per individual screened £1.29 m/100 000	13
Cost per ovarian cancer £1.29 m/40	32 250
Cost per ovarian cancer detected £1.29 m/30	43 000

hoped to recruit 40 000 women a year for 3 years with a mean duration of follow-up of 6 years. On completion of this trial, it is hoped that the question of outcome benefit in terms of reduced mortality as a result of this ovarian screening strategy will be known.

Endometrial cancer

Introduction

In contrast to other gynaecological malignancies, the indications for screening in endometrial cancer are less certain. The reason for this is that the vast majority of women present with stage I disease with the tumour confined to the uterus with an associated excellent prognosis. In this respect, the potential of screening to produce a stage shift and mortality benefit becomes less relevant. Thus, the role of screening of the general asymptomatic population is not justifiable. However, several high-risk groups have been identified, and it has become apparent that a role for the screening and early detection of endometrial neoplasms in these women may assume greater importance. In considering a potential role for screening in endometrial cancer, the WHO criteria shown on p. 403 may be applied to this disease.

Is the condition an important health problem?

Endometrial cancer is the second most common gynaecological malignancy in the UK, accounting for approximately 4000 new cases per year. Although endometrial cancer has widely been regarded as a cancer with a relatively good prognosis, this is true only for favourable histological types and early-stage disease. Well-differentiated tumours confined to the uterine corpus with minimal myometrial invasion are associated with a 5-year survival in excess of 90%. However, there are certain aspects of this disease that are worthy of consideration and would suggest that endometrial cancer is a more important health problem than is immediately apparent. Poorly differentiated and adenosquamous tumours are frequently associated with deep myometrial invasion, regional lymph node involvement and advanced stage. The 5-year survival rates for stage III and IV

Fig. 31.5   A randomized controlled study of screening for ovarian cancer.

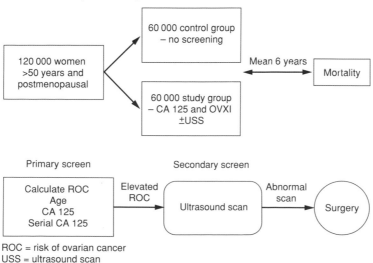

ROC = risk of ovarian cancer
USS = ultrasound scan

disease are only 30% and 10.6%, respectively, and the overall 5-year survival for endometrial cancer is a disappointing 65%. Indeed, 25% of women with endometrial cancer will die of recurrent disease within 5 years.

Is there a recognizable early stage?

In considering the existence of an early/preinvasive stage in endometrial cancer, the role of unopposed oestrogenic stimulation and the concept of progression of simple hyperplasia through atypical hyperplasia to adenocarcinoma are well established in the aetiology of sporadic endometrial cancer [16,17]. It is known that less than 2% of hyperplasia without cytological atypia progresses to carcinoma, no matter how architecturally complex, whereas 23% of hyperplasia with cytological atypia (atypical hyperplasia) progresses to carcinoma [18].

Is treatment at an early stage more beneficial than at a later stage?

The identification and treatment of atypical hyperplasia should have an impact on decreasing the incidence of invasive disease. However, it should be noted that, as illustrated in Figure 31.6, it is likely that at least some poorly differentiated endometrial cancers may be unrelated to endometrial hyperplasia and to oestrogen exposure, and may have a more direct route from benign to malignant epithelium [19,20].

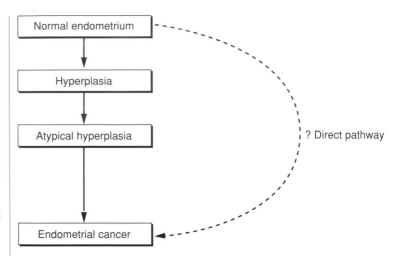

Fig. 31.6   The majority of cases of endometrial cancer are thought to develop in a background of hyperplasia. It is possible that direct transformation of benign endometrium to less well differentiated and more aggressive phenotypes of endometrial cancer may also occur.

Is there a suitable test?

Transvaginal ultrasound

Using transvaginal ultrasound to measure the endometrial thickness, it has been shown that a thickness of greater than 5 mm in a postmenopausal woman is strongly associated with endometrial pathology, including endometrial hyperplasia and cancer [21,22]. However, the specificity for the preclinical diagnosis of endometrial cancer is limited and may in part be due to the focal development of some lesions in an otherwise thin endometrium.

The use of transvaginal colour Doppler for the diagnosis of endometrial cancer has been described [23]. In a study that attempts to screen asymptomatic women for ovarian and endometrial cancer with transvaginal colour and pulsed Doppler sonography, Kurjak et al. demonstrated that it was indeed possible to diagnose early endometrial cancers using this technique [24]. The sensitivity and specificity of this strategy has not been evaluated.

Outpatient endometrial sampling

A variety of sampling devices are available that may be passed through an undilated cervix into the endometrial cavity. In a study assessing the efficacy of the Pipelle endometrial biopsy device, a disappointingly low sensitivity for the detection of endometrial hyperplasia and early stage, small volume, well-differentiated tumours with minimal myometrial invasion was encountered [25]. However, other studies have shown that the Pipelle is just as effective as curettage at obtaining a tissue specimen [26]. The Vabra and Novak curette vacuum aspirator's have been shown to be as accurate when endometrial histology results are compared [27].

Hysteroscopy and curettage

This has been the standard method of sampling the

endometrium. There is evidence to suggest that curettage may not be any more reliable than outpatient biopsy techniques at obtaining an accurate histological diagnosis. Hysteroscopy increases the sensitivity and specificity of dilatation and curettage. The advantage of direct visualization of the endometrial cavity is that focal areas of hyperplasia or carcinoma may be visualized and biopsied under direct vision. It is now possible to perform hysteroscopy as an outpatient procedure utilizing fine-diameter hysteroscopes and fibreoptic technology. The sensitivity of cervical smears for the detection of endometrial pathology is insufficient to consider it as a potential screening method.

How often should screening take place?

The optimal time interval between screens is unknown but is unlikely to be more than 1 year.

Which subgroups should be screened?

Women being treated with tamoxifen

Antioestrogens have a role in the treatment of breast cancer and are potentially useful in the treatment of other oestrogen-dependent neoplasms such as endometrial cancer. However, an excess of endometrial malignancies has been documented in patients taking tamoxifen for the prevention of recurrent breast cancer [28]. This observation is consistent with the partial agonist activity of tamoxifen in endometrial tissue [29]. Other

histopathological changes in the uterus associated with tamoxifen have been described, including polyps, proliferative and hyperplastic endometrium [30]. Tamoxifen causes a significant increase in endometrial thickness measured ultrasonographically, which correlates with an increase in abnormal endometrial histology including adenocarcinoma [31].

Women with a family history of endometrial cancer

The best documented form of familial endometrial cancer occurs as part of the Lynch II syndrome. The Lynch II syndrome describes a subgroup of the hereditary non-polyposis colorectal cancer (HNPCC) syndrome in which colorectal, endometrial, breast and ovarian tumours are inherited in an autosomal dominant fashion [32,33]. Table 31.1 illustrates the increase in risk associated with carriers of a mutation predisposing to HNPCC and also that of first-degree relatives. As can be seen, screening may be justified in this group of the population.

This syndrome only accounts for a small proportion of endometrial cancers but recent studies raise the possibility that a

further group of endometrial cancers may have a hereditary basis. The relative risk of endometrial cancer is also significantly elevated in the family members of probands with breast cancer [34].

Women with a high risk profile

It is well recognized that the triad of diabetes, hypertension and obesity are risk factors for the development of endometrial cancer. There have been suggestions that such women should be screened for the development of endometrial neoplasms. Gronroos et al. screened 597 asymptomatic women with the above risk factors by Vabra aspiration [35]. They found that regular mass screening of asymptomatic women with diabetes over the age of 45 years was indicated. The study did not indicate that similar screening would be effective for women with hypertension.

Given that the indications for screening the general population for endometrial cancer are debatable, it would appear that efforts should be directed at the detection of atypical hyperplasia and/or more accurate assessment of the symptomatic woman. It is well recognized that only 15% of

Table 31.1 Risk of endometrial cancer in putative gene carriers of mutations may justify screening measures or prophylactic hysterectomy. A detailed family history is essential for accurate risk assessment

	Mean age at diagnosis	Cumulative risk to age 50 years	Cumulative risk to age 70 years
General population	61 years	1%	3%
Putative carriers of mutation predisposing to HNPCC	46 years	15%	30%
First-degree relative of putative gene carrier		5%	15%

HNPCC = hereditary non-polyposis colorectal cancer.

women who present with postmenopausal bleeding eventually have a diagnosis of endometrial cancer. More efficient subselection of women who are actually at risk based on nulliparity and other personal details combined with ultrasound and outpatient biopsy information may lead to a decrease in the proportion of women subjected to an 'unnecessary' general anaesthetic.

Is the test acceptable to the general population?

The techniques used are eminently acceptable to most women. Transvaginal ultrasound is often preferred to abdominal ultrasound owing to the fact that a full bladder is not required. Outpatient sampling devices can be easily passed through an undilated cervix even in nulliparous patients with minimum discomfort. Very occasionally in postmenopausal women with atrophic changes, difficulty may be encountered in obtaining an adequate sample.

Are there adequate facilities for diagnosis and treatment?

Transvaginal ultrasound and endometrial sampling devices are available in most general hospitals and thus are easily provided to a wide section of the population. Doppler equipment is expensive and the skills required are rather specialized, thus limiting the potential for the widespread use of this modality.

What are the costs and benefits?

No information is available regarding the potential cost–benefit aspects of screening for endometrial cancer.

Future directions

It is expected that in the future it will be possible to screen for genetic changes associated with premalignant conditions, e.g. atypical hyperplasia and early invasive disease. At present the Ki-*ras* oncogene provides the best

model for this approach to screening for endometrial cancer. Although Ki-*ras* mutations only occur in 15–30% of endometrial cancers, they do appear to be early events in endometrial carcinogenesis [36]. The uterine cavity is easily sampled and it may be feasible to use the power of molecular genetic techniques, such as the polymerase chain reaction, to identify early cancers by detecting a small number of mutated copies of a gene from cancer cells in a background of many thousand-fold excess wild-type copies of the gene in normal cells.

Acknowledgements

The authors are indebted to Mr Ian Jacobs, Consultant Gynaecological Oncologist and co-director of the Ovarian Cancer Screening Unit at St Bartholomew's Hospital, for the use of data from the unit. We also wish to thank previous research fellows in the unit, Ann Prys-Davis and Robert Woolas, whose MD theses have been an invaluable reference source in the preparation of this chapter.

References

1. Wilson JMG, Jungner G. Principles and practice of screening for disease. Public Health Papers no. 34. Geneva: World Health Organisation, 1968.

2. Cramer DW, Hutchinson GB, Welch WR, et al. Determinants of ovarian cancer risk 1: reproductive experiences and family history. *J Natl Cancer Inst* 1983;71:711–6.

3. Young RC, Walton LA, Ellenberg SS, et al. Adjuvant therapy in stage I and stage II epithelial ovarian cancer. *N Engl J Med* 1990;322:1021–7.

4. Zurawski VR, Orjaseter H, Andersen A, et al. Elevated serum CA 125 levels prior to diagnosis of ovarian neoplasia: relevance for early detection of ovarian cancer. *Int J Cancer* 1988; 42:677–80.

5. Campbell S, Bhan J, Royston, et al. Transabdominal ultrasound screening for early ovarian cancer. *Br Med J* 1989;299:1363–7.

6. van Nagell JR, DePriest PD, Puls LE, et al. Ovarian cancer screening in asymtomatic postmenopausal women by transvaginal sonography. *Cancer* 1991;68:458–62.

7. Bourn TH, Campbell S, Reynolds KM, et al. Screening for early familial ovarian cancer with transvaginal ultrasonography and colour flow imaging. *Br Med J* 1993;306:1025–9.

8. Bast RC, Klug TL, St John E, et al. A radioimmunoassay using a monoclonal antibody to monitor the course of epithelial ovarian cancer. *N Engl J Med* 1983; 309:169–71.

9. Redman C, Blackledge GR, Kelly K, et al. Early serum CA 125 response and outcome in epithelial ovarian cancer. *Eur J Cancer* 1990;26:593–6.

10. Vergote I, Bormer O, Abeler VM. Evaluation of serum CA 125 levels in the monitoring of ovarian cancer. *Am J Obstet Gynecol* 1987;157:88–92.

11. Jacobs IJ, Oram DH, Fairbanks J, et al. A risk of malignancy index incorporating CA 125, ultrasound and menopausal status for the accurate preoperative diagnosis of ovarian cancer. *Br J Obstet Gynaecol* 1990;97:922–9.

12. Jacobs IJ, Bast RC. The CA 125 tumour-associated antigen: a review of the literature. *Hum Reprod* 1989;4:1–12.

13. Jacobs IJ, Prys Davies A, Bridges J, et al. Prevelence screening for ovarian cancer in postmenopausal women by CA 125 measurement and ultrasonography. *Br Med J* 1993;306:1030–4.

14. Woolas RP, Xu FJ, Jacobs IJ, et al. Elevation of multiple serum markers in patients with stage I ovarian cancer. *J Natl Cancer Inst* 1993;85:1748–52.

15. Skates SJ, Xu FJ, Yu YH, et al. Toward an optimal algorithm for ovarian cancer screening with longitudinal tumor markers. *Cancer* 1995;76(10 Suppl.): 2004–10.

16. Kurman RJ, Kaminski PF, Norris HJ. The behavior of endometrial hyperplasia. A long-term study of 'untreated' hyperplasia in 170 patients. *Cancer* 1985;56:403–12.

17. Gordon MD, Ireland K. Pathology of hyperplasia and carcinoma of the endometrium (review). *Semin Oncol* 1994; 21:64–70.

18. Hunter JE, Tritz DE, Howell MG, et al. The prognostic and therapeutic implications of cytologic atypia in patients with endometrial hyperplasia. *Gynecol Oncol* 1994;55:66–71.

19. Deligdisch L, Cohen CJ. Histologic correlates and virulence implications of endometrial carcinoma associated with adenomatous hyperplasia. *Cancer* 1985; 56:1452–5.

20. Deligdisch L, Holinka CF. Progesterone receptors in two groups of endometrial carcinoma. *Cancer* 1986;57:1385–8.

21. Nasri MN, Shepherd JH, Setchell ME, et al. The role of vaginal scan in measurement of endometrial thickness in postmenopausal women. *Br J Obstet Gynaecol* 1991;98:470–5.

22. Sheth S, Hamper UM, Kurman RJ. Thickened endometrium in the postmenopausal woman: sonographic–pathologic correlation. *Radiology* 1993; 187:135–9.

23. Kurjak A, Shalan H, Sosic A, et al. Endometrial carcinoma in postmenopausal women: evaluation by transvaginal color Doppler ultrasonography. *Am J Obstet Gynecol* 1993;169: 1597–603.

24. Kurjak A, Shalan H, Kupesic S, et al. An attempt to screen asymptomatic women for ovarian and endometrial cancer with transvaginal colour and pulsed doppler sonography. *J Ultrasound Med* 1994; 13:295–301.

25. Ferry J, Farnsworth A, Webster M, et al. The efficacy of the pipelle endometrial biopsy in detecting endometrial carcinoma. *Austl NZ J Obstet Gynaecol* 1993;33:76–8.

26. Stovall TG, Photopulos GJ, Poston WM, et al. Pipelle endometrial sampling in patients with known endometrial carcinoma. *Obstet Gynecol* 1991;77:954–6.

27. Stovall TG, Solomon SK, Ling FW. Endometrial sampling prior to hysterectomy [published erratum appears in *Obstet Gynecol* 1989;74:105]. *Obstet Gynecol* 1989;73:405–9.

28. Fornander T, Rutqvist LE, Cederrnark B, et al. Adjuvant tamoxifen in early breast cancer: occurrence of new primary cancers. *Lancet* 1989;1:117–20.

29. Lyman SD, Jordan VC. Possible mechanisms for the agonist actions of tamoxifen and the antagonist actions of MER-25 (ethamoxytriphetol) in the mouse uterus. *Biochem Pharmacol* 1985;34:2795–806.

30. Friedl A, Jordan VC. What do we know and what don't we know about tamoxifen in the human uterus (review). *Breast Cancer Res Treat* 1994;31:27–39.

31. Kedar RP, Bourne TH, Powles TJ, et al. Effects of tamoxifen on uterus and ovaries of postmenopausal women in a randomised breast cancer prevention trial. *Lancet* 1994;343:1318–21.

32. Lynch HT, Watson P, Kriegler M, et al. Differential diagnosis of hereditary nonpolyposis colorectal cancer (Lynch syndrome I and Lynch syndrome II). *Dis Colon Rectum* 1988; 31:372–7.

33. Watson P, Lynch HT. Extracolonic cancer in hereditary nonpolyposis colorectal cancer. *Cancer* 1993;71:677–85.

34. Tulinius H, Egilsson V, Olafsdottir GH, et al. Risk of prostate, ovarian, and endometrial cancer among relatives of women with breast cancer. *Br Med J* 1992; 305:855–7.

35. Gronroos M, Salmi TA, Vuento MH, et al. Mass screening for endometrial cancer directed in risk groups of patients with diabetes and patients with hypertension. *Cancer* 1993;71:1279–82.

36. Jeyarajah AR, Oram DH, Jacobs IJ. Molecular events in endometrial carcinogenesis. *Int J Gynecol Cancer* 1996;6:425–38.

Appendix

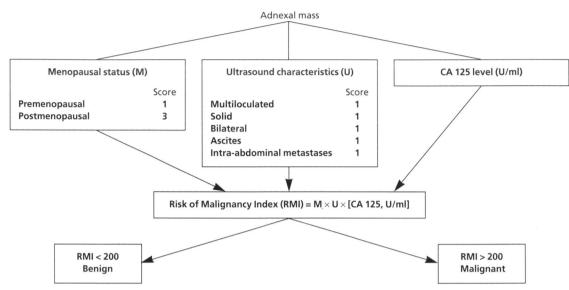

Fig. 31.A1   Flow chart for the management of adnexal masses.

Screening issues in male genital tract cancer

John P Pryor MS FRCS

Introduction

The goal of screening for cancer is the detection of the tumour before there are symptoms in the expectation that early treatment will reduce mortality and morbidity. At present there are no screening programmes for male genital cancers and it is for this reason that this chapter is concerned with screening issues.

The relative incidence of tumours of the penis, testis and prostate is shown in Table 32.1. Malignant tumours of the penis and testis are uncommon, treatment is often effective and, whilst early detection improves the prognosis for the individual, the incidence of the tumours is too low for this to affect overall population mortality rates. Carcinoma of the prostate is common, more new cases being diagnosed each year than carcinoma of the lung. It is readily diagnosed, but there is still controversy as to whether early treatment is beneficial and the cost of screening may be too high.

Carcinoma of the penis

Squamous cell carcinoma of the penis usually occurs in the preputial groove or inner surface of the prepuce of an uncircumcized man with a phimosis. The tumours are uncommon (Table 32.1) and there is a good deal of geographical variation in the incidence. In the past it was rare before the sixth decade but younger men are now being seen with this tumour. Its rarity precludes screening programmes but the following issues are highlighted.

Aetiological factors

Penile hygiene

Poor penile hygiene is the traditional cause for carcinoma of the penis. All men should be encouraged to retract the foreskin when bathing or showering. Failure to retract the foreskin in adult life is an indication for circumcision. It is thought that smegma might contain a carcinogen but this has never been proven.

Circumcision

This is one of the oldest operations and is depicted in ancient Egyptian hieroglyphs. It may be performed for religious (in Jews and Muslims), social or medical reasons. In 1975 the American Academy of Paediatrics determined that the procedure offered no medical benefit and should be discontinued, but in 1989 it revised its opinion and stated that newborn circumcision has 'potential medical benefits and advantages as well as disadvantages and risks'. This change of opinion was based upon a 10% increase in the risk of upper urinary tract infections in uncircumcised infants when compared to those who had been circumcised. Subsequent studies [1] have shown a 5–89-fold increased risk of infection in the uncircumcised and none have shown a decreased risk. Circumcision for religious reasons is not funded by the UK National Health Service.

Table 32.1 Incidence and mortality of male genital cancers in England and Wales (1989)

	Incidence (per 100 000)	Mortality (per 100 000)
Prostate	50.7	33.5
Testis	5.1	0.4
Penis	1.5	<0.5

It has been suggested that the risk of sexually transmitted diseases is less in circumcised men [2] but the evidence for this is not conclusive [3,4]. Carcinoma of the penis is almost unheard of in those circumcised at birth, rare in those circumcised during childhood and uncommon in those who have not been circumcised. The disadvantages of circumcision are small when the operation is performed by a physician at the time of birth using specially devised devices. Substandard circumcision – particularly when performed by non-medical personnel – is on rare occasions fatal (death from the anaesthetic or haemorrhage) and more frequently associated with excision of too much skin, amputation of the glans penis or fistula formation.

Some men suffer a great deal of stress on account of what they consider to be a mutilation carried out at birth and without their consent. They seek conservative (preferable) or surgical means of uncircumcision and such operations were common in the early years of Christianity.

In England, circumcision is currently performed on religious grounds or medical indications, but, in the USA, social circumcision remains common [5].

Viral infection

The clinical association between carcinoma of the penis and cervix was noted in 1969, and there is now evidence that human papillovirus (HPV) may cause penile tumours [6]. Condyloma acuminatum (HPV types 6 and 11) are common and occasionally form the large exuberant cauliflower-like growth known as the Buscke–Lowenstein tumour. This tumour has malignant features and may be locally invasive, but it rarely metastasizes and may be treated by local excision.

Squamous carcinoma of the penis in younger men may be the result of HPV 16, 18 or 33, and probably explains the association with carcinoma of the cervix. Kaposi's sarcoma of the penis is sometimes associated with human immunodeficiency virus (HIV) infections.

Premalignant lesions

Bowen's disease, erythroplasia of Queyrat and Paget's disease are all flat velvety lesions that may occur on the glans penis or elsewhere on the penile shaft. They are considered to be premalignant, and clinical and histopathological differentiation of these lesions may be difficult. Paget's disease may occasionally be associated with an underlying carcinoma of the prostate or bladder, but otherwise the aetiology of these lesions is unknown.

Diagnosis and treatment

The clinical presentation of a blood-stained discharge and a phimosis should alert the clinician to the possibility of a penile tumour. Unfortunately, many of the men presenting with carcinoma of the penis present late and they are often sexually inactive, elderly and shy.

A dorsal slit or circumcision is performed to enable the lesion to be biopsied and with small tumours, circumcision may be curative. The local tumour may be controlled surgically by either direct excision, Mohs' micrographic excision or by laser. Radiotherapy – external beam, mould or radioactive implantation – is often effective in controlling the tumour and has the advantage of preserving the organ for sexual function. Extensive tumours involving the corpora cavernosa require radical amputation of the penis but the prognosis is poor once the disease has spread to the vascular erectile tissue. Tumour spread is initially to the regional lymph nodes (inguinal). Treatment of suspicious nodes is surgical but should be delayed until any infection associated with the primary lesion has settled. Radiotherapy and chemotherapy are used for palliative purposes.

Prognosis

Early tumours have a relatively good prognosis with a 70–95% 5-year disease-free survival. If there is extensive invasion of the corpora, 5-year survival falls to 30–50% and death is inevitable with soft tissue or bony metastases.

Good sexual function is possible [7] provided that the penile length remains greater than 7 cm but phalloplasty is necessary for young men with a shorter stump.

Testicular tumours

Malignant tumours of the testis are rare but they are the most common solid tumours in men aged 15–35. The prognosis has improved dramatically over the past three decades owing to a better understanding of the tumour and the advent of effective chemotherapy. There are differences of nomenclature (Box 32.1) and treatment of testicular tumours between Europe and the USA, but although differences in terminology remain, the treatment policy has become more similar.

For practical purposes all testicular tumours are considered to be malignant as the 'benign' Sertoli cell and Leydig cell tumours are very uncommon. Bilateral tumours in elderly men are usually lymphomas and the remaining tumours, which occur predominantly in 15–50-year-old men, are classified as germ cell tumours.

Incidence

The incidence of germ cell tumours of the testis has doubled in Europe during the past 30 years and continues to rise [8,9]. This increase has not been observed in the USA. Despite this, such tumours remain uncommon with an incidence of 2–5 per 100 000 men and it is much lower in both American

and African Blacks (0.9:100 000). A man has been calculated as having a lifetime risk of 1:500 of developing a testicular tumour [8]. However, in young adult men, germ cell tumours are the most common cancers encountered.

Aetiological factors
(Table 32.2)

Testicular maldescent
The incidence of testicular maldescent is increasing. The increased risk of malignancy in undescended testis is well recognized and is thought to be 1:100 for a unilateral maldescent and 1:50 for bilateral maldescent, accounting for 10% of testicular cancer. The risk is highest with an intra-abdominal testis, particularly when associated with XY dysgenesis. Orchidopexy lowers the risk of a testicular tumour developing but does not remove it completely, and there is also a risk of tumour occurring in the contralateral testis.

Testicular atrophy
This is often stated to be a factor and may account for germ cell tumours occurring after mumps

orchitis, epididymo-orchitis or testicular torsion. Testicular carcinoma *in situ* (intratubular germ cell neoplasia) is a premalignant lesion found in 0.5% of the testicular biopsies of infertile men but only when there is evidence of impaired spermatogenesis. Such testes are usually atrophic but a testicular biopsy is not a good screening test [10].

Familial predisposition
There is a small but definite risk of occurrence in the offspring of men with testicular tumours. Foreman [11] calculated a 10% relative risk of a brother of an index case developing a testicular germ cell tumour.

Oestrogen exposure In utero
The administration of oestrogens to the mother increases the risk of testicular neoplasm in the offspring by 2–5 times. More recently, a Swedish study [12] showed that indicators of high levels of pregnancy oestrogens such as maternal age, high placental weight and low parity, imparted an increased risk of testicular cancer, which was mainly the occurrence of seminoma. Neonatal jaundice was also associated with an increased risk of testicular tumours.

Environmental oestrogen exposure
The harmful effect of oestrogen exposure on spermatogenesis was highlighted by Carlsen in 1992 [13] and, since that time, evidence has accumulated that environmental oestrogens may be responsible for the increasing incidence of testicular abnormalities including cancer

---

Box 32.1 Classification and relative incidence of testicular tumours (US nomenclature in brackets)

Usually benign
- Sertoli cell tumour — 1.2%
- Leydig (interstitial) cell tumour — 1.6%

Malignant
- Seminoma — 39.5%
- Non-seminomatous germ cell tumours — 47.0%
  - Malignant teratoma intermediate
  - Malignant teratoma undifferentiated (embryonal carcinoma)
  - Yolk sac tumour
  - Combined seminoma/teratoma
  - Malignant teratoma (trophoblastic chorioncarcinoma)
- Malignant lymphoma — 6.7%

Miscellaneous — 4.0%

Table 32.2 Risk factors for testicular tumours

Factor	Relevance
Testicular maldescent	Definite – even in contralateral testis
Testicular atrophy	Probable – worth self-examination
Familial incidence	Uncommon but does occur
Intrauterine oestrogen exposure	Likely but significance uncertain now that oestrogens not prescribed to pregnant women
Environmental oestrogen exposure	An increasing cause for concern
Vasectomy	No proven association

[14]. It is now thought that the problem is not confined to oestrogenic steroids but applies also to phytoestrogens or to environmental oestrogens that affect the oestrogen receptor mechanisms but whose structure differs from that of the classical steroid hormones. The term 'oestrogen disruptors' [15] has been coined for this activity. The antiandrogen activity of a metabolite of dichlorodiphenyl trichloroethane (DDT) may also act as an endocrine distruptor [15].

Vasectomy and testis cancer

In 1987 it was suggested that testicular cancer might be associated with vasectomy [16]. Two Scottish studies of 1764 and 3079 vasectomized men suggested that there was a relative risk of testis cancer of 2.1 and 4.2, respectively, compared with controls. However, larger studies in Oxford and the USA of 13 246 and 14 607 vasectomized men showed no increase in testicular cancer [17,18].

Diagnosis of testicular germ cell tumours

The traditional teaching that all tumours of the testis itself are malignant still holds true and young men should be encouraged to examine themselves. Delay in diagnosis increases the risk of metastatic disease [19]; all adolescents should be taught to self-examine the testes and alerted to the significance of painless enlargement. A total of 80% of patients present with symptoms of enlarged, heavy and/or painful testes. Confusion may arise from other scrotal swellings such as chronic epididymo-orchitis or cystic swellings, such as spermatocoeles, epididymal cysts or a hydrocoele, although the latter may be associated with a tumour. Some cases present with an 'acute' orchitis picture or post-traumatic 'haematoma'. Most testicular tumours are pain free and only rarely would a patient present with lumbar or abdominal pain, cough or haemoptysis. Gynaecomastia may occur as a result of hormonal production in an undifferentiated malignant teratoma.

Scrotal ultrasound is a rapid, available and non-invasive means of confirming the diagnosis of a testicular tumour with good sensitivity and specificity. Blood should also be taken for testicular tumour markers: β-HCG, alphafetoprotein, lactate dehydrogenase or placental alkaline phosphatase. These may not be positive in all patients but a fall to zero following orchidectomy is a good omen, and a subsequent rise indicative of metastatic disease.

Management of germ cell tumours of the testis

This is a highly specialized area and, after the initial inguinal orchidectomy, treatment is best carried out in a multispecialty setting. Inguinal orchidectomy is the primary treatment of choice and the subsequent management depends upon the histology and stage of the tumour. Monitoring tumour marker levels is used to predict metastatic disease. The prognosis is excellent for seminoma and even with bulky metastases 90% of patients survive. These tumours are sensitive to both chemotherapy and radiotherapy.

The prognosis is not so good for non-seminomatous germ cell tumours and more aggressive chemotherapy is indicated. Patients with stage I disease and testicular histology associated with poor prognosis require early prophylactic chemotherapy. The advent of effective chemotherapy has improved survival with metastatic teratoma by 70% over the past two decades. Earlier arguments over the relative merits of radiotherapy (European) or retroperitoneal node dissection (North American) have been largely abandoned and lymph node dissection is now reserved for residual masses.

The reduction of treatment morbidity and maintaining quality of life are now even more important as survival is assured for most patients. Sperm banking should be considered in those patients without children before orchidectomy or chemotherapy. Semen quality may be impaired at the time of presentation but in some patients it improves following orchidectomy. Retroperitoneal node dissection or the excision of residual masses should be 'nerve sparing' so that ejaculation is not abolished. Ejaculatory failure following retroperitoneal node dissection is best treated by the surgical retrieval of sperm from the vas deferens and these may be used in assisted conception therapy protocols.

The loss of a testis in young single men may be associated with impairment of body image and it is worthwhile implanting a testicular prosthesis for such men. Finally, men with bilateral orchidectomy will require long-term hormone replacement therapy with androgen patches, tablets, monthly injections or a 6-monthly hormone implant.

Prostate cancer

Adenocarcinoma of the prostate is an important public health problem as it is a common tumour and its incidence is increasing. It is already more common than lung cancer and it is estimated that it will soon cause more deaths (Table 32.3). It would therefore seem sensible to screen for prostate cancer but this is not done because of the costs and lack of agreement as to the relative merits of radical treatment or watchful waiting for early disease. These issues will be examined in this section but readers are also referred to one of several recent monographs for further information [20].

Table 32.3 Total cases of and mortality from carcinoma of lung and prostate in the US Cancer Registry

Year	Lung		Prostate	
	Cases	Deaths	Cases	Deaths
1992	102 000	93 000	132 000	34 000
1994	96 000	95 400	244 000	40 400
1995	98 900	94 400	317 000	41 400

Incidence

The incidence of prostate cancer increases with age (Table 32.4) and the classical autopsy study of Franks in 1954 [21] found evidence of prostate cancer in 30% of 50–59-year-old men and 67% of 80–90-year-old men dying of other causes. In the USA, 75 000 men were diagnosed as having prostate cancer in 1983, there were 132 000 new cases in 1992 and it was estimated that there would be 317 000 in 1996 owing to widespread prostate cancer screening in the USA. In total, 2–3% of all men will die from the disease.

The increasing number of men being diagnosed as having prostate cancer is due to a combination of better detection – by the measurement of prostate specific antigen and due to more frequent surgery for benign prostatic hypertrophy – and an ageing population. It remains to

Table 32.4 Age-specific incidence of prostate cancer in England and Wales [22]

Age group (years)	Incidence (per 100 000 population)
50–54	7.5
55–59	29.7
60–64	80.9
65–69	158.9
70–74	315.1
75–79	468.3
70–84	621.3
85+	723.5

be seen whether the increased detection will change mortality rates [22].

Aetiological factors
(Table 32.5)

Genetic

There is good evidence to suggest that there is a 5–10-fold increased risk of prostate cancer in those men with a family history. The tumour may develop at an earlier age and a good case could be made for screening the sons of men with prostate cancer with regular prostate specific antigen assays. Screening should start after the age of 40 years. There have been some recent observations to suggest that there may be genetic changes in prostatic cancer. Such abnormalities may in future serve to identify a group of susceptible men who should be screened.

Hormones

Carcinoma of the prostate is dependent on circulating androgens and the mainstay of treatment has been androgen deprivation. Prostate cancer does not occur in men with severe hypogonadism and isolated case reports have appeared of 30–40-year-old men on high doses of testosterone who have developed prostate cancer at a young age. The precise role of androgens in initiating prostatic cancer remains unclear and the relevance of a

Table 32.5 Aetiological factors in prostate cancer

Factor	Comment
Genetic	Men with a close family history should have a regular PSA screening when 40 years old
Hormones	Tumour is androgen dependent; rare in castrate; recorded in body builders on androgens
Diet	Possible benefits from low animal fat diet with plenty of yellow or green vegetables
Sexual activity	Avoid early sexual intercourse, sexually transmitted diseases and multiple partners?
Environmental factors	Industrialization may lead to increased exposure to oestrogen-like activity
Vasectomy	Link not proven
Benign prostatic hypertrophy	No proven link

PSA = prostate specific antigen.

recent study suggesting a connection with perinatal hormonal exposures is uncertain [23].

Diet
Differences in the geographical incidence of prostate cancer have been related to diet. American and European men on diets that are rich in animal fats and relatively low in vegetables have a much higher incidence of the tumour than that found in Asia, where the diet contains less animal fat and a higher content of yellow and green vegetables.

Sexual activity and sexually transmitted diseases
There is some evidence to suggest that sexual activity commencing at a younger age, a history of sexually transmitted disease and multiple sexual partners are all risk factors associated with prostate cancer. The significance of these factors is uncertain and they may be related to other hormonal or social factors.

Environmental factors
Prostate cancer is more common in urban than rural life, and men of the same ethnic group who move from a low-risk to a high-risk environment have an increased risk of prostatic cancer. These factors, operating in this instance, may be similar to those discussed under testicular tumours.

Vasectomy
The possibility that sterilization by vasectomy might predispose to prostate cancer caused widespread alarm when the studies were first published [24,25]. The methodology of these studies was questioned and it was with some relief that subsequent studies have been unable to show such an association [26,27]. It has been suggested that changes in hormonal levels after vasectomy might occur and be an aetiological factor. Numerous studies performed over the past 20 years have failed to show any consistent alteration in hormonal levels, particularly when allowance is made for the increasing age of the individuals.

Benign prostatic hypertrophy
Benign prostatic hypertrophy and prostatic cancer are both common in ageing men and it is therefore to be expected that they will often coexist. The conditions arise in different parts of the prostate gland and there is no good evidence to show that one predisposes to the other.

Diagnosis

Clinical presentation
Deterioration in the urinary stream occurs as men age and is usually due to benign prostatic hypertrophy. The symptoms of prostatism (hesitancy, poor stream, terminal dribbling and nocturia) may also occur in men with prostatic cancer. Additional symptoms due to complications of outflow obstruction – bladder instability and urinary incontinence, retention of urine or chronic renal failure – may also occur. In many men the prostatic neoplasm is asymptomatic and all the symptoms are due to benign hypertrophy.

Local invasion by the tumour may cause haematuria, haemospermia and/or decreased semen volume. Local nerve invasion may cause perineal pain or ureteric obstruction can cause loin pain. Erectile failure and rectal symptoms may also occur as a result of local invasion.

Carcinoma of the prostate metastasizes readily to both the pelvic lymph nodes (usually silent), to bone to cause osteosclerotic deposits – a common cause of backache in the elderly and a rare cause of paraplegia – and may also produce anaemia, weight loss and cachexia.

Digital rectal examination (DRE)
This is the traditional method of diagnosing prostatic cancer and is

clearly dependent on the skill and experience of the examiner [28]. Overall detection rates of 5% have been reported and as a screening test the sensitivity is between 55% and 69%, with a specificity of 89–97% and positive predictive values of between 11% and 26%.

Many of the tumours detected by digital rectal examination are too advanced for curative treatment and tumours detected at repeat examination have a worse prognosis, probably because they are growing more rapidly. Digital rectal examination alone is an unsatisfactory method of screening for prostate cancer and there is no evidence to suggest that annual screening by this method will lower the mortality of the disease.

Transrectal ultrasound

Transrectal ultrasound (TRUS) of the prostate was introduced in the mid-1970s and has been used extensively in clinical practice. The more recent introduction of high-frequency transducers and colour Doppler has improved the resolution and provides better images. This, together with ultrasound-directed needle biopsy, has led to better appreciation of the ultrasound appearances of prostate cancer.

The overall usefulness of TRUS for screening is hampered by the fact that it is relatively invasive, time consuming and requires skill. Overall cancer detection rates vary from 2.6% to 22% and the positive values range from 17% to 54%. The sensitivity values have been estimated at 71–92% for prostate cancer and 60–85% for subclinical tumours. Specificity values range from 41% to 79%.

Prostate specific antigen

Prostate specific antigen (PSA) is a glycoprotein produced by the prostate gland, but not specifically by prostate cancer. Benign prostatic hypertrophy (BPH) can cause raised PSA levels. In screening asymptomatic men, a PSA level above 4 ng/ml is a more sensitive test than digital rectal examination (DRE) or TRUS; the accuracy of PSA may be improved by age-specific cut-off values.

An assay of the PSA level has replaced measurement of acid phosphatase as a marker for prostate cancer. It has the potential to be used as a screening test as it is relatively simple and inexpensive. The estimated sensitivity appears to be about 70% and positive predictive values of between 26% and 52% have been found. Higher PSA levels are found with increasing age, benign enlargement of the prostate or in urinary tract infection. It is therefore necessary to have an age-specific reference range [29].

Screening studies diagnose prostate cancer in 2–3% of men (Table 32.6) [30–32]. The initial level for normality was 10 μg/l or below but, although this level has good specificity, few of the tumours detected were potentially curable by radical prostatectomy. In Catalona's study [30], 107 men

had a PSA in the range of 4–9.9 μg/l and 85 were biopsied. Cancer was detected in 19 men (22%) but, at the time of radical prostatectomy, the tumour was only confined to the prostate in 59% of the 17 operations. Of the 30 patients with a PSA greater than 10 μg/l, a cancer was diagnosed in 18 (67%) of the 27 biopsied but the tumour was organ confined in only 13% of the 16 patients having radical prostatectomy. In a later study of 6630, the same group claimed that PSA + DRE improved detection of prostate cancer confined to the gland by 78% over DRE alone, with 71% of 114 men having histological evidence of gland-confirmed cancer.

Perhaps even more worrying was a prospective study of 22 000 physicians. There was a failure of the PSA level to diagnose prostate cancer early, as 47% of the 366 men who developed a tumour within 4 years had a PSA of less than 4 μg/l [33].

As there is 30% test variation, an abnormal PSA must be repeated. If the second test is abnormal, ultrasound-guided transrectal needle biopsy should be carried out. Biopsy can be uncomfortable and is complicated by infection in 5% of men. A total of 70% of those investigated will not have prostate cancer.

Table 32.6 Screening studies for prostate cancer with prostate specific antigen (PSA) Levels

Study	Number of men screened	PSA 4.1–9.9 μg/l n	PSA >10.0 μg/l n (%)[a]	Tumours detected n (%[a])
Catalona et al. [30]	1653	107	30 (1.8)	37 (2.2)
Brawer et al. [31]	1249	149	38 (3.0)	32 (2.6)
Shroder et al. [32]	4724		47 (1.0)	151 (3.2)

[a] % screened.

Feasibility of routine screening for prostate cancer (Box 32.2)

Prostate cancer is characterized by slow but at times unpredictable progression. There is no agreement on the optimal treatment of early disease. However, it is clear that the incidence of prostate cancer makes it an ideal target for screening but the overall detection of prostate cancer must depend upon a combination of 'tests'; digital rectal examination, PSA and TRUS. This concept was appraised in a European study [32]. In Antwerp, 4724 men were studied and prostate cancer was diagnosed in 3.2%. The positive predictive values of the three screening modalities either alone or in combination are shown in

Table 32.7. Random prostatic biopsies were performed on all suspicious lesions, even if the PSA was less than 4 µg/l and a third of all tumours were in the latter group. The TNM staging of 18 tumours found in this study showed that half of the tumours were organ confined. It has therefore been suggested that, at the present time, screening

should be considered in the following groups.

1. Healthy men aged 45–70 years having an annual digital rectal examination and PSA. Although the mean age of presentation is 73 years, it is believed that localized tumours are present up to 20 years earlier. Men with a life expectancy of less than 10 years would be excluded as there would be no benefit from early diagnosis and radical treatment.
2. TRUS should be performed for any abnormality found on digital rectal examination.
3. TRUS should be performed when the digital rectal examination was normal but the PSA was greater than 4 µg/l, although it could be argued that this level should be corrected for age and prostate volume [29].

The implementation of such screening would certainly increase the number of tumours diagnosed, but would it lower mortality rate?

Table 32.7 Positive Predictive Values of Screening Tests used in the Diagnosis of Prostate Cancer in a European Study Performed in Antwerp (31 Tumours) and Rotterdam (41 Tumours) [32]

Screening test	Positive predictive value (%)	
	Antwerp	Rotterdam
TRUS	7	4
DRE alone	2	8
PSA alone	50	12
TRUS + DRE	40	19
TRUS + PSA	50	38
DRE + PSA	75	57
TRUS + DRE + PSA	75	63

DRE = digital rectal examination; TRUS = transrectal ultrasound; PSA = prostate specific antigen.

Box 32.2 The prostate cancer 'screening' debate

- Prostate cancer is the third most common cause of cancer death in men in developed countries
- The incidence of prostate cancer justifies the search for a screening strategy
- DRE + PSA can detect prostate cancer earlier and detect more gland-confined disease
- The majority of prostate cancer has locally metastasized at the time of diagnosis by DRE alone
- There is no curative therapy for advanced disease

But
- No single screening test is adequate on its own
- The natural history of the disease is of slow progression, but can be unpredictable. This means that as many as 50% of men with prostate cancer will die of other intercurrent disease
- The evidence that screening saves lives is lacking (no RCTs)
- No optimal treatment regimen exists
- Many 'occult' cancers will never harm their owners
- PSA has a low predictive value but picks up 'significant' disease
- The progression potential for biopsy-proven prostate cancer has not been predicted

Therefore, screen/test
- Those with a family history
- Those aged 45–70 year requesting screenings
- Opportunistically those who present with lower urinary tract symptoms and who request screening/testing. Men with lower urinary tract symptoms are not at increased risk of prostatic cancer
- US Food and Drugs Administration recommended a combination of DRE + PSA in the detection of prostatic cancer [40].

DRE = digital rectal examination; PSA = prostate specific antigen; RCT = randomized controlled trial.

Treatment

Carcinoma of the prostate was one of the first tumours shown to be hormone dependent and amenable to treatment by orchidectomy or oestrogen therapy. Testosterone deprivation remains the standard treatment for advanced disease but debate continues over when to commence treatment – before or after the patient has symptoms. There has also been an increase in the choices of androgen ablation with the objective of increasing efficacy and reducing morbidity. However, these alternatives are more costly and have little or no benefit over bilateral orchidectomy [34].

The best option for the management of early prostate cancer is also unresolved (Table 32.8). The American Urological Association considered the evidence for radical prostatectomy, radical radiotherapy or surveillance, and considered all of 'these interventions to be options because data from the literature do not provide clear-cut evidence for the superiority of any one treatment' [35]. Treatment therefore depends upon the informed choice of the patient, which in turn will be influenced by the clinician's bias.

Comparing the results of different treatment modalities has been particularly difficult, owing to small sample sizes, difficulties and differences in staging techniques, exclusions and a tendency to use ancillary forms of treatment (and not only for relapses). The survival of men with untreated T1 tumours is similar to that of age-matched controls and this may be because of the high incidence of unsuspected disease in the control group. Chodak et al. [36] analysed the outcome of six clinical trials for men who were either observed or received hormonal treatment for T1 or T2 tumours. They found the disease-specific survival to be 87% for men with grade I and II tumours, but only 34% with grade III tumours. Unfortunately, there is much intratumour variation in histological grading of prostate tumours. The use of Gleason scores (grading on a 1–10 scale) was introduced to further refine, or complicate, the histological grading.

Radical prostatectomy offers the man a chance to have the tumour removed and good results are obtained with small tumours

that are organ confined. The cause-specific 10-year survival is approximately 90%. The operative mortality of radical prostatectomy is less than 1% with experienced surgeons and, apart from the immediate postoperative complications, the main morbidity is due to urinary incontinence (up to 20%) or erectile dysfunction. Better understanding of the anatomy has led most surgeons to attempt a nerve-sparing radical prostatectomy and Walsh was able to preserve potency in 68% of men who were potent preoperatively [37]. It must be noted that many men with prostate cancer are more distressed about the loss of sexual function than they are by other symptoms [38].

The great advantage of radical prostatectomy is that it offers a chance to completely remove the tumour. Preoperative staging of the disease is essential and this includes histological sampling of the pelvic lymph nodes, which may be obtained by open operation or laparoscopically.

Radical radiotherapy offers an equally good chance of 10-year disease-free survival and is preferred by many men. The treatment is associated with less immediate mortality and morbidity, although there may be considerable local irritative bladder and rectal symptoms. There is also an appreciable risk of incontinence and impotence. It is probable that radiotherapy is less likely to prevent metastatic disease than radical surgery and the late relapse is possibly higher.

In conclusion, it is not possible to give definitive advice as to the best treatment for a fit man aged less than 70 with a small tumour

Table 32.8 Treatment options of early prostate cancer

Option	Issues to consider
Surveillance (watchful waiting)	Patient anxiety about 'living with cancer' Not curative Avoids postsurgical morbidity
Radical prostatectomy	Mortality up to 1% Postoperative morbidity of incontinence (up to 27%) and/or impotence (up to 85%) Not curative if metastatic disease
Radical radiotherapy	Common first-line treatment in USA Postradiation morbidity (cystitis, proctitis, etc.) Incontinence (1–6%) and impotence (40%)
Antiandrogen therapy	Role in management of early cancer not fully appraised Early disease more hormone-sensitive and less bulky, therefore may respond better

confined to the prostate. The 10-year survival rates are similar with all modalities of treatment and, if the man is free of disease at 10 years, he is less likely to die of prostate cancer after radical surgery than after radiotherapy or surveillance.

Cost effectiveness of screening

It has been estimated that the cost of screening and treating American men aged 50–70 would be $27.9 billion in the first year [39]. This would mean an increase in the amount spent on prostate cancer from 0.6% ($255 million) of the health budget to 5%. Similarly, it has been estimated [39] that to screen and then treat

the 800 000 men aged 50–68 years in one Health Region in the UK would cost £95 million. At present, the total budget available for all screening programmes in the UK is £300–400 million.

Conclusion

Malignant tumours of the penis and testis are too uncommon to warrant screening programmes. The overall success in treating these conditions is good and, although early diagnosis improves an individual's chance of survival, it will make little impact on overall cancer mortality figures. Resources should therefore be concentrated on encouraging penile hygiene and the early diagnosis of

testicular tumours by self-examination. The latter is of importance in those men who have been operated upon for testicular maldescent or who are known to have an atrophic testis. Adults with an absent testis require further investigation as intra-abdominal testes are particularly prone to neoplasia.

Screening methods are already available for carcinoma of the prostate and PSA estimation is the method of choice. It should only be performed in those men with a family history of prostate cancer until there is evidence that early treatment offers better survival and quality of life than watchful surveillance. Radical prostatectomy for healthy men aged less than 70 may prove to be beneficial for long-term survival.

Resources

UK

- Leaflet for men – Screening for prostate cancer.

Information for men considering or asking for PSA tests. University of York, 1997.

- National Health Information Service (Freephone 0800 66 55 44).

References

1. Wiswell TE. Circumcision and urinary tract infection. *Curr Opin Urol* 1994;4:50–3.

2. Cameron DW. Female to male transmission of human immunodeficiency virus type 1: risk factors for seroconversion in men. *Lancet* 1989;342:403–7.

3. Cook LS, Koutsky LA, Holmes KK. Clinical presentation of genital warts among circumcised and uncircumcised homosexual men attending an urban STD clinic. *Genito-Urinary Med* 1993;69:262–4.

4. Maden C, Sherman KJ, Beckmann AM, et al. History of circumcision, medical conditions and sexual activity

and risk of penile cancer. *J Natl Cancer Inst* 1993;85:19–24.

5. Gonik B, Barrett K. The persistence of new born circumcision: an American perspective. *Br J Obstet Gynaecol* 1995;102:940–1.

6. McCance DJ, Kalache A, Ashdown K, et al. HPV types 16 and 18 in carcinoma of the penis from Brazil. *Int J Cancer* 1986;37:55–9.

7. Opjordsmoen S, Fossa FD. Quality of life in patients treated for penile cancer. *Br J Urol* 1993;71:208–13.

8. Senturia YD. The epidemiology of testicular cancer. *Br J Urol* 1987;60:285–91.

9. Moller H. Clues to the aetiology of testicular germ cell tumours from descriptive epidemiology. *Eur Urol* 1993;23:8–16.

10. Pryor JP, Bettocchi C, Deacon J, Parkinson MC. The value of testicular biopsy as a screening procedure for future malignant germ cell tumours in infertile men. In: Jones WG, Hearnden P, Appleyard I (eds) Germ cell tumours III. Oxford: Pergamon 1994:87.

11. Foreman D, Oliver RJD, Brett AR, et al. Familial testicular cancer: a report of the UK Family Register, estimation of risk and HLA Class 1 subpair analysis. *Br J Cancer* 1992;65:255–62.

12. Ahre O, Ekbom A, Hsieh CC, Trichopoooulos D, Adami HO. Testicular non-seminoma and seminoma in relation to preinatal characteristics. *J Natl Cancer Inst* 1996;88:883–9.

13. Carlsen E, Giwerlman A, Keilding N, Skakkebaekk NE. Evidence for decreasing quality of semen during past 50 years. *Br Med J* 1992;305:609–13.

14. Sharpe RM. Could environmental oestrogenic chemicals be reponsible for some disorders of human male reproductive development? *Curr Opin Urol* 1994;4:295–301.

15. Ginsberg J. Tackling environmental endocrine disrupters. *Lancet* 1996;347:1501–2.

16. Thornhill JA, Butler M, Fitzpatrick JM. Could vasectomy accelerate testicular cancer? The importance of prevasectomy examination. *Br J Urol* 1987;59:367.

17. West RR. Vasectomy and testicular cancer. *Br Med J* 1992;304:729–30.

18. Lynge E, Knudsen LB, Moller H. Vasectomy and testicular cancer: epidemiological evidence of association. *Eur J Cancer* 1993;29a:1064–6.

19. Oliver RTD, Ong JP, Blandy JP, Altman DG. Testis conservation studies in germ cell cancer justified by improved primary chemotherapy response and reduced delay 1978–1994. *Br J Urol* 1996;78:119–24.

20. Peeling WB (ed.). Questions and uncertainties about prostate cancer. Oxford: Blackwell Science, 1996.

21. Franks LM. Latent carcinoma of the prostate. *J Pathol Bacteriol* 1954;68:603–16.

22. George NJR. Incidence of prostrate cancer will double by the year 2030: the argument against. *Eur Urol* 1996;29(Suppl 2):1–136.

23. Ekbom A, Hsieh C-C, Lipworth L, et al. Perinatal characteristics in relation to incidence and mortality from prostate cancer. *Br Med J* 1996;313:337–41.

24. Rosenbert L, Palner JR, Zamber AG, Warshauer ME, Stolley PD, Shapiro S. Vasectomy and the risk of prostate cancer. *Am J Epidemiol* 1990;132:1051–55.

25. Giovannucci E, Tosteson TD, Speizer FE, Ascherro A, Vessey MP, Colditz GA. A retrospective cohort study of vasectomy and prostate cancer in US men. *JAMA* 1993;269:878–82.

26. Guess HA. Is vasectomy a risk for prostate cancer? *Eur J Cancer* 1993;233:1055–60.

27. John EM, Whittemore AS, Wu AH, et al. Vasectomy and prostate cancer: results from a multiethnic case-control study. *J Natl Cancer Inst* 1995;87:662–9.

28. Smith DS, Catalona WJ. Interexaminer variability of digital rectal examination in detecting prostate cancer. *Urology* 1995;45:70–4.

29. Oesterling JE. Using prostate specific antigen to eliminate unnecessary diagnostic tests: significant worldwide economic implications. *Urology* 1995;46 (Suppl 3):4–11.

30. Catalona WJ, Smith DS, Ratliff TL, et al. Measurement of prostate specific antigen in serum as a screening test for prostate cancer. *N Engl J Med* 1991;324:1156–61.

31. Brawer MK, Chetner MP, Beckie J, Buchner DM, Vewwella RL, Lange PH. Prostate specific antigen and early detection of prostate carcinoma. *J Urol* 1992;147:841–5.

32. Schroder FH, Denis LJ, Kirkels W, de Koning HJ, Standaert B. European randomised study of screening for prostate cancer. *Cancer* 1995;76:129–34.

33. Gann PH, Hennekens CH, Stampfer MJ. A prospective evaluation of plasma prostate specific antigen for detection of prostate cancer. *JAMA* 1995;273:289–94.

34. Denis L. Commentary on maximal androgen blockade in prostate cancer: a theory to put into practice? *Prostate* 1995;27:233–40.

35. Middleton RG. The management of clinically localised prostate cancer: guidelines from the American Urological Association. *CA Cancer Clin J* 1996;46:249–53.

36. Chodak GW, Thisted RA, Gerber GS, et al. Results of conservative management of clinically localised prostate cancer. *N Engl J Med* 1994;330:242–8.

37. Walsh PC, Parkin AW, Epstein J. Cancer control and quality of life following anatomical radical retropubic prostatectomy: results at 10 years. *J Urol* 1994;152:1831–6.

38. Helgason AR, Adolfsson J, Dickman P, Frederikson M, Arder S, Steineck G. Waning sexual function – the most important disease-specific distress for patients with prostate cancer. *Br J Cancer* 1996;73:1417–21.

39. Peeling WB, Neal DE, Byrne RL. Screening for prostate cancer – is it affordable? In: Peeling WB (ed.). Questions and uncertainties about prostate cancer. Oxford: Blackwell Science, 1996;299–304.

40. Schoder FH. Detection of prostate cancer. *Br Med J* 1995;310:140–41.

Anesthesia, analgesia and resuscitation

Linda F Lucas BS MD
Benjamin M Rigor MD

Introduction

Ambulatory surgery and outpatient office procedures have many advantages over hospital procedures for the following reasons:

- patients have shorter separation from their families and usual surroundings;

- less likelihood of hospital-acquired infection;

- decreased analgesic requirement;

- fewer postoperative complications;

- increased flexibility of scheduling and efficiency for patient and medical personnel;

- generally decreased costs.

They account for more than 60% of all elective operations performed. Efficiency and flexibility for the patient and physician appear to be improved.

Patient selection, evaluation and monitoring

Patient selection
Careful selection of patients and procedures is crucial for safety and efficiency. Short procedures not associated with excessive blood loss, fluid shifts or extensive postoperative care (including pain management) are most effectively performed as ambulatory or office procedures. Previously only young, healthy patients were considered for outpatient procedures, since a higher incidence of complications and hospital admissions was reported in patients older than 65 years of age and in the presence of pre-existing disease. More recently, it has been shown that patients with chronic, but stable, medical conditions can safely undergo ambulatory procedures with proper preoperative assessment and postoperative supervision. Regional or local anesthetic techniques are often preferable to general anesthesia in elderly or debilitated patients, since recovery of fine motor skills and cognitive function is improved.

Preoperative evaluation and preparation

Appropriate patient selection is dependent on reliable preoperative assessment. The same criteria for preoperative assessment apply to general, regional and local anesthesia. Preoperative evaluation is ideally performed well in advance of the procedure date to allow for optimization of patient condition and medications (Box 33.1). If the patient is to receive major regional or general anesthesia, preoperative evaluation is best performed by an anesthesiologist immediately after scheduling the procedure. This, however, is frequently impractical. Often, the

---

Box 33.1   Criteria for selecting patients for day/outpatient surgery

If procedure planned under general anesthesia, exclude patients:
- With chronic cardiorespiratory disease
- Who are obese
- With diabetes
- If significant postoperative pain is anticipated
- If inadequate post-discharge arrangements (no telephone, no escort, too far from hospital)

Patients with the following history are not suitable for day surgery:
- Uncontrolled hypertension
- Ischemic heart disease
- Previous anesthetic complications/reactions
- Bleeding disorders

gynecologist or family practitioner will see the patient in the office preoperatively and may administer local anesthetics at the time of the procedure, with or without sedation and without the assistance of an anesthesiologist. The family practitioner or gynecologist, as the patient's primary healthcare provider, may be the most appropriate individual to assess the patient preoperatively. Various means of acquiring preoperative information have been employed:

- a visit to the facility for interview and laboratory screening;

- an office visit prior to the surgery date;

- a telephone interview only;

- a review of health questionnaire;

- a preoperative evaluation at the surgical site prior to the procedure;

- computer-assisted input of patient information.

Assessment should include a history of chronic medical conditions, medications, allergies, previous surgical procedures and anesthetics, and personal or family adverse events during surgery or anesthesia. Physical examination should assess the patient's airway, pulmonary and circulatory status and any aspect of the patient's condition related to the procedure.

In the past, 'nil per os status' has not been considered for patients undergoing minor procedures under local anaesthesia. Restriction of oral intake was challenged for its contribution to perioperative dehydration, hypoglycemia and patient discomfort. Risk of aspiration is determined by both gastric volume and pH. Oral ingestion of small amounts of clear liquids prior to surgery may not increase residual gastric volume or decrease pH, the mechanisms responsible for increasing the risk of vomiting and aspiration. Increasingly, more complex procedures requiring sedation combined with larger doses of local anesthetics are being performed in higher risk patients in a variety of outpatient settings. Elderly, obese and uncooperative patients, diabetics, and patients with abnormal airway anatomy should, however, be considered for restriction of oral intake and for premedication with histamine (H_2) antagonists and metoclopramide (Reglan/Maxolon) to increase gastric pH and improve gastric emptying.

Monitoring

Continuous patient assessment is essential during any procedure where sedation or analgesia is employed or where hemodynamic variability is anticipated. All procedure areas should have monitoring capability for continuous electrocardiography, pulse oximetry, blood pressure and temperature. Consideration should be given to the availability of end-tidal carbon dioxide analysis in the event that respiratory compromise would necessitate intubation. Economical, reliable, pH-sensitive disks are commercially available for emergency use. The procedure area should include a readily available source of 100% oxygen, nasal cannulae, face mask and endotracheal tubes of various sizes, means of positive-pressure ventilation, laryngoscopy equipment, electrical defibrillator and emergency medications. If sedatives or anesthetics are to be used, a cart similar to the anesthesia carts used in operating rooms should be assembled and available.

Use of local anesthesia

Improvements in ambulatory anesthesia

Until recently, many procedures were limited to hospital inpatient or ambulatory surgery centers owing to the need for adequate anesthesia and analgesia. General and major regional anesthesia may produce significant hemodynamic and/or respiratory effects and should be reserved for a hospital or ambulatory center surgical suite. In addition, the investment in anesthesia equipment is generally beyond the scope of community clinic and office budgets. Increasingly, however, procedures traditionally performed under general anesthesia are being performed with a combination of local or regional anesthesia and sedation with greater patient and physician acceptance in office and clinic settings. Used correctly, local anesthesia is safe. In the UK over 10 million dental procedures take place with only one death per year reported. As examples, dilation and curettage and sterilizations were once performed under general or major regional anesthesia in a hospital setting. The combination of paracervical block and sedation can be used for dilation and curettage. For sterilization, sedation combined with local infiltration, with or without uterine instillation of local anesthetic and/or paracervical block, is a successful anesthetic technique. These alternatives compare favourably with general or spinal anesthesia when the properties of the ideal anesthetic for outpatient procedures are considered. These are as follows:

- it is cost effective;
- it has a rapid, effective onset of action;
- it produces sedation, hypnosis, amnesia and analgesia;
- it has no intraoperative side effects;
- it has a rapid recovery profile without adverse postoperative side effects.

Combinations of regional or local anesthesia and sedation have been increasingly used (up to 60%) for ambulatory surgery owing to a rapid recovery profile, minimal residual analgesic effects and a lack of significant side effects.

Choice of local anesthetic agents

The choice of local anesthetic agents for regional anesthesia, peripheral nerve block or infiltration must take into consideration the duration of surgery, the technique used, and the potential for local and systemic toxicity. Physiochemical factors such as lipid solubility, protein binding, pK_a of the agent, and the pH of surrounding tissues affect the potency, duration of action, speed of onset and quality of the block, respectively (Table 33.1).

Local anesthetics are generally divided into two classes based on the presence of an ester (–CO–) or an amide (–NHC–) bond, linking the hydrocarbon chain to the lipophilic, aromatic ring of the molecule. The clinically important differences between ester and amide local anesthetics relate to their site of metabolism and potential for producing allergic reactions. Ester local anesthetics are metabolized by plasma cholinesterase. They have a very short half-life, limiting their toxicity. Patients with reduced plasma cholinesterase activity (as occurs in newborns, pregnancy and certain hereditary conditions) may, however, have an increased potential for toxicity. The major metabolite of ester local anesthetics is para-aminobenzoic acid, which may produce allergic reactions, particularly in patients sensitive to certain antibiotics, sulfonamides or thiazide diuretics.

Amide derivatives are metabolized primarily in the liver by N-dealkylation followed by hydrolysis. Patients with liver disease may be more sensitive to the toxic effects of amide local anesthetics, although they have

Table 33.1 Characteristics of commonly used local anesthetics

Generic name	Trade name	Potency	Onset	Duration	Toxicity	Primary use
Esters						
Procaine	Novocaine	Low	Fast	Short	Low	Spinal infiltration
Chloroprocaine	Nesacaine	Low	Fast	Short	Low	Nerve blocks, epidural infiltration
Tetracaine/ Amethocaine	Pontocaine/ Ametop®	High	Slow	Long	Moderate	Spinal
Amides						
Lidocaine (lignocaine)	Xylocaine®	Moderate	Rapid	Moderate	Moderate[a]	Nerve blocks, spinal, epidural, local, topical
Mepivacaine	Carbocaine Scandonest Polocaine	Moderate	Moderate	Moderate	Moderate	Nerve blocks, epidural, spinal infiltration
Bupivacaine	Marcaine® Sensorcaine®	High	Slow	Long	High[b]	Nerve blocks, epidural, spinal infiltration
Etidocaine	Duranest	High	Rapid	Long	Moderate	Nerve blocks, epidural
Ropivacaine	Naropin	High	Slow	Long	Moderate	Nerve blocks, epidural

[a]Standard doses are unlikely to induce cardiac arrhythmias, but higher doses can decrease cardiac output.
[b]For use only by anesthesiologists.
Prilocaine (Citanest, Xylonest) is equipotent with lidocaine with lower toxicity and lower vasodilative properties. Instillagel® is lignocaine hydrochloride 2% gel with chlorhexidine solution preloaded in disposable syringe used for cervical and uterine surface anesthesia.

little, if any, intrinsic allergic potential. Solutions of these agents frequently contain methylparaben as a preservative. Methylparaben may produce an allergic reaction in patients sensitized to para-aminobenzoic acid. The commonly used local anesthetics (prilocaine and lignocaine) are medium-acting amides.

Toxicity of local anesthetics

Systemic toxicity usually results from accidental intravascular injections or use of excessive doses that are absorbed into the circulation from the tissues, producing central nervous system (CNS) and/or cardiovascular effects. Concentrations, doses and dosage limits for commonly used local anesthetics used are listed in Table 33.2. Drugs that may increase toxicity include phenytoin and pethidine (being highly protein bound, these increase free plasma levels of local anesthetics), antiarrhythmic drugs (being related amides) and anticoagulants. Treatment for local anesthetic toxicity is essentially supportive (Box 33.2) with treatment for seizures, arrhythmias and respiratory and circulatory depression. For most local anesthetics, CNS toxicity occurs at lower plasma concentrations than cardiovascular toxicity, and may occur alone or precede cardiovascular symptoms. The exception is bupivacaine, where the patient may have sudden cardiovascular collapse without prior evidence of CNS toxicity. Pregnant women are particularly susceptible to the cardiodepressant effects of bupivacaine and its use is contraindicated in the pregnant patient. Resuscitation of local anesthetic toxicity is dependent upon drug redistribution, and resuscitative efforts for several hours may be required for a successful outcome. Patients with liver disease, cardiac failure or on concurrent medication are also at high risk for toxicity.

Systemic toxicity can be minimized with the use of appropriate doses (see Table 33.2), injection of small incremental volumes (slow gradual injection), especially when injecting into highly vascular areas, aspiration prior to all injections and use of solutions containing a vasoconstrictor. Vasoconstrictors such as epinephrine (adrenaline), phenylephrine or norepinephrine not only decrease toxicity but also prolong the duration and improve the quality of the block. The addition of a small amount of vasoconstrictor allows for the use of lower concentrations, higher doses, and less total volume of local anesthetic solutions. It also decreases surgical blood loss. Most commonly, epinephrine in a concentration of 1:200 000 (0.1 ml of 1:1000 epinephrine in 20 ml of plain local anesthetic solution) to 1:400 000 (0.05 ml epinephrine in 20 ml) is added

Table 33.2 Infiltration Anesthesia

Drug	Concentration (%)	Plain solution		Epinephrine-containing solution	
		Maximum dosage (mg)	Duration of action (min)	Maximum dosage (mg)	Duration of action (min)
Short duration					
Procaine	0.5–2	500	15–30	1000	30–75
Chloroprocaine	1.0–2.1	800	15–30	1000	30–90
Moderate duration					
Lidocaine (lignocaine)	0.5–1.0	200	30–60	500	120–360
Mepivacaine	0.5–1.0	300	45–90	500	120–360
Prilocaine (Citanest)	0.5–1.0	400	30–90	600	120–360
Long duration					
Bupivacaine (Marcaine)	0.25–0.5	175	120–240	175	180–420
Bidocaine	0.5–1.0	300	120–180	400	180–420

Reproduced with permission from Strichartz GR, Covino BG. Local anesthetics. In: Miller RD (ed.) Anesthesia, 3rd edn. New York: Churchill Livingstone, 1990:454.
The lowest concentrations are adequate for infiltration anesthesia. The higher concentrations more appropriate for nerve blocks. Lignocaine (2%) has higher potential toxicity.

Box 33.2 Central nervous system toxicity

Symptoms/signs
- Dizziness
- Light-headedness
- Tinnitus
- Metallic taste
- Tongue and circumoral numbness
- Visual and auditory disturbance
- Restlessness
- Aggression
- Muscle twitching
- Unconsciousness
- Seizure/convulsions
- Coma

Predisposing factors
- Acidosis
- Hypoxia and hypercarbia

Treatment
1. Stop the injection
2. Administer oxygen via face mask at onset of symptoms. Observe patient until fully alert
3. Treat seizures with benzodiazepines (e.g. diazepam 2–5 mg (used as Diazemuls²), midazolam 1–2 mg) or barbiturates (e.g. thiopental 50–200 mg or methohexital 20–50 mg)
4. Support oxygenation and ventilation, provide suction if required; tracheal intubation may be facilitated with succinylcholine 0.5–1 mg/kg
5. Start intravenous line, monitor blood pressure

Cardiovascular toxicity (follows CNS toxicity)

Symptoms/signs
- Decreased blood pressure
- Arrhythmias due to decreased peripheral vascular resistance
- Decreased ventricular contractility and conduction delays
- Cardiovascular collapse

Treatment
1. Administer oxygen, intubate, if necessary, for control of airway
2. Cardiopulmonary resuscitation (may be prolonged), intravascular volume support, vasopressors, inotropes, as necessary
3. Cardioversion for ventricular fibrillation, tachycardia
4. Bretylium may be more effective than lidocaine for ventricular arrythmias
5. Atropine for bradycardia

² Drug of choice for non-anesthologists – note long duration of action, therefore, patient must be kept under observation.

just prior to injection. The maximum permitted dose is 0.2 mg. Epinephrine should not be used in areas with poor collateral blood flow and should be used with caution in patients with hypertension, arrhythmias, coronary artery disease and certain endocrine disorders.

Vasovagal reactions present as pallor, sweating, bradycardia, hypotension, nausea and vomiting and loss of consciousness. They can be avoided by reassurance and 'talking through' the procedure with anxious patients. Sedation may be required for very anxious patients. If it occurs, a vasovagal reaction is treated by elevation of the foot of the bed, maintaining an airway and managing bradycardia. In severe cases, oxygen administered by mask and fluid infusion may be necessary.

Techniques of administration

Topical anesthesia

Local anesthetics can be applied topically, as liquids, sprays, creams or gels, and are most effective when applied to mucous membranes or abraded skin. While the onset of effect is around 60 min for skin, it is only 2–3 min for mucosal surfaces. Lidocaine, dibucaine and benzocaine are commonly used (Table 33.3). When applied to mucous membranes in vascular areas, such as the genitourinary tract, the rate of uptake of local anesthetic solutions approaches that of vascular injection and may result in toxic plasma concentrations. Recently, a eutectic mixture of lidocaine and prilocaine (EMLA) has been formulated for cutaneous analgesia. It must be applied approximately 60 min prior to the procedure and covered by an occlusive bandage. It is most effective for minimizing the pain associated with percutaneous injections and placement of intravenous cannulae. For mucosal anesthesia, lidocaine 2%, 4% or 10% is used as a spray or ointment. Topical uterine anesthesia has been used for a range of procedures from intrauterine device (IUD) placement to hysteroscopy. A quill or tuberculin needle is used to inject a small volume of local anesthetic into the uterus. Agents used included mepivacaine 2% (2 ml).

Local infiltration

For many minor ambulatory surgical and office procedures, the most appropriate anesthetic is direct local infiltration or field

Table 33.3 Topical anesthetics

Anesthetic ingredient	Concentration (%)	Form of application	Intended area of use
Benzocaine	1–5	Cream	Skin and mucous membrane
	20	Ointment	Skin and mucous membrane
	20	Aerosol	Skin and mucous membrane
Dibucaine	0.25–1	Cream	Skin
	0.25–1	Ointment	Skin
	0.25–1	Aerosol	Skin
	0.25	Solution	Ear
	2.5	Suppositories	Rectum
Cyclonine	0.5–1	Solution	Skin, oropharynx, tracheobronchial tree, urethra, rectum
Lidocaine	2	Jelly	Urethra
	2.5–5	Ointment	Skin, mucous membrane, rectum
	10	Suppositories	Rectum
Tetracaine	0.5–1	Ointment	Skin, rectum, mucous membrane
	0.5–1	Cream	Skin, rectum, mucous membrane

Modified from Covino BG, Vassallo HG. Local anesthetics: mechanisms of action and clinical use. Orlando: Grune and Stratton, 1976.

block of the affected area. For direct infiltration, 0.5–1% lidocaine or prilocaine is used, administered in a fanwise infiltration for skin anesthesia. Longer acting agents, such as bupivacaine, may be used to reduced immediate postoperative pain, such as follows certain types of female sterilization. For field blocks (e.g. paracervical block), the two-point entry technique at both sides of the operative field is recommended using lower concentrations of lidocaine. Advantages include ease of administration, postoperative analgesia, more rapid recovery profile, early discharge and generally reduced side effects. Local anesthetics are often used with sedative and anxiolytic medications. Although this may improve patient comfort and acceptance, it may also delay recovery and produce nausea and vomiting.

Regional blocks

Paracervical block is useful for cervical biopsy, conization, first-trimester termination of pregnancy and hysteroscopy. It anesthetizes the lower two-thirds of the uterus and is useful for intrauterine procedures. Paracervical block involves the transvaginal deposition of a local anesthetic, usually at the 3 o'clock and 9 o'clock positions of the cervical rim to a depth of 10 mm using a pudendal block needle or a long 22-gauge needle. Its advantages include ease of administration, rapid onset, and absence of sympathetic blockade and the hemodynamic effects that occur with spinal or epidural anesthesia. The usual volume of 10–20 ml of local anesthetic solution is well within the toxic limits of clinically useful concentrations of chloroprocaine, lidocaine (1%) and etidocaine, which are approved for use in the USA. Prilocaine (3%) is very popular in the UK. Toxic vascular injection, however, can occur. In addition, one disadvantage of this technique is the short duration of action, which may increase the need for repeated injections and potential toxicity. The addition of epinephrine does not increase the quality or duration of the block, since its effectiveness is dependent upon adequate local spread.

Pudendal nerve blocks can be used for anesthesia of the lower genital tract. The sensory fibers are derived from the ventral branches of the 2nd, 3rd and 4th sacral nerves and provide peripheral branches that innervate the perineum, anus, and the more medial and inferior parts of the vulva and clitoris. Pudendal nerve block involves the injection of approximately 10 ml of local anesthetic solution over the pudendal nerve (Figure 33.1). For most procedures, bilateral block is performed.

Pudendal block should provide adequate analgesia for procedures such as treatment of vulvar or lower vaginal lesions, biopsies or repair of lacerations, etc. Its usefulness is limited by the delay of onset, which may be as long as 15 min for adequate analgesia, and the frequency of patchy or inadequate analgesia. Inadequate blocks may, however, be augmented by the use of sedative analgesics to produce a successful result for many procedures. Abdominal pain following laparoscopic procedures can be minimized using a rectus sheath block. A mesosalpinx block may reduce the deep pelvic pain that occurs after tubal ligation.

Sedation and analgesia

The objective of reducing the volumes of local anesthetic solutions administered, and increasing patient acceptance of outpatient procedures, can be achieved with the judicious use of sedative, analgesic and anxiolytic

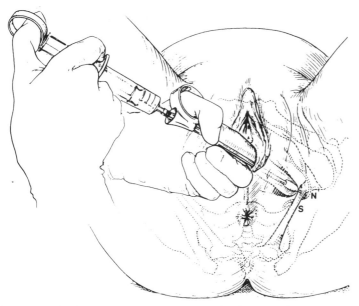

Fig. 33.1 Local infiltration of the pudendal nerve – transvaginal technique showing the needle extended beyond the needle guard and passing through the sacrospinous ligament (S) to reach the pudendal nerve (N). Reproduced with permission from Cunningham FG, MacDonald PC, Gant NF (eds). Williams obstetrics, 18th edn. East Norwalk: Appleton and Lange, 1989.

pharmacologic agents. The recovery profile and time to discharge for patients receiving 'monitored anesthesia care' with intravenous sedatives and analgesics with local anesthesia and/or peripheral nerve blocks are generally improved over those receiving major regional or general anesthesia. Oversedation, nausea and vomiting may, however, limit patient comfort and delay ambulation and discharge.

The most widely used intraoperative, intravenous, sedative–hypnotic for ambulatory anesthesia is propofol (Diprivan). It is a short-acting non-barbiturate with antiemetic effects and a rapid recovery profile. Alternatively, local anesthetic administration combined with short-duration narcotics, such as fentanyl (Sublimaze) or alfentanil (Alfenta), and/or

benzodiazepines, allows for invasive procedures such as dilation and curettage, hysteroscopy and sterilization to be performed with a comfortable, awake patient. Methohexital and ketamine can also be used successfully for intraoperative sedation. Although ketamine is a powerful analgesic and amnestic, its cardiovascular, cholinergic and psychomimetic effects limit its usefulness. Hypertensive or elderly patients suspected of having coronary artery disease may be particularly susceptible to adverse, ketamine-induced cardiovascular effects.

Dexmedetomidine is a potent, highly selective alpha-2-adrenoceptor agonist with sedative–hypnotic and anesthetic-sparing properties. However, it produces a dose-related bradycardia and hypotension. In large doses, it may also cause myocardial ischemia. It has been

shown to produce sedative and anxiolytic effects similar to midazolam with less ventilatory depression and delay in recovery of psychomotor function. It reduces the anesthetic requirements for intravenous and inhalational anesthetics and opioids in ambulatory surgery patients, and may prove useful for gynecologic procedures.

For children, chloral hydrate (20–50 mg/kg orally or rectally) or methohexital (Brevital, 20–30 mg/kg rectally) is frequently used for sedation or as a premedicant for minor procedures. Chloral hydrate is administered 30–60 min prior to the procedure. Rectal methohexital has an onset time of 5–10 min. While chloral hydrate has a higher incidence of inadequate sedation, rectal barbiturates may produce loss of consciousness and general anesthesia. Rectal methohexital should, therefore, only be administered by an anesthesiologist with adequate monitoring and preparation for airway control.

Premedication

Careful choice of medications and premedicants may reduce unwanted side effects (Table 33.4). Premedication alone may be adequate for sedation and analgesia when combined with local anesthetic infiltration or nerve block. Although barbiturates were once widely used as perioperative oral and intravenous medications, benzodiazepines have become the mainstay of preoperative anxiolytic and sedative therapy. Midazolam (0.025–0.1 mg/kg iv or im) or diazepam (0.1–0.2

Table 33.4 Analgesics and antiemetics for premedication and intraoperative use (common adult dosages)

Generic name	Proprietary name	Typical oral dose (mg)	Typical parenteral dose (mg)
Opioids – agonists[a]			
Morphine		30–60 q.6–12 h	10 q.2–6 h
Codeine		180 q.4–6 h	120 q.2–3 h
Oxycodone	Percocet, Tylox	30 q.4–6 h	
Hydromorphone	Dilaudid	7.5 q.4–6 h	1.5 q.2–4 h
Methadone	Dolophine	20 q.24 h	2.5–10 q.4–6 h
Meperidine	Demerol	300 q.4–6 h	50–150 q.2–6 h
Fentanyl	Sublimaze		0.05–0.1 q.30–60 min
Opioids – agonist–antagonists			
Butorphanol	Stadol		2 q.3–4 h
Nalbupine	Nubain		10 q.3–6 h
Pentazocine	Talwin	180	60 q.3–6 h
Opioids – partial agonist			
Buprenorphine	Buprenex		0.4 q.4–6 h
Dezocine	Dalgan		5 q.2–4 h
NSAIDs			
Aspirin		650 q.3–4 h	
Ibuprofen	Motrin, Advil	200–800 q.6 h	
Naproxen	Naprosyn	250–500 q.12 h	
Choline magnesium trisalicylate	Trilisate	1000–1500 q.12 h	
Ketorolac	Toradol	10 q.4–6 h	15–60 im/iv q.6 h
Diclofenac	Voltaren	50–75 q.8–12 h	
Sulindac	Clinoril	150–200 q.12 h	
Piroxicam	Feldene	20 q.24 h	
Etodolac	Lodine	200–400 q.6–8 h	
Acetaminophen	Tylenol	325–650 q.4–6 h	
Anxiolytics, antispasmodics[a]			
Diazepam	Valium	2.5–10.0 q.6–8 h	5–10 iv q.4–6 h
Alprazolam	Xanax	0.5–1.0 q.8 h	
Midazolam	Versed		2.5–10 im q.15–90 min
			0.5–5 iv q.15–90 min
Hydroxyzine	Vistaril, Atarax	50–100 q.6 h	50–100 im q.4–6 h
Antiemetics[a]			
Prochlorperazine	Compazine	5–10 q.8 h	5–10 im q.3–4 h
Metoclopramide	Reglan	10–15 q.6–8 h	10 im/iv q.4–6 h
Promethazine	Phenergan	25–50 q.4–6 h	12.5–25.0 im q.4–6 h
Droperidol	Inapsine	5–15 q.8 h	0.625–1.25 q.6 h
Ondansetron	Zofran		4 iv – may repeat x1
Histamine (H_2) antagonists[a]			
Cimetidine	Tagamet	300 q.6–8 h	300 slowly q.6–8 h
Ranitidine	Zantac	150 q.12 h	50 q.6–8 h
Famotidine	Pepcid	20 q.12 h	20 q.12 h
Nizatidine	Axid	300 qhs	

[a]Commonly used for premedication. Modified with permission from Davison JK, et al. Clinical anesthesia procedures of the Massachusetts General Hospital, 4th edn. Boston: Little, Brown and Company, 1993:586–8.

inhibitors, such as ibuprofen or mefenamic acid, provide variable intraoperative but adequate postoperative analgesia, and may be used as premedicants prior to the patient's arrival for the procedure. These non-steroidal anti-inflammatory agents have been shown to be as effective for postoperative pain as narcotic analgesics for many minor gynecological procedures and produce fewer side effects.

Other premedications that may be considered include metoclopramide (Reglan/Maxolon), droperidol (Inapsine) and other butyrophenones, phenothiazines and antihistamines (H_1 and H_2 antagonists). Agents such as hydroxyzine (Vistaril) or promethazine (Phenergan) are useful throughout the perioperative period for sedation, the prevention or treatment of nausea and vomiting, and to decrease the incidence and severity of allergic reaction. Consideration should be given to the possibility that any patient undergoing sedation could develop unconsciousness, apnea or airway compromise with the risk of vomiting and pulmonary aspiration. For this reason, it is recommended that restriction of oral intake be considered in patients receiving sedation. Those patients at particular risk (elderly, obese and uncooperative patients, diabetics and patients with abnormal airway anatomy) should be considered for premedication with H_2 antagonists and/or metoclopramide (Reglan/ Maxolon) to reduce gastric acidity and promote gastric emptying. Premedication with metoclopramide, nizatidine

mg/kg po or iv) provide excellent anxiolysis and amnesia, and may be augmented with additional incremental intravenous doses as required throughout the procedure without significantly delaying recovery. An additional advantage of benzodiazepines is their anticonvulsive effect, which may raise the seizure threshold

for toxic doses of local anesthetic solutions. Midazolam is probably the optimal choice for sedation. Given intravenously via an indwelling cannula, midazolam is non-irritant to veins and has a short half-life of 2 h. Its main drawback is respiratory and cardiac depression in the elderly.

For minor procedures, such as IUD placement, prostaglandin

(Axid), famotidine (Pepcid), ranitidine (Zantac), cimetidine (Tagamet) or a non-particulate antacid, such as sodium citrate (Bicitra), may reduce the risks associated with unanticipated or unrecognized aspiration of gastric contents (Table 33.4). Diabetics should receive reduced insulin doses preoperatively and have serum glucose concentrations monitored perioperatively, since their oral intake may be compromised.

Postoperative analgesia

Analgesics should be titrated throughout the perioperative period to maintain patient comfort and to avoid the need for excessive doses of narcotic analgesics postoperatively. Although small doses of parenteral analgesics may be used early in the recovery period, the patient should be able to maintain adequate pain control with oral medications prior to discharge. Frequently administered oral medications include acetaminophen (Tylenol, 975 mg), oxycodone (Percocet, 1–2 tablets) and ibuprofen (600–800 mg). Many patients who receive local or regional anesthetics have residual sensory nerve block and only small to moderate doses of oral analgesics are necessary for postoperative pain management.

Fentanyl (Sublimaze) and alfentanil (Alfenta) are parenteral opioids frequently used for ambulatory procedures, owing to their potency and short duration of action. Morphine sulfate and meperidine (Demerol) may be used in small doses if longer duration is required but may delay recovery. Requirements

vary depending on age, weight, type of procedure and the presence of pre-existing tolerance (Table 33.4).

Non-steroidal anti-inflammatory drugs (NSAIDs) provide effective analgesia by inhibiting the enzyme cyclooxygenase, thereby preventing the synthesis of prostaglandins that act to mediate pain associated with many gynecologic procedures. NSAIDs are used alone to treat mild to moderate pain or to act synergistically when combined with other types of analgesics for more severe pain. They are effective in reducing narcotic requirements and their concomitant respiratory and CNS depression. Ketorolac (Toradol), the first parenteral NSAID, is particularly useful in the treatment of acute postoperative pain. Although premedication with NSAIDs prior to gynecologic procedures may provide superior pain relief when compared to postoperative administration, concerns about ketorolac's effect on platelet aggregation preclude its use prior to procedures where blood loss is anticipated.

Mixed opioid agonist–antagonists and partial agonists such as butorphanol (Stadol), nalbuphine (Nubain) and buprenorphine (Buprenex) are administered parenterally for relief of mild to moderate pain. Although they are less predictable in controlling pain than narcotics, they are less likely to cause nausea, vomiting and respiratory depression. Many antiemetics, including promethazine (Phenergan), contribute to pain control, but they also produce sedation and must be used

sparingly to avoid delayed recovery. Ondansetron (Zofran) is a potent, parenteral antiemetic with no significant side effects. Its use can significantly reduce nausea, vomiting and time to discharge (Table 33.4).

General anesthesia

Procedures requiring general anesthesia, postoperative analgesia and prolonged recovery have been restricted to hospital or ambulatory surgery centers. Although the use of bolus or continuous infusions of short-acting, intravenous anesthetics has made it possible to perform many plastic surgery and gynecologic procedures in office and clinic settings, many patients and procedures require deeper planes of anesthesia. The introduction of the short-duration inhalational agents desflurane (Suprane) and sevoflurane (Sevoflurane) has significantly reduced the time to recovery and improved 'street-fitness' for patients requiring general anesthesia. The use of the laryngeal mask airway as an alternative to endotracheal intubation in suitable patients may also reduce time to recovery and the anesthetic requirement as a result of decreased sympathetic stimulation.

Procedures such as diagnostic laparoscopy require brief but significant muscle relaxation. Until recently, however, there were no muscle relaxants devoid of significant side effects suitable for these procedures. With the introduction of short-duration, non-depolarizing muscle relaxants, such as mivacurium (Mivacron) and rocuronium bromide (Zemuron), rapid onset and reversal of surgical muscle relaxation for 15–20 min cases is now safe and effective.

Discharge criteria

Prior to discharge, it is important to confirm the patient's adequate recovery (Box 33.3). Unanticipated hospital admission rates after outpatient procedures range from 0.1% to 5.0%. Although more than half are related to minor complications, such as nausea, vomiting or inadequate pain relief, serious complications, including respiratory depression and anaphylaxis, may also occur.

Complications

Respiratory depression

Respiratory depression most commonly results from administration of anesthetic agents, narcotics and/or benzodiazepines. Although most agents used today for outpatient procedures provide remarkable cardiovascular stability in the sedated or anesthetized patient, almost all result in additive or synergistic depression of ventilatory drive and sedation that can lead to hypoventilation, apnea and/or airway obstruction. Any procedure requiring significant sedation should only be performed by experienced anesthesia personnel who can provide endotracheal intubation and general anesthesia if necessary.

Emergency treatments for narcotic–induced respiratory depression (Box 33.4) include administration of 100% oxygen, bag and mask ventilation (or

> **Box 33.3 Discharge criteria and instructions**
>
> - The patient should be alert and oriented with stable vital signs for 1 h.
> - There should be no abnormal bleeding, edema or circulatory compromise at the surgical site.
> - Analgesia should be controlled with oral medications. Prescriptions with clear instructions should be provided. The patient should be warned against using alcohol, making important decisions or resuming activities requiring alertness and concentration until at least the next day, and while taking analgesics.
> - The patient should be able to ambulate without undue difficulty or support.
> - The patient should be able to take oral fluids without nausea or vomiting. The patient should be instructed to begin resumption of oral intake with clear liquids and gradually progress to a normal diet.
> - The patient should be able to urinate.
> - The patient should be informed of possible complications and given adequate instructions concerning emergencies, telephone numbers and follow-up appointments.

intubation, if necessary) and reversal with the antagonist naloxone (Narcan). A mixed agonist–antagonist, such as nalbuphine, may be used for reversal in less urgent situations with the advantages of longer duration of action, minimal effects on analgesia, and decreased incidence of nausea, vomiting and renarcotization. Benzodiazepine-induced respiratory depression and oversedation may be similarly reversed with flumazenil (Romazicon). Flumazenil may produce seizures, particularly in those patients habituated to benzodiazepines or treated with tricyclic antidepressants. Patients receiving reversal agents should be observed for recurrent respiratory depression and

sedation for at least 2 h following the last dose of the reversal drug. If treatment is delayed or inadequate, cardiac arrest requiring cardiopulmonary resuscitation may occur.

Anaphylaxis

Anaphylaxis is another life-threatening emergency that may occur in any medical setting (see details of treatment in Box 33.5). In general, anesthetic agents used today are less likely to produce histamine release and allergic reactions than their predecessors; local anesthetics of the ester group are more likely to cause adverse reactions. Premedication the night before and just prior to

> **Box 33.4 Treatment of sedation-induced respiratory depression**
>
> - Administer 100% oxygen.
> - Check for and, if necessary, establish airway patency.
> - For narcotic-induced depression, administer naloxone (Narcan) 0.04–0.4 mg iv for adults (1–10 µg/kg for pediatric patients) q 2–3 min until responsive and adequate respiration is restored. May need to repeat q 10–60 min.
> - For benzodiazepine-induced depression, administer flumazenil (Romazicon) 0.2–1.0 mg iv q 20 min at 0.2 mg/min. Be prepared to treat CNS excitation and/or seizures.
> - Observe for recurrent respiratory depression for at least 2 h and repeat treatment as necessary.

Box 33.5   Treatment of anaphylaxis

1. Discontinue possible pharmacologic causes, including anesthetic agents.
2. Administer 100% oxygen. Control the airway; intubate, if necessary.
3. Treat hypotension with intravascular balanced salt solutions and/or colloids (volume replacement).
4. Administer:
   - Histamine antagonists (diphenhydramine, 50 mg iv for adults) may be used for very mild reactions, but do not delay administration of epinephrine for more severe reactions.
   - Epinephrine (adrenaline) 50–100 µg iv (0.5–1.0 mg for cardiovascular collapse[a]), or 0.5 ml of 1:1000 solution im, or 3–5 ml of 1:1000 solution im or slow iv. This may be repeated to 3.0 mg. Norepinephrine, isoproterenol (dopamine) or other vasopressors or inotropes may also be used.
   - For bronchospasm, epinephrine is the first choice. Aminophylline and/or salbutamol may be added.
   - Steroids (hydrocortisone 250 mg–1.0 g iv or methylprednisolone 1–2 g iv).
5. Begin resuscitative efforts according to ACLS guidelines, if indicated.
6. Ensure follow-up, and accurate communication to patient regarding the cause, to prevent recurrence.

[a]In the absence of high-level monitoring, im adrenaline would be safer.

the procedure with H_1 and H_2 antagonists, such as diphenhydramine hydrochloride (Benadryl) and famotidine (Pepcid) may significantly reduce allergic reaction. Prompt recognition of the problem and swift intervention are the key to successful management. Hypotension and tachycardia should alert the physician to the possibility of anaphylaxis.

Resuscitation

Personnel and equipment

All physicians should be trained to administer cardiopulmonary resuscitation as the necessity may occur in any setting. Even simple office procedures or patient anxiety alone can precipitate vasovagal bradycardia and circulatory depression that may progress to cardiac arrest. Use of sedative and anesthetic agents increases the likelihood of respiratory and cardiac depression, particularly when administered to

elderly patients or those with concurrent medical conditions and pharmacologic treatment. Equipment and medication for resuscitation and monitoring should be readily available. In any medical setting at least two people should be trained in cardiopulmonary resuscitation (CPR) and advanced cardiac life support (ACLS) to ensure availability of qualified personnel and co-ordinated, efficient care.

Respiratory depression and/or cardiac arrest may be sudden or insidious; common causes include airway obstruction, hypoxemia, hypovolemia, arrhythmias, electrocution, acid–base or electrolyte disturbances, adverse drug effects or interactions, trauma or surgery. Correct diagnosis is essential, since performance of resuscitative efforts may result in morbidity or mortality. All patients undergoing procedures, particularly those involving sedative or anesthetic agents, should be appropriately monitored as previously described.

When a person is found to be apneic or unconscious, medical personnel should attempt to arouse the patient and summon assistance (Figure 33.2). If the patient is unarousable, the 'ABCs' of resuscitation, as established by the American Heart Association (AHA), should be initiated. Breathing should be assessed by listening and feeling over the patient's mouth for air movement, and observing the patient's chest for respiratory effort. Airway patency should be assessed. If the airway appears to be obstructed, it should be cleared and opened with the 'head tilt/chin lift' or 'jaw thrust' maneuver. The patient should then be reassessed. If effective respiratory effort is absent, assistance with a bag and mask and 100% oxygen should be initiated until breathing is restored or intubation equipment is available. Oxygenation should be established with a good mask airway and low airway pressure prior to intubation. Positive-pressure ventilation with 100% oxygen should be maintained throughout the resuscitation and early recovery periods. For hemodynamically stable patients being treated for arrhythmias in whom spontaneous ventilation is adequate, supplemental oxygen may be delivered with a face mask.

Circulation is assessed by palpating for a carotid or femoral pulse, electrocardiogram (ECG) and blood pressure monitoring. If no pulse can be palpated, particularly if there is asystole or ventricular fibrillation by electrocardiography, chest compressions should be performed at a rate of 80–100 min with the patient on a firm surface.

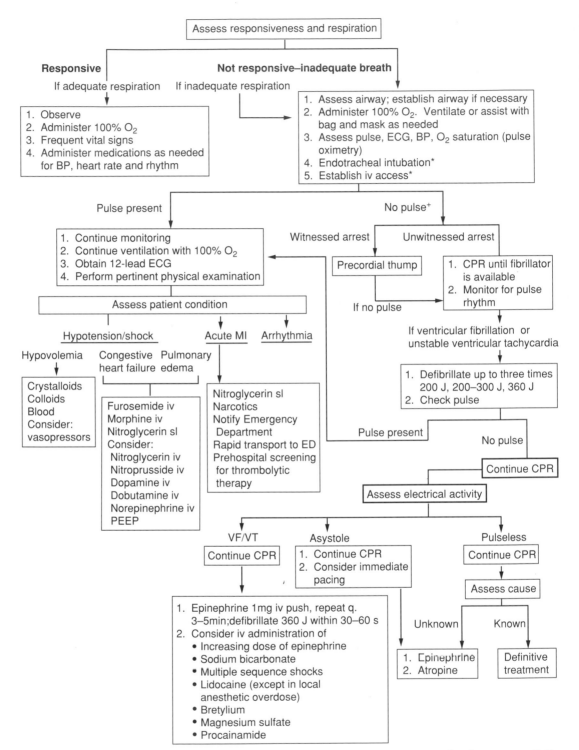

Fig. 33.2 Resuscitation in a medical setting. BP = blood pressure; ECG = electrocardiogram; CPR = cardiopulmonary resuscitation; PEEP = positive end-expiratory pressure; ED = Emergency Department; VF = ventricular fibrillation; VT = ventricular tachycardia. * Do not delay defibrillation to intubate trachea or establish iv access – these may be performed after defibrillation attempts. † CPR should be continued throughout until the return of spontaneous circulation. If spontaneous circulation returns, monitor, administer 100% O_2 and medications as indicated.

If cardiac arrest is witnessed and an electrical defibrillator is not readily available, a precordial thump is first delivered and the patient reassessed for return of circulation prior to institution of chest compressions.

Vital organ oxygenation and perfusion should be maintained with endotracheal intubation, electrical defibrillation and pharmacologic intervention. Endotracheal intubation should be performed as quickly as possible by experienced personnel while other resuscitative efforts continue. Intravenous access should be established as soon as possible. If intravenous access is not immediately available, lidocaine, epinephrine and atropine may be delivered through the endotracheal tube. Absorption and therapeutic plasma concentrations are aided by dilution of these drugs in 10 ml of sterile saline prior to endotracheal instillation.

Early electrical defibrillation is essential to successful outcome for patients in cardiac arrest, since the cardiac rhythm tends to become more resistant to conversion as the duration of arrest increases. The cardiac rhythm should be evaluated as soon as possible by ECG or with the 'analyze' capabilities of the defibrillator. As soon as the defibrillator is available, everyone involved in the resuscitation should be 'cleared' of contact with the patient and three shocks delivered rapidly at 200, 300 and 360 J. If an effective rhythm returns, the patient should be continuously observed for recurrent deterioration with support of respiration and circulation as required, and immediate transport to an acute care facility. If an effective rhythm or pulse is not restored, subsequent shocks should be delivered at 360 J. Shocks should be repeatedly administered after each pharmacologic intervention.

Intravenous access should be established as quickly as possible after oxygenation is restored, and chest compressions and/or defibrillation attempts begun. The most effective intravenous routes are internal or external jugular, subclavian, femoral or long peripheral lines into the central venous circulation. If cannulation of these vessels cannot be achieved quickly with minimal disruption of resuscitative efforts, antecubital or even more peripheral veins can be used. Intravenous lines should be maintained with crystalloid solutions delivered only at the minimal rate necessary to flush medications into the central circulation. Only patients with known intravascular volume depletion should receive replacement of crystalloids or colloids at more rapid rates.

Pharmacologic agents as recommended by the AHA for use during ACLS should be administered as indicated, with continuous monitoring. The patient should be evaluated for the causes of respiratory and/or cardiac instability as quickly as possible, with the recognition that the patient's condition can change abruptly.

For high-grade heart block with hemodynamically significant bradycardia, atropine (0.5–1.0 mg) should be administered intravenously and repeated if necessary. If unsuccessful, isoproterenol 2–10 μg/min may be infused. If atropine and/or isoproterenol administration does not produce a hemodynamically effective heart rate, temporary pacing should be initiated. Transcutaneous pacemakers are the fastest, most effective way to achieve temporary pacing in most patients. If unavailable or ineffective, transvenous pacing wires should be positioned and transvenous pacing performed through a central venous catheter while CPR continues. Arrhythmias causing hypotension or a change in level of consciousness should be dealt with promptly to avoid progression to more refractory malignant rhythms.

Patients presenting with chest pain, shortness of breath or other symptoms of acute myocardial ischemia or infarction should have ECG, blood pressure monitoring and pulse oximetry at the onset of symptoms. A 12-lead ECG should be obtained as soon as available. Oxygen should be administered at 4 l/min by face mask or nasal cannula. Intravenous access should be obtained. Nitroglycerin can be administered by paste, spray or sublingually if the systolic blood pressure is greater than 90 mmHg, and is followed by intravenous nitroglycerin at a rate adequate to maintain systolic blood pressure at 90 mmHg or 10–30% below the patient's preoperative blood pressure. Morphine sulfate in small doses (1–3 mg) should be administered intravenously and repeated at 5-min intervals as needed for pain relief. If signs or symptoms of heart failure are present, furosemide (Lasix) 0.5–1.0 mg/kg iv may be given. If symptoms of myocardial ischemia persist after initiation of therapy or there is ECG evidence of myocardial infarction, the patient should be urgently transported to an acute care facility. Transfer to an acute care facility and/or thrombolytic therapy should not be delayed for further therapeutic management in a patient stable enough for transport.

Termination of CPR

Although studies indicate that patients undergoing resuscitation for greater than 30 min have a probability of survival and discharge from the hospital that approaches zero, there are no absolute guidelines for termination of unsuccessful attempts at resuscitation. The individual physician is left to decide when the patient is not responding to resuscitative efforts and cannot survive.

In the outpatient and community office or clinic setting, it is probably wise to plan for transport to an acute care facility early in the course of any significant hemodynamic deterioration in a patient's condition. When at all possible, patients should be stabilized prior to transport. The physician, or at least other trained personnel from the outpatient facility, should accompany the patient on transfer. As soon as possible, the physician should carefully document the resuscitative efforts and the reasons for their termination should it become necessary.

Bibliography

- Aho M, Lehtinen A-M, Erkola O, Kallio A, Kortilla K. The effect of intravenously administered dexmedetomidine on perioperative hemodynamics and isoflurane requirements in patients undergoing abdominal hysterectomy. *Anesthesiology* 1991;73:997–1002.

- Cummins RO (ed.). Textbook of advanced cardiac life support. Dallas, TX: American Heart Association, 1994.

- Cunningham FG, MacDonald PC, Gant NF. Williams Obstetrics, 18th edn. East Norwalk, CT: Appleton & Lange, 1989;332–35.

- Davison JK, Eckhardt WF III, Perese DA. Clinical anesthesia procedures of the Massachusetts General Hospital, 4th edn. Boston: Little, Brown and Company, 1993:476–81, 582–600.

- Miller RD (ed.). Anesthesia, Vol. 1, 4th edn. New York: Churchill Livingstone, 1994.

- Omoigui S (ed.). The anesthesia drugs handbook, 2nd edn. St Louis, MO: Mosby-Year Book Inc. 1995.

- Stoelting RK, Miller RD (eds). Basics of anesthesia, 3rd edn. New York: Churchill Livingstone, 1994:103–12.

Section 6:
Education and management

The theory and practice of medical education

Athol Kent MBChB MPhil FRCOG

Introduction

- What should be learnt?

- Who decides the aims and objectives of medical education?

- Are there modern theories and practical strategies for achieving new goals?

With so many of our medical schools reviewing their medical education curricula, it is appropriate to consider these questions in the light of educational development. Ideally, medical education should be seen as a continuum from the undergraduate curriculum, through postgraduate training, to lifelong continuing medical education (CME).

Most countries have given critical attention to postgraduate specialist education with rigorous theoretical and practical training plus examinations providing both audit and standardization. These same specialist organizations are now pushing hard for ongoing quality control and recertification while practice continues. The term continuing professional development (CPD) has replaced CME.

It is, however, the development of undergraduate education that is catching the profession's attention and imagination. Learning has been viewed as a passive process with teaching too long relegated to an unimportant, albeit interesting, part of academic obligations [1]. Medical education is clearly an area of expertise that is evolving into a discipline in its own right. Medical education now occupies a central place in our professional lives.

The responsibility for medical education

The real responsibility for becoming and remaining educated is ours, and ours alone. We are all ultimately responsible for the standard of care which we provide for our patients and this is based on the knowledge, skills and attitudes we have acquired.

At the undergraduate level, it takes time for this realization to dawn on us. We carry secondary education expectations with us in our minds and our hearts, but eventually we make the pedagogic switch from being taught to learning. This is as much an emotional and attitudinal change as it is an intellectual one.

At medical school the syllabus, the teachers, the examinations, the university and the licensing authorities conjure up a structure of responsibility outside ourselves that tends to obscure personal obligations. The shift in emphasis as to where the obligations correctly lie underpins much of modern thinking in medical education. Changes in the curriculum, setting goals, learning strategies, assessments and teaching techniques, as well as CPD, are all moving to accommodate this shift in emphasis and theory.

- Does teaching cause learning [2]?

- You can't teach anybody anything.

- Teaching as a subversive activity [3].

These are statements designed to challenge the Luddite mind-set that has resisted change and retarded the application of up-to-date principles of education in the medical domain.

Responsibility for developing educational activities has devolved from statutory bodies, such as medical councils, and licensing boards to universities and colleges who are the examiners and, more often than not, the teachers. They seldom have educational training [4] and often no incentive to explore the world of adult learning.

The requirements at undergraduate level are dependent on each university and, ultimately, the standards set by each department. Although there is usually a strong tradition of distilled wisdom, few interuniversity objective comparisons are made [5]. Although we like to think the exchange of external examiners maintains standards, there is little evidence to support this notion. The boon of information exchange over the Internet will, no doubt, rapidly change this situation to a more illuminated future. The lead given by postgraduate examinations along multicentre or national lines may well filter to the undergraduate level and lead to interuniversity papers being set. Apprenticeship requirements, practical experience and formative assessments, together with new types of summative examinations, all point towards a more rigorous academically approved system [6,7].

Evidence-based medicine (EBM) [8], driven by databases such as the Cochrane Collaboration electronic linkage, is leading to objective comparisons of management. This logically leads to more objective and verifiable knowledge, which can be combined with increasingly valid examination techniques, such as structured orals, simulated patients, gynaecological teaching associates, and objective structured clinical examinations (OSCEs).

New undergraduate educational strategies may well positively affect attitudes towards lifelong learning and boost a culture of the reflective doctor.

Curriculum reform

Medical education at the undergraduate level changed little during the first three-quarters of the 20th century. Since Flexner pioneered the change from apprenticeship to scientifically oriented education, questioning the system was rare. Control of the curriculum classically resided in the hands of the clinical heads of departments who saw little reason to change teaching – or learning.

Scant attention has been paid to educational progress, with an ever-burgeoning mass of factual information ladled on to undergraduates' plates. Clear lessons from the behavioural sciences have been slow to be incorporated into undergraduate programmes and preclinical tuition has remained out of context.

The situation changed in the 1960s with moves towards a more professional approach to teaching. Implementation has been slow, but is now gathering momentum influenced by the following:

Dissatisfaction with the product

All in-depth reviews of what we want our graduates to be, and what they actually are, reveal a substantial discrepancy between theory and reality. Most frequently, the product is defined as someone who should be an independent lifelong learner having the knowledge, skills and attitudes to be a competent intern. Scrutiny of the traditional medical graduate shows that we have been focusing on the student's knowledge and facts with insufficient attention to skills and attitudes [9].

The product is profoundly influenced by the examination process, which should be congruent with the stated aims and objectives of each medical school. Too often these aims and objectives are not stated or, if they are, not adhered to in the assessment process.

Powerful arguments are now available to attest that the skill to look up something or to know who to ask is of greater value than the ability to regurgitate facts. The attributes of a reflective practitioner with communication skills and a compassionate attitude are being seen as more important qualities than the ability to answer multiple choice questions.

Hills [10], in his delightful vignette 'The knowledge disease', and Popper [11], discussing the value of mistakes, make persuasive arguments that we are too precious in our present teaching philosophies.

The process

The process of becoming an accomplished practitioner is a continuum from undergraduate to postgraduate and CPD [12]. The undergraduate facet of this training is the aspect most in need of change. The focus needs to shift from what we teach to what they learn. If students can be motivated to learn independently of their teachers, then we have indeed made a contribution to their education.

This shift in responsibility is fundamental to the ongoing transformation from traditional to innovative learning strategies that began in the 1990s, preparing students for lifelong learning.

Politics

Politicians and purse-string holders have affected teaching in every country of the world. Fewer resources allocated to health in the face of increasing consumer expectations have precipitated rethinking and research. This has not always been destructive, and critical reviews of what is taught and how it is taught have increased efficiency and shaken intransigence.

Strong pressures are required to force change in teaching philosophies and learning strategies. Reports such as the General Medical Council's (GMC's) 'Tomorrow's doctors' [13] in the UK, the Robert Wood-Johnson review of undergraduate education in the USA [14], and the leadership of innovative medical schools in Canada as well as in The Netherlands, Israel and Australia, have all provided strong incentives for curriculum transformation.

Changing the curriculum

There is innate resistance to changing the curriculum at any medical school. All those participating in or observing this process will realize the powerful emotions and reactions it unleashes.

It challenges traditions, strongly held views, territories, mind sets, behaviours and existing values. It provokes strong antipathy because it suggests that the very people who are being asked to change are 'doing it wrong at present'. It is a poor principle to ask for change by starting with an insult.

It also requires time – which few people have – energy which is required for other endeavours, and money which always has to be acquired from 'somewhere else'.

Academics who concentrate on teaching and medical education are notoriously under-rewarded for their efforts [15]. Reformers are seen as reactionaries and the whole exercise seldom perceived to be beneficial – other than in the distant future.

If institutions choose to ignore the thrust for change in this dynamic field, then they run the risk of being left behind [16]. Change is surrounded by many myths, and requires vision and courage to invest in a complex process that takes many years to provide its ultimate benefit.

The learning process

Medical students are expected to acquire knowledge, skills and attitudes. Their education must, therefore, contain a mix of intellectual, practical and behavioural qualities. At secondary school, aspiring medical students are rewarded for factual recall (dualistic responses). Considerably more emphasis on deductive thinking, reasoning, problem solving and coping with ambiguity is expected in tertiary education (relativistic learning). Box 34.1 shows the bases and stages of intellectual and ethical development.

Knowledge

The accumulation and retention of medical facts has long been the focus of medical examinations. In turn, examinations and assessments drive the direction of student learning [19] and there is something of a collusion between examiners and students which pretends that if 'the student knows enough, they will be alright'. The move towards evidence-based medicine and the availability of the Cochrane

> **Box 34.1 The bases and stages of intellectual and ethical development**
> 1. A dualistic position expecting the 'right' answers to be presented by the teacher and reproduced by the student.
> 2. Diversity of opinion is perceived but seen as part of an exercise to encourage students to find the 'right' answers.
> 3. Diversity and uncertainty are recognized but only as temporary. Grades are seen as relating to 'good expression'.
> 4. Diversity is interpreted as indicating 'everyone has a right to his/her own opinion'. Relativistic reasoning is recognized as 'what they want', but without understanding why.
> 5. A recognition that all knowledge and values are relativistic, leading to the understanding of the interpretation of evidence.
> 6. An acceptance of the need to make some personal commitment based on a careful examination of the available evidence.
> Adapted from Perry by Entwistle [17,18].

Database on many aspects of obstetrics and gynaecology are useful in synthesizing information, and this constant reviewing of our knowledge epitomizes the need to instil a culture of ongoing learning.

It is impossible for students to acquire all the facts necessary to sustain them for the rest of their professional lives. Even if they could, the information would soon become obsolete. Students, being young adults, learn appropriately. If they see the application of the knowledge and the context in which it will be used, then they can make a rational judgement whether to commit this to short-term or long-term memory. This subconscious adoption of learning techniques runs concomitant with the rites of passage and maturation described earlier. The learning approaches as enunciated by Marton and Saljo use the terms 'deep' and 'surface' to describe qualitative differences in the manner in which students describe their own learning [20,21]. Later, Entwistle and Ramsden [22] added the strategic approach and these have been summarized in Box 34.2.

Many factors drive the learner at undergraduate, postgraduate or CPD level in the approach adopted to learning. These include personal goals, motivation and anxieties, and the perceived magnitude of the task. Also involved are the learner's intrinsic abilities and skills. Learning skills are often taken for granted but seldom formulated, taught and capitalized on in the traditionally based medical schools. The observation by students of their peers using different learning techniques is one of the many spin-offs of small group teaching.

Skills

Apart from 'knowing things', medical graduates are expected by their mentors, colleagues, prospective patients and themselves to be 'able to do things'. The search for and retrieval of information is a basic skill required for communicating to and about patients. Notes about admissions, procedures and referral letters are frequently shown to be inadequate. This can lead at best to irritation and, at worst, to litigation. More obviously, the taking of histories, examining competently, presenting cases, choosing investigations and constructing cost-effective lines of management are too often passive elements in teaching programmes.

Skills acquisition is intimately bound with experiential learning. How to listen, communicate and handle people are behavioural skills. Inspecting, palpating, percussing and auscultating are examining skills. Deducing, reasoning and reflecting are intellectual skills.

Skills required in medical education or of competent doctors, must be defined, encouraged and examined if their acquisition is genuinely expected.

Attitudes

Attitudes are acquired from parents, families, schools, communities, cultures and religious backgrounds. These are modified and added to by the observation of peers' and colleagues' attitudes towards patients as reflected in their empathy and kindness, or lack thereof. Work ethics, standards of behaviour, courtesy, manners, honesty and intellectual rigour are all assimilated through experience.

Moral reasoning and the formulation of one's own ethical attitudes are subjects which are best approached in small group situations. Open discussion with a skilled facilitator is the most fruitful way of exploring attitudinal beliefs. The wisdom of skilled minds is helpful, as are intellectual writings, but these are no substitute for experiential small group learning.

Holistic approaches,

Box 34.2   Learning approaches

Surface (Recognition)
- Learner focuses on details and information
- Completing task requirements in a minimal way – levels of processing are not required
- Reproducing from memory
- Memory involvement is short term and its embedding shallow

Deep (Understanding)
- The student seeks understanding and meaning of the message
- More processing and reflection is used relating the ideas together
- Information is committed to long-term memory
- Own experience is used in the process

Strategic
- Getting the highest possible marks in whatever way is necessary

community sensitivity, the ability to work as a team member and an awareness of social responsibilities are highly desirable qualities in graduates.

A crucial attitude a student has to develop is his or her approach towards learning. If it is seen as intriguing, stimulating and fun, this will be more important than all the so-called facts learned in medical school. Most of us were trained in traditional methodologies and remember with misgiving the slog and angst of student life, rather than its stimulation and exhilaration. Have our personal attitudes to learning changed?

Teaching strategies

We have examined where the responsibility for medical education should lie and the pressures – scientific, clinical, educational and political – that are obliging medical schools to relook at their teaching strategies.

A better understanding of the learning process and how the attitudes and habits of undergraduate education affect postgraduate and continuing education all reinforce the need for radical change at medical schools and in professional organizations.

The explosion of medical information at the preclinical and clinical levels, technologies, therapies and informatics requires teachers to become better educationalists. We cannot simply 'add on' and must therefore look at more efficient ways of learning as well as what syllabi contain. The syllabus for a medical course has to be built on robust principles that are auditable (Box

> **Box 34.3 The principles of syllabus/course design**
> - A syllabus is a contract between teacher and learner.
> - It is based on the learner's 'needs' providing opportunities to learn.
> - It is set with stated, measurable aims and objectives that are clear cut to both the teacher and the learner. Behavioural objectives are required, e.g. 'to have a working knowledge' is not a measurable objective, while to be able to list, identify, criticize or demonstrate are.
> - It motivates the student to learn in an environment of enthusiasm and fun.
> - It employs appropriate teaching aids and identifies key resource materials/handouts.
> - It encourages feedback/evaluation.
> - The core matrix should be components of ethics, communication, public health and community perspective.
> - It incorporates fair and objective-derived assessment with clear information about the number, timing and nature of each 'test'.

34.3). Delivering a particular syllabus can employ a number of formats (Box 34.4).

Traditional versus innovative curricula

Traditional schools base their training on the acquisition of, first of all, basic sciences, including the normal and abnormal, and then move on to their application in the clinical years.

Innovative schools, on the other hand, employ problem-based learning (PBL) with community orientation throughout their curricula, with early patient contact, horizontal and vertical integration of disciplines, group work and community interaction as crucial aspects of their students' learning.

> **Box 34.4 The teaching formats**
> - Classroom teaching
> - Workshop/tutorial
>   - System based
>   - Problem based (problem solving)
> - Small group work (see Box 34.5)
> - Role play/video feedback
> - Collaborative project work
> - Computer-assisted learning

Supporters of the innovative philosophy see as progressive the revising of Flexnerian notions of basic science building blocks, the de-Balkanizing of instruction, subject by subject, and the motivational impetus achieved when learning takes place in context.

Fundamental to the innovative principles is the motivation of the learner. Many personal qualities of young adults are brought to the learning situation, such as intrigue, curiosity, competitiveness and the need to conform to peer pressures. These positive factors can be woven into the curriculum with advantage to all.

In the UK, the GMC's 'Tomorrow's doctors' and 'The new doctor' have catapulted forward the reform process. They have precipitated an exciting, if somewhat traumatic, evolution in British medical schools that is being followed with considerable interest.

The vast majority of North American schools are involved in educational transformation, with each being asked to review where they stand on the continuum between traditional and innovative extremes. The

Box 34.5   Facilitating small group learning – the facilitator's role

- To set and explain the task
- To choose a rapporteur
- To introduce the subject and set a framework
- To draw group members into the discussion/listening
- To prevent domination by a group member
- To identify obstacles to progress/deal with conflict
- To test and challenge the validity of arguments
- To summarize

Table 34.1   Curriculum assessment – the SPICES model

Innovative	Traditional
Student-centred	Teacher-centred
Problem-based	Information gathering
Integrated	Discipline-based
Community-based	Hospital-based
Electives	Standard programme
Systematic	Apprenticeship-based or opportunistic

SPICES model (Table 34.1) compiled by Harden [23] is a logical start to this process.

Student-centred

Young adults take new knowledge and experiences, and weight these against what they already know and feel. They use intrinsic and extrinsic thinking processes [24] and conclude the value of the information to them. The more this is devolved to them, the more empowered they will be and the more their learning will be driven in desirable directions. Teachers have to co-operate in this process and facilitate rather than 'teach' (Box 34.5).

Problem-based learning

The perceived advantages of PBL are often seen as the onus being placed on the student to be responsible for his or her own learning, the recognition of the power of small groups and the motivation of early clinical contact.

Together with appropriate learning contexts and progressive assessment systems, the philosophy has much to recommend it. It also claims to be fun. This simple characteristic may turn out to be far more important than anyone has realized [25]. PBL is not 'problem solving'. In PBL the subject is 'learned' through tackling the problem.

Box 34.6   Learning unit (session) components

- Title of session, e.g. new intrauterine devices (IUDs)
- Objectives, e.g. to identify the role of and demonstrate the fitting of new IUDs
- Content, e.g. improve skills in selecting the right IUD and fitting it
- Activity, e.g. lecture, discussion, demonstration on model
- Teaching aids, e.g. slides, flip charts, pelvic models
- Evidence of mastery, e.g. able to demonstrate on a pelvic model

Integrated

In traditional medical schools, 'chunks' of teaching material are learnt without necessarily matching with what is being offered in other disciplines. Horizontal integration combines the learning of the anatomy and physiology of organs at the same time. This brings added meaning to both aspects of the work. If the third factor, that of the pathology and – better still – the clinical picture, are addressed at the same time, then this is vertical integration (Box 34.6).

PBL takes this process one step further, and includes holistic family and community factors, such as the contributions of professions allied to medicine. The teacher–learner relationship applied to a holistic integrated approach would progress gradually through to independent learning by:

- observation;
- partial care;
- collaborative care;
- supervised care;
- facilitation.

(Taken from 'Teaching in General Practice' – see 'Resources'.)

Systems-based curricula do integrate disciplines with time tabling, allowing systems to be covered sequentially. In the early years, the anatomy, physiology and pathology of various systems are tackled at the same time. This adds logic and meaning to the student's grasp and, if combined with clinical application, makes for even more relevance. Integration is part of problem-based learning.

Community-based

The tertiary referral hospital is becoming an increasingly less appropriate venue for medical student learning. Expedience, cost and subspecialization all militate against generalist and holistic experiences.

Trends towards preventative rather than curative approaches, plus the rise of primary health care, make non-hospital-based teaching more attractive. This trend calls for imaginative associations being formed between the rigid academic institutions and their partners in health care – be they in the professions allied to medicine or community-based organizations.

Electives

The elective theme has been developed by the introduction of the core curriculum and special study modules. The core must be based on three specific considerations:

- prevalence;
- dangerous conditions;
- instructive examples.

Each discipline, in concert with multidisciplinary committees, must work out the prevalence of conditions in its geographical area. They must also know what rare but life-threatening conditions exist. Some esoteric conditions do need to be studied to demonstrate and reinforce pathophysiological conditions.

Electives excite interest, promote in-depth thought and scientific rigour, and also allow domains of personal interest to be pursued. They complement the core curriculum. Students delve into subjects of their own choice which stimulate their development and challenge their intellect.

Systematic

A strong central curriculum committee, with power to oversee the entire learning process, will ensure that agreed essential knowledge, skills and attitudes are systematically taught, learnt and examined. Covering the entire syllabus in a systematic way is essential if the core curriculum philosophy is used. Subjects falling into the 'must know' category are seen as essential and opportunistic learning from whatever the student encounters in the wards is insufficient.

The SPICES model, together with appropriate, valid and reliable assessment systems, provides the means for a quantum leap forward in medical education, producing the type of graduate that academics and the public want.

Feedback/assessment

Giving and receiving feedback is integral in the further development and refinement of a curriculum. The learner can give feedback anonymously through prepared evaluation forms (questionnaires/surveys) and through regular review meetings with an external advisor (someone within the department who is not directly 'responsible' for the course or module in question). Indirect feedback can be given through the ongoing assessment of the learner by his/her mentor or advisor.

Timetabled reviews of the learning experience should be built into the curriculum, and based on the attainment of objectives set by the learner/teacher unit at the beginning of the course and at pre-agreed milestones during the course. A hierarchy of supradepartmental or regional advisors must be in place in case of disputes, genuine learner problems or personality clashes.

One to one teaching is the hallmark of practical postgraduate training of family planning and reproductive health care in the UK. The training is structured along the teacher–learner relationship (see 'Integrated learning') but by its nature allows a two-way feedback process. The availability of check lists helps both the learner and teacher to achieve the covering of a particular curriculum, especially when more than one trainer is involved.

Assessment can be formative and/or summative. Formative assessment is an ongoing, participative process achieved through preplanned reviews of accumulated experience and attainment of learning objectives aided by log books of experience. The assessment environment should be open, supportive and non-judgmental. No mark is awarded for these assessments. Formative assessment assists students to evaluate their understanding and define their teachers' expectations. Summative assessment tests knowledge, skills and attitudes through one, but more likely several, formats (Box 34.7). It occurs at the end of the course.

Box 34.7   Summative assessment

- Multiple choice questions (MCQs)
- Long essays/dissertations
- Critical reading tests (CRQs)
- Modified essay questions (MEQs)
- Objective, structured clinical examination (OSCE) – based on 'stations' through which students move; these can include clinical skill stations, counselling stations, clinical problem stations and knowledge-based stations
- Vivas
- Use of skills laboratories and virtual reality (skills testing)
- Gynaecology teaching associates – use of real 'surrogate' patients who themselves will contribute to the educational process

The bright future

The bright future of medical education shines through on our computer screens. It is logical to co-opt the power of information technology to the information transfer we call teaching.

As typewriters have become obsolete, teaching and learning without computers will become archaic. Word processing, e-mail, the Internet and the World Wide Web have catapulted this medium into our everyday lives, and now into education. CD ROMs with their prodigious storage capacity have opened up multimedia possibilities and teleconferencing is here to stay. Teleconferencing saves time and travel, and allows meetings to be held at short notice and facilitates faster decision making.

Word processing and e-mail

It would be unthinkable to produce any teaching material without a word processor. Manuals, lecture notes, guidelines and examinations are all generated and stored on our computers. Using e-mail, we can send this information to each other if we wish. The concept of electronic information exchange has considerable attraction for those working in undergraduate, postgraduate and CPD spheres [26].

The Internet

More sophisticated linkages to the Information Highway have opened several communication doors for educational access. One of the earliest innovations has been the development of news groups to provide forums for like-minded people to leave messages, pose questions and help each other. These are run by list servers, who are usually university-based, with the membership and content being monitored. A moderator controls who joins the group and reviews the messages sent and received. The exchanges that take place are usually academically erudite, have a truly international flavour and are very popular. A good example of such a group focusing on problem-based learning is the PBL List [27]. Similarly, a group exists for those involved in undergraduate education in obstetrics and gynaecology [28].

The World Wide Web is a free international electronic library for medical education. Web sites can easily be accessed through standard browser software, allowing viewing by anyone. These sites contain vast stores of 'information and resources for helping educators in all the health professions, enhance their instructional leadership/management and research skills, with additional resources that can help them with career development' [29].

Other electronic linkages provide informal publication of academic material, research or preliminary results, which is an exciting, if somewhat controversial, development that established journals have viewed with scepticism [30]. The legitimacy and citability of on-line publications will undoubtedly be unravelled and find its place in people's academic lives – and curricula vitae [31].

Already Web pages contain courses available for undergraduates, postgraduates and CPD. These will be engaged by students before, during or after their formal medical school training, and there is no reason why this concept should not be taken further. Banks of multiple choice questions, OSCE stations, lecture notes and manuals can be pooled to prevent reduplication and tedious examination setting.

Textbooks are available from these sources, which should provide standardized management and cheap text that will be of particular advantage to developing countries. A 'virtual textbook' [32] will be readily updatable and adaptable to the local practices and prevalences of different communities.

Computer-assisted learning

Computer-assisted learning (CAL) started off as a series of question and answer exercises that were similar to multiple choice examinations. With sophistication, information is now presented in the form of text, diagrams and flow charts. CAL packages can be used in formal teaching, in 'testing' or for self-learning. Better resolution screens and more powerful computers provide video material with audio options that make multimedia the medium of the future. Case studies, interactive videos (skills teaching) and electronic care plans allowing e-mail communications between professionals, with down loading of text and video, are all possible. CAL assessment packages with audit trails allow student-directed learning at the learner's pace which is especially suited for CPD.

The World Wide Web with its hypertext linkages allows entire courses to be found on Web pages complete with modules and assignments, as well as hints and self-testing for subscribers.

What started as undergraduate computer laboratories are now becoming university courses available wherever the consumer's computer is stationed.

Distance learning

Distance learning has arrived in the form of laptops that medical students either carry with them or have available at home or at medical school. They can access CAL programmes, lectures, teaching material and references wherever they are. Factual learning can be done at their own pace and at all times that suit them either socially or when appropriate for their clinical experience.

It has also arrived across the Internet. Undergraduate and postgraduate courses are available, but most of these do not allow free access and can only be reached by people approved of by their creators. Such postgraduate 'membership-style' courses are becoming commonplace for those in training for higher degrees in obstetrics and gynaecology, and cover the subspecialties of feto-maternal medicine, infertility, endocrinology and oncology [33].

Continuing medical education for practising obstetricians and gynaecologists is also available on the Internet and will surely become part of the way specialists can accumulate credit points as part of recertification programmes. The Royal College of Obstetricians and Gynaecologists of the UK is developing its education resources, and these include considerable electronic media facilities such as CD ROM archives and interactive programmes.

The speciality of obstetrics and gynaecology has distance learning available commercially. The Higher Education Resource Organisation (hero@ct.lia.net) has been established to allow practitioners to update their knowledge on a regular basis [26]. The convenience of learning from home or the workplace will greatly enhance the standardization of practice and will hopefully result in better obstetric services for individuals and the community [34].

Conclusion

The three tiers of medical education, those of undergraduate, postgraduate and continuing learning, are more exciting now than they have been at any time. The emphasis on a better type of learning rather than increasing the amount of teaching augurs well for the medical profession in the new millennium. Improved teaching strategies, innovative technology and, most of all, a renewed interest in adult education offers real prospects of advancement. Obstetrics and gynaecology as a discipline has taken the lead and now it is up to all of us in the specialty to maintain the momentum.

Resources

Further reading

- Barrows HS, Tamblyn RN. Problem-based learning: an approach to medical education. New York: Springer 1980.

- Beard R, Hartley J. Teaching and learning in higher education. London: Harper and Row, 1984.

- Medical Teacher. This is a quarterly journal published by Carfax Publishing Company: PO Box 25, Abingdon, Oxfordshire OX14 3UE, UK; or 875–81 Massachusetts

Avenue, Cambridge, MA 02139, USA; or PO Box 352, Cammeray, NSW 2026, Australia.

- Cormack J, Marinker M, Morrell D (eds). Teaching in general practice. London: Kluwer Publishing Co., 1981.

References

1. Pitkin RM. But isn't that your job, son? Presidential address. *Am J Obstet Gynecol* 1996;174:1083–8.

2. Purdie DW. Does teaching cause learning? In: Training in obstetrics and gynaecology: the time for change. London: RCOG Press, 1993.

3. Postman N, Weingartner C. Teaching as a subversive activity. Harmondsworth: Penguin, 1971.

4. Newble DI, Cannon. A handbook for clinical teachers. Lancaster: MTP Press, 1983.

5. Godfrey RC. Undergraduate examinations – the continuing tyranny. *Lancet* 1995;345:765–7.

6. Rolfe I, McPherson J. Formative assessment: How am I doing? *Lancet* 1995;345:837–9.

7. Collins JP, Gamble GD. A multi-format interdisciplinary final examination. *Med Educ* 1996; 30:259–65.

8. Evidence-Based Medicine Working Group. Evidence-based medicine. A new approach to the teaching of medicine. *JAMA* 1992;268:2420–5.

9. Clack GB. Medical graduates evaluate the effectiveness of their education. *Med Educ* 1994; 28:418–31.

10. Hills G. The knowledge disease. *Br Med J* 1993;307:1578.

11. McIntyre N, Popper K. The critical attitude in medicine: the need for a new ethic. *Br Med J Clin Res Ed* 1983,287:1919–23.

12. Purdie DW. Royal College of Obstetricians and Gynaecologists Year Book 1993 Continuing Medical Education. London: RCOG.

13. General Medical Council. Tomorrow's doctors: recommendations on undergraduate medical education. London: GMC, 1993.

14. Marston RQ, Jones RM (eds). Medical education in transition. Commission on Medical Education: the science of medical Practice. Princeton, New Jersey: The Robert Wood Johnson Foundation, 1992.

15. Biggs JSG, Price DA. Sustaining and rewarding clinical teaching. *Med Educ* 1992;26:264–8.

16. Lennox B. Editorial: The editor regrets and the Hawthorne effect. *Med Educ* 1983;17:347–8.

17. Perry WG. Forms of intellectual and ethical development in the college years A scheme. New York: Holt, Rinehart & Winston, 1970.

18. Entwistle NJ. Influences on the quality of student learning – implications for medical education. *S Afr Med J* 1992; 81:596–606.

19. Newble DI, Jaeger K. Effect of assessments and examinations on the learning of medical students. *Med Educ* 1983;28:418–31.

20. Marton F, Saljo R. On qualitative differences in learning. 1. Outcome and process. *Br J Educ Psychol* 1976a;46:4–11.

21. Marton F, Saljo R. On qualitative differences in learning. 2. Outcome as a function of the learner's conception of the task. *Br J Educ Psychol* 1976b; 46:115–27.

22. Entwistle NJ, Ramsden P. Understanding student learning. London: Croom Helm, 1983.

23. Harden RM, Howden S, Dunn WR. Educational strategies in curriculum development: the SPICES model. *Med Educ* 1984;18:284–97.

24. Boreham NC. The dangerous practice of thinking. *Med Educ* 1994;28:172–9.

25. Bligh J. Problem based, small group learning. *Br Med J* 1995;311:342–3.

26. Journal Article Summary Service. <hero@ct.lia.net.>

27. Internet. Problem-based learning Listserve. <pblist@sparky.uthscsa.edu>

28. Internet. Undergraduate education in O&G Listserve. <doogie-l@uct.ac.za>

29. Internet. The Centre for Instructional Support. Web site for health profession educators. <http://www.sls.org/CIS>

30. Kazera JP, Angel M. The Internet and the journal. *N Engl J Med* 1995;332:1707–10.

31. Internet. Medical education online. Solomon D (ed.). <http://www.utmb.edu/meo>

32. Ingils TJJ, Fu B, Kwok-Chan L. Teaching microbiology with hypertext: first steps towards a virtual textbook. *Med Educ* 1995;29:393–6.

33. Dracott T. SWOT-education for specialist registrars. *J Audiovis Media Med* 1997;3:135–8.

34. Kent AP. Medical schools without walls. *Med Educ* 1997;31:157–8.

Effective management options in women's healthcare

Charles DA Wolfe MD FRCOG FFPHM
Roger Beech BSc(Hons) MSc PhD MFPHM(Hons)

Introduction

Previous chapters of this book have outlined the evidence for optimal delivery of family planning and reproductive health practice, and given an overview of the epidemiology of the topic. This chapter outlines the context in which policies and priorities for family planning and reproductive health services are determined by society, and by purchasers and providers of healthcare.

First, the global approach to determining health policy is described in order to illustrate the complex range of factors that influence policy and the logicality, or otherwise, of decisions made about healthcare priorities and the introduction of new technologies or innovative methods of service provision. Although political and subjective values influence policy, the use of objective information is vital. Second, approaches are described that should be used to generate objective information for informing policy and priority setting. These approaches generate information about the healthcare need for a given service, its impact or outcome, and its costs and cost-effectiveness. The final section of the chapter then describes the ways in which target setting and audit can be used to implement and monitor agreed healthcare priorities and policies.

Global approaches to determining health policies and priorities

The patterns of health service organization adopted in different countries are the result of the interaction between historical, political, cultural and socioeconomic factors. These reflect broader societal values and the relative weights assigned to different social objectives, such as equity and efficiency. The level of healthcare expenditure, and how and where services are provided, reflects the relative value politicians, managers and healthcare professionals assign to healthcare compared with competing public sector interests. They also reflect the differing priorities placed on different healthcare services and client groups by policy makers.

Health policy is the decision-making process concerning resource expenditure on competing health programmes in relation to anticipated benefits/outcomes (i.e. health status or quality of life). A decision regarding one aspect of healthcare has to be made in the context of all the other healthcare options. Cultural, social, economic and political influences, as well as individual interests, all influence the decision process. Some, but not many, policy decisions are rational processes, and are often taken incrementally. A complex political process replaces any formal comparison of costs and outcomes, and this is particularly so, for example, with the debates over tobacco and alcohol.

In Europe, healthcare coverage is mainly financed by taxation with predominantly public sector providers in countries such as the UK, Spain, Portugal and Greece. In Germany, France, Belgium and Luxembourg, the services are mainly financed by social insurance with mixed public and private providers. In The Netherlands, the health services are financed by a mixture of social and private insurance with mainly private providers [1].

As a proportion of the gross domestic product, the cost of health services varies from 5.2% in Greece through 7% in the UK (6% public sector) to 13.5% in the USA (6.5% public). The highest public sector funding is in Canada, Belgium and Finland, which is between 7% and 8%. The

USA and Canada, as well as most of Western Europe, are spending an increasing proportion of their economic wealth on healthcare, and it is estimated in the USA that, by the year 2000, healthcare will consume over 16% of the gross domestic product, having been 12.2% in 1990. This projected rise is due principally to an ageing population, development of new technologies and, in some countries, supplier-induced demand and rapidly rising consumer demand. Increasing age will mean in reproductive health more resource for diseases related to the menopause and hormone replacement therapy. New technologies include the emergence of genetic prenatal screening, ultrasound surveillance in pregnancy, and minimal access surgical techniques. In the USA and the UK, pregnant women have increasing representation on maternity health policy bodies and Governments have specifically requested consumer-led services. Governments can respond to these financial pressures in several ways: by increasing the proportion of the gross domestic product spent on health; by controlling the demand through private insurance incentives; by controlling prices with pay freezes or price controls; by making cost-effective choices; and by priority setting and rationing.

The healthcare system in the USA gives neither the providers of healthcare nor patients an incentive to control expenditures, since insurers pay the majority of the bills. Public expectations for health and healthcare play a major role in increasing healthcare costs. Fixes to control expenditure have included improved management and efficiency, increasing competition, price control programmes using diagnostic-related groups to shift costs outside the hospital, auditing and rationing services. These fixes are potentially effective in the short term but are unlikely to have long-term effects on the growth of expenditure. In the UK, funding healthcare places a ceiling on overall expenditure. However, health sector reform has been used to introduce a quasi market for healthcare, aiming among other things to increase the efficient delivery of care.

Healthcare management

With finite resources, new technologies and diseases, clinicians and managers need to streamline services to provide the most cost-effective options. There are a variety of ways of managing services with a burgeoning lexicon of terms. Like clinical practice, systems of management come and go, and are rarely subject to evaluation. One such example is 'managed care', which seeks to cut the costs of healthcare whilst maintaining quality, but the evidence that it is able to achieve these aims is mixed [2]. Managed care is a spectrum of activities carried out in a range of organizational settings to produce cost-effective care, many of the elements of which will be discussed in this chapter.

The as yet unproven implications of such organizational strategies are numerous. It has restricted patients' choice of doctors and limited their access to specialists, reduced the professional autonomy and earnings of doctors, shifted power from the non-profit to the for-profit sectors, and from hospitals and doctors to private corporations. It has also raised issues about the future structuring and financing of medical education and research. It has, however, accorded greater prominence to the assessment of patient satisfaction, profiling and monitoring of doctors' work, the use of guidelines and quality assurance procedures, and indicated the potential to improve the integration and outcome of care [3].

The health sector is only one among many sectors of society demanding available finite resources and it seems unlikely that there will be major shifts from, say, defence to health. Controlling the escalating costs by rationing healthcare services is a consequence. Making decisions on health priorities has become more explicit, open and democratic, especially when they are likely to be controversial. The UK Government, via its policy, providers and purchasers by their business plans and purchasing intentions, along with the public, all contribute to the priority setting. The relative contribution of each is hard to determine (Box 35.1). The extent to which a government is involved in priority setting varies considerably around Europe and is greatest in those countries where the health services are funded out of taxation. Beyond the health services, the wider determinants of health are influenced by different ministries, such as social services, education and the police. Some countries have created bodies with wider responsibilities for public health and which undertake activities such as health promotion and screening. In the UK, there is now a Minister for Public Health. Health action zones, involving health and social services, are also being developed.

Health policy and cost

Rationing refers to the distribution of resources to services or individuals according to rules based on one or more characteristics: demography, socioeconomic status, disease status, costs and outcomes. In the USA, the explicit criteria include, for example, Medicaid eligibility based on the federal poverty level. Explicit rationing, based on costs and outcomes, is increasingly being used around Europe and the USA as outlined in the Oregon experience [4]. However, the debates centre on assumptions and estimates, the relationship between costs and outcome, and do not provide a watertight methodology.

No comprehensive plan for controlling healthcare costs exists between the various commissioners and providers of healthcare. A major ethical challenge to health resource allocation is how to involve the community in making difficult healthcare decisions. In Europe, there are three main ways of involving the public in health

policy: the democratic process of election; organized interest groups; and the direct involvement of individuals. In the Oregon Health Services Judgement, reproductive services ranked sixth and were considered most important or essential [4].

One particular theoretical model for policy decision making is suggested by Patrick and Erickson [5]. The health resource allocation strategy involves the following eight steps:

- specifying the health decision within a sociocultural context, identifying the stakeholders and the budgetary constraints;

- classifying the health outcome;

- assigning values to the health states;

- measuring the health-related quality of life of the target population;

- estimating the prognosis and years of healthy life;

- estimating the direct and indirect healthcare costs;

- ranking costs and outcome of healthcare alternatives by calculating the ratio of costs per year of healthy life gained for each alternative course of action;

- revising the ranking of costs and outcomes with stakeholders and

recommending the revised rank order to political decision makers.

In order to determine what the priorities for health are and to place them in the wider context of policy decision making, various aspects need to be considered at a population level. The next few sections discuss how the need for services is assessed, how the evidence on effectiveness and health economic aspects of effectiveness/efficiency is considered, what the main issues concerning quality and audit are, and how targets can be set to improve the reproductive health of populations.

'Objective' approaches to generating information for policy and priority setting

Needs assessment

Previous chapters have outlined the epidemiology relevant to family planning and reproductive health. Extrapolation from the epidemiological evidence should enable the health gain from various family planning and reproductive health interventions to be estimated. The need depends on the potential of preventive or treatment services to remedy the health problems. Population healthcare needs assessment includes on the one hand the incidence and prevalence of the problem, and on the other the efficacy and effectiveness of whatever the health (or other) services can do for them. Need, as the ability to benefit from healthcare, is distinct from demand and supply, although there is a relationship between the three (Figure 35.1). Both demand and supply are based on the market paradigm of microeconomics within which individuals buy (demand) products, so as to maximize their utility, while firms sell (supply) products so as to maximize their profits. The equilibration of healthcare supply and demand has never been shown to approximate to need for healthcare at a population level. Healthcare is seldom organized as a market and its products are heavily subsidized and regulated.

Defining need for services as 'what people can benefit from' leads to questions on the definition of benefit and who interprets the information and sets the rules. Benefits can be clinical and non-clinical, and accrue to both patient and carer. The range of problems will also

change over time, reflecting the cultural background of the day.

Lay demand is unlikely to match the scientific evidence of the need and this desired demand is heavily influenced by political, social and educational factors. The supply of health services is unlikely to match population need, owing to the constraints of policy decisions and financial influences. Supply may be aimed at maintaining the status quo or rationing services. Figure 35.1 outlines the relationship between supply, need and demand.

The approach to needs assessment, based on incidence and prevalence on the one hand, and the effectiveness of healthcare on the other, has been developed by Stevens and Raftery [6]. It aims to make incremental changes to the health services which may be at the edges, rather than complete service reconfigurations. The

components of such an assessment are outlined below:

- definition of the healthcare problem/disease;

- estimates of incidence/prevalence of the conditions in question;

- estimates of current health service provision;

- evidence of effectiveness;

- development of new models of service based on the above;

- measurement of health outcome and setting targets;

- information requirements to monitor service;

- research and development strategy.

In the UK, Ashton et al. [7] undertook a population-based assessment of the need for family planning and fertility services. They stressed that, while there is no substitute for local epidemiologically based assessments, their template could be successfully applied across countries. The needs assessment illustrates the need for various services for a typical population of 250 000 and is a useful resource to those planning services.

In a reference population of 250 000 there would be 53 639 women in the reproductive age group 15–44 years. Contraception will be used by 72%, i.e. 35 000, of whom 12 000 will use the oral contraceptive. There is little detailed information concerning the level and type of provision, and referral patterns for abortion and fertility services by family doctors. Issues relating

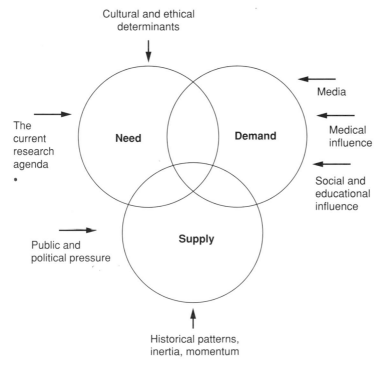

Fig. 35.1   Need, supply and demand for health services.

to planning contraceptive services are outlined in Box 35.2.

Outcome assessment

Outcomes are all the possible results that may stem from exposure to a causal factor, or from preventive or therapeutic interventions. Although it has become fashionable to measure outcome, it is worth considering what is meant by outcome and whether what we measure actually achieves its aim, in terms of measuring health status or informing decisions in healthcare. Outcome measures should be valid, reliable, readily collectable and the outcome of concern identifiable, measurable and most importantly modifiable. Identifiable outcomes come under the umbrella of mortality, morbidity and quality of life:

- death;
- impairment (morbidity);
- disability;
- handicap/quality of life;
- satisfaction with services.

There are significant differences in mortality and morbidity from various diseases around the world, although it has been difficult to establish the significance of health service provision in this variation. Morbidity and quality of life data are not readily available for family planning and reproductive health other than in the research setting. When assessing outcome, it is necessary to distinguish measures that are person centred from those that are population based. The factors that influence outcome other than health service intervention need to be understood. These are the effects of social, political, cultural and economic factors. It is worthwhile asking the question of whose outcome is being measured and from what perspective, as a good outcome for politicians and society may be a poor outcome for individuals or their carers.

Many of the outcomes in the area of reproductive health and family planning are actually process measures (such as attendances and coverage) that should lead to reduced unplanned pregnancy rates, but do not address physical, psychological or social outcomes. McColl and Gulliford [8] outlined possible routine UK National Health Service (NHS) outcome measures for reproductive health, in their population indicators. These included the following.

- The total-period abortion rate, defined as the average number of abortions that would occur per woman resident in the district if women experienced the current age-specific abortion rates throughout their childbearing span from the age of 15 to 44 years;

- The total-period abortion rate as a percentage of the crude potential fertility rate, which is an age-standardized measure of the percentage of known pregnancies that end in abortion.

- Conception rates in the under 16s.

- The uptake of contraceptive services divided by the conception rate.

The strength of the last measure is that it controls for the variation in the proportion of the female population that is at risk of pregnancy. This is particularly important when evaluating contraceptive services for teenagers, among whom the prevalence of sexual activity may be very varied.

Economic evaluation

Why economic evaluations are needed

Economists take the view that, as outlined previously, there are unlikely to be sufficient funds to meet all of the healthcare needs of society. Hence choices have to be made about both the nature and the scale of the types of health services to be provided. These choices should depend not only upon the relative effectiveness of

---

Box 35.2   Planning contraceptive services

- Services for contraception should cater for various age and ethnic groups within the local population
- Young people require easily accessible specific youth-orientated services, which provide health education and advice about AIDS, safe sex, sexually transmitted diseases and pregnancy
- There should be a full range of contraceptive methods
- A choice of services for older women needs to be developed
- Contraceptive advice postpartum to be incorporated in the plan
- Outreach services for people unable to access the established service
- Special advice and services from healthcare workers for people with disabilities, both physical and mental

alternative health interventions, but also on consideration of their relative costs. This is because providing funds for one type of service means less are available for another.

To inform decisions regarding the allocation of funds and the prioritization of health interventions, health economists use the techniques of economic evaluation. These techniques compare the costs and consequences of alternative types of health models.

The issues covered by economic evaluations

Economic evaluations usually take a broad perspective in terms of the assessment of costs and consequences. Hence the costs considered might include, for example, those incurred by:

- health services, e.g. the costs of doctors, nurses and primary practice staff and the costs of diagnostic and therapeutic interventions;

- social services, e.g. the costs of home cleaning, catering and nursing services;

- patients, e.g. loss of earnings and travel for treatment costs;

- the carers of patients, e.g. loss of earnings, or time away from normal daily activities, by a relative who has to take time out to care for an individual.

Likewise, a broad perspective can be taken of the consequences of health services. Outcomes can include:

- clinical outcomes, e.g. mortality and morbidity;

- patient outcomes, e.g. satisfaction with care and quality of life;

- carer outcomes, e.g. morbidity incurred by carers because they are having to take care of a sick relative or friend.

The techniques that are used in economic evaluations

The four types of economic evaluation that are available are described below.

- Cost-minimization is used where the consequences of the alternatives are thought to be the same. An example might be day surgery versus inpatient surgery for minor surgical interventions. Here the favoured intervention is the one with the lowest cost.

- Cost-effectiveness analysis is used where the alternatives achieve the same type of outcome but to differing degrees. An example might be lithotripsy versus percutaneous surgery for the treatment of kidney stones. Here the favoured option is the one with the lowest cost per unit of outcome.

- Cost–benefit analysis is used where it is possible to attach a monetary value to the consequences of an intervention. In practice, this type of economic evaluation is rarely used because of the difficulties of attaching a monetary value to outcomes although the term cost-benefit analysis is commonly misused to describe an economic analysis. An evaluation which compares the costs of 9 prenatal screening programme

to detect fetuses with severe disorders with the savings on the costs of caring for the individuals whose birth the programme prevents might be thought of as a limited type of cost–benefit analysis. In cost–benefit analysis, the best alternative is the one which gives the greatest payback on the cost input.

- Cost–utility analysis is used when the consequences of an intervention can be valued using measures of utility, such as quality adjusted life years (QALYs). The QALY concept takes account of the impact of a health intervention on both quantity and quality of life in terms of disability and distress. Studies in the UK have compared hip replacements (£1180 per QALY) and hospital haemodialysis (£21 970 per QALY), with the implication being that investments in hip replacements represent better value for money. Hence, in this type of economic evaluation, the favoured option is the one with the lowest cost per QALY generated.

A more comprehensive review of economic studies and techniques is to be found in the *Oxford Textbook of Public Health* [9].

The types of decision supported by the results of an economic evaluation

Because cost–benefit and cost–utility analyses use generic measures to value consequences, they allow health interventions which have a different purpose to be compared. Hence, the results of these types of economic evaluation have the potential to inform decisions about the appropriate balance of healthcare spending between different types of healthcare programme, e.g. the proportionate spending on family planning services and services for care of the elderly. However, their use in this way remains largely theoretical at present because of the difficulties of generating the data on outcomes that the techniques require. Currently, cost–effectiveness analysis is the most commonly used type of economic evaluation. Results of this type of economic evaluation have the aim of informing decisions about the appropriate balance of spending within a specific healthcare programme.

The potential role of cost-effectiveness analysis in informing choices in family planning and reproductive health is now considered using as examples studies of contraceptive services and services for *in vitro* fertilization.

Examples of economic evaluations covering family planning services

Studies in the USA by Trussell et al. [10] and in the UK by Hughes and McGuire [11] have assessed the cost–effectiveness of alternative methods of contraception. The healthcare consequences of contraception were taken as the number of unwanted pregnancies avoided. Costs included those of the contraceptive method, the costs of terminating unwanted pregnancies, and the costs of delivering babies, where couples opt to proceed with the pregnancy to full term.

Trussell et al. [10] estimated that attempts to avoid conception without the use of contraception would have an 85% annual failure rate and result in 4.25 unwanted pregnancies per couple over a 5-year time horizon. Amongst the methods of contraception considered, vasectomy had the lowest annual failure rate (0.04%), and the cervical cap and the sponge the highest (30%). Five-year costs for the various methods ranged from $540 for the Copper-T intrauterine device (IUD) to $5730 for the cervical cap in an insurance-based method of reimbursement. In a public-funded system 5-year costs ranged from $357 for vasectomy to $2682 for the cervical cap. Not using contraception had a 5-year cost of $14 663 in the insurance-based system and $6490 in the public funding system, meaning that all of the methods of contraception were estimated to achieve a cost saving and to be cost effective. The most cost-effective methods of contraception, i.e. having the lowest cost per unwanted pregnancy, were male and female sterilization, with the Copper-T IUD, the implant and the injectable contraceptive being the most cost-effective of the reversible methods in that order.

Hughes and McGuire [11] used the effectiveness data of Trussell et al. [10], but added UK data on costs. Again they found that family planning services are highly cost effective, with savings per unwanted pregnancy avoided ranging from £634 for the diaphragm (assumes contraceptive services provided in a family planning clinic) to £780 and £783 for female and male sterilization, respectively (assumes

service provided in a hospital setting).

It could be argued that, to some extent, contraception delays rather than avoids pregnancies. However, when the above researchers extended their analysis to consider this, they still concluded that family planning services were highly cost effective, resulting in savings in health service costs.

Such findings provide strong evidence in favour of the provision of family planning services. In the UK, contraceptive services are largely free to users, a policy that creates little debate. Although economic considerations are not the sole reason for this strategy, it is in keeping with that which would be recommended by the results of economic evaluations.

In the case of family planning services, the findings of economic evaluations provide clear evidence in favour of a particular choice of strategy. Often the choice of 'best' strategy is less clear-cut, as is the case in investment decisions surrounding the supply of programmes for *in vitro* fertilization.

In the UK, Page [12] assessed the health service costs and consequences of an *in vitro* fertilization unit. The cost per couple treated was estimated as £1100, the cost per maternity as £11 000 and per baby delivered as £8800. Achieving each of these outcomes requires an increase in expenditure, unlike family planning services, which save money. Hence the choice of policy is less obvious, depending upon the subjective valuations that health service funders attach to the healthcare consequences of the service. In the UK, although there is some public provision of *in vitro* fertilization, the service is largely provided by the private sector. Redmayne and Klein [13] compared the policies of six health authorities, three that had chosen to purchase *in vitro* fertilization services and three that had not. The reasons for purchase included the views that infertility can have harmful psychological effects and adverse consequences for the stability of a marriage, and that it is contradictory to purchase termination and sterilization services but not services for fertility. Reasons for not purchasing the service included the views that it is inappropriate to provide services for people who are not 'ill', the costs of the services are too high, the services are ineffective and, in affluent populations, it is reasonable for individuals to purchase these services privately.

It is impossible to say which of the choice of strategies is correct, with the above example illustrating that economic considerations are only one component of policy making. However, they are an important component which should not be ignored. Given that healthcare resources are scarce, the results of economic evaluations have a key role in informing choices about the provision of health services.

Evaluating the evidence of the effectiveness of interventions/services

Effectiveness is the extent to which a specific intervention procedure, regimen or service, when deployed in the field, does what it is intended to

do for a defined population. There is an increasing move to implement evidence-based medicine in Europe. In the UK, effectiveness bulletins [14–16] have been produced for subfertility, menorrhagia and teenage pregnancy, outlining effective and ineffective interventions. The US task force on preventive healthcare has classified interventions on two scales with a rating on both the direction of the evidence in support of a procedure and the quality of that evidence. The strength of the recommendation ranges from good evidence to support it to good evidence to support the rejection of the procedure. The quality of the evidence ranges from grade one, which includes evidence obtained from at least one properly randomized controlled trial or meta-analysis (I), through evidence obtained from well-designed controlled trials without randomization (II-1), evidence from well-designed cohort or case-controlled analytic studies, preferably from more than one centre or research group (II-2), evidence from multiple time series with or without intervention, from dramatic results in uncontrolled experiments (II-3), opinions of respected authorities (III) and,

lastly, inadequate evidence owing to problems of methodology (IV) [17].

There are variations on this form of classification used in different countries and institutions. For example, the NHS Executive [18] in the UK categorizes evidence as:

A. based on randomized controlled trials (RCTs);

B. based on other robust experimental or good observational studies;

C. more limited evidence, but the advice relies on expert opinion and has the endorsement of respected authorities.

The review by Ashton et al. [7] outlines the strength of evidence for a broad spectrum of services associated with family planning and reproductive health. Box 35.3 gives examples of level of evidence that is appropriate for audit.

Implementing and monitoring policy

Targets

A strategic approach to healthcare planning requires the

Box 35.3   Examples of the levels of incidence which are eminently auditable

- Second-trimester abortion by dilation and evacuation (D&E), preceded by cervical preparation is safe and effective providing the operator has appropriate training and experience (A)
- Abortion care should encompass a strategy for minimizing the risk of postabortion infective morbidity. Appropriate strategies include antibiotic prophylaxis (A) or screening for lower genital tract organisms and treatment in positive cases (B)
- Women presenting early in pregnancy (at < 9 weeks' gestation) should have access to a choice of surgical or medical methods of abortion (C)

identification of specific long-term goals for improvements in the population's health. However, in order to chart progress towards such long-term goals, it is often necessary to identify intermediate goals not only for health, but also for the important determinants of health, and the processes that lead to change in those factors. In other words, the intermediate determinants such as levels of smoking and the processes such as attendances at health promotion clinics are proxies for longer term health gains. The measures need to be credible, clear, selective, compatible, achievable, balanced, quantifiable and ethical [19].

The World Health Organization Health For All [20] strategy has the following principles:

- equity;
- health promotion;
- community participation;
- multisectoral collaboration;
- primary healthcare;
- international co-operation.

The most comprehensive national objective setting exercise to date has been in the USA [21]. Two hundred and twenty-six objectives were set to achieve the five main goals. The objectives covered improved health status (to reduce death, disability), reduced risk (to reduce the prevalence of risks to health or to increase behaviours known to reduce such risk), and improved services and protection (coverage, access, quality). In addition, surveillance and data needs were identified in a separate section. The objectives were repeated and a new set produced for the year 2000 [22]. These were arrived at after extensive process of consultation which included many public hearings.

The disadvantages of numerical targets are that they can lead to spurious priority being given to that which is measurable. Moreover, if taken in isolation, numerical targets may represent an oversimplification of policy. The other danger is that, unless the target levels are carefully chosen, they can appear unrealistic and be easily dismissed as unattainable.

The UK Faculty of Public Health Medicine [19] also set targets for birth control. Family planning has a direct impact on a range of health outcomes. Higher than average rates of maternal/infant mortality and morbidity are associated with conceptions in teenagers, older women and high-parity women. An individual's 'sexual lifestyle' can also affect the transmission of human immunodeficiency virus (HIV) and other sexually transmitted organisms, and the incidence of precancer and cancer of the cervix. It was considered that, when setting national targets, the following societal considerations should be taken into account: the basic right of any woman to control her own fertility and, on the other hand, the burden of global overpopulation. Data on abortion are included in this section as evidence of failed contraception. The targets set included the following:

- By the year 2000, conception rates in teenage girls aged 15 years should be reduced to below 10 per 1000 and in girls under 10 to zero.

- By the year 2000, 90% of legal abortions performed on girls aged 15 years should be carried out before 13 weeks gestation and 98% before 20 weeks.

- By the year 2000, no offences of procuring an illegal abortion should be recorded by the police in the UK.

- There should be an appropriate, accessible and comprehensive service based on need of the local population.

- There should be a free source of condoms.

- There should be a free provision of abortion services. Currently, in the UK, 52% of abortions are performed by NHS staff and a further 20% are funded by the NHS through contracts with non-NHS providers.

- Sterilization services should be based on local needs.

In 1992, 'The Health of the Nation' White Paper was published in the UK covering targets for health across five areas: coronary heart disease and stroke, cancers, mental illness, accidents and HIV/AIDS and sexual health. The general objectives for sexual health include the reduction of the number of unwanted pregnancies and ensuring the provision of effective family planning services for those people that want them. The specific targets include the reduction of the rate of conceptions amongst the under 16s by at least 50% by the year 2000 (from 9.5 per 1000 girls aged 13–15 in 1989 to no more than 4.8). A Key Area Handbook [23] outlines how to develop services to achieve these targets. Figure 35.2 demonstrates a structure to develop family planning services to achieve 'Health of the Nation' targets.

The International Planned Parenthood Federation (IPPF) has produced a charter on sexual and reproductive rights, providing an ethical framework within which IPPF carries out its mission [24]. These are basic human rights (life, liberty, equality, privacy) and broad objectives rather than measurable targets over a specific time period.

Quality and audit

Quality of care can be defined as a level of performance or accomplishment that characterizes the healthcare provided. Ultimately, measures of the quality of care always depend upon value judgements, but there are ingredients and determinants of quality that can be measured objectively: structure (e.g. manpower, facilities), process (e.g. diagnostic and therapeutic procedures) and outcome (e.g. case fatality rates, disability rates and levels of patient satisfaction with the service).

In the USA, the external monitoring of quality is complex and fragmented. Not only are there multiple and overlapping systems, but each of them is constantly evolving. It is a mixture of public and private systems with the principal objectives being split between public protection, quality improvement and cost containment.

While the central tenet of the British system is that healthcare should be delivered equally to all according to need, the concept of quality in the USA is restricted to considering the attributes of care that is provided rather than the broader consideration of the system in which it is delivered.

In the UK, the Family Planning Association's family planning service group [25] thought that a definition of quality for family planning services might usefully be that of their fitness for their purposes: the prevention of unwanted pregnancy and sexually transmitted diseases and the promotion of sexual health. The group identified the following key issues to be addressed in tailoring services:

- tailoring services for particular groups;
- making a range of methods and providers available in each designated geographic area;
- effective advertisement;
- appropriate negotiation on confidentiality;
- information leaflets;
- training and support of staff;
- collecting and incorporating audit material;
- developing and implementing practice guidelines;
- joint working between providers;
- encouraging outreach and development work.

Clinical audit has been defined in many ways, depending on the perspective taken. One of the definitions used in the UK has been the systematic, critical analysis of the quality of care, including the

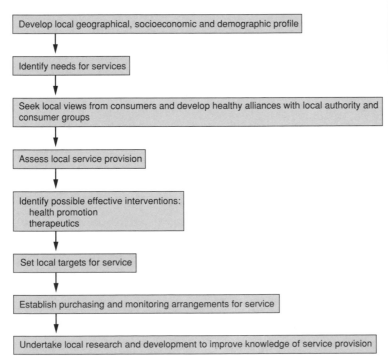

Develop local geographical, socioeconomic and demographic profile

Identify needs for services

Seek local views from consumers and develop healthy alliances with local authority and consumer groups

Assess local service provision

Identify possible effective interventions:
    health promotion
    therapeutics

Set local targets for service

Establish purchasing and monitoring arrangements for service

Undertake local research and development to improve knowledge of service provision

Fig. 35.2 Developing family planning services to achieve 'Health of the Nation' targets.

procedures used for the diagnosis and treatment, the use of resources and the resulting outcome and quality of life for the patient.

The purpose of audit is to identify opportunities and to implement improvements in the quality of medical care, medical training and continuing education, and the effective use of resources. It involves abstracting information from patient records and making judgements about the quality of care given. These judgements are made by considering indicators of structure (the quantity and type of resources), process (what is done to the patient) and outcome (results of clinical intervention). Audit can be retrospective or prospective. The success of its implementation depends on a basic understanding of the principles of the audit cycle (Box 35.4).

First, standards are set and compared with the practice already in place. If any differences are noted, recommendations for change are made and subsequently implemented. Then, after a specific period of time, the cycle can be repeated to ensure that either the desired standards

have been achieved and maintained or, on reflection, the standards themselves need to be changed. The differences between audit and traditional review include the use of explicit criteria for measurement rather than implicit judgement, numerical comparisons of current practice patterns against the criteria, comparison of practice among peers, formal identification of action required to resolve any discrepancy disclosed, and recording the process to retain information and increase the impact of audit on future management. How audit has improved outcome has not been documented in the medical literature to a great extent because of several factors. Firstly, audit may not be effective and, secondly, the audits are not undertaken correctly.

Scott and Jackson [26] illustrate how audit can help manage a service and give an example using dilation and curettage in the under–50s. Their suggested key points for successful audit include:

- a problem that is of clinical relevance and which is also a

health service delivery/ management issue;

- both clinicians and managers wish to see the audit undertaken;

- the audit group is multidisciplinary;

- guidelines are developed locally;

- the audit group should facilitate the collection of notes/data, as this is an important component of the audit which needs organizational support;

- care needs to be taken to ensure appropriate linkages are made between clinical peer review and management mechanisms to ensure the full benefit to the organization;

- improvements depend on learning from information about performance, and feedback and revisiting the issue.

Strategies such as development and dissemination of practice guidelines/protocols have become fashionable. Grimshaw et al. [27] have undertaken systematic reviews of rigorous evaluations of clinical guidelines published between 1976 and 1992. One study was on infertility and referral to hospital by general practitioners [28]. A total of 81 out of 87 studies reported significant improvements in the adherence to guidelines over the study period and 12 of the 17 studies which assessed patient outcomes reported significant improvements. The behavioural factors which influence adherence to clinical guidelines are very

Box 35.4 The audit cycle

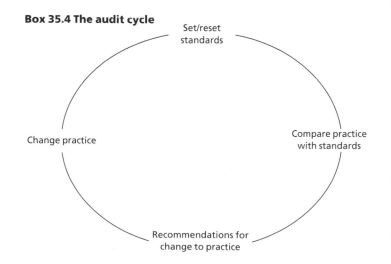

Set/reset standards

Compare practice with standards

Recommendations for change to practice

Change practice

complex. Although it is thought that local development and ownership is important, this was not found to be the case for all studies. Educational interventions involving more active participation by professionals (including seminars, educational outreach visits and the involvement of opinion leaders) are more likely to lead to change in behaviour. Guidelines based on reviews that identify, synthesize and interpret evidence systematically are, therefore, more likely to be valid. These guidelines need to be 'evidence-based', using the strengths of evidence discussed earlier. The skills for understanding the principles of 'evidence-based' medicine are taught in epidemiology and consist of: healthcare evaluation methods (randomized controlled trials, case series, consensus); synthesis of information (systematic reviews of literature, e.g. Cochrane Collaboration in UK, including meta-analysis); and the ability to access literature databases such as Medline and Web-sites to assimilate current evidence [29]. A philosophy of evidence-based medicine and skills needs to be incorporated into audit.

References

1. Abel-Smith B, Figueras J, Holland W, McKee M, Mossialos E. Choices in health policy. An agenda for the European Union. Dartmouth: Office for Official Publications of the European Communities, 1995.

2. Fairfield G, Hunter DJ, Mechanic D, Rosleff F. Managed care. Origins, principles and evolution. *Br Med J* 1997; 314:1823–6.

3. Fairfield G, Hunter DJ, Mechanic D, Rosleff F. Managed care implications of managed care for health systems, clinicians and patients. *Br Med J* 1997; 314:1895–8.

4. Oregon Health Service Commission. Prioritisation of health services; a report to the governor and legislature. Salem: Oregon Health Services Commission, 1991.

5. Patrick DL, Erickson P. Health status and health policy. Allocating resources to health policy. Oxford: Oxford University Press, 1993.

6. Stevens A, Raftery J. Health care needs assessment, Vol. 1. Oxford: Radcliffe Medical Press, 1994.

7. Ashton JR, Marchbank A, Mawle P, Hotchkiss J. Family planning, abortion and fertility services. In: Stevens A, Raftery J (eds). Health care needs assessment, Vol. 2. Oxford: Radcliffe Medical Press, 1994.

8. McColl AJ, Gulliford MC. Population health outcome indicators for the NHS. A feasibility study. London: Faculty of Public Health Medicine, 1993.

9. Drummond M. Economic studies. In: Holland WW, Detels R, Knox G (eds) Oxford textbook of public health medicine, 2nd edn. Oxford: Oxford Medical Publications, 1991.

10. Trussell J, Leveque JA, Koenig JD, et al. The economic value of contraception: a comparison of 15 methods. *Am J Public Health* 1995;85:494–503.

11. Hughes D, McGuire A. The cost-effectiveness of family planning service provision. *J Public Health Med* 1996;18:189–96.

12. Page H. An economic appraisal of in-vitro fertilisation. *J Roy Soc Med* 1988;88:99–102.

13. Redmayne S, Klein R. Rationing in practice: the case of in-vitro fertilisation. *Br Med J* 1993;299:1521–3.

14. Effective Health Care Bulletin, Vol. 1, no. 3. The management of subfertility. Leeds: University of Leeds School of Public Health, 1992.

15. Effective Health Care Bulletin, Vol. 1, no. 9. The management of menorrhagia. Leeds: University of Leeds School of Public Health, 1995.

16. Effective Health Care Bulletin, Vol. 3, no. 1. Preventing and reducing the adverse effects of unintended teenage pregnancies. Leeds: University of Leeds School of Public Health, 1997.

17. Report of the US Preventive Services Task Force. Guide to clinical preventive services. An assessment of the effectiveness of 169 interventions. Baltimore: Williams and Wilkins, 1989.

18. NHS Executive Clinical Guidelines. Using clinical guidelines to improve patient care within the NHS. London: Department of Health, 1996.

19. The Faculty of Public Health Medicine. UK Levels of Health. London: Faculty of Public Health Medicine First Report, June, 1991.

20. World Health Organisation (WHO) Regional Office for Europe. Targets for health for all: targets in support of the European Regional strategy for health for all. Copenhagen: WHO, 1985.

21. US Department of Health and Human Services. Healthy people: the Surgeon General's report on health promotion and disease prevention. Washington, DC: US GPO, 1979.

22. US Department of Health and Human Services, Public Health Service. Healthy People 2000. Washington, DC:US GPO, 1990.

23. Department of Health. The Health of the Nation Key Area Handbook: HIV/AIDS and sexual health. London: Department of Health, 1993.

24. Sexual and Reproductive Rights Charter. International Planned Parenthood Federation, London, 1996.

25. Smith C. Family planning services. *Qual Health Care* 1992;1:197–201.

26. Scott T, Jackson P. Using information for managing clinical services effectively. *Br Med J* 1995;310:848–50.

27. Grimshaw J, Freemantle N, Wallace S, et al. Developing and implementing clinical practice guidelines. *Qual Health Care* 1995;4:55–64.

28. Emslie CJ, Grimshaw J, Templeton A. Do clinical guidelines improve general practice management and referral of infertile couples? *Br Med J* 1993;306:1728–31.

29. Sackett DL, Richardson WS, Rosenberg W, Haynes RB. Evidence-based medicine. How to practice and teach EBM. Edinburgh: Churchill Livingstone, 1997.

Additional Resources

Unless stated all postal addresses are in the UK.

Abortion

Abortion Law Reform Association
11–13 Charlotte Street
London
W1P 1HD

Birth Control Trust
3rd Floor
16 Mortimer Street
London
W1N 7RD
Tel: + 44 207 580 9360
Fax: + 44 207 637 1378
E-mail *bct@birthcontroltrust.org.uk*

National Abortion Campaign
The Print House,
18 Ashwin Street
London
E8 3DL

AIDS/HIV

AIDS Care Education and Training (ACET)
PO Box 3693
London
SW15 2BQ
Tel: + 44 208 780 0400
Fax: + 44 208 780 0450

AIDS Education and Research Trust (AVERT)
11 Denne Parade
Horsham
West Sussex
RH12 1JD
Tel: + 44 1403 210202
Fax: + 44 1403 211011

Body Positive – self help group
51b Philbeach Gardens
London SW5 9EB
Tel: + 44 207 835 1045
Fax: + 44 207 373 5237

National AIDS Helpline
PO Box 5000
Glasgow
G12 9BL
Helpline: 0800 567123

National HIV Prevention Information Service (NHPIS)
30 Great Peter Street
London
SW1P 2HW
www.hea.org.uk/nhpis

Positively Women
347–349 City Road
London
EC1V 1LR
Tel: + 44 207 713 0444
Helpline: + 44 207 713 0222
Fax: + 44 207 713 1020

The Centre for AIDS Prevention Studies (CAPS)
www.epibiostat.ucsf.edu/capsweb
HIV .net
http://hiv.net/hiv/us/index.htm

The Terence Higgins Trust
52–54 Grays Inn Road
London
WC1X 8JU
Tel: +44 207 831 0330
Helpline: +44 207 242 1010
www.tht.org.uk

UK Department of Health
(The Communicable Diseases Branch)
Wellington House
135–155 Waterloo Road
London
SE1 8UG
Tel: + 44 207 972 2000; 207 972 4440

AIDS
http://www.iohk.com/
UserPages/mlau/aidshome.html

AIDS Resource List
http://www.teleport.com/
~celinec/aids.shtml

AIDS Virtual Library
http://planetq.com/aidsvl/
index.html

JAMA HIV/AIDS Information Center
http://www.ama-assn.org/
special/hiv/hivhome.htm

Just Say Yes
http://www.positive.org/cps/
jsy/jsy.html

NIH Safer Sex Documents
http://gopher.niaid.nih.gov:70/
11/aids/comm/teach

The Center for AIDS Prevention Studies (CAPS)
http://www.epibiostat.ucsf.edu/
capsweb

The Safer Sex Page
http://www.safersex.org/

Cancer

American Cancer Society
1599 Clifton Road
NE Atlanta
GA 30329
USA
Tel: + 800 ACS 2345

Breast Cancer Care
Kiln House
210 New Kings Road
London
SW6 4NZ
Helpline tel: (020) 7 384 2344
Admin tel: (020) 7 384 2984

Breast Cancer Care
13a Castle Terrace
Edinburgh
EH1 2DP
Helpline tel: 0131 221 0407
Admin tel: 0131 221 0407
Admin fax: 0131 221 0407

Breast Care Campaign
Number 1
St Mary Abbots Place
London
W8 6LS
Admin tel: (020) 7 371 1510
Admin fax: (020) 7 371 4598

British Association of Cancer
United Patients (BACUP)
3 Bath Place
Rivington Street
London
EC2A 3JR
Helpline tel: 0800 208199
Admin tel: (020) 7 696 9003
Admin fax: (020) 7 696 9002
Opening times: 9am–7pm

Cancer Research Campaign
10 Cambridge Terrace
London
NW1 4JL
Admin tel: (020) 7 224 1333
Admin fax: (020) 7 935 1546

Cancer You Are Not Alone
(CYANA)
31 Church Road
Manor Park
London
E12 6AD
Helpline tel: (020) 8 553 5366
Admin tel: (020) 8 553 5366

National Cancer Institute
Rockville Park
Building 31 4A–21
Bethesda
MD 20892
USA
Tel: + 800 4 CANCER 900

Womens Nationwide Cancer Control Campaign (WNCCC)
Suna House
128–130 Curtain Road
London
Helpline tel: (020) 7 729 2229
Admin tel: (020) 7 729 4688;
(020) 7 729 1735
Admin fax: (020) 7 613 0771

The Breast Cancer Compendium
http://www.microweb.com/clg/
index.html

The Breast Cancer Roundtable
http://www.seas.gwu.edu/
student/tlooms/MGT243/
bcr.html

Breast Disease – Multimedia Course Work: McGill
http://mystic.biomed.mcgill.ca/
MedinfHome/MedInf/Breastcou
rse/htmltext/
home/BreastHome.html

CancerNet
http://wwwicic.nci.nih.gov/
CancerNet.html

Community Breast Health Project (CBHP)
http://www-med.stanford.edu/
CBHP/

National Cancer Institute
http://www.nci.nih.gov/
Oncology Online
http://medserv.com/

Ovacome
St Bartholomew's Hospital, West
Smithfields, London
EC1A 7BA, UK

Prostate Cancer Home Page
http://www.cancer.med.umich.
edu/prostcan/prostcan.html

General

Brook Advisory Centres
165 Grays Inn Road
London
WC1X 8VD
Helpline tel: (020) 7 713 9000;
(020) 7 713 8000
Admin tel: (020) 7 833 8488
Admin fax: (020) 7 833 8182

Family Planning Association
2–12 Pentonville Road
London
N1 9FP
Helpline tel: (020) 7 837 4044
Admin tel: (020) 7 837 5432
Admin fax: (020) 7 837 3042

Family Planning Association Scotland
Unit 10
Firhill Business Centre
Glasgow
G20 7BA
Helpline tel: 0141 676 5088
Admin tel: 0141 676 5088
Admin fax: 0141 576 5006

Family Planning Association Wales
Grace Phillips House
4 Museum Place
Cardiff
CF1 3BG
Helpline tel: 01222 342766
Admin tel: 01222 644034
Admin fax: 01222 644306

Health Education Authority
Hamilton House
Mabledon Place
London
WC1M 9TX
Admin tel: (020) 7 383 3833

Healthwise Helpline
First Floor
Cavern Walks
8 Mathew Street
Liverpool
L2 6RE
Helpline tel: 0800 665544
Admin tel: 0151 227 4150
Admin fax: 0151 227 4019
Opening times:
Every day 9am–9pm

**International Planned
Parenthood Federation**
Regent's College
Inner Circle
Regent's Park
London
NW3 4NS
Admin tel: (020) 7 486 0741
Admin fax: (020) 7 487 7950

**Irritable Bowel Syndrome
Network (IBS Network)**
St John's House
Hither Green Hospital
Hither Green Lane
London
SE13 6RU
Helpline tel: (020) 8 698 4611 ext.
8194
(enquiries)
Admin tel: (020) 8 698 4611 ext.
8194
Admin fax: (020) 8 698 5655
Opening times: Mon, Wed, Fri
10.30am–1.30pm

Migraine Trust, The
45 Great Ormond Street
London
WC1N 3HZ
Helpline tel: (020) 7 278 2676
Admin tel: (020) 7 278 2676
Admin fax: (020) 7 831 5174

National Women's Register
3a Vulcan House
Vulcan Road
Norwich
NR6 5LX
Admin tel: 01603 406767
Admin fax: 01603 407003

NHS Helpline
PO Box 5000
Glasgow
G12 9JQ
Helpline tel: 0800 224488

Public Health Alliance, The
138 Digbeth
Birmingham
B5 6DR
Admin tel: 0121 643 7628
Admin fax: 0121 643 4541

Scottish Women's Aid
12 Torphichen Street
Edinburgh
EH3 8JQ
Helpline tel: 0131 221 0401
Admin tel: 0131 221 0481
Admin fax: 0131 221 0402

**Women's Environmental
Network (WEN)**
Aberdeen Studios
22 Highbury Grove
London
N5 2EA
Admin tel: (020) 7 354 8823
Admin fax: (020) 7 354 0464

**Women's Environmental
Network Directory of
Information (WENDI)**
Aberdeen Studios
22 Highbury Grove
London
N5 2EA
Helpline tel: (020) 7 704 6800

Women's Health
52 Featherstone Street,
London
EC1Y 8RT
Tel: +44 207 251 6580
E-mail:
womenshealth@pop3.poptel.org.uk

*The American College of
Obstetricians and Gynecologists*
http://www.acog.com/

*Centers for Disease Control and
Prevention*
http://www.cdc.gov/

*Centers for Disease Control and
Publications*
http://www.bioreg.com/
cdcpubs.html

Internet FDA
http://www.fda.gov/

MD InterActive
http://www.business1.com/
mdinteract

The National Institutes of Health
http://www.nih.gov/

*Planned Parenthood Federation of
America*
http://www.ppfa.org/ppfa/
index.html

World Health Organization
http://www.who.org/

General Gynaecology

**National Association for
Premenstrual Syndrome
(NAPS)**
PO Box 72
Sevenoaks
Kent
TN13 1XQ
Helpline tel: 01732 741709
Admin tel: 01732 459378

**National Endometriosis
Society**
Suite 50
Westminster Palace Gardens
1–7 Artillery Row
London
SW1P 1RL
Helpline tel: (020) 7 222 2776
Admin tel: (020) 7 222 2781

PMS Help
PO Box 83
Hereford
HR4 8YB
Admin tel: 01432 760993
Admin fax: 01432 760993

Premenstrual Society
PO Box 429
Addlestone
Surrey
KT15 1DZ
Admin tel: 01932 872560
(Mon–Fri 11am–6pm)

The Museum of Menstruation
http://www.mum.org/

The Pap Test
http://www.erinet.com/fnadoc/
fpap.htm

PMS Center
http://www.bairpms.com/

*The Women's Health Care Advocacy
Service*
http://www.2cowherd.net/
findings/

Guide to Women's Health Issues
http://asa.ugl.lib.umich.edu/
chdocs/womenhealth/
womens_health.html

Infertility

Child
Charter House
43 St Leonards Road
Bexhill on Sea
East Sussex
TN40 1JA
Helpline tel: 01424 732361
Admin tel: 01424 732361
Admin fax: 01424 731858

**Donor Insemination
Network**
PO Box 265
Sheffield
S3 7YX
Admin tel: 0114 231 3812

**Fertility Awareness and
Natural Family Planning**
Clitherow House
1 Blythe Mews
Blythe Road
London
W14 0NW
Helpline tel: (020) 7 371 1341
Admin tel: (020) 7 371 1341
Admin fax: (020) 7 371 1341

**Human Fertilisation and
Embryology Authority**
Paxton House
30 Artillery Lane
London
E1 7LS
Admin tel: (020) 7 377 5077
Admin fax: (020) 7 377 1871

**Issue (The National Fertility
Association)**
509 Aldridge Road
Great Barr
Birmingham
B44 8NA
Helpline tel: 0121 344 4414
Admin fax: 0121 344 4336

*International Council on Infertility
Information Dissemination
(INCIID)*
http://www.inciid.org

Menopause and Osteoporosis

**National Osteoporosis
Society**
PO Box 10
Radstock
Bath
BA3 3YB
Helpline tel: 01761 472721
Admin tel: 01761 471771
Admin fax: 01761 471104

Power Surge
http://www.members.aol.com/
dearest/index.html

*Menopause: Another Change in
Life*
http://www.ppfa.org/ppfa/
menopub.html

*North American Menopause Society
Website*
http://www.menopause.org

Post Partum

Breastfeeding Articles and Resources
http://www.parentsplace.com/
readroom/bf.html

Breastfeeding Resources
http://users.aol.com/kristachan/
brstres.htm

Preconception

Maternity Alliance, The
45 Beech Street
London
EC2P 2LX
Helpline tel: (020) 7 588 8582
Admin tel: (020) 7 588 8582
Admin fax: (020) 7 588 8584

Miscarriage Association, The
c/o Clayton Hospital
Northgate
Wakefield
West Yorkshire
WF1 3JS
Helpline tel: 01924 200799
Admin tel: 01924 200795; 01924
200799
Admin fax: 01924 298834

National Childbirth Trust
Alexandra House
Oldham Terrace
Acton
London
W3 6NH
Helpline tel: (020) 8 992 8637
Admin tel: (020) 8 992 8637
Admin fax: (020) 8 992 5929

Support Around Termination For Abnormality (SATFA)
73 Charlotte Street
London
W1P 1LB
Helpline tel: (020) 7 631 0285
Admin tel: (020) 7 631 0280
Admin fax: (020) 7 631 0280

Support Organisation For Trisomy (UK) (SOFT)
48 Froggatts Ride
Walmley
Sutton Coldfield
West Midlands
B76 2TQ
Admin tel: 0121 351 3122

Support Organisation For Trisomy 13/18 and Related Disorders (SOFT)
Tudor Lodge
30 Redwood
Ross-on-Wye
Herefordshire
HR9 5UD
Helpline tel: 01989 567480

Toxoplasmosis Trust, The
61–71 Collier Street
London
N1 9BE
Helpline tel: (020) 7 713 0599
Admin tel: (020) 7 713 0663
Admin fax: (020) 7 715 0611

Teenage Parenthood Network
Govanhill Neighbourhood Centre
6 Daisy Street
Glasgow
G42 8JL
Admin tel: 0141 424 0448

Sexuality

Albany Trust
Art of Health and Yoga
280 Balham High Road
London
SW17 7AL
Helpline tel: (020) 8 767 1827
Admin tel: (020) 8 767 1827

Impotence Information Centre
PO Box 1130
London
W3 OBB

Impotence World Service (IWS)
119 South Ruth Street
Maryville
USA
TN 37803

Ask NOAH About: Sexuality
http://www.noah.cuny.edu/
sexuality/sexuality.html

Coalition for Positive Sexuality Resources
http://www.positive.org/
%7Ecps/cps/resources.html

Complete Internet Sex Resource Guide
http://sleepingbeauty.com/
world/netsex.html

The Sex Directory
http://www.u-net.com/
~healthdv/sexweb/

Sexuality Information and Education Council
http://www.siecus.org/

The Society for Human Sexuality
http://weber.u.washington.edu/
~sfpse/

STIs

Herpes Viruses Association
41 North Road
London
N7 9DP
Helpline tel: (020) 7 609 9061
Admin tel: (020) 7 607 9661

Communicable Disease Surveillance Centre (CDSC) Home Page
http://www.open.gov.uk/cdsc/
cdschome.htm

Complete Facts on STDs
http://med-www.bu.edu/
people/sycamore/std/std.htm

The Herpes Zone
http://www.worldpassage.net/
herpeszone/

Sexually Transmitted Disease (STD) (Venereal Disease) Prevention for Everyone
http://www.iacnet.com/health/
09112524.htm

Index